P9-DBY-525

Contents

Contributors and consultants

Louise A. Aurilio, RN,C, PhD, CAN
Assistant Professor
Nursing Department
Youngstown (Ohio) State University

Cynthia Chatham, RN,C, DSN
Associate Professor
University of Southern Mississippi
Long Beach

Marsha L. Conroy, RN, BA, MSN, APN
Instructor of Nursing
Cuyahoga Community College
Cleveland

Cheryl DeGraw, RN, MSN, CRNP
Instructor
Florence-Darlington Technical College
Florence, S.C.

Patricia Greer, RN
Practical Nursing Intermediate Instructor
Tennessee Technology Center
Paris

Shelton M. Hisley, RNC, PhD, WHNP
Assistant Professor, Graduate Clinical Coordinator
School of Nursing
The University of North Carolina at Wilmington

Randy Sue Miller, RN, BS
Registered Nurse
Orlando (Fla.) Regional Healthcare System

Kristi Robinia, RN, MSN, RN,C
Assistant Professor, Practical Nursing
Northern Michigan University
Marquette

Linda S. Wood, RN, MSN
Director of Practical Nursing
Massanutten Technical Center
Harrisonburg, Va.

Foreword

To paraphrase Shakespeare, brevity is the soul of nursing. Every nurse recognizes the importance of brevity, of communicating information simply and clearly. This skill is vital in the patient-care setting, where minutes can mean the difference between life and death.

Maternal-Neonatal Nursing Made Incredibly Easy was put together with this consideration in mind. This handy reference does what every capable, busy nurse knows how to do—convey important information clearly and succinctly in an organized manner, without losing the essence of what needs to be told. The facts are all here; they're interesting and relevant and covered in appropriate but not excessive detail. Unnecessary verbiage has been eliminated, and the pitfall of overexplaining has been avoided. Above all, the content is easy to understand!

Everyone can benefit from a textbook that makes information easy to comprehend, from the student enrolled in her first course in maternity nursing to the experienced nurse who can benefit from refreshing her knowledge of maternal-neonatal nursing. *Maternal-Neonatal Nursing Made Incredibly Easy* makes that easy to do by providing the fundamentals in a back-to-the-basics approach that emphasizes the important and essential aspects of maternal-neonatal nursing—from conception to birth to postpartum care and complications.

Maternal-Neonatal Nursing Made Incredibly Easy provides the information needed for competent and safe nursing practice. This delightful reference provides information about culture and family, legal and ethical issues, anatomy and physiology, all aspects of nursing care, and all of the roles of maternity nurses. This book also includes the latest information on dozens of maternal-neonatal complications—such as those relating to addiction, multiple gestation, preeclampsia, and adolescent pregnancy—and how to manage them, including collaborative care issues that are essential in nursing practice today.

Some additional features of this book include:
• exquisite organization that makes it easy to follow the flow of ideas and find information without reading through long tracts of text
• clear, simple explanations of concepts and procedures
• scores of tables and charts that focus on key information and make it easy to find
• a multitude of illustrations that clarify difficult concepts and help you visualize what's going on
• a quiz at the end of each chapter that includes the correct answers and an explanation of the correct answer.

In addition, icons throughout the text attract your attention to important information, including:

- *Take charge!* — sidebars that point out potentially lethal situations and steps to take when they occur, encouraging vigilance by the nurse

- *Education edge* — patient-teaching tips and checklists that help the nurse pass along the information that can be vital to promoting a healthy pregnancy and preventing complications

- *Bridging the gap* — details on cultural differences that may affect care

- *Advice from the experts* — tips and tricks for maternal-neonatal nurses provided by the people who know best — other maternal-neonatal nurses.

Finally, *Maternal-Neonatal Nursing Made Incredibly Easy* conveys the enthusiasm about maternal-neonatal nursing that I initially felt while taking my first course in maternity nursing. This book makes learning about maternal-neonatal nursing interesting and easy. Enjoy!

Janet Engstrom, PhD, APN, CNM
Associate Professor and Program Director
Nurse-Midwifery and Women's Health Nurse Practitioner Programs
University of Illinois at Chicago

Introduction to maternal-neonatal nursing

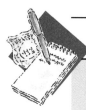

Just the facts

In this chapter, you'll learn:

♦ roles of maternal-neonatal nurses

♦ dynamics of family-centered nursing care

♦ structures and functions of families

♦ factors that influence a family's response to pregnancy

♦ legal and ethical issues associated with maternal-neonatal nursing.

A look at maternal-neonatal nursing

In North America, nurses care for more than four million pregnant patients each year. Providing this care can be challenging and rewarding. After all, you must use technology efficiently and effectively, offer thorough patient teaching, and remain sensitive to and supportive of patients' emotional needs.

In recent decades, infant and maternal mortality rates have progressively declined, even among women older than age 35. Factors responsible for this decline include the availability of antibiotics for controlling infection, the use of blood and blood substitutes for treating hemorrhage, the legalization of and decreased risks associated with abortion, the increased use of sophisticated diagnostic techniques and genetic testing, and enhanced education and professional training in obstetrics.

Room for improvement

Despite these advances, improving maternal and neonatal health care is still a concern. Infant and maternal mortality rates remain high for poor patients, minorities, and teenage mothers—largely because of a lack of good prenatal care.

> Your goal is to provide comprehensive care to patients and their families.

Maternal-neonatal nursing goals

The primary goal of maternal-neonatal nursing is to provide comprehensive family-centered care to the pregnant patient, the family, and the baby throughout pregnancy. (See *Three pregnancy periods.*)

Setting the standards

In 1980, the American Nurses Association's Maternal Child Health Nursing Practice division set standards for maternal-neonatal nursing. These standards provided guidelines for planning care and formulating desired patient outcomes. Later, the Association of Women's Health, Obstetric, and Neonatal Nurses (AWHONN) built upon these standards to create the current practice standards.

Three pregnancy periods

Pregnancy can be broken down into three periods:

The *antepartum period* refers to the period from conception to the onset of labor.

The *intrapartum period* extends from the onset of contractions that cause cervical dilation to the first 1 to 4 hours after the birth of the neonate and the placenta.

The *postpartum period* refers to the 6 weeks after delivery of the neonate and the placenta. Also known as the *puerperium,* this stage ends when the reproductive organs return to the nonpregnant state.

Practice settings

Maternal-neonatal nurses practice in various settings. These include community-based health centers, doctors' offices, hospital clinics, acute care hospitals, maternity hospitals, birthing centers, and patient's homes.

There's no place like home...

Up until the year 2000, 98% of all births occurred in hospital labor and delivery suites or birthing units. Today, an increasing number of families are choosing to have their babies in alternative birth settings, such as birthing clinics or their homes. These alternative settings may give families more control over their birth experiences by allowing them to become more involved in the process.

...or a home away from home

In response to consumer demands for more relaxed, family-friendly birthing environments, many hospitals have revamped their labor and delivery units to create more natural childbirth environments. Labor, delivery, and recovery rooms or labor, delivery, recovery, and postpartum suites are now found in most hospitals. In these homelike settings, partners, family members, and other support people may remain in the room throughout the birth experience. The patient then stays in the same room where she gave birth during the recovery and postpartum period. These home-style environments allow for a more holistic and family-centered approach to maternal and neonatal health care.

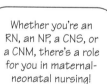

Today, many families are choosing to have their babies in alternative settings, such as birthing clinics or their homes.

Maternal-neonatal nursing roles and functions

Nurses involved in maternal-neonatal nursing assume many roles. These may include care provider, educator, advocate, and counselor. The functions involved for each of these roles depend on the nurse's level of education. Nurses involved in maternal-neonatal nursing may be registered nurses (RNs), certified nurse-midwives (CNMs), nurse practitioners (NPs), or clinical nurse specialists (CNSs).

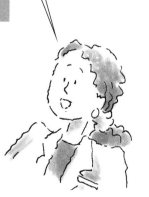

Whether you're an RN, an NP, a CNS, or a CNM, there's a role for you in maternal-neonatal nursing!

Registered nurse

An RN is a graduate of an accredited nursing program who has successfully passed the National Council Licensure Examination and is licensed by the state in which she works. To work in a maternal-neonatal department, an RN goes through extensive on-site training, including competency checks and ongoing education. She plays a vital role in providing direct patient care, meeting the educational needs of the patient and her family, and functioning as an advocate and counselor.

Certified nurse-midwife

A CNM is an RN who has achieved advanced education at a master's level or has obtained certification. A CNM works independently and is able to care for a low-risk obstetric patient throughout her pregnancy. A CNM is also licensed to deliver a neonate.

Nurse practitioners

An NP is also an RN who has received advanced education at a master's level or has obtained certification. An NP performs in an expanded advanced practice role. She obtains histories, performs physical examinations, and manages care (in consultation with a doctor) throughout the pregnancy and the postpartum period. She may practice as a women's health, family, neonatal, or pediatric NP.

Women's health nurse practitioner

A women's health NP plays a vital role in educating women about their bodies and offering information on preventive health care. She cares for women with sexually transmitted diseases and counsels them about reproductive issues and contraceptive choices. A women's health NP helps women remain well so that they can experience a healthy pregnancy and maintain good health throughout life.

Family nurse practitioner

A family nurse practitioner (FNP) provides care to all patients throughout the life cycle. She performs health physicals, prepares pregnancy histories, orders and performs diagnostic and obstetric examinations, plans care for the family throughout pregnancy and after birth, and can provide

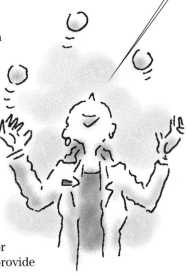

An NP juggles many responsibilities. She obtains histories, performs physicals, and manages care in consultation with a doctor.

prenatal care in an uncomplicated pregnancy. An FNP cares for the entire family, focusing on health promotion, wellness, and optimal family functioning.

Neonatal nurse practitioner

A neonatal nurse practitioner (NNP) is highly skilled in the care of neonates and can work in practice settings with various care levels, from well-baby term nurseries to high-level intensive care and preterm nurseries. She can also work in neonatal intensive care units (NICUs) or neonatal follow-up clinics. An NNP's responsibilities include normal neonate assessment and physical examination as well as high-risk follow-up and discharge planning.

Pediatric nurse practitioner

A pediatric nurse practitioner (PNP) provides well-baby counseling and care, performs physical assessments, and obtains detailed patient histories. The PNP serves as a primary health care provider. She can order diagnostic tests and prescribe appropriate drugs for therapy, although prescribing privileges depend on individual state regulations. If the PNP determines that the child has a major illness, such as heart disease, she may collaborate with a pediatrician or other specialists.

Clinical nurse specialist

A CNS is an RN who has received education at a master's level. The CNS focuses on health promotion, patient teaching, direct nursing care, and research activities. A CNS serves as a role model and teacher of quality nursing care. She may also serve as a consultant to RNs working in the maternal-neonatal field.

Training day

A CNS may be trained:
• to provide care in NICUs
• as a childbirth educator who develops and provides childbirth education programs, prepares the expectant patient and her family for labor and birth, and cares for the patient and her family in normal birth situations
• as a lactation consultant who teaches and assists the woman as she learns about breast-feeding.

Family-centered care

Maternal-neonatal nurses are responsible for providing comprehensive care—including ethical and legal care—to the pregnant mother, her fetus, and family members. This approach is known as *family-centered care*. Understanding the makeup and function of the family is essential to delivering family-centered care.

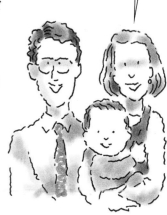

Family-centered care is a cornerstone of maternal-neonatal nursing.

Family ties

A family is a group of two or more persons who possibly live together in the same household, perform certain interrelated social tasks, and share an emotional bond. Families can profoundly influence the individuals within them. Therefore, care that considers the family—not just the individual—has become a focus of modern nursing practice.

Changes such as the addition of a new family member alter the structure of the family. If one family member is ill or is going through a rough developmental period, other family members may feel a tremendous strain. Family roles must be flexible enough to adjust to the myriad changes that occur with pregnancy and birth.

Family structure

Several different family structures exist today. These structures may change over the life cycle of the family because of such factors as work, birth, death, and divorce. Family structures may also differ based on the family roles, generation issues, means of family support, and sociocultural issues.

Types of family structures include:
- nuclear family
- cohabitation family
- extended or multigenerational family
- single-parent family
- blended family
- communal family
- gay or lesbian family
- foster family
- adoptive family.

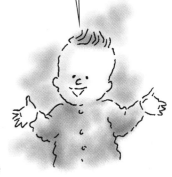

I may be small, but I have a big effect on my family's structure!

Nuclear family

A nuclear family is traditionally defined as a family consisting of a wife, a husband, and children. A nuclear family can provide support to and feel affection for family members because of its size. However, small family size may also be a weakness for the nuclear family. For example, when a crisis arises, such as an illness, there are fewer family members to share the burden and provide support.

Cohabitation family

A cohabitation family is composed of a heterosexual couple who live together but aren't married. The living arrangement may be short- or long-term. A cohabitation family can offer psychological and financial support to its members in the same way as a traditional nuclear family.

Extended or multigenerational family

Extended or multigenerational families include members of the nuclear family and other family members, such as grandparents, aunts, uncles, cousins, and grandchildren. In this type of family, the main support person isn't necessarily a spouse or intimate partner. The primary caregiver may be a grandparent, an aunt, or an uncle. This type of family may experience financial problems because the family's income must be stretched to accommodate more people.

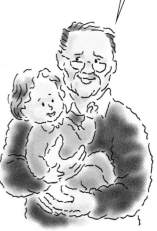

In an extended family, I may be the primary caregiver.

Single-parent family

Today, single-parent families account for 50% to 60% of families with school-age children. Although in many of these families the mother is the single parent present, an increasing number of fathers are also rearing children alone. Single-parent families occur for many reasons, including divorce, death of a spouse, and the decision to raise children outside of marriage.

Working hard for the money

Financial problems such as low income can be an issue for single parents. Even though an increasing number of single parents are fathers, most are mothers. Traditionally, women's salaries have been lower than men's salaries. This situation poses a problem when a mother's salary is the only source of income for the family.

Flying solo

Another difficulty for the single-parent family is the lack of family support for childcare, which can be problematic if the single parent becomes ill. A single parent may also have difficulty fulfilling the multitude of parental roles that are required of her, such as being a mother and a father in addition to being the sole income provider for the family.

Blended family

In a blended family, two separate families have joined as one as a result of remarriage. Many times, conflicts and rivalries develop in these families when the children are exposed to new parenting methods. Jealousy and friction between family members may be an issue, especially when the new blended family has children of their own. On the other hand, children of blended families may also be more adaptable to new situations.

Communal family

A communal family is a group of people who have chosen to live together who aren't necessarily related by marriage or blood. Instead, they may be related by social or religious values. People in communal families may not adhere to traditional health care procedures, but they may be proactive in participating in their health care and be receptive to patient teaching.

Gay or lesbian family

Some gay and lesbian couples choose to include children in their families. These children may be adopted, or they may come from surrogate mothers, artificial insemination, or previous unions or marriages.

Foster family

Foster parents provide care for children whose biological parents can no longer care for them. Foster family situations are usually temporary arrangements until the biological parents can resume care or until a family can adopt the foster child. Foster parents may or may not have children of their own.

Adoptive family

Families of all types can become adoptive families. Families adopt children for various reasons, which may include the inability to have children biologically. In some cases, families choose to adopt foster children whose parents are unable to provide care and are willing to have their children adopted. Sometimes, adoptive parents are the child's biological siblings or a relative of the parent. This type of family poses many challenges to the family unit, especially if biological children also live in the family. Adoptions can be arranged through an agency, an international adoption program, or private resources.

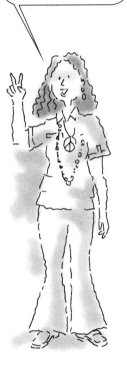

C'mon people now, smile on your brother. A communal family is a group of people who aren't related by blood or marriage but choose to live together. That's groovy!

Family tasks

A healthy family typically performs eight tasks to ensure its success as a working unit and the success of its members as individuals. These include:
- distribution of resources
- socialization of family members
- division of labor
- physical maintenance
- maintenance of order
- reproduction, release, and recruitment of family members
- placement of members into society
- safeguarding of motivation and morale.

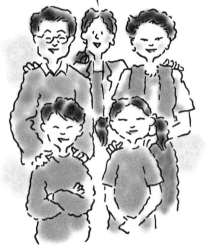

You work together as a family to perform a number of tasks that make you successful as a unit and as individuals.

Distribution of resources

Because each family has limited resources, the family needs to decide how those resources should be distributed. In some cases, certain family needs will be met and others won't. For example, one child may get new shoes whereas another gets hand-me-down shoes.

Money isn't everything

Money isn't the only resource. Such resources as affection and space must also be distributed. For example, the eldest child may get his own room whereas younger children have to share a room. Most families can make these decisions well. Dysfunctional families or those with financial problems may have problems completing these tasks.

Socialization of family members

Preparing children to live in society and to socialize with other individuals in their society is another important family task. If the culture of the family differs from the community in which it lives, this may be a difficult task.

Division of labor

Division of labor is the family task that involves assignment of responsibilities to each family member. For example, family members must decide who provides the family with monetary resources, who manages the home, and who cares for the children. The division of labor may change within a family when a new baby arrives, especially if both parents work full-time.

Physical maintenance

The task of physical maintenance includes providing for basic needs, such as food, shelter, clothing, and health care. The family fulfills these needs by finding and maintaining employment and securing housing. It's important to have enough resources to complete these tasks or the family may find itself in crisis. Improper distribution of resources can also lead to problems related to providing for basic needs. Physical maintenance also includes providing emotional support and caring for family members who are ill.

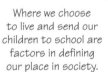

Hold it right there. Someone has to maintain order in the family, especially when a new member is on the way.

Maintenance of order

The task of maintenance of order includes communication among family members. It also involves setting rules for family members and defining each individual's place within the family. For example, as a new baby comes into the family, a family with a healthy maintenance of order and well-defined rules and roles knows where that new member belongs. Family members welcome the new baby as a part of the family unit and understand the baby's role as a family member. An unhealthy family may find this task difficult. Members of a family without a healthy maintenance of order may feel threatened that the baby will change or take their place in the family. They may see the new baby as an intruder.

Reproduction, release, and recruitment of family members

Reproduction, release, and recruitment of family members can occur several ways. For example:
- a new child is born (reproduction)
- a child leaves home for college (release)
- a child is adopted (recruitment)
- elderly parents come to live with the nuclear family (recruitment).

Even though family members don't always control reproduction, release, and recruitment, accepting any of these life changes is a family task. A healthy family accepts the change and understands the effects that the change will have on family roles and functions.

Where we choose to live and send our children to school are factors in defining our place in society.

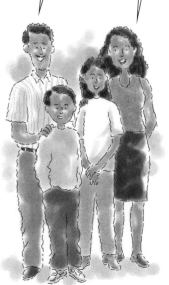

Placement of members into society

Families also make decisions that define their place in society. In other words, when parents choose where to live and where to send their children to school, the family becomes part of a particular community within society. The activities they choose to participate in—such as church or synagogue, physical activities, and clubs—also define the family's place within the social community.

Safeguarding of motivation and morale

The task of safeguarding of motivation and morale is achieved though the development of family pride. Much of this is achieved through emotional encouragement and support. If family members are proud of their accomplishments, a sense of pride for each other and the family as a unit develops. This makes them more likely to care about each other and to defend the family and what the family does. They're also more likely to support each other during crises.

The nursing process

Maternal-neonatal nurses provide care following the nursing process steps, which are:
- assessment
- nursing diagnosis
- planning
- implementation
- outcome evaluation.
  These steps help to ensure quality and consistent care.

Assessment

Assessment involves continually collecting data to identify a patient's actual and potential health needs. According to the American Nurses Association guidelines, data should accurately reflect the patient's life experiences and patterns of living. To accomplish this, assume an objective and nonjudgmental approach when gathering data. Data can be obtained through a nursing history, physical examination, and review of pertinent laboratory and medical information. A maternal-neonatal nursing assessment should include an assessment of the patient and her family.

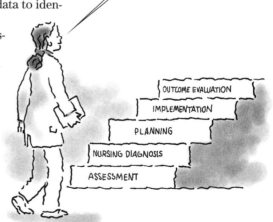

Adhering to the nursing process helps me provide quality care. And because we nurses are all following the same steps, the care our patients receive is also consistent.

OUTCOME EVALUATION
IMPLEMENTATION
PLANNING
NURSING DIAGNOSIS
ASSESSMENT

Mommy factors

During pregnancy, assess such maternal factors as:
- patient's age
- past medical, pregnancy, and birth history
- reaction to fetal movement
- nutritional status.

Remember that the mother's health directly affects the well-being of the fetus.

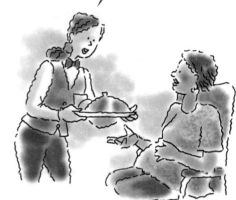

Remember that maternal factors such as nutritional status directly affect the well-being of the fetus.

Baby factors

After birth, assess such neonatal factors as:
- Apgar score
- gestational age
- weight in relation to gestational age
- vital signs
- feeding patterns
- muscle tone
- condition of the fontanels
- characteristics of the neonate's cry.

Family factors

Assessment should always reflect a family-centered approach. Be sure to assess family status, and note how it's affected by the pregnancy and birth. Be aware of how the family is coping with the new arrival and how parents, siblings, and other family members are affected. Also, assess how the mother, father, siblings, and other family members bond with the neonate.

Nursing diagnosis

In 1990, the North American Nursing Diagnosis Association (NANDA) defined a nursing diagnosis as, "a clinical judgment about individual, family, or community responses to actual or potential health problems or life processes." It went on to say that nursing diagnoses provide the basis for the selection of nursing interventions to achieve outcomes for which the nurse is accountable.

Diagnosis: mother

In maternal-neonatal nursing, you'll develop nursing diagnoses for the patient, family, and neonate that are appropriate for the prenatal, intrapartum, and postpartum periods. The information gathered during your nursing assessment can be used to help you formulate appropriate nursing diagnoses. For example, a new mother might experience frustration because her neonate is fussing and crying within the first hour after breast-feeding. Based on this assessment data, the patient would be assigned a nursing diagnosis of *Ineffective breast-feeding.*

Planning

After establishing a nursing diagnosis, you'll develop a care plan. A care plan serves as a communication tool among health care team members that helps ensure continuity of care. The plan consists of expected outcomes that describe behaviors or results to be achieved within a specified time as well as the nursing interventions needed to achieve these outcomes.

Keep it in the family

Be sure to include the patient and her family when planning and implementing the care plan. For example, when you're developing a care plan for a patient who has a nursing diagnosis of *Interrupted family process,* you should make sure that the care plan encourages family members to express their feelings about the pregnancy. Be aware of the family's changing needs and be aware of the new mother's sensitivity and emotional concerns. (See *Ensuring a successful care plan.*)

Advice from the experts

Ensuring a successful care plan

Your care plan must rest on a solid foundation of carefully chosen nursing diagnoses. It also must fit your patient's needs, age, developmental level, culture, strengths, weaknesses, and willingness and ability to take part in her care. Your plan should help the patient attain the highest functional level possible while posing minimal risk and not creating new problems. If complete recovery isn't possible, your plan should help the patient cope physically and emotionally with her impaired or declining health.

Use the following guidelines to help ensure that your care plan is effective.

Be realistic
Avoid setting a goal that's too difficult for the patient to achieve. The patient may become discouraged, depressed, and apathetic if she can't achieve expected outcomes.

Tailor your approach to each patient's problem
Individualize your outcome statements and nursing interventions. Keep in mind that each patient is different; no two patient problems are exactly alike.

Avoid vague terms
It's best to use precise, quantitative terms rather than vague ones. For example, if your patient seems ambivalent toward her neonate, describe this behavior: "doesn't respond when the baby cries," "watches television when changing the baby's diaper," or "frequently asks to take the baby back to the nursery so she can talk on the phone." To indicate that the patient's vital signs are stable, document specific measurements, such as "heart rate less than 100 beats/minute" or "systolic blood pressure greater than 100 mm Hg."

Implementation

During the implementation phase of the nursing process, you put your care plan into action. Implementation encompasses all nursing interventions directed at solving the patient's problems and meeting her health care needs. When you're coordinating implementation, seek help from the patient as well as the patient's family and other caregivers.

Anticipate adjustments

After implementing the care plan, continue to monitor the patient to gauge the effectiveness of interventions and to adjust them as the patient's condition changes. Expect to review, revise, and update the entire care plan regularly, according to facility policy.

Expect to review, revise, and update the care plan regularly.

Outcome evaluation

The outcome evaluation step of the nursing process evaluates how well the patient met her care plan goals, or outcomes. It also evaluates the effectiveness of the care plan. To evaluate the plan effectively, you must establish criteria for measuring the goals and the outcomes of the plan. Then you must assess the patient's responses to these interventions. These responses help determine whether the care plan should be continued, discontinued, or changed. Inevitably, this evaluation brings about new assessment information, which necessitates the creation of new nursing diagnoses and a modification of the plan.

Follow up

Evaluate the care plan frequently. This allows for changes and revisions as the needs of the patient and her family change, ensuring that the care plan accurately reflects the family's current needs.

Family response to pregnancy

Several factors can influence a family's response to pregnancy. These factors include:
- maternal age
- cultural beliefs
- whether the pregnancy was planned
- family dynamics

- social and economic resources
- age and health status of other family members
- mother's medical and obstetric history.

Maternal age

The mother's age can affect how family members respond to a pregnancy. Whether the mother is nearing menopause or just a teenager, family members may respond negatively to the pregnancy.

Waiting it out

Today, more families are waiting to have children until later in life. The number of women age 40 and older having children has risen dramatically in the past 10 years. The number of women who have their first child after age 40 has also increased. If an older woman becomes pregnant, especially one who's already a mother, the family may react unfavorably. For example, older children may be disgusted by the idea that their parents are having sex or by the pregnancy itself. Also, some family members may perceive pregnancy as the role of a young mother—not one nearing menopause.

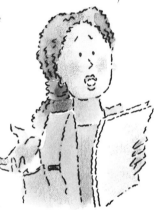

An increasing number of women are waiting until after age 40 to have their first child.

Aren't you a little young?

Teenage pregnancy rates have also changed dramatically. According to the Centers for Disease Control and Prevention, the birth rate for teenagers in the United States declined steadily throughout the 1990s, falling from 62.1 births per 1,000 teenagers ages 15 to 19 in 1991 to 48.5 births in 2000—a reduction of 22%.

If the mother is a young teenager who isn't married, the family may view the pregnancy unfavorably for several reasons. For example, family members may fear that the single mother won't be able to provide for her baby or that the mother won't finish her schooling. Family members may also be concerned about how their own roles will change as a result of the pregnancy. They may fear that they'll become full-time caregivers for the child. In addition, the family's religious beliefs may lead them to view the pregnancy as unacceptable or sinful; they may reject the pregnant teenager as well as the child she carries.

Cultural beliefs

Cultural values can influence how a family plans for or reacts to childbearing. Some cultures view childbearing as something to be shared with others as soon as the pregnancy is known. Other cultures, such as the Jewish culture, shy away from being public about pregnancy until the pregnancy has reached a certain gestation.

Woman's work

Cultural norms impact family roles, behaviors, and expectations. For example, culture may influence how a man participates in the pregnancy and childbirth. Members of some cultures, such as Mexican-Americans and Arab-Americans, allow only women in the birthing room during childbirth. In some cases, childbirth is considered a woman's place—not a man's.

Cultural cues

Cultural values can also influence your care. Acknowledging the cultural characteristics and beliefs of a patient and her family is an important part of family-centered care. To provide culturally competent care for women during pregnancy, a nurse needs to familiarize herself with the practices and customs of various cultures. (See *Childbearing practices of selected cultures*.)

> *Being sensitive to the patient's cultural needs is an important part of family-centered care.*

Planned versus unplanned pregnancy

Some women view pregnancy as a natural and desired outcome of marriage. To them, having children is a natural progression after marriage. They may plan to have children, or they may not plan the pregnancy but are accepting when it happens. Women who are prepared to accept a pregnancy seek medical validation at some of the first signs of pregnancy.

For other women, pregnancy may be unplanned. In some cases, especially in some adolescents, pregnancy may be an unwanted result of sexual experimentation without contraception. In cases where the pregnancy wasn't planned, the woman may react with ambivalence or she may deny her symptoms and postpone seeking medical validation.

Family matters

Just because a pregnancy is planned, however, doesn't mean that no family member will have trouble accepting it—possibly, even the mother or father. For example, if the pregnancy is unplanned and the father doesn't want a child or the parents are having other difficulties in their relationship, family upheaval can result. The mother may initially want the pregnancy but may be ambivalent about how the pregnancy is changing her body. The parents as a

Childbearing practices of selected cultures

A patient's cultural beliefs can affect her attitudes toward illness and traditional medicine. By trying to accommodate these beliefs and practices in your care plan, you can increase the patient's willingness to learn and comply with treatment regimens. Because cultural beliefs may vary within particular groups, individual practices may differ from those described here.

Culture	Childbearing practices
Asian-American	• View pregnancy as a natural process • Believe mother has "happiness in her body" • Omit milk from diet because it causes stomach distress • Believe inactivity and sleeping late can result in difficult birth • Believe childbirth causes a sudden loss of "yang forces," resulting in an imbalance in the body • Believe hot foods, hot water, and warm air restore the yang forces • Are attended to during labor by other women (usually patient's mother)—not the father of the baby • Have stoic response to labor pain • May prefer herbal medicine • Restrict activity for 40 to 60 days postpartum • Believe that colostrum is harmful (old, stale, dirty, poisonous or contaminated) to baby so may delay breast-feeding until milk comes in
Native-American	• View pregnancy as a normal, natural process • May start prenatal care late • Prefer a female birth attendant or a midwife • May be assisted in birth by mother, father, or husband • View birth as a family affair and may want entire family present • May use herbs to promote uterine contractions, stop bleeding, or increase flow of breast milk • Use cradle boards to carry baby and don't handle baby much • May delay breast-feeding because colostrum is considered harmful and dirty • May plan on taking the placenta home for burial
Hispanic-American	• View pregnancy as normal, healthy state • May delay prenatal care • Prefer a "patera," or midwife • Are strongly influenced by the mother-in-law and mother during labor and may listen to them rather than the husband during birth • View crying or shouting out during labor as acceptable • Bring together mother's legs after childbirth to prevent air from entering uterus • May wear a religious necklace that's placed around the neonate's neck after birth • Believe in hot and cold theory of disease and health • Restricted to boiled milk and toasted tortillas for first 2 days after birth • Must remain on bed rest for 3 days after birth • Delay bathing for 14 days after childbirth • Delay breast-feeding because colostrum is considered dirty and spoiled • Don't circumcise male infants • May place a bellyband on the neonate to prevent umbilical hernia

(continued)

Childbearing practices of selected cultures *(continued)*

Culture	Childbearing practices
Arab-American	• May not seek prenatal care • Seek medical assistance when medical resources at home fail • Fast during pregnancy to produce a son • May labor in silence to be in control • Limit male involvement during childbirth
Black-American	• View pregnancy as a state of well-being • May delay prenatal care • Believe that taking pictures during pregnancy may cause stillbirth • Believe that reaching up during pregnancy may cause the umbilical cord to strangle the baby • May use self-treatment for discomfort • May cry out during labor or may be stoic • May receive emotional support during birth from mother or another woman • May view vaginal bleeding during postpartum period as sickness • May prohibit tub baths and shampooing hair in the postpartum period • May view breast-feeding as embarrassing and, therefore, bottle-feed • Consider infant who eats well "good" • May introduce solid food early • May oil the baby's skin • May place a bellyband on the neonate to prevent umbilical hernia

unit may feel they aren't prepared to be parents or that they don't have enough experience around children. In addition, one family member may feel that the family's resources can't provide for a new addition. This too can lead to turmoil over the pregnancy.

Family dynamics

Family dynamics—including a family's structure and how it functions—also affect how a new pregnancy is perceived. Family members are influenced by their changing roles as well as by the physical and emotional changes the pregnant woman experiences. Some family members accept the pregnancy as a part of the family's growth. Other family members may view the pregnancy as a stressor and consider the new member an intruder.

For many families, pregnancy causes career and lifestyle changes that must be made to accommodate the new addition. The parent's ability to meet the physical and emotional needs of existing children in the family also changes.

Coping or moping?

The family support system may be affected as it attempts to cope with the pregnancy. Effective coping methods are demonstrated by the family's participation in parenting classes, childbirth education classes, and prenatal care. Ineffective coping mechanisms are evidenced by delaying confirmation of the pregnancy, hiding the pregnancy, or delaying prenatal care.

> Because you're all participating in parenting and childbirth education classes, I can tell that you're coping well with your pregnancies.

Social and economic resources

Economic status can also affect how a family responds to pregnancy. A pregnant woman living in a family whose financial responsibilities are stretched may delay prenatal care or chose not to take prenatal vitamins because of financial issues. Many families are barely able survive on two incomes; a pregnancy may reduce that income, which places emotional and financial strain on the family.

Age and health status of other family members

The health of other family members is another factor that can affect how a family views a pregnancy. If one family member is sick or has a long-term illness that requires a lot of family time and support, the addition of another family member may not be viewed favorably. It also affects the time family members have available to spend with the sick family member. As a result, family roles may have to change.

Sibling rivalry

Siblings may also be influenced by the arrival of a new member. Some siblings may perceive the new addition as a threat to their position in the family and become jealous. Such threats can be real or perceived, especially when the sibling experiences separation from the mother when she's hospitalized.

What a difference a year makes

Sibling reaction depends on the child's age. For instance, toddlers are aware of the mother's changing appearance and may have difficulty with separation when the mother leaves. A toddler exhibits this stress by showing signs of regression. Preschoolers and school-age children are likely to be interested in the pregnancy and may ask a lot of questions. They may also express a willingness to participate in childcare. Adolescents, on the other hand, are more likely to be embarrassed by the mother's pregnancy because it represents sexual activity between their parents. However, they may also be very attentive to the needs of the mother.

Medical and obstetric history of the mother

Ideally, a woman should be in good health when she begins her pregnancy. Sometimes, however, a woman with an ongoing illness (such as cardiac disease) becomes pregnant. Such an illness can complicate the pregnancy and cause problems for the woman, affecting how the mother and other members of the family respond to the news. Family members may be concerned that a pregnancy could jeopardize the mother's health. Likewise, if a woman has an obstetric history that includes some difficult labors or births, the family may react unfavorably out of concern for the mother's health.

> It says here that you two may be affected when a new baby is born. How you respond depends on your age.

Ethical and legal issues

Some of the most difficult decisions made in the health care setting are those that involve children and their families. Because maternal-neonatal nursing is so family centered, conflicts commonly arise because family members don't agree on how a situation should be handled. In addition, the values of the health care provider may conflict with those of the family. Legal and ethical issues that may arise in maternal-neonatal care include abortion, prenatal screening, in vitro fertilization (IVF), fetal tissue research, eugenics and gene manipulation, and treatment of preterm and high-risk neonates. (See *Dealing with ethical and legal issues.*)

Abortion

Abortion can pose a complex ethical dilemma for a nurse and her patients. A nurse who's ethically or morally opposed to abortion can't be forced to participate in the procedure. However, the nurse's employer can insist that she provide nursing care to all patients.

Practice, don't preach

No matter what your opinions are regarding abortion, don't allow personal feelings to interfere with your care for a postabortion patient, and don't try to impose your values on the patient. A nurse's role is to provide the best possible care, not to judge or make comments about a patient's personal decision.

Dealing with ethical and legal issues

When you're faced with an ethical or a legal issue in your practice, such as abortion or in vitro fertilization, be sure to follow these guidelines to ensure that you're providing the best care to your patient and fulfilling your nursing duties.

Inform and be informed

Nurses can help their patients make informed decisions by providing factual information and supportive listening and by helping the family clarify its values.

Be self-aware

To reach your own resolutions about legal and ethical issues, you'll need to examine your views honestly and carefully. You'll want to periodically reevaluate your position in light of new medical information and your own experi-

ence. If you feel strongly about a particular issue, you should consider working for a facility that matches your views.

Remember your role

Every nurse has an ethical obligation to provide competent, compassionate care. Even if your views on a particular issue differ greatly from those of your patient, don't allow your personal feelings to interfere with the quality of care you provide.

Prenatal screening

Thanks to such diagnostic procedures as amniocentesis, ultrasound, alpha-fetoprotein screening, and chorionic villi sampling, it's now possible to detect inherited and congenital abnormalities long before birth. In a few cases, the diagnosis has paved the way for repair of a defect in utero. However, because it's easier to detect genetic disorders than to treat them, prenatal screening commonly forces a patient to choose between having an abortion and taking on the emotional and financial burden of raising a severely disabled child.

Benefits vs. risks

Prenatal diagnostic procedures involve some risk to the fetus. Amniocentesis, for example, causes serious complications or death in about 0.5% of patients. Some people feel that this risk creates a conflict between the rights of the fetus and the parents' right to know his health status.

Knowing is half the battle

If testing is to be considered ethically by patients and their families, the nurse must take steps to help the patients fully understand the procedure. Patients must also comprehend what the test can and can't tell them and be informed about other available options. Thus, effective pretest and posttest counseling sessions are essential parts of an ethical prenatal screening program.

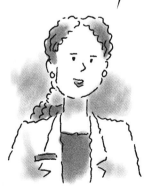

Effective pretest and posttest counseling sessions are essential parts of an ethical prenatal screening program.

In vitro fertilization

Infertility can have devastating effects on the emotional well-being of a couple who yearns for children. As a result, many couples spend time and money to conceive or adopt a child. When medical procedures (such as fertility medications, hysterosalpingostomy, and artificial insemination) fail and adoption isn't an option, infertile couples may turn to IVF.

In IVF, ova are removed from a woman's ovaries, placed in a petri dish filled with a sterilized growth medium, and covered with healthy motile spermatozoa for fertilization. Three to five embryos are then implanted in the woman's uterus 10 to 14 days after fertilization, and the remaining fertilized ova are frozen for future use or discarded. IVF can be performed using the partner's sperm (homologous) or a donor's sperm (heterologous).

Conception controversy

Some people hail the scientific manipulation of ova and sperm as a medical miracle. Others are concerned that IVF circumvents the natural process of procreation. Another IVF issue involves leftover embryos. About 15 to 20 embryos may result from a single fertilization effort, but only 3 to 5 of them are implanted in the woman's uterus. Some individuals question whether it's ethical to discard these leftover embryos, destroy them, or use them for scientific study.

No matter what your values are concerning IVF, keep in mind that your goal is to provide the best nursing care possible to your patients.

Surrogate motherhood

A surrogate mother is a woman who gives birth after carrying the fertilized ovum of another woman or, more commonly, after being artificially inseminated with sperm from the biological father. In the latter case, the biological father then legally adopts the infant.

Offering hope

Surrogate motherhood offers hope for the 60% to 70% of infertile couples in which the woman is the infertile partner. It's also an option for a woman whose age or health makes pregnancy risky. A surrogate birth poses no greater risk to the fetus (or surrogate mother) than any average birth.

Whose rights are right?

One of the ethical concerns about surrogate motherhood involves the potential conflicts concerning the rights of the surrogate mother, the infertile couple, the fetus, and society. The basic dispute involves who has the strongest claim to the child. Does the surrogate mother have rights by virtue of her biological connection? Does the surrogate contract guarantee the infertile couple the right to the child? Courts of law usually rule in favor of the infertile couple.

Support systems

In a surrogate mother situation, the nurse's role is to support her patient. If the patient is the surrogate mother, collaboration with a social worker or a psychologist may be necessary.

Fetal tissue research

Although still in the early stages, transplants using tissue from aborted fetuses offer new hope for treating Parkinson's disease, Alzheimer's disease, diabetes, and other degenerative disorders. Transplanted fetal nerve cells help to generate new cells in a patient with a degenerative disorder, which somehow reduce the symptoms of the disorder. The immaturity of the fetal immune system reduces the chances of the recipient rejecting the tissue, making fetal tissue ideally suited to transplantation. However, such treatment is controversial and may conflict with your values or those of your patient. As a nurse, you'll need to stay informed about developing research so that you can provide your patients with the most current information.

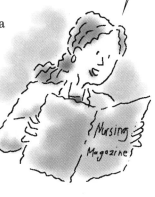

You need to keep up with current research in order to provide the most up-to-date information to your patients.

Eugenics and gene manipulation

Eugenics is the science of improving a species through control of hereditary factors — in other words, by manipulating the gene pool. In the past, medical research has been limited to efforts to repair or halt the damage caused by disease and injury. Today, however, genetic manipulation and engineering have tremendous potential for altering the course of human development.

It's all in the genes

Using current techniques, researchers can learn many things about a fetus before it's born, including its sex or whether it suffers from certain serious medical conditions. Deoxyribonucleic acid (DNA) can even tell parents what color hair their child will have or how tall he'll be.

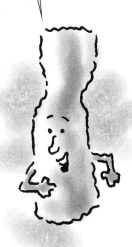

More and more, scientists are using genes like me to screen for disease.

Mr. Screen Genes

The identification of the genes responsible for inherited diseases and congenital malformations has spurred the development of new screening tests. Genetic testing is now a fairly common component of prenatal care, facilitating the identification of fetuses with such disorders as Down syndrome and Tay-Sachs disease. The screening of neonates for phenylketonuria is legally required in most states.

Harnessing the power of heredity

Many medical conditions don't have safe and effective treatments. In some cases, gene therapy can change that. Gene therapy using DNA can be used to:
- increase the activity of a gene in the body
- decrease the activity of a gene in the body
- introduce a new gene into the body.

Genetic engineering can even give science the ability to recreate the human body. Scientists frequently discover new ways to identify and manipulate the genetic material of everything from single-cell organisms to human beings.

Designer genes

There's little controversy about the ethics of gene therapy as it's currently practiced. However, some groups express concerns about the future. Genetic engineering can potentially allow parents to choose what traits they want their child to have. These "designer babies" may pose ethical dilemmas for some health care practitioners. Although enormous advances in technology are still needed before selecting such complicated traits as hair color, intelligence, and height becomes a reality, it's possible that these choices will be available to parents in the future.

Genetic manipulation and gene therapy are still experimental in some cases. As a result, few nurses are directly involved in these aspects of genetic research. Nonetheless, you have an ethical obligation to stay informed and to support efforts to establish legal and technological safeguards.

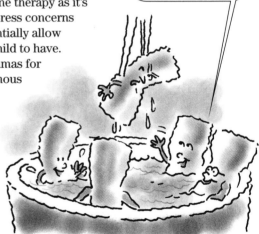

Eugenics is a controversial issue. However, when a bad gene is fished out of the pool, it could potentially prevent fatal diseases.

Preterm and high-risk neonates

Twenty years ago, an infant born at 26 weeks' gestation had almost no chance of survival. Today, this is no longer the case. Advances in neonatology, such as intrauterine surgery, synthetic lung surfactant, and new antibiotics, help save increasingly smaller and sicker infants.

Matters of life and death

When you care for an extremely premature or a critically ill infant and his mother, family members look to you to assist them with life-and-death decisions. To help the parents of an extremely premature or critically ill neonate reach ethically sound decisions, you'll need to present all available options in a compassionate, unbiased manner using simple terms. By carefully helping family members consider the pros and cons of both initiating and withholding treatment, you can help them come to terms with the neonate's condition and reach a decision with which they'll be able to live.

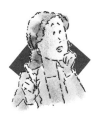

Quick quiz

1. The intrapartum period starts:
    A.   after delivery of the neonate and placenta.
    B.   at the onset of contractions.
    C.   at conception.
    D.   during the second trimester.

Answer: B. The intrapartum period starts at the onset of contractions that cause cervical dilation and lasts through the first 1 to 4 hours after the birth of the neonate and placenta.

2. An RN who has achieved advanced education at a master's level or through certification, cares for low-risk obstetric patients, and is licensed to deliver a neonate is called a:
    A.   nurse practitioner.
    B.   clinical nurse specialist.
    C.   pediatric nurse practitioner.
    D.   certified nurse-midwife.

Answer: D. A certified nurse-midwife is an RN with advanced education who cares for low-risk obstetric patients and is licensed to deliver a neonate.

3. A family that consists of parents, grandparents, and grandchildren is known as:
    A.   a cohabitation family.
    B.   an extended family.
    C.   a blended family.
    D.   a communal family.

Answer: B. An extended or multigenerational family consists of the nuclear family as well as other family members, such as grandparents, aunts, uncles, cousins, and grandchildren.

4.   When a woman gives birth after carrying the fertilized ovum of another woman, it's called:

    A.   in vitro fertilization.
    B.   cesarean birth.
    C.   surrogate motherhood.
    D.   gamete fertilization.

Answer: C. Surrogate motherhood involves one woman giving birth after carrying the fertilized ovum of another woman or after being inseminated with sperm from the biological father.

5.   The science of improving a species through control of hereditary factors by manipulation of the gene pool is called:

    A.   eugenics.
    B.   in vitro fertilization.
    C.   fetal tissue research.
    D.   genealogy.

Answer: A. Eugenics is the science of improving a species through control of hereditary factors by manipulation of the gene pool.

Scoring

☆☆☆ If you answered all five questions correctly, fantastic! Your labor is paying off!

☆☆ If you answered four questions correctly, good work! You're sure to reproduce these results in later chapters.

☆ If you answered fewer than four questions correctly, don't worry! Take a deep breath and then take a moment to review the chapter.

Conception and fetal development

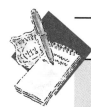

Just the facts

In this chapter, you'll learn:

♦ anatomic structures and functions of the male and female reproductive systems

♦ effects of hormone production on sexual development

♦ the process of fertilization

♦ stages of fetal development

♦ structural changes that result from pregnancy.

A look at conception and fetal development

Development of a functioning human being from a fertilized ovum involves a complex process of cell division, differentiation, and organization. Development begins with the union of spermatozoon and ovum (conception) to form a composite cell containing chromosomes from both parents. This composite cell (called a *zygote*) divides repeatedly. Finally, groups of differentiated cells organize into complex structures, such as the brain, spinal cord, liver, kidneys, and other organs that function as integrated units.

To fully understand the dramatic physical changes that occur during pregnancy, you must be familiar with reproductive anatomy and physiology and the stages of fetal development. Let's start with the male reproductive system.

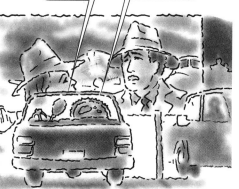

Male reproductive system

Anatomically, the main distinction between a male and a female is the presence of conspicuous external genitalia in the male. In contrast, the major reproductive organs of the female lie within the pelvic cavity.

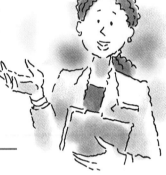

Here's the main difference — males have external genitalia, whereas most female reproductive organs are inside the pelvic cavity.

Making introductions

The male reproductive system consists of the organs that produce, transfer, and introduce mature sperm into the female reproductive tract, where fertilization occurs. (See *Structures of the male reproductive system.*)

Extra work

In addition to supplying male sex cells (spermatogenesis), the male reproductive system plays a part in the secretion of male sex hormones.

Penis

The organ of copulation, the penis deposits sperm in the female reproductive tract and acts as the terminal duct for the urinary tract. The penis also serves as the means for urine elimination. It consists of an attached root, a free shaft, and an enlarged tip.

What's inside

Internally, the cylinder-shaped penile shaft consists of three columns of erectile tissue bound together by heavy fibrous tissue. Two corpora cavernosa form the major part of the penis. On the underside, the corpus spongiosum encases the urethra. Its enlarged proximal end forms the bulb of the penis.

The glans penis, at the distal end of the shaft, is a cone-shaped structure formed from the corpus spongiosum. Its lateral margin forms a ridge of tissue known as the *corona*. The glans penis is highly sensitive to sexual stimulation.

What's outside

Thin, loose skin covers the penile shaft. The urethral meatus opens through the glans to allow urination and ejaculation.

In a different vein

The penis receives blood through the internal pudendal artery. Blood then flows into the corpora cavernosa through the penile artery. Venous blood returns through the internal iliac vein to the vena cava.

Structures of the male reproductive system

The male reproductive system consists of the penis, the scrotum and its contents, the prostate gland, and the inguinal structures.

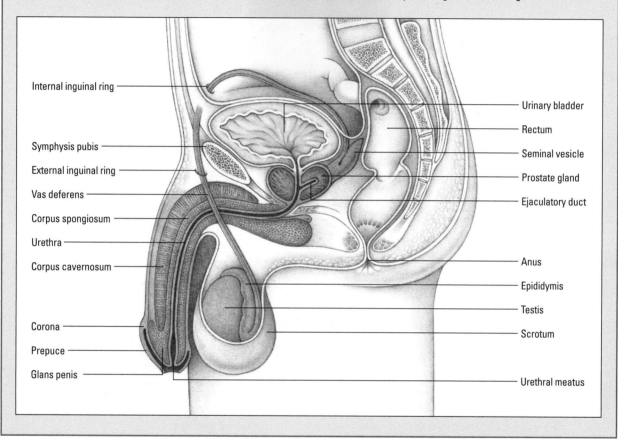

Internal inguinal ring

Symphysis pubis

External inguinal ring

Vas deferens

Corpus spongiosum

Urethra

Corpus cavernosum

Corona

Prepuce

Glans penis

Urinary bladder

Rectum

Seminal vesicle

Prostate gland

Ejaculatory duct

Anus

Epididymis

Testis

Scrotum

Urethral meatus

Scrotum

The penis meets the scrotum, or scrotal sac, at the penoscrotal junction. Located posterior to the penis and anterior to the anus, the scrotum is an extra-abdominal pouch that consists of a thin layer of skin overlying a tighter, musclelike layer. This musclelike layer, in turn, overlies the tunica vaginalis, a serous membrane that covers the internal scrotal cavity.

Canals and rings

Internally, a septum divides the scrotum into two sacs, which each contain a testis, an epididymis, and a spermatic cord. The spermatic cord is a connective tissue sheath that encases autonomic nerve fibers, blood vessels, lymph vessels, and the vas deferens (also called the *ductus deferens*).

The spermatic cord travels from the testis through the inguinal canal, exiting the scrotum through the external inguinal ring and entering the abdominal cavity through the internal inguinal ring. The inguinal canal lies between the two rings.

Loads of nodes

Lymph nodes from the penis, scrotal surface, and anus drain into the inguinal lymph nodes. Lymph nodes from the testes drain into the lateral aortic and pre-aortic lymph nodes in the abdomen.

> An important function of the scrotum is to keep the testes cooler than the rest of the body.

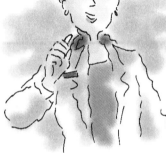

Testes

The testes are enveloped in two layers of connective tissue: the *tunica vaginalis* (outer layer) and the *tunica albuginea* (inner layer). Extensions of the tunica albuginea separate the testes into lobules. Each lobule contains one to four seminiferous tubules, small tubes where spermatogenesis takes place.

Climate control

Spermatozoa development requires a temperature lower than that of the rest of the body. The dartos muscle, a smooth muscle in the superficial fasciae, causes scrotal skin to wrinkle, which helps regulate temperature. The cremaster muscle, rising from the internal oblique muscle, helps to govern temperature by elevating the testes.

Duct system

The male reproductive duct system, consisting of the epididymis, vas deferens, and urethra, conveys sperm from the testes to the ejaculatory ducts near the bladder.

Swimmer storage

The epididymis is a coiled tube that's located superior to and along the posterior border of the testis. During ejaculation, smooth muscle in the epididymis contracts, ejecting spermatozoa into the vas deferens.

> During ejaculation, smooth muscle in the epididymis contracts, sending spermatozoa into the vas deferens.

Descending tunnel

The vas deferens leads from the testes to the abdominal cavity, extends upward through the inguinal canal, arches over the urethra, and descends behind the bladder. Its enlarged portion, called the *ampulla*, merges with the duct of the seminal vesicle to form the short ejaculatory duct. After passing through the prostate gland, the vas deferens joins with the urethra.

Tube to the outside

A small tube leading from the floor of the bladder to the exterior, the urethra consists of three parts:
• prostatic urethra, which is surrounded by the prostate gland and drains the bladder
• membranous urethra, which passes through the urogenital diaphragm
• spongy urethra, which makes up about 75% of the entire urethra.

Accessory reproductive glands

The accessory reproductive glands, which produce most of the semen, include the seminal vesicles, bulbourethral glands (Cowper's glands), and prostate gland.

A pair of pairs

The seminal vesicles are paired sacs at the base of the bladder. The bulbourethral glands, also paired, are located inferior to the prostate.

Improving the odds

The walnut-size prostate gland lies under the bladder and surrounds the urethra. It consists of three lobes: the left and right lateral lobes and the median lobe.

The prostate gland continuously secretes prostatic fluid, a thin, milky, alkaline fluid. During sexual activity, prostatic fluid adds volume to semen. It also enhances sperm motility and improves the odds of conception by neutralizing the acidity of the man's urethra and the woman's vagina.

Slightly alkaline

Semen is a viscous, white secretion with a slightly alkaline pH (7.8 to 8) that consists of spermatozoa and accessory gland secretions. The seminal vesicles produce roughly 60% of the fluid portion of semen, whereas the prostate gland produces about 30%. A viscid fluid secreted by the bulbourethral glands also becomes part of semen.

Spermatogenesis

Sperm formation, or *spermatogenesis*, begins when a male reaches puberty and usually continues throughout life.

Divide and conquer

Spermatogenesis occurs in four stages:

Memory jogger

To remember the meaning of spermatogenesis, keep in mind that genesis means "beginning" or "new." Therefore, spermatogenesis means beginning of new sperm.

☝ In the first stage, the primary germinal epithelial cells, called *spermatogonia*, grow and develop into primary spermatocytes. Both spermatogonia and primary spermatocytes contain 46 chromosomes, consisting of 44 autosomes and the two sex chromosomes, X and Y.

✌ Next, primary spermatocytes divide to form secondary spermatocytes. No new chromosomes are formed in this stage; the pairs only divide. Each secondary spermatocyte contains one-half of the number of autosomes, 22; one secondary spermatocyte contains an X chromosome; the other, a Y chromosome.

☟ In the third stage, each secondary spermatocyte divides again to form spermatids (also called *spermatoblasts*).

🖐 Finally, the spermatids undergo a series of structural changes that transform them into mature spermatozoa, or sperm. Each spermatozoa has a head, neck, body, and tail. The head contains the nucleus; the tail, a large amount of adenosine triphosphate, which provides energy for sperm motility.

Queuing up

Newly mature sperm pass from the seminiferous tubules through the vasa recta into the epididymis. Only a small number of sperm can be stored in the epididymis. Most of them move into the vas deferens, where they're stored until sexual stimulation triggers emission.

Check the expiration date?

After ejaculation, sperm can survive for 24 to 72 hours at body temperature. Sperm cells retain their potency and can survive for up to 4 days in the female reproductive tract.

The number of sperm and their motility affect fertility. A low sperm count (less than 20 million per milliliter of semen) may be a cause of infertility.

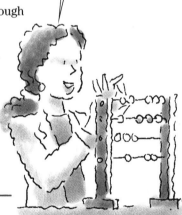

Hormonal control and sexual development

Androgens (male sex hormones) are produced in the testes and adrenal glands. Androgens are responsible for the development of male sex organs and secondary sex characteristics. One major androgen is testosterone.

The captain of the team

Leydig's cells, located in the testes between the seminiferous tubules, secrete testosterone, the most significant male sex hormone. Testosterone is responsible for the development and maintenance of male sex organs and secondary sex characteristics, such as facial hair and vocal cord thickness. Testosterone is also required for spermatogenesis.

Just call me the captain of team testosterone!

Calling the plays

Testosterone secretion begins approximately 2 months after conception, when the release of chorionic gonadotropins from the placenta stimulates Leydig's cells in the male fetus. The presence of testosterone directly affects sexual differentiation in the fetus. With testosterone, fetal genitalia develop into a penis, scrotum, and testes; without testosterone, genitalia develop into a clitoris, vagina, and other female organs.

During the last 2 months of gestation, testosterone usually causes the testes to descend into the scrotum. If the testes don't descend after birth, exogenous testosterone may correct the problem.

Other key players

Other hormones also affect male sexuality. Two of these, luteinizing hormone (LH) — also called *interstitial cell-stimulating hormone* — and follicle-stimulating hormone (FSH), directly affect secretion of testosterone.

Time to grow

During early childhood, a boy doesn't secrete gonadotropins and thus has little circulating testosterone. Secretion of gonadotropins from the pituitary gland, which usually occurs between ages 11 and 14, marks the onset of puberty. These pituitary gonadotropins stimulate testis functioning as well as testosterone secretion.

From boy to man

During puberty, the penis and testes enlarge and the male reaches full adult sexual and reproductive capability. Puberty also marks the development of male secondary sexual characteristics, including:
- distinct body hair distribution
- skin changes (such as increased secretion by sweat and sebaceous glands)
- deepening of the voice (from laryngeal enlargement)
- increased musculoskeletal development
- other intracellular and extracellular changes.

Reaching the plateau

After a male achieves full physical maturity, usually by age 20, sexual and reproductive function remain fairly consistent throughout life.

Subtle changes

With aging, a man may experience subtle changes in sexual function but he doesn't lose the ability to reproduce. For example, an elderly man may require more time to achieve an erection, experience less firm erections, and have reduced ejaculatory volume. After ejaculation, he may take longer to regain an erection.

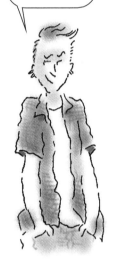

> I've reached puberty. Now can I borrow the car?

Female reproductive system

Unlike the male reproductive system, the female system is largely internal, housed within the pelvic cavity.

External genitalia

The vulva, or external female genitalia, include the mons pubis, labia majora, labia minora, clitoris, and adjacent structures. These structures are visible on inspection. (See *Structures of the female reproductive system*, pages 36 and 37.)

Mons pubis

The mons pubis is a rounded cushion of fatty and connective tissue covered by skin and coarse, curly hair in a triangular pattern over the symphysis pubis (the joint formed by the union of the pubic bones anteriorly).

Labia majora

The labia majora are two raised folds of adipose and connective tissue that border the vulva on either side, extending from the mons pubis to the perineum. After *menarche* (onset of the first menses), the outer surface of the labia is covered with pubic hair. The inner surface is pink and moist.

Labia minora

The labia minora are two moist folds of mucosal tissue, dark pink to red in color, that lie within and alongside the labia majora. Each upper section divides into an upper and lower lamella. The two upper lamellae join to form the prepuce, a hoodlike covering over

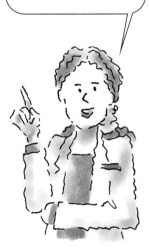

> The labia are highly vascular and have many nerve endings — making them sensitive to pain, pressure, touch, sexual stimulation, and temperature extremes.

the clitoris. The two lower lamellae form the frenulum, the posterior portion of the clitoris.

The lower labial sections taper down and back from the clitoris to the perineum, where they join to form the fourchette, a thin tissue fold along the anterior edge of the perineum.

Minor in name only

The labia minora contain sebaceous glands, which secrete a lubricant that also acts as a bactericide. Like the labia majora, they're rich in blood vessels and nerve endings, making them highly responsive to stimulation. They swell in response to sexual stimulation, a reaction that triggers other changes that prepare the genitalia for coitus.

Clitoris

The clitoris is the small, protuberant organ just beneath the arch of the mons pubis. It contains erectile tissue, venous cavernous spaces, and specialized sensory corpuscles, which are stimulated during sexual activity.

Adjacent structures

The vestibule is an oval area bounded anteriorly by the clitoris, laterally by the labia minora, and posteriorly by the fourchette.

Featuring glands

The mucus-producing Skene's glands are found on both sides of the urethral opening. Openings of the two mucus-producing Bartholin's glands are located laterally and posteriorly on either side of the inner vaginal orifice.

The urethral meatus is the slitlike opening below the clitoris through which urine leaves the body. In the center of the vestibule is the vaginal orifice. It may be completely or partially covered by the hymen, a tissue membrane.

Not too simple

Located between the lower vagina and the anal canal, the perineum is a complex structure of muscles, blood vessels, fasciae, nerves, and lymphatics.

Internal genitalia

The female internal genitalia are specialized organs; their main function is reproduction.

(Text continues on page 38.)

Structures of the female reproductive system

The female reproductive system consists of external and internal genitalia. These structures include the vagina, cervix, uterus, fallopian tubes, ovaries, and other structures. Reproductive, urinary, and GI structures are housed in the female pelvis. These include the bladder, anus, and rectum.

View of external genitalia in lithotomy position

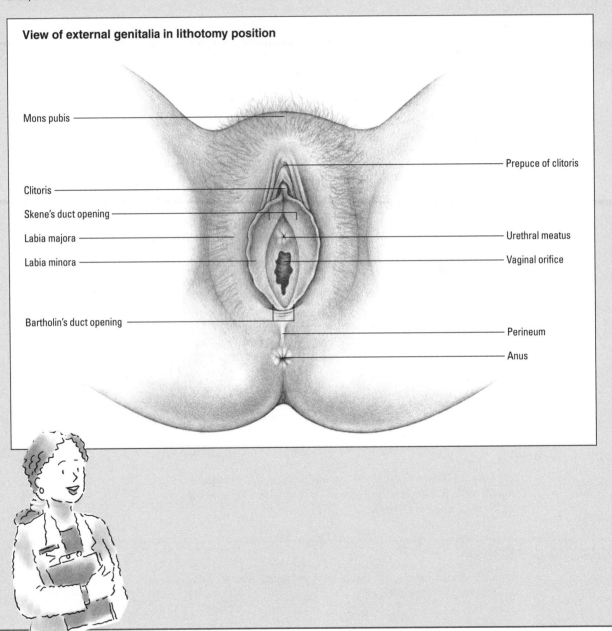

Lateral view of internal genitalia

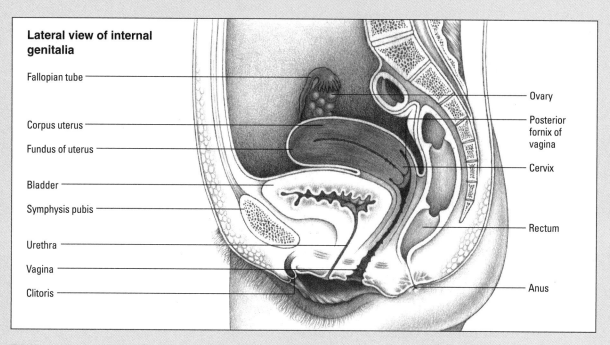

Fallopian tube

Corpus uterus

Fundus of uterus

Bladder

Symphysis pubis

Urethra

Vagina

Clitoris

Ovary

Posterior fornix of vagina

Cervix

Rectum

Anus

Anterior cross-sectional view of internal genitalia

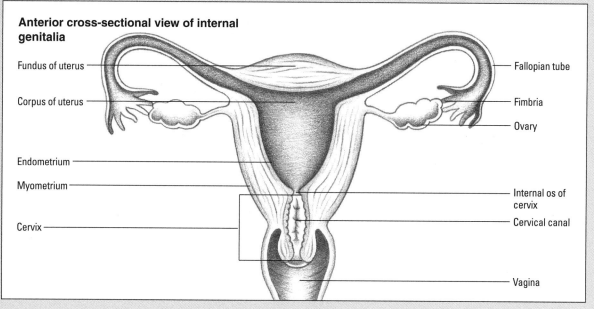

Fundus of uterus

Corpus of uterus

Endometrium

Myometrium

Cervix

Fallopian tube

Fimbria

Ovary

Internal os of cervix

Cervical canal

Vagina

Vagina

The vagina, a highly elastic muscular tube, is located between the urethra and the rectum.

Three layers...

The vaginal wall has three tissue layers: epithelial tissue, loose connective tissue, and muscle tissue. The uterine cervix connects the uterus to the vaginal vault. Four fornices, recesses in the vaginal wall, surround the cervix.

...three functions

The vagina has three main functions:

 to accommodate the penis during coitus

 to channel blood discharged from the uterus during menstruation

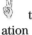 to serve as the birth canal during childbirth.

Supplied separately

The upper, middle, and lower vaginal sections have separate blood supplies. Branches of the uterine arteries supply blood to the upper vagina, the inferior vesical arteries supply blood to the middle vagina, and the hemorrhoidal and internal pudendal arteries feed into the lower vagina.

Blood returns through a vast venous plexus to the hemorrhoidal, pudendal, and uterine veins and then to the hypogastric veins. This plexus merges with the vertebral venous plexus.

Cervix

The cervix is the lowest portion of the uterus. It projects into the upper portion of the vagina. The end that opens into the vagina is called the *external os;* the end that opens into the uterus, the *internal os.* The cervix is sealed with thick mucus. This prevents sperm from entering except for a few days around ovulation when the plug becomes thinner.

Permanent alterations

Childbirth permanently alters the cervix. In a female who hasn't delivered a child, the external os is a round opening about 3 mm in diameter; after the first childbirth, it becomes a small transverse slit with irregular edges.

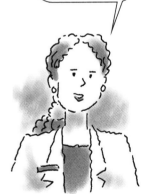

Over a woman's lifetime, the size and shape of her cervix change.

Uterus

The uterus is a small, firm, pear-shaped, muscular organ situated between the bladder and rectum. It typically lies at almost a 90-degree angle to the vagina. The mucous membrane lining of the uterus is called the *endometrium*, and the muscular layer of the uterus is called the *myometrium*.

Fundamental fundus

During pregnancy, the elastic, upper portion of the uterus, called the *fundus*, accommodates most of the growing fetus until term. The uterine neck joins the fundus to the cervix, the uterine part extending into the vagina. The fundus and neck make up the *corpus*, the main uterine body.

Fallopian tubes

Two fallopian tubes attach to the uterus at the upper angles of the fundus. These narrow cylinders of muscle fibers are where fertilization occurs.

Riding the wave

The curved portion of the fallopian tube, called the *ampulla*, ends in the funnel-shaped infundibulum. Fingerlike projections in the infundibulum, called *fimbriae*, move in waves that sweep the mature ovum (female gamete, or sex cell) from the ovary into the fallopian tube.

Ovaries

The ovaries are located on either side of the uterus. The size, shape, and position of the ovaries vary with age. Round, smooth, and pink at birth, they grow larger, flatten, and turn grayish by puberty. During the childbearing years, they take on an almond shape and a rough, pitted surface; after menopause, they shrink and turn white.

400,000 follicles

The ovaries' main function is to produce mature ova. At birth, each ovary contains approximately 400,000 graafian follicles. During the childbearing years, one graafian follicle produces a mature ovum during the first half of each menstrual cycle. As the ovum matures, the follicle ruptures and the ovum is swept into the fallopian tube.

The ovaries also produce estrogen and progesterone as well as a small amount of androgens.

Fingerlike projections called fimbriae move in waves, sweeping the ovum from the ovary to the fallopian tube.

Mammary glands

The mammary glands, located in the breast, are specialized accessory glands that secrete milk. Although present in both sexes, they typically function only in the female.

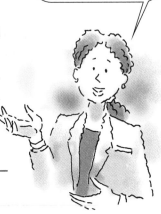

Both males and females have mammary glands — but they function only in the female.

Thanks for the mammaries

Each mammary gland contains 15 to 25 lobes that are separated by fibrous connective tissue and fat. Within the lobes are clustered acini — tiny, saclike duct terminals that secrete milk during lactation.

The ducts draining the lobules converge to form excretory (*lactiferous*) ducts and sinuses (*ampullae*), which store milk during lactation. These ducts drain onto the nipple surface through 15 to 20 openings. (See *The female breast.*)

Hormonal function and the menstrual cycle

Like the male body, the female body changes as it ages in response to hormonal control. When a female reaches the age of menstruation, the hypothalamus, ovaries, and pituitary gland secrete hormones — estrogen, progesterone, FSH, and LH — that affect the buildup and shedding of the endometrium during the menstrual cycle. (See *Events in the female reproductive cycle*, pages 42 and 43.)

A sometimes shocking development

During adolescence, the release of hormones causes a rapid increase in physical growth and spurs the development of secondary sex characteristics. This growth spurt begins at approximately age 11 and continues until early adolescence, or about 3 years later.

Irregularity of the menstrual cycle is common during this time because of failure of the female to ovulate. With menarche, the uterine body flexes on the cervix and the ovaries are situated in the pelvic cavity.

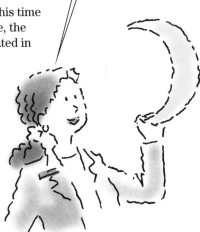

The menstrual cycle may range from 22 to 34 days, although a typical cycle lasts 28 days.

A monthly thing

The menstrual cycle is a complex process that involves both the reproductive and endocrine systems. The cycle averages 28 days.

Supply exhausted

In contrast to the slowly declining hormones of the aging male, the aging female's hormones decline rapidly in a process called *menopause*. Although the pituitary gland

The female breast

The breasts are located on either side of the anterior chest wall over the greater pectoral and the anterior serratus muscles. Within the areola, the pigmented area in the center of the breast, lies the nipple. Erectile tissue in the nipple responds to cold, friction, and sexual stimulation.

Support and separate

Each breast is composed of glandular, fibrous, and adipose tissue. Glandular tissue contains 15 to 20 lobes made up of clustered acini, tiny sac-like duct terminals that secrete milk. Fibrous Cooper's ligaments support the breasts; adipose tissue separates the two breasts.

Produce and drain

Milk glands in each breast produce milk by acini cells and then deliver it to the nipple by a lactiferous duct.

Sebaceous glands on the areolar surface, called Montgomery's tubercles, produce sebum, which lubricates the areola and nipple during breast-feeding.

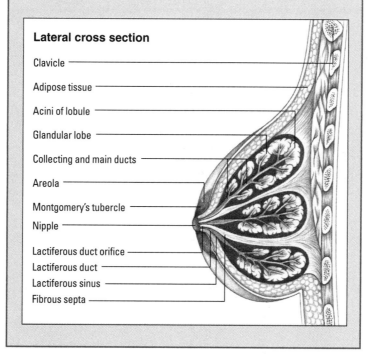

Lateral cross section

Clavicle
Adipose tissue
Acini of lobule
Glandular lobe
Collecting and main ducts
Areola
Montgomery's tubercle
Nipple
Lactiferous duct orifice
Lactiferous duct
Lactiferous sinus
Fibrous septa

still releases FSH and LH, the body has exhausted its supply of ovarian follicles that respond to these hormones and menstruation no longer occurs.

(Text continues on page 44.)

Events in the female reproductive cycle

The female reproductive cycle usually lasts 28 days. During this cycle, three major types of changes occur simultaneously: ovulatory, hormonal, and endometrial (involving the lining [endometrium] of the uterus).

Ovulatory

• Ovulatory changes, which usually last 5 days, begin on the 1st day of the menstrual cycle.
• As the cycle begins, low estrogen and progesterone levels in the bloodstream stimulate the hypothalamus to secrete gonadotropin-releasing hormone (Gn-RH). In turn, Gn-RH stimulates the anterior pituitary gland to secrete follicle-stimulating hormone (FSH) and luteinizing hormone (LH).
• Follicle development within the ovary (in the follicular phase) is spurred by increased levels of FSH and, to a lesser extent, LH.
• When the follicle matures, a spike in the LH level occurs, causing the follicle to rupture and release the ovum, thus initiating ovulation.
• After ovulation (in the luteal phase), the collapsed follicle forms the corpus luteum, which degenerates if fertilization doesn't occur.

Hormonal

• During the follicular phase of the ovarian cycle, the increasing FSH and LH levels that stimulate follicle growth also stimulate increased secretion of the hormone estrogen.
• Estrogen secretion peaks just before ovulation. This peak sets in motion the spike in LH levels, which causes ovulation.
• After ovulation (about day 14), estrogen levels decline rapidly. In the luteal phase of the ovarian cycle, the corpus luteum is formed and begins to release progesterone and estrogen.
• As the corpus luteum degenerates, levels of both of these ovarian hormones decline.

Endometrial

• The endometrium is receptive to implantation of an embryo for only a short time in the reproductive cycle. Thus, it's no accident that its most receptive phase occurs about 7 days after the ovarian cycle's release of an ovum—just in time to receive a fertilized ovum.
• In the first 5 days of the reproductive cycle, the endometrium sheds its functional layer, leaving the basal layer (the deepest layer) intact. Menstrual flow consists of this detached layer and accompanying blood from the detachment process.
• The endometrium begins regenerating its functional layer at about day 6 (the proliferative phase), spurred by rising estrogen levels.
• After ovulation, increased progesterone secretion stimulates conversion of the functional layer into a secretory mucosa (secretory phase), which is more receptive to implantation of the fertilized ovum.
• If implantation doesn't occur, the corpus luteum degenerates, progesterone levels drop, and the endometrium again sheds its functional layer.

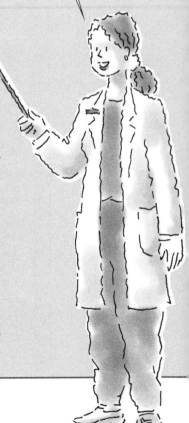

Three major types of changes occur during the reproductive cycle: ovulatory, hormonal, and endometrial.

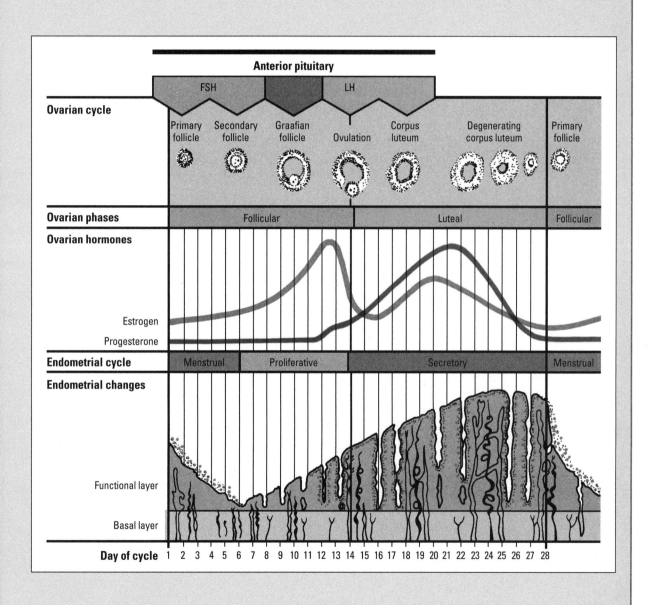

Cessation of menses usually occurs between ages 45 and 55. Some women experience menopause early, possibly as a result of genetics, ovarian damage, autoimmune disorders, or surgical interventions such as hysterectomy. When menopause occurs before age 45, it's known as *premature menopause.*

Menopause can be broken down into three stages (perimenopause, menopause, and postmenopause).

A time of decline

Perimenopause consists of the 8 to 10 years (called the *climacteric years*) of declining ovarian function that occur before menopause. During this time, the ovaries gradually begin to produce less estrogen and the woman may experience irregular menses that become further apart and produce a lighter flow. As menopause progresses, the ovaries stop producing progesterone and estrogen altogether.

1-year marker

A woman is considered to have reached the menopause stage after menses are absent for 1 year. At this stage, the ovaries have stopped producing eggs and have almost completely stopped producing estrogen.

Signs and symptoms of menopause include:
• hot flashes (sudden feelings of warmth that spread throughout the upper body and may be accompanied by blushing or sweating)
• irregular or skipped menses
• mood swings and irritability
• fatigue
• insomnia
• headaches
• changes in sex drive
• vaginal dryness.

Menopause can be confirmed through analysis of FSH levels or a Pap-like test that assesses for vaginal atrophy.

One thing leads to another

Postmenopause refers to the years after menopause. During this stage, the symptoms of menopause cease for most women. However, the risk of other health problems increases as a result of declining estrogen levels. These problems include:
• osteoporosis
• heart disease
• decreased skin elasticity
• vision deterioration.

Fertilization

Production of a new human being begins with *fertilization*, the union of a spermatozoon and an ovum to form a single new cell. After fertilization occurs, dramatic changes begin inside a woman's body. The cells of the fertilized ovum begin dividing as the ovum travels to the uterine cavity, where it implants itself in the uterine lining. (See *How fertilization occurs*, page 46.)

One in a million

For fertilization to take place, however, the spermatozoon must first reach the ovum. Although a single ejaculation deposits several hundred million spermatozoa, many are destroyed by acidic vaginal secretions. The only spermatozoa that survive are those that enter the cervical canal, where cervical mucus protects them.

Timing is everything

The ability of spermatozoa to penetrate the cervical mucus depends on the phase of the menstrual cycle at the time of transit:
• Early in the cycle, estrogen and progesterone levels cause the mucus to thicken, making it more difficult for spermatozoa to pass through the cervix.
• During midcycle, however, when the mucus is relatively thin, spermatozoa can pass readily through the cervix.
• Later in the cycle, the cervical mucus thickens again, hindering spermatozoa passage.

Help along the way

Spermatozoa travel through the female reproductive tract by means of flagellar movements (whiplike movements of the tail). After spermatozoa pass through the cervical mucus, however, the female reproductive system assists them on their journey with rhythmic contractions of the uterus that help the spermatozoa to penetrate the fallopian tubes. Spermatozoa are typically viable (able to fertilize the ovum) for up to 2 days after ejaculation; however, they can survive in the reproductive tract for up to 4 days.

Success becomes a zygote

Before a spermatozoon can penetrate the ovum, it must disperse the granulosa cells and penetrate the zona pellucida, the thick, transparent layer surrounding the incompletely developed ovum. Enzymes in the acrosome (head cap) of the spermatozoon permit this penetration. After penetration, the ovum completes its second

It's a lot of work for one sperm! After I make my way through the cervical mucus, uterine contractions help me to penetrate the fallopian tubes.

How fertilization occurs

Fertilization begins when the spermatozoon is activated upon contact with the ovum. Here's what happens.

The spermatozoon, which has a covering called the *acrosome,* approaches the ovum.

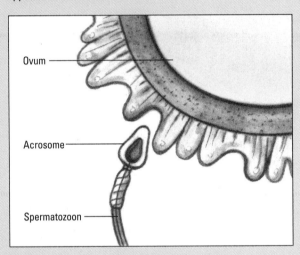

The acrosome develops small perforations through which it releases enzymes necessary for the sperm to penetrate the protective layers of the ovum before fertilization.

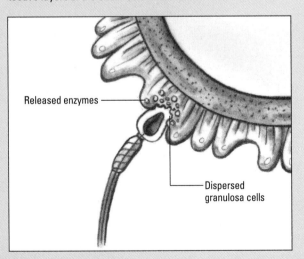

The spermatozoon then penetrates the zona pellucida (the inner membrane of the ovum). This triggers the ovum's second meiotic division (following meiosis), making the zona pellucida impenetrable to other spermatozoa.

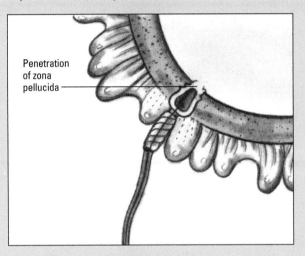

After the spermatozoon penetrates the ovum, its nucleus is released into the ovum, its tail degenerates, and its head enlarges and fuses with the ovum's nucleus. This fusion provides the fertilized ovum, called a *zygote,* with 46 chromosomes.

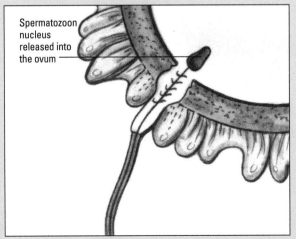

meiotic division and the zona pellucida prevents penetration by other spermatozoa.

The spermatozoon's head then fuses with the ovum nucleus, creating a cell nucleus with 46 chromosomes. The fertilized ovum is called a *zygote*.

Pregnancy

Pregnancy starts with fertilization and ends with childbirth; on average, its duration is 38 weeks. During this period (called *gestation*), the zygote divides as it passes through the fallopian tube and attaches to the uterine lining by implantation. A complex sequence of pre-embryonic, embryonic, and fetal developments transforms the zygote into a full-term fetus.

Nägele's rule can't predict the future, but it can provide a good estimation of when a baby will be born.

Making predictions

Because the uterus grows throughout pregnancy, uterine size serves as a rough estimate of gestation. The fertilization date is rarely known, so the woman's expected delivery date is typically calculated from the beginning of her last menses. The tool used for calculating delivery dates is known as *Nägele's rule.*

Here's how it works: If you know the first day of the last menstrual cycle, simply count back 3 months from that date and then add 7 days. For example, let's say that the first day of the last menses was April 29. Count back 3 months, which gets you to January 29, and then add 7 days for an approximate due date of February 5.

Stages of fetal development

During pregnancy, the fetus undergoes three major stages of development:

 pre-embryonic period (fertilization to week 3)

 embryonic period (weeks 4 through 7)

 fetal period (week 8 through birth).

The first 3 weeks

The pre-embryonic phase starts with ovum fertilization and lasts 3 weeks. As the zygote passes through the fallopian tube, it undergoes a series of mitotic divisions, or cleavage. (See *Pre-embryonic development.*)

The next month

During the embryonic period (the fourth through the seventh week of gestation), the developing zygote starts to take on a human shape and is now called an *embryo.* Each germ layer—the ectoderm, mesoderm, and endoderm—eventually forms specific tissues in the embryo. (See *Embryonic development*, page 50.)

Organ systems form during the embryonic period. During this time, the embryo is particularly vulnerable to injury by maternal drug use, certain maternal infections, and other factors.

The rest of the way

During the fetal stage of development, which extends from the eighth week until birth, the maturing fetus enlarges and grows heavier. (See *From embryo to fetus*, page 51.)

Two unusual features appear during this stage:

☝ The fetus' head is disproportionately large compared to its body. (This feature changes after birth as the infant grows.)

✌ The fetus lacks subcutaneous fat. (Fat starts to accumulate shortly after birth.)

Structural changes in the ovaries and uterus

Pregnancy changes the usual development of the corpus luteum and results in the development of the following structures:
• decidua
• amniotic sac and fluid
• yolk sac
• placenta.

Corpus luteum

Normal functioning of the corpus luteum requires continuous stimulation by LH. Progesterone produced by the corpus luteum suppresses LH release by the pituitary gland. If pregnancy occurs, the corpus luteum continues to produce progesterone until the placenta takes over. Otherwise, the corpus luteum atrophies 3 days before menstrual flow begins.

> The fetus isn't the only thing changing during pregnancy—the mother's reproductive system undergoes changes as well.

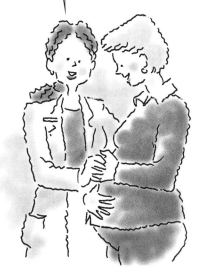

(Text continues on page 52.)

Pre-embryonic development

The pre-embryonic phase lasts from conception until approximately the end of the 3rd week of development.

Zygote formation...

As the fertilized ovum advances through the fallopian tube toward the uterus, it undergoes mitotic division, forming daughter cells, initially called *blastomeres,* that each contain the same number of chromosomes as the parent cell. The first cell division ends about 30 hours after fertilization; subsequent divisions occur rapidly.

The *zygote,* as it's now called, develops into a small mass of cells called a *morula,* which reaches the uterus at about the 3rd day after fertilization. Fluid that amasses in the center of the morula forms a central cavity.

...into blastocyst

The structure is now called a *blastocyst.* The blastocyst consists of a thin trophoblast layer, which includes the blastocyst cavity, and the inner cell mass. The trophoblast develops into fetal membranes and the placenta. The inner cell mass later forms the embryo *(late blastocyst).*

Getting attached: Blastocyst and endometrium

During the next phase, the blastocyst stays within the zona pellucida, unattached to the uterus. The zona pellucida degenerates and, by the end of the 1st week after fertilization, the blastocyst attaches to the endometrium. The part of the blastocyst adjacent to the inner cell mass is the first part to become attached.

The trophoblast, in contact with the endometrial lining, proliferates and invades the underlying endometrium by separating and dissolving endometrial cells.

Letting it all sink in

During the next week, the invading blastocyst sinks below the endometrium's surface. The penetration site seals, restoring the continuity of the endometrial surface.

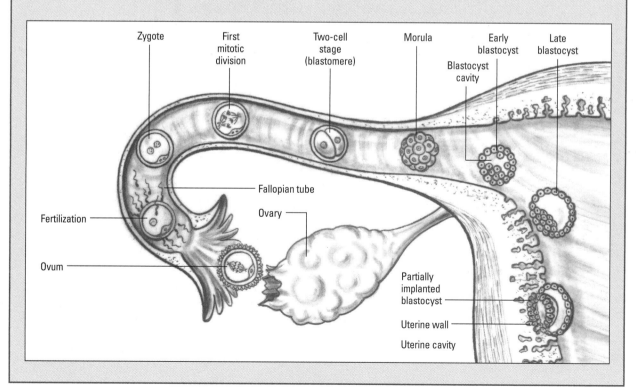

Zygote — First mitotic division — Two-cell stage (blastomere) — Morula — Early blastocyst — Late blastocyst — Blastocyst cavity — Fallopian tube — Ovary — Fertilization — Ovum — Partially implanted blastocyst — Uterine wall — Uterine cavity

Embryonic development

Each of the three germ layers—ectoderm, mesoderm, and endoderm—forms specific tissues and organs in the developing embryo.

Ectoderm

The ectoderm, the outermost layer, develops into the:
• epidermis
• nervous system
• pituitary gland
• tooth enamel
• salivary glands
• optic lens
• lining of lower portion of anal canal
• hair.

Mesoderm

The mesoderm, the middle layer, develops into:
• connective and supporting tissue
• the blood and vascular system
• musculature
• teeth (except enamel)
• the mesothelial lining of pericardial, pleural, and peritoneal cavities
• the kidneys and ureters.

Endoderm

The endoderm, the innermost layer, becomes the epithelial lining of the:
• pharynx and trachea
• auditory canal
• alimentary canal
• liver
• pancreas
• bladder and urethra
• prostate.

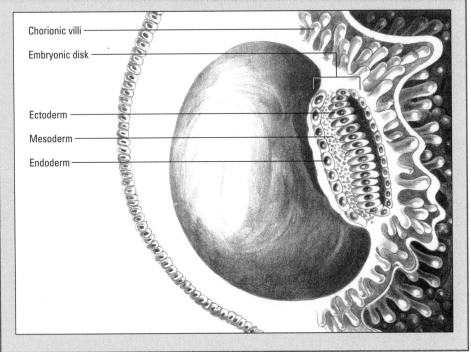

Chorionic villi

Embryonic disk

Ectoderm

Mesoderm

Endoderm

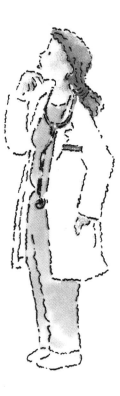

From embryo to fetus

Significant growth and development take place within the first 3 months following conception, as the embryo develops into a fetus that nearly resembles a full-term neonate.

Month 1

At the end of the first month, the embryo has a definite form. The head, the trunk, and the tiny buds that will become the arms and legs are discernible. The cardiovascular system has begun to function, and the umbilical cord is visible in its most primitive form.

Month 2

During the second month, the embryo—called a *fetus* from the 8th week—grows to 1" (2.5 cm) and weighs $\frac{1}{30}$ oz (1 g). The head and facial features develop as the eyes, ears, nose, lips, tongue, and tooth buds form. The arms and legs also take shape. Although the gender of the fetus isn't yet discernible, all external genitalia are present. Cardiovascular function is complete, and the umbilical cord has a definite form. At the end of the second month, the fetus resembles a full-term neonate except for size.

Month 3

During the third month, the fetus grows to 3" (7.6 cm) and weighs 1 oz (28.3 g). Teeth and bones begin to appear, and the kidneys start to function. The fetus opens its mouth to swallow, grasps with its fully developed hands, and prepares for breathing by inhaling and exhaling (although its lungs aren't functioning). At the end of the first *trimester* (the 3-month periods into which pregnancy is divided), its gender is distinguishable.

Months 3 to 9

Over the remaining 6 months, fetal growth continues as internal and external structures develop at a rapid rate. In the third trimester, the fetus stores the fats and minerals it will need to live outside the womb. At birth, the average full-term fetus measures 20" (50.1 cm) and weighs 7 to 7½ lb (3 to 3.5 kg).

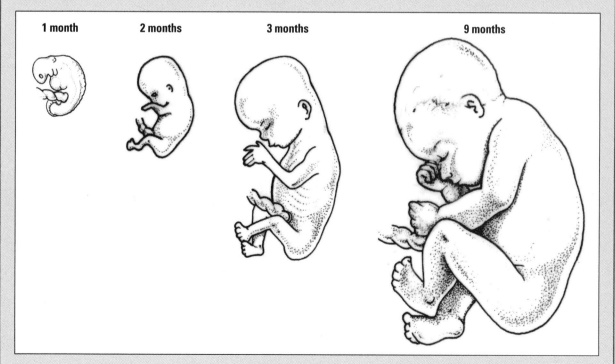

1 month   2 months   3 months   9 months

Hormone soup

With age, the corpus luteum grows less responsive to LH. There-fore, the mature corpus luteum degenerates unless stimulated by progressively increasing amounts of LH.

Pregnancy stimulates the placental tissue to secrete large amounts of human chorionic gonadotropin (HCG), which resem-bles LH and FSH. HCG prevents corpus luteum degeneration, stimulating the corpus luteum to produce large amounts of estro-gen and progesterone.

Early detection through HCG

The corpus luteum, stimulated by the hormone HCG, produces the estrogen and progesterone needed to maintain the pregnancy dur-ing the first 3 months. HCG can be detected as early as 9 days af-ter fertilization and can provide confirmation of pregnancy even before the woman has missed her first menses.

The HCG level gradually increases during this time, peaks at about 10 weeks' gestation, and then gradually declines.

Decidua

The decidua is the endometrial lining of the uterus that undergoes hormone-induced changes during pregnancy. Decidual cells se-crete the following three substances:
• the hormone *prolactin*, which promotes lactation
• a peptide hormone, *relaxin*, which induces relaxation of the connective tissue of the symphysis pubis and pelvic ligaments and promotes cervical dilation
• a potent hormonelike fatty acid, *prostaglandin*, which mediates several physiologic functions.

(See *Development of the decidua and fetal membranes.*)

Amniotic sac and fluid

The amniotic sac, enclosed within the chorion, gradually grows and surrounds the embryo. As it enlarges, the amniot-ic sac expands into the chorionic cavity, eventually filling the cavity and fusing with the chorion by the 8th week of gesta-tion.

A warm, protective sea

The amniotic sac and amniotic fluid serve the fetus in two impor-tant ways, one during gestation and the other during delivery. Dur-ing gestation, the fluid gives the fetus a buoyant, temperature-con-trolled environment. Later, amniotic fluid serves as a fluid wedge that helps to open the cervix during birth.

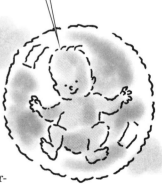

Amniotic fluid protects me during pregnancy — and later helps open the cervix for delivery.

Development of the decidua and fetal membranes

Specialized tissues support, protect, and nurture the embryo and fetus throughout its development. Among these tissues, the decidua and fetal membranes begin to develop shortly after conception.

Decidua

During pregnancy, the endometrial lining is called the *decidua*. It provides a nesting place for the developing ovum and has some endocrine functions.

Based primarily on its position relative to the embryo, the decidua may be known as the *decidua basalis,* which lies beneath the chorionic vesicle; the *decidua capsularis,* which stretches over the vesicle; or the *decidua parietalis,* which lines the remainder of the endometrial cavity.

Fetal membranes

The *chorion* is a membrane that forms the outer wall of the blastocyst. Vascular projections, called *chorionic villi,* arise from its periphery. As the chorionic vesicle enlarges, villi arising from the superficial portion of the chorion, called the *chorion laeve,* atrophy, leaving this surface smooth. Villi arising from the deeper part of the chorion, called the *chorion frondosum,* proliferate, projecting into the large blood vessels within the decidua basalis through which the maternal blood flows.

Blood vessels that form within the growing villi become connected with blood vessels that form in the chorion, body stalk, and within the body of the embryo. Blood begins to flow through this developing network of vessels as soon as the embryo's heart starts to beat.

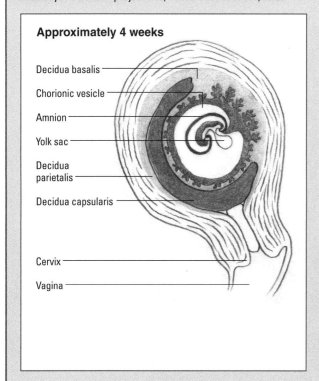

Approximately 4 weeks

- Decidua basalis
- Chorionic vesicle
- Amnion
- Yolk sac
- Decidua parietalis
- Decidua capsularis
- Cervix
- Vagina

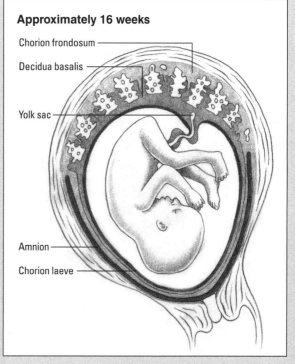

Approximately 16 weeks

- Chorion frondosum
- Decidua basalis
- Yolk sac
- Amnion
- Chorion laeve

Some from the mother, some from the fetus

Early in pregnancy, amniotic fluid comes chiefly from three sources:
- fluid filtering into the amniotic sac from maternal blood as it passes through the uterus
- fluid filtering into the sac from fetal blood passing through the placenta
- fluid diffusing into the amniotic sac from the fetal skin and respiratory tract.

Later in pregnancy, when the fetal kidneys begin to function, the fetus urinates into the amniotic fluid. Fetal urine then becomes the major source of amniotic fluid.

Every sea has its tides

Production of amniotic fluid from maternal and fetal sources balances amniotic fluid that's lost through the fetal GI tract. Typically, the fetus swallows up to several hundred milliliters of amniotic fluid each day. The fluid is absorbed into the fetal circulation from the fetal GI tract; some is transferred from the fetal circulation to the maternal circulation and excreted in maternal urine.

Yolk sac

The yolk sac forms next to the endoderm of the germ disk; a portion of it is incorporated in the developing embryo and forms the GI tract. Another portion of the sac develops into primitive germ cells, which travel to the developing gonads and eventually form *oocytes* (the precursor of the ovum) or *spermatocytes* (the precursor of the spermatozoon) after gender has been determined.

Not a permanent addition

During early embryonic development, the yolk sac also forms blood cells. Eventually, it undergoes atrophy and disintegrates.

Placenta

Using the umbilical cord as its conduit, the flattened, disk-shaped placenta provides nutrients to and removes wastes from the fetus from the 3rd month of pregnancy until birth. The placenta is formed from the chorion, its chorionic villi, and the adjacent decidua basalis.

A fetal lifeline

The umbilical cord contains two arteries and one vein and links the fetus to the placenta. The umbilical arteries, which transport blood from the fetus to the placenta, take a spiral course on the

Picturing the placenta

At term, the placenta (the spongy structure within the uterus from which the fetus derives nourishment) is flat, cakelike, and round or oval. It measures 6″ to 7¾″ (15 to 19.5 cm) in diameter and ¾″ to 1¼″ (2 to 3 cm) in breadth at its thickest part. The maternal side is lobulated; the fetal side is shiny.

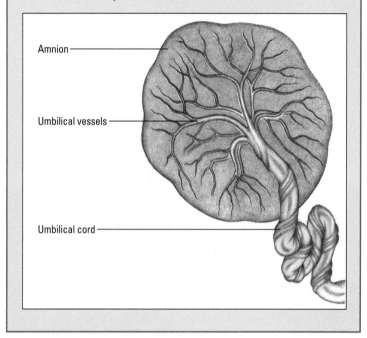

Amnion

Umbilical vessels

Umbilical cord

cord, divide on the placental surface, and branch off to the chorionic villi. (See *Picturing the placenta*.)

In a helpful vein

The placenta is a highly vascular organ. Large veins on its surface gather blood returning from the villi and join to form the single umbilical vein, which enters the cord, returning blood to the fetus.

Specialists on the job

The placenta contains two highly specialized circulatory systems:
• The *uteroplacental* circulation carries oxygenated arterial blood from the maternal circulation to the intervillous spaces—large spaces separating chorionic villi in the placenta. Blood enters the intervillous spaces from uterine arteries that penetrate the basal

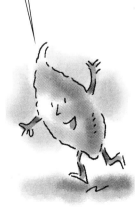

The placenta has two circulation systems — one involving maternal blood and another transporting fetal blood.

part of the placenta; it leaves the intervillous spaces and flows back into the maternal circulation through veins in the basal part of the placenta near the arteries.

• The *fetoplacental* circulation transports oxygen-depleted blood from the fetus to the chorionic villi by the umbilical arteries and returns oxygenated blood to the fetus through the umbilical vein.

Placenta takes charge

For the first 3 months of pregnancy, the corpus luteum is the main source of estrogen and progesterone—hormones required during pregnancy. By the end of the 3rd month, however, the placenta produces most of the hormones; the corpus luteum persists but is no longer needed to maintain the pregnancy.

Hormones on the rise

The levels of estrogen and progesterone, two steroid hormones, increase progressively throughout pregnancy. Estrogen stimulates uterine development to provide a suitable environment for the fetus.

Progesterone, synthesized by the placenta from maternal cholesterol, reduces uterine muscle irritability and prevents spontaneous abortion of the fetus.

Keep those acids coming

The placenta also produces human placental lactogen (HPL), which resembles growth hormone. HPL stimulates maternal protein and fat metabolism to ensure a sufficient supply of amino acids and fatty acids for the mother and fetus. HPL also stimulates breast growth in preparation for lactation. Throughout pregnancy, HPL levels rise progressively.

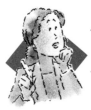

Quick quiz

1. Spermatogenesis is:
    A. the growth and development of sperm into primary spermatocytes.
    B. the division of spermatocytes to form secondary spermatocytes.
    C. the structural changing of spermatids.
    D. the entire process of sperm formation.

Answer: D. Spermatogenesis refers to the entire process of sperm formation—from the development of primary spermatocytes to the formation of fully functional spermatozoa.

2.   The primary function of the scrotum is to:
    A.   provide storage for newly developed sperm.
    B.   maintain a cool temperature for the testes.
    C.   deposit sperm in the female reproductive tract.
    D.   provide a place for spermatogenesis to take place.

Answer: B. The function of the scrotum is to maintain a cool temperature for the testes, which is necessary for spermatozoa formation.

3.   The main function of the ovaries is to:
    A.   secrete hormones that affect the buildup and shedding of the endometrium during the menstrual cycle.
    B.   accommodate a growing fetus during pregnancy.
    C.   produce mature ova.
    D.   channel blood discharged from the uterus during menstruation.

Answer: C. The main function of the ovaries is to produce mature ova.

4.   The corpus luteum degenerates in which phase of the female reproductive cycle?
    A.   Luteal
    B.   Follicular
    C.   Proliferative
    D.   Ovarian

Answer: A. The corpus luteum degenerates in the luteal phase of the ovarian cycle of reproduction.

5.   The four hormones involved in the menstrual cycle are:
    A.   LH, progesterone, estrogen, and testosterone.
    B.   estrogen, FSH, LH, and androgens.
    C.   estrogen, progesterone, LH, and FSH.
    D.   LH, estrogen, testosterone, and androgens.

Answer: C. The four hormones involved in the menstrual cycle are estrogen, progesterone, LH, and FSH.

6.   Each of the three germ layers forms specific tissues and organs in the developing:
    A.   zygote.
    B.   ovum.
    C.   embryo.
    D.   fetus.

Answer: C. Each of the three germ layers (ectoderm, mesoderm, and endoderm) forms specific tissues and organs in the developing embryo.

7.   The structure that guards the fetus is the:
  A.   decidua.
  B.   amniotic sac.
  C.   corpus luteum.
  D.   yolk sac.

Answer: B. The structure that guards the fetus by producing a buoyant, temperature-controlled environment is the amniotic sac.

Scoring

☆☆☆   If you answered all seven questions correctly, fabulous! You're first-rate with the physiology of fertilization.

☆☆   If you answered five or six questions correctly, excellent! You're looking good in the areas of reproduction and conception.

☆   If you answered fewer than five questions correctly, don't fear! A little review will deliver positive results.

3

Family planning, contraception, and infertility

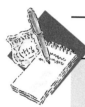

Just the facts

In this chapter, you'll learn:

♦ goals of family planning

♦ various methods of contraception, including the advantages and disadvantages of each

♦ surgical methods of family planning

♦ issues related to elective termination of pregnancy

♦ causes of infertility

♦ treatments and procedures used to correct infertility.

A look at family planning

Family planning involves the decisions couples or individuals make regarding when (and if) they should have children, how many children to have, and how long to wait between pregnancies. Family planning also consists of choices to prevent or achieve pregnancy and to control the timing and number of pregnancies. Family planning is a personal topic that has many ethical, physical, emotional, religious, and legal implications. Effectiveness, cost, contraindications, and adverse effects for all contraceptives should be presented to the patient and her partner so that they can make an informed decision.

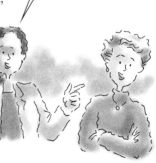

Family planning involves a lot of decision making. Be sure to keep couples informed so they can decide what's best for themselves.

A look at contraception

Contraception is the deliberate prevention of conception, using a method or device to avert fertilization of an ovum.

Choosing a contraceptive

When discussing with a patient the contraceptive methods that are most appropriate for her and her partner, remember that a contraceptive should be safe, easily obtained, free from adverse effects, affordable, acceptable to the user and her partner, and free from effects on future pregnancies. In addition, couples should use a contraceptive that's as close as possible to being 100% effective.

History lesson

Information from the patient's menstrual and obstetric history should be used to determine which contraceptive method is best for her. The patient's history is also used to plan appropriate patient teaching.

An assessment for family planning involves collecting a reproductive history, including:
- interval between menses
- duration and amount of flow
- problems that occur during menses
- number of previous pregnancies
- number of previous births (and date of each)
- duration of each pregnancy
- type of each delivery
- gender and weight of children when delivered
- problems that occurred during previous pregnancy
- problems that occurred after delivery.

Scope out potential complications

The patient's health history may also identify potential risks of complications and help to determine if hormonal contraceptives are safe for the patient to use. For example, a breast-feeding patient may be prescribed progesterone alone or a low-dose combination of hormonal contraceptives, which may cause her milk supply to decrease.

Factor in the partner factor

In some cases, the health of the patient's sexual partner influences which contraception method is used. For example, if the patient's

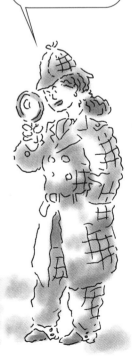

Identifying potential risks of complications is an important part of determining which method of contraception is best for the patient.

Education edge

Teaching tips on contraception

Here are some points you should cover when teaching a patient about contraception:
• Teach proper use of the selected contraceptive, and describe the procedure for the chosen method accurately.
• Discuss possible adverse reactions. Direct the patient to report adverse reactions to her health care provider.
• Stress the importance of keeping follow-up appointments. During follow-up visits, contraceptive use and adverse reactions are evaluated and a repeat Papanicolaou test is performed. Follow-up visits also provide an opportunity to address any questions the patient may have.
• Answer all questions in a manner that's easily understood by the patient.

sexual partner is infected with human immunodeficiency virus (HIV), ideally, she should exercise abstinence. If this isn't an option for your patient, encourage her to use a condom to prevent contraception as well as infection transmission.

Implementing the chosen contraceptive

The effectiveness and safety of any contraceptive depends greatly on the patient's knowledge of and compliance with the chosen method. The patient's inability to understand proper use of the contraceptive device or an unwillingness to use it correctly or consistently may result in pregnancy. That's why patient teaching is such an important component of family planning. (See *Teaching tips on contraception.*)

With proper instruction and information, the patient should be able to:
• describe the use of the selected contraceptive correctly
• describe adverse reactions to the selected contraceptive and state her responsibility to report any that occur
• state that she'll make an appointment for her next visit (if indicated)
• express that the current method of birth control is an acceptable method for her.

Methods of contraception

Contraceptive methods include abstinence, natural family planning methods, oral contraceptives, transdermal contraceptive patches, intramuscular (I.M.) injections, intrauterine devices, and mechanical and chemical barrier methods. A once-a-month intravaginal contraceptive device is also available. (See *Vaginal contraceptive ring.*)

Abstinence

Abstinence, or refraining from having sexual intercourse, has a 0% failure rate. It's also the most effective way to prevent the transmission of sexually transmitted diseases (STDs). However, most individuals—especially adolescents—don't consider it an option or a form of contraception. Abstinence should always be presented as an option to the patient in addition to information about other forms of contraception.

The plus side

Here are the advantages of abstinence:
• It's the only method 100% effective against pregnancy or STDs.
• It's free.
• There are no contraindications.

The minus side

The only disadvantage to abstinence is that partners and peers may have negative reactions to it.

Natural family planning methods

Natural family planning methods are contraceptive methods that don't use chemicals or foreign material or devices to prevent pregnancy. Religious beliefs may prevent some individuals from using hormonal or internal contraceptive devices. Others just prefer a more natural method of planning or preventing pregnancy. Natural family planning methods include the rhythm, or calendar, method; basal body temperature method; cervical mucus, or Billings, method; symptothermal method; ovulation awareness; and coitus interruptus.

Keeping count

For most natural family planning methods, the woman's fertile days must be calculated so that she can abstain from intercourse

---

Vaginal contraceptive ring

The newest form of contraception on the market is a vaginal contraceptive ring called the NuvaRing. It consists of a flexible, colorless, transparent ring that contains the hormones estrogen and progestin. These hormones stop ovulation and thicken the cervical mucus, which blocks sperm from reaching the egg and fertilizing it.

How to use it
The vaginal contraceptive ring is inserted into the vagina during the first 5 days of the woman's menses and remains in place for 21 days. The ring is removed and a new ring is inserted 1 week later.

Adverse effects
Possible adverse effects include:
• breast tenderness
• headache
• irregular bleeding
• mood changes
• nausea
• weight gain
• vaginal discharge
• vaginal irritation.

on those days. Various methods are used to determine the woman's fertile period. The effectiveness of these methods depends on the patient's and partner's willingness to refrain from sex on the female partner's fertile days. Failure rates vary from 10% to 20%.

Rhythm method

The rhythm, or calendar, method requires that the couple refrain from intercourse on the days that the woman is most likely to conceive based on her menstrual cycle. This fertile period usually lasts from 3 or 4 days before until 3 or 4 days after ovulation.

For the record

Teach the woman to keep a diary of her menstrual cycle to determine when ovulation is most likely to occur. She should do this for 6 consecutive cycles. To calculate her safe periods, tell her to subtract 18 from the shortest cycle and 11 from the longest cycle that she has documented. For instance, if she had 6 menstrual cycles that lasted 26 to 30 days, her fertile period would be from the 8th day (26 minus 18) to the 19th day (30 minus 11). To ensure that pregnancy doesn't occur, she and her partner should abstain from intercourse during days 8 to 19 of her menstrual cycle. During those fertile days, she and her partner may also choose to use contraceptive foam. (See *Using the calendar method*, page 64.)

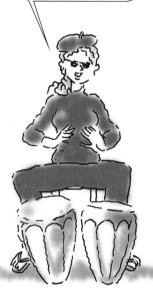

I've got rhythm, I've got music...but that won't necessarily keep me from getting pregnant. The rhythm method requires meticulous record keeping and the ability to monitor body changes.

The plus side

Here are the advantages of the rhythm method:
• No drugs or devices are needed.
• It's free.
• It may be acceptable to members of religious groups that oppose birth control.
• It encourages couples to learn more about how the female body functions.
• It encourages communication between partners.
• It can also be used to plan a pregnancy.

The minus side

Here are the disadvantages of the rhythm method:
• It requires meticulous record keeping as well as an ability and willingness for the woman to monitor her body changes.
• It restricts sexual spontaneity during the woman's fertile period.
• It requires extended periods of abstinence from intercourse.
• It's only reliable for women with regular menstrual cycles.
• It may be unreliable during periods of illness, infection, or stress.

Using the calendar method

This illustration demonstrates how the calendar method would be used to determine the woman's fertile period (ovulation) and when she should abstain from coitus.

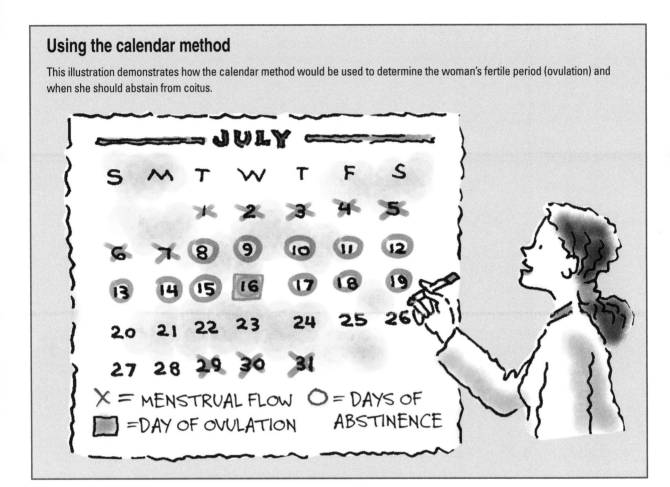

Basal body temperature

Just before the day of ovulation, a woman's basal body temperature (BBT) falls about one-half of a degree. At the time of ovulation, her BBT rises a full degree because of progesterone influence.

Recording the highs and lows

To use the BBT method of contraception, a woman must take her temperature every morning before sitting up, getting out of bed, or beginning her morning activity. (See *Teaching a patient how to take BBT*, pages 66 and 67.) By recording this daily temperature, she can see a slight dip and then an increase in body temperature. The increase in temperature indicates that she has ovulated. She should refrain from intercourse for the next 3 days. Three days is significant because this is the life of a discharged ovum. Because sperm can survive in the female reproductive tract for 4 days, the BBT method of contraception is typically combined with the calendar method so that the couple can abstain from intercourse a few days before ovulation as well.

Avoiding various variables

One problem with this method is that many things can affect BBT. The woman may forget and take her temperature after rising out of bed or she may have a slight illness. These situations cause a rise in temperature. If the woman changes her daily routine, the change in activity could also affect her body temperature, which may lead her to mistakenly interpret a fertile day as a safe day and vice versa.

The plus side

Here are the advantages of using BBT for family planning:
• It's inexpensive. The only expense involved is the cost of a BBT thermometer, which is calibrated in tenths of a degree.
• No drugs are needed.
• It may be acceptable to members of religious groups that oppose birth control.
• It encourages couples to learn more about how the female body functions.
• It encourages communication between partners.
• It can also be used to plan a pregnancy.

The minus side

Here are the disadvantages of BBT:
• It requires meticulous record keeping and an ability and willingness to monitor the woman's body changes.
• It restricts sexual spontaneity during the woman's fertile period.
• It requires extended periods of abstinence from intercourse.
• It's reliable only for women with regular menstrual cycles.
• It may be unreliable during periods of illness, infection, or stress.
• It's contraindicated in women who have irregular menses.

Cervical mucus

The cervical mucus method (also known as the Billings method) predicts changes in the cervical mucus during ovulation. Each month, before a woman's menses, the cervical mucus becomes thick and stretches when pulled between the thumb and forefinger. The normal stretchable amount of cervical mucus (also known as *spinnbarkeit*) is 8 to 10 cm (3″ to 4″). Just before ovula-

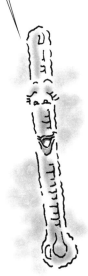

To obtain an accurate reading, a patient should take her basal body temperature before rising out of bed.

Education edge

Teaching a patient how to take BBT

Here are tips to help you teach your patient about recording basal body temperature (BBT). Remind the patient that BBT is lower during the first 2 weeks of the menstrual cycle, before ovulation. Immediately after ovulation, the temperature begins to rise. It continues to rise until it's time for the next menses. This rise in temperature indicates that progesterone has been released into the system, which, in turn, means that the woman has ovulated.

Charting BBT doesn't predict the exact day of ovulation; it just indicates that ovulation has occurred. However, this can be used to help the patient to monitor her ovulatory pattern and gives the patient a timeframe during which ovulation occurs that she can use in her planning.

Getting started

Tell your patient to follow these instructions for taking BBT:
• Advise the patient to chart the days of menstrual flow by darkening the squares above the 98° F (36.7° C) mark. She should start with the first day of her menses (day 1) and then take her temperature each day after her menses ends.
• Tell the patient to use a thermometer that measures tenths of a degree.
• Instruct the patient to take her temperature as soon as she wakes up. Tell her that it's important to do this at the same time each morning.

• The patient should now place a dot on the graph's line that matches the temperature reading. (Tell her not to be surprised if her waking temperature before ovulation is 96° or 97° F [35.6° or 36.1° C].) If she forgets to take her temperature on one day, instruct her to leave that day blank on the graph and not to connect the dots.
• Instruct her to make notes on the graph if she misses taking her temperature, feels sick, can't sleep, or wakes up at a different time. Advise her also that if she's taking any medicine—even aspirin—it may affect her temperature. Remind her to mark the dates when she had sexual relations.

Sample chart

Look over this sample temperature chart, recorded by Susan Jones. Ms. Jones used an S to record sexual relations and made notes showing she had insomnia on September 27. She forgot to take her temperature on September 19. Notice that she didn't connect the dots on this day. Her temperature dipped on September 24 (day 15 of the cycle). Then it began rising.

Of course, your patient's chart will be larger and will probably include temperatures over 99.3° F (37.4° C) and under 97° F.

tion, the cervical mucus becomes thin, watery, transparent, and copious.

Slippery peaks

During the peak of ovulation, the cervical mucus becomes slippery and stretches at least 2.5 cm (1″) before the strand breaks. Breast tenderness and anterior tilt of the cervix also occur with ovulation. The fertile period consists of all the days that the cervical mucus is copious and the 3 days after the peak date. During these days, the woman and her partner should abstain from intercourse to avoid conception.

Sample temperature chart

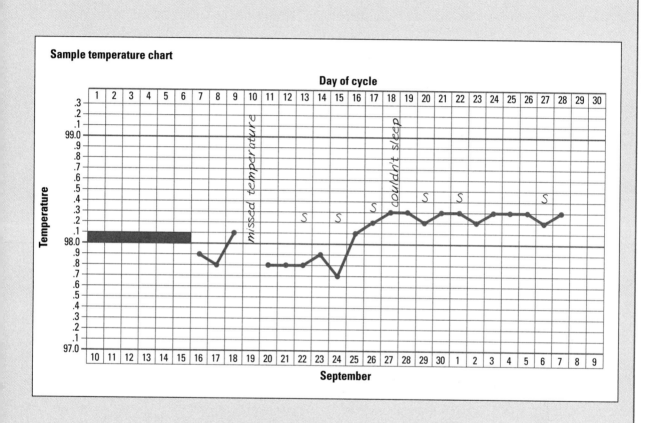

Consistently checking consistency

Cervical mucus must be assessed every day to note changes in the consistency and amounts if the woman is to be sure of the changes that signify ovulation. Assessing cervical mucus after intercourse is unreliable because seminal fluid has a watery, post-ovulatory consistency, which can be confused with ovulatory mucus.

The plus side

Here are the advantages of using the cervical mucus method:
• No drugs or devices are needed.
• It's free.
• It may be acceptable to members of religious groups that oppose birth control.
• It encourages couples to learn more about how the female body functions.
• It encourages communication between partners.
• It can also be used to plan a pregnancy.
• There are no contraindications.

The minus side

Here are the disadvantages:
• It requires meticulous record keeping and an ability and willingness to monitor the woman's body changes.
• It restricts sexual spontaneity during the woman's fertile period.
• It requires extended periods of abstinence from intercourse.
• It's reliable only for women with regular menstrual cycles.
• It may be unreliable during periods of illness, infection, or stress.

Combining the BBT and cervical mucus methods is more effective than using just one method.

Symptothermal method

The symptothermal method combines the BBT method with the cervical mucus method. The woman takes her daily temperature and watches for the rise in temperature that signals the onset of ovulation. She also assesses her cervical mucus every day. The couple abstains from intercourse until 3 days after the rise in basal temperature or the fourth day after the peak day (indicating ovulation) of cervical mucus because these symptoms indicate the woman's fertile period. Combining these two methods is more effective than if either is used alone.

The plus side

Here are the advantages of using the symptothermal method of family planning:
• It's inexpensive. The only expense involved is the cost of a BBT thermometer, which is calibrated in tenths of a degree.
• No drugs are needed.
• It may be acceptable to members of religious groups that oppose birth control.
• It encourages patients and their partners to learn more about how the female body functions.
• It encourages communication between partners.
• It can also be used to plan a pregnancy.

The minus side

Here are the disadvantages of the symptothermal method:
- It requires meticulous record keeping and ability and willing-ness of a woman to monitor body changes.
- It restricts sexual spontaneity during the woman's fertile period.
- It requires extended periods of abstinence from intercourse.
- It's reliable only for women with regular menstrual cycles.
- It may be unreliable during periods of illness, infection, or stress.

> Phew! The symptothermal method certainly requires meticulous record keeping!

Ovulation awareness

Over-the-counter ovulation detection kits determine ovulation by measuring luteinizing hormone (LH) in the urine. Usually, during each menstrual cycle, LH levels rise suddenly (called an *LH surge*), causing an ovum to be released from the ovary 24 to 36 hours later (ovulation). This test determines the midcycle surge of LH, which can be detected in the urine as early as 12 to 24 hours after ovulation. These kits are about 98% to 100% accurate, but they're fairly expensive to use as a primary means of birth control. (See *Performing a home ovulation test*, page 70.)

The plus side

Here are the advantages of the ovulation awareness method:
- It's an easier way to determine ovulation than the BBT or cervi-cal mucus methods.
- It may be less offensive to a woman than the cervical mucus method.
- It has a high rate of accuracy.
- There are no contraindications.

The minus side

Here are the disadvantages:
- It's expensive.
- It requires extended periods of abstinence from intercourse.
- It's reliable only for women with regular menstrual cycles.

Coitus interruptus

Coitus interruptus, one of the oldest known methods of contra-ception, involves withdrawal of the penis from the vagina during intercourse before ejaculation. However, because pre-ejaculation

Education edge

Performing a home ovulation test

A home ovulation test helps the patient determine the best time to try to become pregnant or to prevent pregnancy by monitoring the amount of luteinizing hormone (LH) that's found in her urine. These test kits can be purchased over-the-counter.

Normally, during each menstrual cycle, levels of LH rise suddenly, causing an egg to be released from the ovary 24 to 36 hours later.

Getting ready
Tell your patient to follow these instructions before performing a home ovulation test:
• Read the kit's directions thoroughly before performing the test.
• Before testing, calculate the length of the menstrual cycle. Count from the beginning of one menses to the beginning of the next menses. (The patient should count her first day of bleeding as day 1. She can use a chart such as the one shown at right to determine when to begin testing.)
• This test can be performed any time of the day or night, but it should be performed at the same time every day.
• Don't urinate for at least 4 hours before taking the test, and don't drink a lot of fluids for several hours before the test.

Taking the test
Tell your patient to follow these instructions for performing a home ovulation test:

• Remove the test stick from the packet.
• Sit on the toilet and direct the absorbent tip of the test stick downward and directly into the urine stream for at least 5 seconds or until it's thoroughly wet.
• Be careful not to urinate on the window of the stick.
• Alternatively, urinate in a clean, dry cup or container and then dip the test stick (absorbent tip only) into the urine for at least 5 seconds.
• Lay the stick on a clean, flat, dry surface.

Reading the results
Explain to your patient the following instructions for reading home ovulation test results:
• Wait at least 5 minutes before reading the results. When the test is finished, a line appears in the small window (control window).
• If there's no line in the large rectangular window (test window) or if the line is lighter than the line in the small rectangular window (control window), the patient hasn't begun an LH surge. She should continue testing daily.
• If she sees one line in the large rectangular window that's similar to or darker than the line in the small window, she's experiencing an LH surge. This means that ovulation should occur within the next 24 to 36 hours.
• Once the patient has determined that she's about to ovulate, she'll know

she's at the start of the most fertile time of her cycle and should use this information to plan accordingly.

Length of cycle	Start test this many days after your last menses begins	Length of cycle	Start test this many days after your last menses begins
21	5	31	14
22	5	32	15
23	6	33	16
24	7	34	17
25	8	34	18
26	9	36	19
27	10	37	20
28	11	38	21
29	12	39	22
30	13	40	23

fluid that's deposited outside the vagina may contain spermatozoa, fertilization can occur.

The plus side

Here are some advantages of coitus interruptus:
- It's free.
- It doesn't involve record keeping.
- There are no contraindications.

The minus side

The major disadvantage of this method is that it isn't reliable.

> What a team! The estrogen in oral contraceptives suppresses ovulation and the progesterone decreases the permeability of cervical mucus.

Oral contraceptives

Oral contraceptives (birth control pills) are hormonal contraceptives that consist of synthetic estrogen and progesterone. The estrogen suppresses production of follicle-stimulating hormone (FSH) and LH, which, in turn, suppresses ovulation. The progesterone complements the estrogen's action by causing a decrease in cervical mucus permeability, which limits sperm's access to the ova. Progesterone also decreases the possibility of implantation by interfering with endometrial proliferation.

Fixed vs. varying doses

There are two types of oral contraceptives:
- *Monophasic* oral contraceptives provide fixed doses of estrogen and progesterone throughout a 21-day cycle. These preparations provide a steady dose of estrogen but an increased amount of progestin during the last 11 days of the menstrual cycle.
- *Triphasic* oral contraceptives maintain a cycle more like a woman's natural menstrual cycle because they vary the amount of estrogen and progestin throughout the cycle. Triphasic oral contraceptives have a lower incidence of breakthrough bleeding than monophasic oral contraceptives.

Small but powerful

A mini pill is available for women who can't take estrogen-based pills because of a history of thrombophlebitis. This type of pill is taken every day — even when the woman has her menses. Progestins in the pill inhibit the development of the endometrium, thus preventing implantation.

21- or 28-day package deals

Monophasic and triphasic oral contraceptives are dispensed in either 21- or 28-day packs. The first pill is usually taken on the first Sunday following the start of a woman's menses, but it's possible to start oral contraceptives on any day. For a woman who has recently given birth, oral contraceptives can be started on the first Sunday 2 weeks after delivery. Patients should be advised to use an additional form of contraception for the first week after starting an oral contraceptive because the drug doesn't take effect for 7 days. (See *Teaching tips on oral contraceptives*.)

Birth control pills that are prescribed in a 21-day dispenser allow the woman to take a pill every day for 3 weeks. The woman should expect to start her menstrual flow about 4 days after she takes a cycle of pills. The 28-day pills are packaged with 21 days of birth control pills and 7 days of placeboes. With these pills, the woman starts the new pack of pills when she finishes the last pack and eliminates the risk of forgetting to start a new pack.

> Oral contraceptives can help to regulate the menstrual cycle and decrease premenstrual symptoms. However, they need to be taken daily and they don't protect against STDs.

The plus side

Here are the advantages of oral contraceptives:
• Monophasic and triphasic oral contraceptives are 99.5% effective in providing contraception. The failure rate is about 3% and usually occurs because the woman forgot to take the pill or because of other individual differences in the woman's physiology.
• They don't inhibit sexual spontaneity.
• They may reduce the risk of endometrial and ovarian cancer, ectopic pregnancy, ovarian cysts, and noncancerous breast tumors.
• They decrease the risk of pelvic inflammatory disease (PID) and dysmenorrhea.
• They regulate the menstrual cycle and may diminish or eliminate premenstrual tension.

The minus side

Here are the disadvantages:
• They don't protect the woman or her partner from STDs.
• They must be taken daily.
• They can be expensive (from $25 to $45 monthly).
• Illnesses that cause vomiting may reduce their effectiveness.
• They're contraindicated in women who are breast-feeding or pregnant; those who have a family history of stroke, coronary artery disease, thrombohemolytic disease, or liver disease; and those who have undiagnosed vaginal bleeding, malignancy of the reproductive system, malignant cell growth, or hypertension.

Education edge

Teaching tips on oral contraceptives

Be sure to include these tips when teaching patients about oral contraceptives:
• Inform the patient about possible adverse reactions, such as fluid retention, weight gain, breast tenderness, headache, breakthrough bleeding, chloasma, acne, yeast infection, nausea, and fatigue. It may be necessary to change the type or dosage of the contraceptive to relieve these adverse reactions.
• Instruct the patient on the dietary needs of a woman who's taking an oral contraceptive. Tell her to increase her intake of foods high in vitamin B_6 (wheat, corn, liver, meat) and folic acid (liver; green, leafy vegetables). About 20% to 30% of oral contraceptive users have dietary deficiencies of vitamin B_6 and folic acid. Moreover, health care professionals speculate that oral contraceptive users should also increase their intake of vitamins A, B_2, B_{12}, and C and niacin.
• Advise the patient to use an additional form of contraception for the first 7 days after starting the drug because it doesn't take effect for 7 days.

• Women who are older than age 40 and those who have a history of or have been diagnosed with diabetes mellitus, elevated triglyceride or cholesterol level, breast or reproductive tract malignancy, high blood pressure, obesity, seizure disorder, sickle cell disease, mental depression, and migraines or other vascular-type headaches should be strongly cautioned about taking oral contraceptives for birth control.
• A patient older than age 35 is at increased risk for a fatal heart attack if she smokes more than 15 cigarettes per day and takes oral contraceptives.
• Adverse effects include nausea, headache, weight gain, depression, mild hypertension, breast tenderness, breakthrough bleeding, and monilial vaginal infections.
• When a woman wants to conceive, she may not be able to for up to 8 months after stopping oral contraceptives. The pituitary gland requires a recovery period to begin the stimulation of cyclic gonadotropins, such as FSH and LH, which help regulate ovulation. In addition, many doctors recommend that women not become pregnant within 2 months of stopping the drug.

Transdermal contraceptive patches

The transdermal contraceptive patch is a highly effective, weekly hormonal birth control patch that's worn on the skin. A combination of estrogen and progestin is integrated into the patch. The hormones are absorbed into the skin and then transferred into the bloodstream.

Patchwork

The patch is very thin, beige, and smooth and measures 1¾″ (4.4 cm) square. It can be worn on the upper outer arm, buttocks, abdomen, or upper torso. The patch is worn for 1 week and replaced on the same day of the week for 3 consecutive weeks. No patch is worn during the fourth week. Studies have shown that the patch remains attached and effective when the patient bathes, swims, exercises, or wears it in humid weather.

The plus side

Here are the advantages of using a transdermal contraceptive patch:
• It's 99% effective in preventing pregnancy if used exactly as directed.
• It's convenient. No preparation is needed before intercourse.
• It's a good alternative for patients who commonly forget to take oral contraceptives.

The minus side

Here are the disadvantages of a transdermal patch:
• It doesn't protect the woman or her partner from STDs.
• It's contraindicated in women who are breast-feeding; those who have a family history of stroke, coronary artery disease, thrombohemolytic disease, or liver disease; those who have undiagnosed vaginal bleeding; and those who are sensitive to the adhesive used on the patch.
• Women who are over 40; women who have a history of or have been diagnosed with diabetes mellitus, elevated triglycerides or cholesterol level, breast or reproductive tract malignancy, high blood pressure, obesity, seizure disorder, sickle cell disease, mental depression, and migraine or other vascular-type headaches; and women who smoke should be strongly cautioned about using a transdermal contraceptive patch for birth control.

What a trooper! The transdermal contraceptive patch remains attached to the skin, even when the patient bathes, swims, or exercises.

I.M. injections

I.M. injections of medroxyprogesterone (Depo-Provera) are administered every 12 weeks. Depo-Provera stops ovulation from occurring by suppressing the release of gonadotropic hormones. It also changes the cervical mucosa to prevent sperm from entering the uterus.

The plus side

Here are the advantages of using an I.M. injection to prevent conception:
• It doesn't inhibit sexual response.

- Except for abstinence, it's more effective than other birth control methods.
- It helps prevent endometrial cancer.

The minus side

Here are the disadvantages:
- It requires an injection every 12 weeks.
- It can be expensive. Each injection is around $35, including injection fees.
- If the patient wants to become pregnant, it may take 9 to 10 months after the last injection to conceive.
- It doesn't protect against STDs.
- Its effects can't be reversed once injected.
- It may cause changes in the menstrual cycle.
- It may cause weight gain because of an increase in appetite.
- It may cause headache, fatigue, and nervousness.
- It's contraindicated if the patient is pregnant or has liver disease, undiagnosed vaginal bleeding, breast cancer, blood clotting disorders, or cardiovascular disease.

Intrauterine device

The intrauterine device (IUD) is a plastic contraceptive device that's inserted into the uterus through the cervical canal. (See *IUD insertion*, page 76.) The IUD is inserted into and removed from the uterus most easily during the woman's menses, when the cervical canal is slightly dilated. Inserting the device during menses also reduces the likelihood of inserting an IUD into a woman who's pregnant. Two types of IUDs are available in the United States: the ParaGard-T and the Progestasert system.

Copper interference

The ParaGard-T is a T-shaped, polyethylene device with copper wrapped around its vertical stem. The copper interferes with sperm mobility, decreasing the possibility of sperm crossing the uterine space. A knotted monofilament retrieval string is attached through a hole in the stem.

Progesterone reserve

The Progestasert IUD system is a T-shaped device made of an ethylene vinyl acetate copolymer with a knotted monofilament retrieval string attached through a hole in the vertical stem. Progesterone is stored in the hollow vertical stem, suspended in an oil base. The drug gradually diffuses into the uterus and prevents endometrium proliferation. This IUD must be replaced annually to

IUD insertion

An intrauterine device (IUD) is a plastic contraceptive device that's inserted into a woman's uterus through the cervical canal. This is performed most easily during menses. A bimanual examination is performed to determine uterine position, shape, and size.

Before IUD insertion, make sure that the procedure has been explained to the patient and that her questions have been addressed. Also, be sure to obtain informed consent.

How it's done
Here's how the device is inserted.

The movable flange on the inserter barrel of the IUD is set to the depth of the uterus (measured in centimeters). The loaded inserter tube is introduced through the cervical canal and into the uterus.

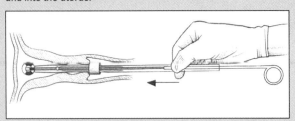

The IUD is inserted by retracting the inserter slowly about ½" (1.3 cm) over the plunger while the plunger is held still. This allows the arms to open.

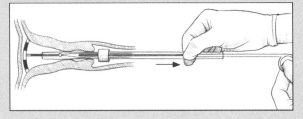

The plunger is gently advanced until resistance is felt. This action ensures high fundal placement of the IUD and may reduce the potential for expulsion.

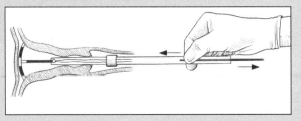

The solid rod is withdrawn while the inserting barrel is held stationary. The insertion barrel is then withdrawn from the cervix. The strings are clipped about 1" to 3" (2.5 to 7.5 cm) from the cervical os. This action leaves sufficient string for checking the placement of and removing the IUD.

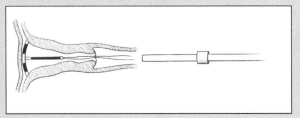

replenish the progesterone. The Progestasert system may relieve excessive menstrual blood loss and dysmenorrhea.

If a woman becomes pregnant with an IUD in place, the device can be left; however, it's usually removed to prevent spontaneous abortion and infection.

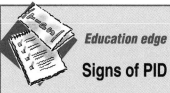

Education edge

Signs of PID

If your patient has an intrauterine device, tell her that untreated vaginal infections can progress to pelvic inflammatory disease (PID). Instruct the patient to watch for signs and symptoms of PID, such as:
• fever of 101° F (38.3° C)
• purulent vaginal discharge
• painful intercourse
• abdominal or pelvic pain
• suprapubic tenderness or guarding
• tenderness on bimanual examination.

The plus side

Here are the advantages of an IUD:
• It doesn't inhibit sexual spontaneity.
• Neither partner feels the device during intercourse.

The minus side

Here are the disadvantages:
• It's expensive.
• It may cause uterine cramping on insertion.
• It may cause infection, especially in the initial weeks after insertion.
• It can be spontaneously expelled in the first year by 5% to 20% of women.
• It doesn't protect against STDs.
• The incidence of PID increases with IUD use. Most cases of PID occur during the first 3 months after insertion. After 3 months, the chance of PID is lower unless preinsertion screening failed to identify a person at risk for STDs. The patient should be instructed to watch for signs of PID. (See *Signs of PID*.)
• It increases the risk of ectopic pregnancy.
• It's contraindicated in women who have Wilson's disease (because of inability to metabolize copper properly).
• It's contraindicated in women who have active, recent, or recurrent PID; infection or inflammation of the genital tract; STDs; diseases that suppress immune function, including HIV; unexplained cervical or vaginal bleeding; previous problems with IUDs; cancer of the reproductive organs; or a history of ectopic pregnancy. In-

sertion is also contraindicated in patients who have severe vaso-vagal reactivity, difficulty obtaining emergency care, valvular heart disease, anatomic uterine deformities, anemia, or nulliparity.

Barrier methods

In the barrier methods of contraception, a chemical or mechanical barrier is inserted between the cervix and the sperm to prevent the sperm from entering the uterus, traveling to the fallopian tubes, and fertilizing the ovum. Because barrier methods don't use hormones, they're sometimes favored over hormonal contraceptives, which can cause many adverse effects. However, failure rates for barrier methods are higher than hormonal contraceptives.

Barrier methods include spermicidal products, diaphragms, cervical caps, vaginal rings, and male and female condoms.

Spermicidal products

Before intercourse, spermicidal products are inserted into the vagina. Their goal is to kill sperm before the sperm enter the cervix. Spermicides also change the pH of the vaginal fluid to a strong acid, which isn't conducive to sperm survival. Vaginally inserted spermicides are available in gels, creams, films, foams, and suppositories.

The gels, foams, and creams are inserted using an applicator and should be inserted at least 1 hour before intercourse. The woman should be instructed not to douche for 6 hours after intercourse to ensure that the agent has completed its spermicidal action in the vagina and cervix.

Spermicidal films are made of glycerin that's impregnated with nonoxynol 9. The film is folded and then inserted into the vagina. When the film makes contact with vaginal secretions or precoital penile emissions, the film dissolves and carbon dioxide foam forms to protect the cervix against invading spermatozoa.

Spermicidal suppositories consist of cocoa butter and glycerin and are filled with nonoxynol 9. The suppositories are inserted into the vagina where they dissolve to release the spermicide. The suppository takes 15 minutes to dissolve, so patients should be instructed to insert it 15 minutes before intercourse.

The plus side

Here are the advantages of spermicidal products:
• They're inexpensive.
• They may be purchased over-the-counter, which makes them easily accessible.
• They don't require a visit to a health care provider.
• Spermicidal films wash away with natural body fluids.
• Nonoxynol 9, one of the most preferred spermicides, may also help prevent the spread of STDs.
• Vaginally inserted spermicides may be used in combination with other birth control methods to increase their effectiveness.
• They're useful in emergency situations such as when a condom breaks.

The minus side

Here are the disadvantages:
• They need to be inserted from 15 minutes to 1 hour before intercourse, so they may interfere with sexual spontaneity.
• Some spermicides may be irritating to the vagina and penile tissue.
• Some women are bothered by the vaginal leakage that can occur, especially after using cocoa- and glycerin-based suppositories.
• The film form's effectiveness depends on vaginal secretions; therefore, it isn't recommended for women who are nearing menopause because decreased vaginal secretions make the film less effective.
• Spermicidal products may be contraindicated in women who have acute cervicitis because of the risk of further irritation.

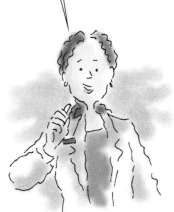

It's better to be safe than sorry. Spermicidal products are useful for added protection during the first several months of oral contraceptive or IUD use.

Diaphragm

The diaphragm is another barrier-type contraceptive that mechanically blocks sperm from entering the cervix. It's composed of a soft, latex dome that's supported by a round, metal spring on the outside. A diaphragm can be inserted up to 2 hours before intercourse. Optimum effectiveness is achieved by using it in combination with spermicidal jelly that's applied to the rim of the diaphragm before it's inserted. Diaphragms are available in various sizes and must be fitted to the individual. (See *Inserting a diaphragm*, page 80.)

The plus side

Here are the advantages of using a diaphragm for contraception:
• It's a good choice for women who choose not to use hormonal contraceptives or don't feel that they can be accurate in using natural family planning methods.

Education edge

Inserting a diaphragm

As you insert a diaphragm, instruct the patient to prepare her for inserting the diaphragm herself. Identify structures and the feelings associated with proper insertion. Follow these steps for insertion.

After putting on gloves, lubricate the rim or dome of the fitting ring or diaphragm to lessen the discomfort of insertion.

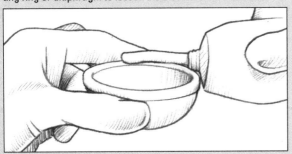

Fold the diaphragm in half with one hand by pressing the opposite sides together. Hold the vulva open with your other hand.

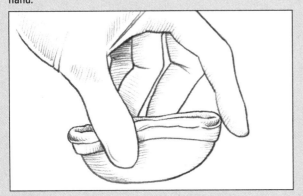

Slide the folded diaphragm into the vagina and toward the posterior cervicovaginal fornix.

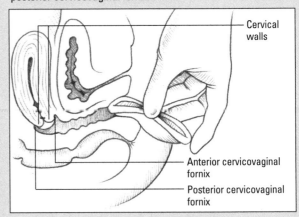

Cervical walls

Anterior cervicovaginal fornix

Posterior cervicovaginal fornix

The diaphragm should fit below the symphysis and cover the cervix. The proximal ring should fit behind the pubic arch with minimal pressure. Note that the cervix is palpable behind the diaphragm. The cervix feels like a "nose."

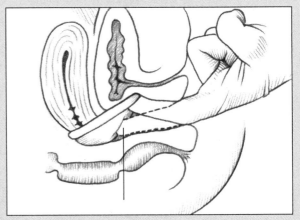

• When combined with spermicidal jelly, its effectiveness ranges from 80% to 93% for new users and increases to 97% for long-term users.
• It causes few adverse reactions.
• It helps protect against STDs when used with spermicide.
• It doesn't alter the body's metabolic or physiologic processes.
• It can be inserted up to 2 hours before intercourse.
• Providing it's correctly fitted and inserted, neither partner can feel it during intercourse.

The minus side

Here are the disadvantages of a diaphragm:
• Some women dislike using a diaphragm because it must be inserted before intercourse.
• Although the diaphragm can be left in place for up to 24 hours, if intercourse is repeated before 6 hours (which is how long the diaphragm *must* be left in place after intercourse) more spermicidal gel must be inserted. The diaphragm can't be removed and replaced because this could cause sperm to bypass the spermicidal gel and fertilization could occur.
• It may cause a higher incidence of upper urinary tract infections (UTIs) caused by the pressure of the diaphragm on the urethra.
• The diaphragm must be refitted after birth, cervical surgery, miscarriage, dilatation and curettage (D&C), therapeutic abortion, or weight gain or loss of more than 15 lb (6.8 kg) because of cervical shape changes.
• It's contraindicated in women who have a history of cystocele, rectocele, uterine retroversion, prolapse, retroflexion, or anteflexion because the cervix position may be displaced making insertion and proper fit questionable.
• It's contraindicated in patients with a history of toxic shock syndrome or repeated UTIs, vaginal stenosis, pelvic abnormalities, allergy to spermicidal jellies or rubber. It's also contraindicated in patients who show an unwillingness to learn proper techniques for diaphragm care and insertion.
• It can't be used in the first 6 weeks postpartum.

Cervical cap

The cervical cap is another barrier-type method of contraception. It's similar to the diaphragm but smaller. It's a thimble-shaped, soft rubber cup that the patient places over the cervix. The cap is held in place by suction. The addition of a spermicide creates a chemical barrier as well. Women who aren't suited for diaphragms may use cervical caps. Failure of the cervical cap is commonly due to failure to use the device or inappropriate use of the device. (See *Recognizing a correct fit*, page 82.)

Advice from the experts

Recognizing a correct fit

With the proper fit, the gap or space between the base of the cervix and the inside of the cervical cap ring should be 1 to 2 mm (to reduce the possibility of dislodgment), and the rim should fill the cervicovaginal fornix.

To verify a good fit, leave the cervical cap in place for 1 to 2 minutes. Then, with the cap in place, pinch the dome until there's a dimple. A dimple that takes about 30 seconds to resume a domed appearance indicates good suction and a good fit. If the cap is too small, the rim leaves a gap where the cervix remains exposed. If the cap is too large, it isn't snug against the cervix and is more easily dislodged.

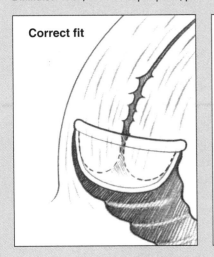

Correct fit

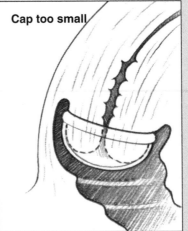

Cap too small

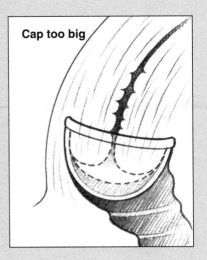

Cap too big

The plus side

Here are the advantages of using a cervical cap:
• The cap requires less spermicide, is less likely to become dislodged during intercourse, and doesn't require refitting with a change in weight.
• It has an efficacy rate of 85% for nulliparous women and 70% for parous women when used correctly and consistently.
• It doesn't alter hormones.
• It can be inserted up to 8 hours before intercourse.
• It doesn't require reapplication of spermicide before repeated intercourse.
• It can remain in place longer than diaphragms because it doesn't exert pressure on the vaginal walls or urethra.

The minus side

Here are the disadvantages:
• It requires possible refitting after weight gain or loss of 15 lb (6.8 kg) or more, recent pregnancy, recent pelvic surgery, or cap slippage.
• It may be difficult to insert or remove.
• It may cause an allergic reaction or vaginal lacerations and thickening of the vaginal mucosa.
• It may cause a foul odor if left in place for more than 36 hours.
• It can't be used during menstruation or during the first 6 post-partum weeks.
• It shouldn't be left in place longer than 24 hours.
• It's contraindicated in patients with a history of toxic shock syndrome, a previously abnormal Papanicolaou smear, allergy to latex or spermicide, an abnormally short or long cervix, history of PID, cervicitis, papillomavirus infection, cervical cancer, or undiagnosed vaginal bleeding.

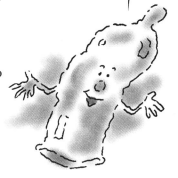

For me to do my job correctly, I need to be positioned properly.

Male condom

A male condom is a latex or synthetic sheath that's placed over the erect penis before intercourse. It prevents pregnancy by collecting spermatozoa in the tip of the condom, preventing them from entering the vagina.

Position is important

The condom should be positioned so that it's loose enough at the penis tip to collect ejaculate but not so loose that it comes off the penis. The penis must be withdrawn before it becomes flaccid after ejaculation or sperm can escape from the condom into the vagina.

The plus side

Here are the advantages of using a male condom:
• Many women favor male condoms because they put the responsibility of birth control on the male.
• No health care visit is needed.
• It's available over-the-counter in pharmacies and grocery stores.
• It's easy to carry.
• It prevents the spread of STDs.

The minus side

Here are the disadvantages of a condom:
• It must be applied before any vulvar penile contact takes place because pre-ejaculation fluid may contain sperm.

Education edge

Inserting a female condom

A female condom is made of latex and lubricated with nonoxynol 9. It has an inner ring that covers the cervix and an outer ring that rests against the vaginal opening, as shown below.

Inserting the condom

Inform your patient to take these steps when inserting the condom:

Fold the inner ring in half with one hand by pressing the opposite sides together, as shown below. When inserted, the inner ring covers the cervix.

After the condom is inserted, the outer ring (open end) rests against the vaginal opening.

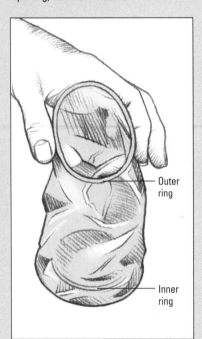

Outer ring

Inner ring

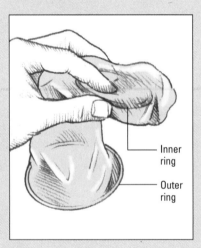

Inner ring

Outer ring

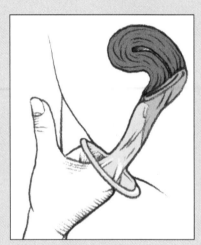

• It may cause an allergic reaction if the product contains latex and the patient or her partner is allergic.
• It may break during use if it's used incorrectly or is of poor quality.
• It can't be reused.
• Sexual pleasure may be affected.

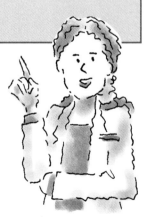

Female condom

A female condom is made of latex and lubricated with nonoxynol 9. The inner ring (closed end) covers the cervix. The outer ring (open end) rests against the vaginal opening. Female condoms are intended for one-time use and they shouldn't be used in combination with male condoms. (See *Inserting a female condom.*)

The plus side

Here are the advantages of using a female condom:
- It's 95% effective.
- It helps prevent the spread of STDs.
- It can be purchased over-the-counter.

The minus side

Here are the disadvantages:
- It's more expensive than the male condom.
- It's difficult to use and hasn't gained as much acceptance as a male condom.
- Pregnancy can occur as a result of failure to use or incorrect use.
- It may break or become dislodged.
- It's contraindicated in patients or partners with latex allergies.

Surgical methods of family planning

Surgical methods of family planning include vasectomy (for men) and tubal ligation (for women). These procedures are the most commonly chosen contraceptive methods for couples over age 30.

Reversal reality

It's possible to reverse these procedures, but it's expensive and isn't always effective. Therefore, surgical sterilization should only be chosen when the patient and her partner, if applicable, have thoroughly discussed the options and know that these procedures are for permanent contraception.

Vasectomy

Vasectomy is a procedure in which the pathway for spermatozoa is surgically severed. Incisions are made on each side of the scrotum, and the vas deferens is cut and tied, then plugged or cauterized. This blocks the passage of sperm. The testes continue to produce sperm as usual, but the sperm can't pass the severed vas deferens. (See *A closer look at vasectomy*, page 86.)

A closer look at vasectomy

In a vasectomy, the vas deferens is surgically altered to prohibit the passage of sperm. Here's how.

① The doctor makes two small incisions on each side of the scrotum.

② He then cuts the vas deferens with scissors.

③ The vas deferens is then cauterized or plugged to block the passage of sperm.

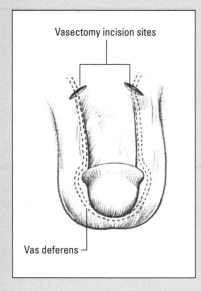

Vasectomy incision sites

Vas deferens

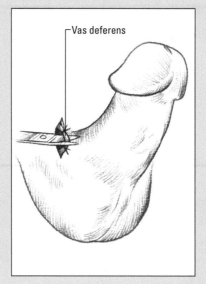

Vas deferens

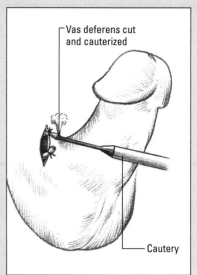

Vas deferens cut and cauterized

Cautery

Postoperative pregnancy potential

The patient should be cautioned that sperm remaining in the vas deferens at the time of surgery may remain viable for as long as 6 months. An additional form of contraception should be used until two negative sperm reports have been obtained. These reports confirm that all of the remaining sperm in the vas deferens has been ejaculated.

To prevent your patients from making a rash decision regarding vasectomy, explain that this procedure should be viewed as irreversible, although reversal is possible in 95% of cases.

The plus side

Here are the advantages of vasectomy:

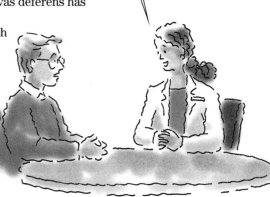

Vasectomy is 99.6% effective, and it can be done as an outpatient procedure with little or no pain.

• It can be done as an outpatient procedure, with little anesthesia and minimal pain.
• It's 99.6% effective.
• It doesn't interfere with male erection and the male still produces seminal fluid — it just doesn't contain sperm.

The minus side

Here are the disadvantages of vasectomy:
• Misconceptions about the procedure may lead some men to resist it.
• Some reports indicate the vasectomy may be associated with the development of kidney stones.
• It's contraindicated in individuals who aren't entirely certain of their decision to choose permanent sterilization and in those with specific surgical risks such as an anesthesia allergy.

Tubal sterilization

In tubal sterilization, a laparoscope is used to cauterize, crush, clamp, or block the fallopian tubes, thus preventing pregnancy by blocking the passage of ova and sperm. The procedure is performed after menses and before ovulation. It can also be performed 4 to 6 hours (although it's usually performed within 12 to 24 hours) after the birth of a baby or an abortion.
    Here's how it works:
• A small incision is made in the abdomen.
• Then carbon dioxide gas is pumped into the abdominal cavity to lift the abdominal wall, providing an easier view of the surgical area.
• A lighted laparoscope is inserted and the fallopian tubes are located.
• An electric current is then used to cauterize the tubes, or the tubes are clamped and cut.
After surgery, patients may notice some abdominal bloating from the carbon dioxide, but this subsides. (See *A closer look at tubal sterilization*, page 88.)

Promoting preoperative protection

Women should be cautioned to not have unprotected intercourse before the procedure because sperm that can become trapped in the tube could fertilize an ovum, resulting in an ectopic pregnancy.
    This procedure should be viewed as irreversible. Although reversal is successful in 40% to 75% of patients, the process is difficult and could cause an ectopic pregnancy.

A closer look at tubal sterilization

In a laparoscopic tubal sterilization, the surgeon inserts a laparoscope and occludes the fallopian tube by cauterizing, crushing, clamping, or blocking. This prevents the passage of ova and sperm.

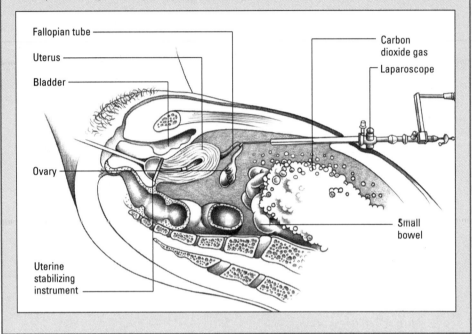

The plus side

Here are the advantages of tubal sterilization:
• It can be performed on an outpatient basis, and the patient is usually discharged within a few hours after the procedure.
• It's 99.6% effective.
• It's been associated with a decreased incidence of ovarian cancer.
• A woman can resume intercourse 2 to 3 days after having the procedure.

The minus side

Here are the disadvantages of this procedure:
• Some woman may be reluctant to choose this type of procedure because it requires a small surgical incision and general anesthesia.

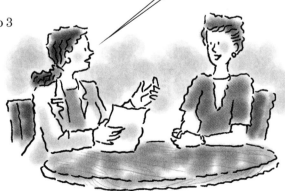

Tubal sterilization is 99.6% effective and can be performed on an outpatient basis.

• Complications include a risk of bowel perforation and hemorrhage and the typical risks of general anesthesia (allergy, arrhythmia) during the procedure.

• Contraindications include umbilical hernia and obesity.

• Posttubal ligation syndrome may occur. This includes vaginal spotting and intermittent vaginal bleeding as well as severe lower abdominal cramping.

• This form of contraception isn't recommended for individuals who aren't certain of their decision to choose permanent sterilization.

Elective termination of pregnancy

A procedure that's performed to deliberately end a pregnancy is known as an *elective termination of pregnancy.* Also known as an *induced abortion,* elective termination of pregnancy can be performed for many reasons, some of which involve:

• pregnancy that threatens a woman's life

• pregnancy in which amniocentesis identifies a chromosomal defect in the fetus

• pregnancy that results from rape or incest

• pregnancy in which the woman chooses not to have a child.

Elective terminations of pregnancy can be medically or surgically induced.

Medically induced abortion

In the medically induced method of abortion, a progesterone antagonist called mifepristone is taken to block the effect of progesterone and prevent implantation of the fertilized ovum. The drug is taken as a single dose at any time within 28 days gestation. If a spontaneous abortion doesn't occur, misoprostol (a prostaglandin E1 analog) is administered 3 days later.

Uterine contractions occur with mild cramping and the products of conception are expelled. One advantage to using this method is that it decreases the risk of damage to the uterus that can occur from instruments used in surgically induced abortions.

Consider this

Disadvantages of medically induced elective termination include the possibility of incomplete abortion as well as prolonged bleeding. Medically induced abortion is contraindicated in patients with suspected or confirmed ectopic pregnancy; hemorrhage disorders; current long-term systemic corticosteroid therapy; history of allergy to mifepristone, misoprostol, or other prostaglandins; an IUD; or chronic adrenal failure.

Surgically induced abortions

Depending on the gestation at the time of the abortion, surgical abortion can be performed several ways. These include D&C, dilatation and vacuum extraction (D&E), saline induction, and hysterotomy.

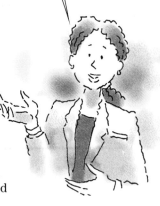

D&E can be performed between 12 and 16 weeks' gestation.

Dilatation and vacuum extraction

D&E uses the same technique as D&C except that the products of conception are removed by vacuum extraction. Some facilities admit the patient the day before the procedure to begin cervical dilation. This is achieved by inserting into the cervix a laminaria tent made of seaweed that has been dried and sterilized. This helps maintain the integrity of the cervix so that future pregnancies aren't threatened. As the seaweed from the laminaria tent absorbs the moisture from the cervix and vagina, it begins to swell and dilate the cervix. Then a small catheter is inserted and the products of conception are extracted by the vacuum over a 15-minute period.

This procedure can be performed between 12 and 16 weeks' gestation as either an outpatient or inpatient procedure. Complications such as uterine puncture and infections can occur.

Saline induction

Saline induction can be performed to terminate pregnancy if gestation is between 16 and 24 weeks. In saline induction, hypertonic saline solution is inserted through the uterine cavity into the amniotic fluid, which forces fluid to shift, causing the placenta and endometrium to slough.

Hysterotomy

A hysterotomy is the removal of the products of conception through a surgical incision in the uterus. This procedure, which is similar to a cesarean birth, can be performed for a pregnancy that's more than 18 weeks' gestation. Hysterotomy is usually performed because the cervix has become resistant to the effect of oxytocin and may not respond to saline induction. When it's determined that an abortion must be performed, gestation is more than 18 weeks, and other methods have failed, this procedure is still possible.

Infertility

Infertility is defined as the inability to conceive after 1 year of consistent attempts without using contraception. As many as 10% to 15% of couples who desire children experience infertility. (See *What's behind rising infertility rates?*)

Infertility can be considered primary or secondary:

• *Primary infertility* refers to infertility that occurs in couples who have had no previous conception.

• *Secondary infertility* refers to infertility that occurs in couples who have previously conceived.

Addressing the topic

Talking to a couple about infertility and its treatment requires many skills. For instance, you need to guide them sensitively through rigorous tests and treatments—some of which may be painful and embarrassing. At the same time, you need to help them deal with their own emotions.

Bittersweet emotions

A diagnosis of infertility may stir up many feelings and conflicts, such as anger, guilt, and blame, which may disrupt relationships and alter self-esteem. What's more, although treatment heightens the hope of conception, it can

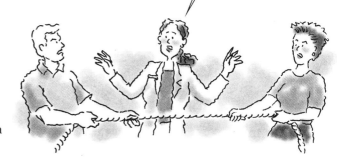

Infertility can be an emotional tug-of-war for many couples. You'll need to guide them sensitively through many tests and treatments.

What's behind rising infertility rates?

Childless couples need to feel that they aren't alone. Let them know that the number of couples dealing with infertility has doubled in recent years. Factors that may contribute to rising infertility rates include:

• aging—more and more couples postpone childbearing until age 30 or older, allowing age and concomitant disease processes to affect fertility

• sexually transmitted diseases, which may be responsible for up to 20% of infertility cases

• intrauterine devices, which can cause pelvic inflammatory disease and consequent infertility

• environmental factors such as toxins

• complications of abortion or childbirth.

There's also a higher incidence of infertility in females who:

• have irregular or absent periods

• experience pain during sexual intercourse

• have had ruptured appendices or other abdominal surgeries.

Education edge

Teaching topics on infertility

When teaching patients about infertility, be sure to cover these topics:
- definition of infertility
- possible causes, such as ovulatory dysfunction and structural abnormalities
- fertility drugs, including menotropins (Pergonal) and clomiphene (Clomid)
- explanation of in vitro fertilization-embryo transfer and gamete intrafallopian transfer, if appropriate
- artificial insemination
- surgery to promote fertility, including varicocelectomy, hysteroscopy, laparoscopy, and laparotomy
- psychological counseling.

also lead to deep disappointment if fertility measures fail. (See *Teaching topics on infertility*.)

Infertile couples need open communication to help build their trust and confidence in the health care team. Understandably, many couples feel uncomfortable discussing their sex life, let alone having intercourse assigned on a rigid schedule that's designed to take advantage of peak fertile days.

Conditions for conception

Many couples think that conception occurs easily when, in fact, certain conditions must be present for conception to occur. These include:
- sufficient and motile sperm
- mucus secretions that promote sperm movement in the reproductive tract
- unobstructed uterus and open fallopian tubes that allow sperm free passage
- regular ovulation and healthy ova
- hormonal sufficiency and balance that support implantation of the embryo in the uterus
- sexual intercourse timed so that sperm fertilize the ovum within 24 hours of the ovum's release.

Sex-specific causes of infertility

Many conditions can cause infertility in men and women.

His

Some causes of male infertility remain unknown, but factors that have been identified include:
• structural abnormalities, such as varicoceles (enlarged, varicose veins in the scrotum that can affect sperm number and motility) and hypospadias
• infection, possibly from an STD
• hormonal imbalances that reduce the amount of spermatozoa produced or disrupt their ability to travel effectively in the female reproductive tract
• heat (produced by wearing tight-fitting underwear or jeans, sitting in a hot tub or hot bath water, or driving long distances) that adversely affects sperm number and motility
• fever-producing illnesses that adversely affect sperm number and motility
• penile or testicular injury or congenital anomalies that diminish sperm
• certain prescription drugs known to affect sperm quality
• use of such substances as alcohol, marijuana, cocaine, and tobacco that are suspected of affecting sperm quality
• coital frequency — either too often or too seldom — which may decrease sperm number and motility
• environmental agents, such as exposure to radiation or other industrial and environmental toxins
• psychological and emotional stress.

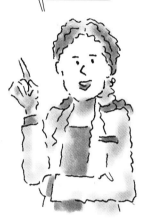

Hormonal imbalances and infections may contribute to male infertility.

Hers

Female infertility usually stems from anovulation (ovulatory dysfunction), fallopian tube obstruction, uterine conditions, or pelvic abnormalities caused by one or more of the following factors:
• hormonal imbalances that prevent the ovary from releasing ova regularly (or at all) or from producing enough progesterone to support growth and maintain the uterine lining needed for implantation of the embryo
• infection or inflammation (past, chronic, or current) that damages the ovaries and fallopian tubes, such as from PID, STDs, appendicitis, childhood disease, or surgical trauma
• structural abnormalities, such as a uterus scarred by infection or one that's abnormally shaped or positioned since birth, deformed by fibroid tumors, exposed to diethylstilbestrol, or injured by conization
• mucosal abnormalities caused by infection, inadequate hormone levels, or antibodies to sperm, which may create a hostile

environment that prevents sperm from entering the uterus and continuing to the fallopian tubes

- endometriosis (in some women), in which the endometrial tissue — usually confined to the inner lining of the uterine cavity — is deposited outside the uterus on such structures as the ovaries or fallopian tubes, causing inflammation and scarring
- endocrine abnormalities, such as elevated prolactin levels and pituitary, thyroid, or adrenal dysfunction
- recreational drug use (including tobacco, marijuana, and cocaine) and environmental and occupational factors (exposure to heat and chemicals).

Normogonadotrophic anovulation

Normogonadotrophic anovulation is usually seen in women with polycystic ovary syndrome and in those who are overweight. Patients with normogonadotrophic anovulation have normal FSH levels but elevated LH levels. They may also bleed in response to a progesterone withdrawal test.

Hyperprolactinemic anovulation

In hyperprolactinemic anovulation, excessive prolactin secretion impairs ovarian function. Elevated levels of prolactin in the blood are normal during lactation but are otherwise pathologic. Hyperprolactinemic anovulation may also be caused by physical or emotional stress, rapid weight loss, or a pituitary adenoma.

Hypogonadotrophic anovulation

Hypogonadotrophic anovulation may be caused by stress, weight loss, or excessive exercise. In many cases, this type of anovulation is functional and transient. An organic cause should be excluded, however, particularly if the patient displays neurologic symptoms. Patients with hypogonadotrophic anovulation typically have low levels of FSH, LH, and estrogen and an absence of withdrawal bleeding after a progesterone challenge test.

Hypergonadotrophic anovulation

Hypergonadotrophic anovulation results from ovarian resistance or failure. It's commonly diagnosed when repeated measurements show plasma levels of FSH are higher than 20 mIU/ml.

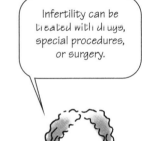

Infertility can be treated with drugs, special procedures, or surgery.

Treatment options

Infertility can be treated with drugs, special procedures, or various types of surgery.

Medications

Drugs can be used in two ways to help treat infertility. First, they may be prescribed to treat certain conditions that inhibit fertility. For example, antibiotics may be prescribed for infections or danazol may be ordered for a patient with endometriosis. (See *Explaining how danazol affects fertility*.) Drugs designed to initiate ovulation, improve cervical mucus, or stimulate sperm production may also be prescribed.

His

For men whose infertility is caused by hypogonadism secondary to pituitary or hypothalamic failure, treatment may include human menopausal gonadotropins (hMGs), human chorionic gonadotropin (HCG), or pulsatile gonadotropin-releasing hormone (Gn-RH). These medications are highly effective in achieving sperm quality that's sufficient to induce pregnancy.

Hers

For women, the type of fertility drug prescribed depends on the type of anovulation.

Normogonadotrophic anovulation

Recommended treatments for normogonadotrophic anovulation include clomiphene (Clomid) or tamoxifen (Nolvadex) combined with weight reduction.

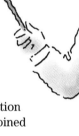

hMGs, HCG, and Gn-RH all help to achieve sperm quality that's sufficient to induce pregnancy.

Education edge

Explaining how danazol affects fertility

If the patient's primary health care provider finds that endometriosis interferes with your patient's ability to conceive, he may recommend treatment with danazol (Danocrine).

Effects of hormonal suppression

Inform the patient that danazol suppresses her hormonal cycle, so she won't menstruate while she's taking it. This gives uterine endometrial tissue, which usually swells and bleeds during menses, a rest. The endometrial implants deposited on her ovaries or fallopian tubes should also recede and refrain from bleeding, helping inflammation subside as well.

The patient can then stop taking the drug and try to become pregnant. Alternatively, the primary health care provider may suggest surgery to remove the implants while they're small.

Adverse reactions

Warn the patient to report adverse reactions, such as voice changes and other signs of virilization, promptly. Some androgenic effects, such as deepening of the voice, may not be reversible after stopping the drug.

Invigorating the ovaries

Clomiphene is an estrogen agonist used to stimulate the ovaries. The drug binds to estrogen receptors, decreasing the number available, and falsely signals the hypothalamus to increase FSH and LH, resulting in the release of more ova.

The drug is taken on cycle days 5 through 10 and may produce ovulation 6 to 11 days after the last dose. The patient needs to have intercourse every other day for 1 week beginning 5 days after she takes her last dose. The initial dose may not cause ovulation, and the dosage may be adjusted later. The patient should document the ovulatory process by keeping a BBT chart or by using an ovulation prediction kit (or both).

Additional effects

> Clomiphene may cause hot flashes in some patients.

The drug may trigger multiple ova development and release, but the incidence of multiple births (mostly twins) stays near 5%. The drug may also make the patient feel moody from fluctuating hormone levels. If the patient fails to have a normal menses, she should contact her primary health care provider, who may withhold the drug and order a pregnancy test.

The patient may experience slight bloating and hot flashes (caused by a release of LH, which indicates that the drug is working). She may also experience dysmenorrhea as a result of the drug triggering the ovulatory cycle (the first cycle the patient has had in a while).

Instruct the patient to report blurred vision; other visual changes, such as spots or flashing lights; and severe headaches that are unrelieved by acetaminophen (Tylenol). Additionally, instruct the patient to tell her primary health care provider if abdominal distention, bloating, pain, or weight gain occurs. These effects may signal ovarian enlargement or ovarian cysts, and treatment may need to be discontinued.

Other options

Another therapy for normogonadotrophic anovulation is the administration of pulsatile Gn-RH or FSH to induce multiple follicular growth, followed by HCG and timed intercourse or assisted reproductive techniques.

Hyperprolactinemic anovulation

Treatment of women with hyperprolactinemic anovulation includes bromocriptine (Parlodel) or chemically related dopamine agonists, such as pergolide (Permax) or cabergoline (Dostinex). If pituitary function is normal, these drugs can be combined with clomiphene or tamoxifen to induce ovulation.

Hypogonadotrophic anovulation

Treatment of hypogonadotrophic anovulation varies depending on the cause. In the presence of primary pituitary failure, ovulation can be induced with pulsatile Gn-RH. In women with suspected luteal phase defects, progesterone may be administered during the luteal phase for 3 to 6 cycles.

Hypergonadotrophic anovulation

No current drug therapy has restored ovulation in patients with hypergonadotrophic anovulation. Adoption or ova donation may be recommended.

Procedures

Such procedures as in vitro fertilization-embryo transfer (IVF-ET), gamete intrafallopian transfer (GIFT), zygote intrafallopian transfer (ZIFT), intracytoplasmic sperm injection (ICSI), embryo donation, and intrauterine insemination (sometimes called *artificial insemination*) may be recommended to help treat infertility.

In vitro fertilization-embryo transfer

IVF-ET refers to the removal of one or more mature oocytes from a woman's ovary by laparoscopy. After removal, these oocytes are fertilized by exposing them to sperm under laboratory conditions outside the woman's body. Embryo transfer (ET) is the insertion of these laboratory-grown fertilized ova (zygotes) into the woman's uterus. This is performed approximately 40 hours after fertilization. Ideally, one or more of the zygotes implant. IVF-ET circumvents the need for a fallopian tube to pick up an ovum or to propel a fertilized ovum to the uterus.

The perfect candidates

IVF-ET is performed for couples who haven't been able to conceive as a result of damaged or blocked fallopian tubes. It can also be used if the man has oligospermia (low sperm count) or if the woman lacks the cervical mucus that enables sperm to travel from the vagina into the cervix.

Agents of ovulation

The woman is given an ovulation drug, such as clomiphene or menotropins (Pergonal). On about the tenth day of her menstrual cycle, the ovaries are examined; when the size of the follicles appears to be mature, the woman is given an injection of HCG hormone. This causes ovulation to occur within 38 to 42 hours. Then the IVF-ET procedure is performed. (See *How IVF works*, page 98.)

How IVF works

For patients who meet the necessary criteria, in vitro fertilization-embryo transfer (IVF-ET) bypasses the barriers to in vivo fertilization.

In IVF-ET, after the ovaries receive hormonal stimulation, laparoscopy may be used to visualize and aspirate fluid (containing eggs) from the ovarian follicles. (To avoid using laparoscopy and a general anesthetic, an ultrasound technique may be used, first to visualize the ovarian follicles and then to guide a needle through the back of the vagina to retrieve fluid and eggs from the ovarian follicles.) The eggs are then placed in a test tube or a laboratory dish containing a culture medium for 3 to 6 hours.

Next, sperm from the patient's husband (or a donor) is added to the dish. Two days after insemination, the now-fertilized egg or embryo is transferred into the patient's uterus, where it may implant and establish a pregnancy.

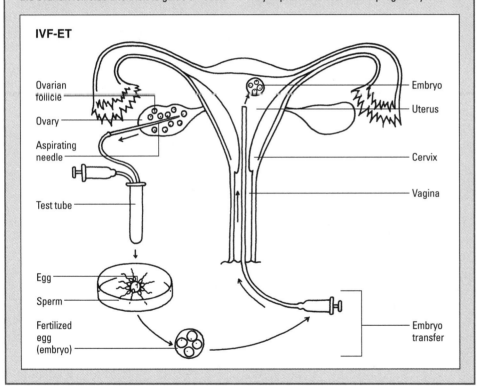

IVF-ET

Ovarian follicle
Ovary
Aspirating needle
Test tube
Egg
Sperm
Fertilized egg (embryo)

Embryo
Uterus
Cervix
Vagina
Embryo transfer

Ova donation

Donor ovum may be used in IVF-ET instead of the woman's ovum if the woman doesn't ovulate or if she carries a sex-linked disease that she doesn't want to pass on to her offspring.

Alternate eggs

In ova donation, ova that are retrieved from a well-screened and hormonally stimulated donor are fertilized in a petri dish by sperm from the recipient's partner or a sperm donor. After an incubation period, the best embryos are transferred into the recipient's uterus. The rest may be frozen for possible use in a second transfer, if necessary or if the recipient desires a second child genetically related to the first. Ova donation is an emotional, expensive, and time-intensive experience. However, it offers a realistic, successful option for couples who otherwise have no way to have a child. Experienced programs report clinical pregnancy rates of 50 percent per egg donation cycle. These success rates are better than pregnancy rates with IVF cycles using a woman's own eggs.

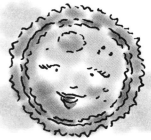

Although it can be expensive, ovum donation may be a good alternative for a woman who doesn't ovulate.

Meet the candidates

Good candidates for egg donation include women who:
• have never had a spontaneous menses
• stopped menstruating at an early age
• produced few or no eggs, or an elevated FSH level, in a previous in vitro fertilization (IVF) cycle
• who have stopped menstruating (usually in their 40s) or don't respond well to fertility drugs
• have an FSH level of 15 or more on day 3 of a Clomiphene Challenge Test. Research suggests these women won't be successful with IVF using their own eggs.
• have had multiple IVF cycles and failed to achieve a pregnancy.

Risky business

In addition to the usual risks of IVF, approximately 15% to 20% of egg donation pregnancies result in miscarriage and 20% to 25% result in multiple births (such as twins, triplets, or more).

Gamete intrafallopian transfer

In GIFT, the ovaries are stimulated with fertility drugs and the results are monitored. Next, ova are collected from the ovaries transvaginally by needle aspiration. They're placed in a catheter with sperm and then transferred into the fallopian tube, allowing fertilization and implantation to occur naturally from that point.

Embryo donation or surrogate embryo transfer

Embryo donation or surrogate embryo transfer can be used when the woman doesn't ovulate or if the woman has ovarian failure but a functioning uterus. The husband's sperm can be used to fertilize a donated ovum so that the embryo contains one-half of the couple's gene pool. The fertilized oocyte is then placed in the woman's uterus by ET or GIFT. Some couples see this option as an advantage over adoption because it allows them to experience pregnancy and they may have a shorter wait for a child.

Surgery

Surgeries for infertility include varicocelectomy, laparoscopy, and laparotomy. If surgery is required to enhance fertility, be sure to explain the procedure to the patients.

Varicocelectomy

A varicocele is a varicosity (abnormality) of the spermatic vein. It allows blood to pool in the scrotum and raises the temperature around the sperm. This, in turn, may reduce sperm production and motility.

A surgery called varicocelectomy can be performed to repair or remove a varicocele. A small incision is made in the scrotum and the enlarged, varicose-like vein that causes this condition is tied off.

I don't function well when the heat is turned up.

Laparoscopy

A female patient may need surgery to treat tubal disease, endometriosis, or such pelvic conditions as adhesions. A laparoscopy is used to visualize the pelvic and upper abdominal organs and peritoneal surfaces. It can also be used to visualize the distance between the fallopian tubes and the ovaries. If this distance is too large, the discharged ovum can't enter the tube. Dye can be injected into the uterus to assess tubal patency. The laparoscope can also be used to examine the fimbria (the fingerlike projections in the fallopian tubes that accept the ovum as it's released from the ovary and heads toward the fallopian tubes). If PID has damaged them, normal conception is unlikely.

Complications of laparoscopy include excessive bleeding, abdominal cramps, and shoulder pain resulting from the abdomen being inflated with carbon dioxide.

Hysteroscopy

A hysteroscopy is the visualization of the uterus through insertion of a hysteroscope. A hysteroscope is a thin, hollow, fiber-optic tube that's inserted through the vagina and cervix into the uterus. This procedure is done to remove uterine polyps and small fibroid tumors.

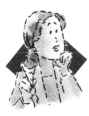

Quick quiz

1. What's one disadvantage of using vaginal spermicides to prevent pregnancy?

    A.   They're difficult to apply.

    B.   The patient must follow detailed instructions to use them.

    C.   Reapplication is necessary each time intercourse occurs.

    D.   They're expensive and require a visit to the doctor.

Answer: C. The patient may feel that having to reapply spermicide each time intercourse occurs is inconvenient. This may decrease the likelihood that the patient will use it regularly.

2. Which family planning method requires assessment of the quality of cervical mucus throughout the menstrual cycle?

    A.   Rhythm method

    B.   Coitus interruptus

    C.   Billings method

    D.   Basal body temperature

Answer: C. The Billings method requires assessment of cervical mucus, which is minimal and not stretchy until ovulation occurs. At the time of ovulation, the cervical mucus is present in greater quantity, stretchy, and more favorable to penetration by sperm.

3. A vasectomy is considered 100% effective after:

    A.   approximately 2 weeks.

    B.   approximately 4 weeks.

    C.   two consecutive sperm counts show zero sperm.

    D.   six consecutive sperm counts show zero sperm.

Answer: C. Some sperm remain in the proximal vas deferens after vasectomy. It may take up to several months to clear the proximal ducts of sperm.

4. Which woman is the best candidate for using an IUD?

    A.   A woman with Wilson's disease

    B.   A mother of two with no history of PID

    C.   A mother of one who has a history of severe dysmenorrhea

    D.   A 35-year-old woman with recent PID

Answer: B. An IUD is an optimal contraceptive for a woman who has had no history of PID, dysmenorrhea, or previous IUD failures.

5. Medically induced abortion is contraindicated in patients who:

    A.   are suspected of having an ectopic pregnancy.

    B.   are tolerant of mifepristone.

    C.   have PID.

    D.   are at 26 weeks' gestation.

Answer: A. Medically induced abortions are contraindicated in women with known or suspected ectopic pregnancy.

6. An ovarian stimulant such as clomiphene may be prescribed for infertility if the cause of infertility is:

    A.   anovulation.

    B.   ovarian cysts.

    C.   ovarian agenesis.

    D.   blocked fallopian tubes.

Answer: A. Clomiphene is given for anovulation.

7. A 38-year-old woman asks about IVF-ET. Which statement is correct about this procedure?

    A.   Oocytes are retrieved from the ovary, placed in a catheter with washed motile sperm, and transferred into the fallopian tube.

    B.   An indication for this procedure would be unexplained infertility with normal tubal anatomy and patency and absence of previous tubal disease.

    C.   The woman's ova are collected from the ovaries, fertilized in the laboratory with sperm, and transferred to her uterus after normal embryo development has occurred.

    D.   Blastocytes are retrieved from the ovary and transferred into the fallopian tube.

Answer: C. VF-ET refers to fertilization of the ovum in a laboratory. The woman's ova are collected from the ovaries, fertilized in the laboratory with sperm, and transferred to her uterus after normal embryo development has occurred.

Scoring

★★★   If you answered all seven questions correctly, super! Your conception of the material is right on target.

★★   If you answered five or six questions correctly, good work! Keep up this rhythm and you'll continue to gestate your knowledge of maternal-neonatal nursing.

★   If you answered fewer than five questions correctly, don't fret. With a little review, you'll master family planning in no time.

Physiologic and psychosocial adaptations to pregnancy

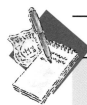

Just the facts

In this chapter, you'll learn:

♦ presumptive, probable, and positive signs of pregnancy

♦ ways in which the major body systems are affected by pregnancy

♦ methods of promoting acceptance of pregnancy

♦ psychosocial changes that occur during each trimester.

A look at pregnancy changes

During pregnancy, a woman undergoes many physiologic and psychosocial changes. Her body adapts in response to the demands of the growing fetus while her mind prepares for the responsibilities that come with becoming a parent. Physiologic changes initially indicate pregnancy; these changes continue to affect the body throughout pregnancy as the fetus grows and develops. Psychosocial changes occur in both the mother and father and may vary from trimester to trimester.

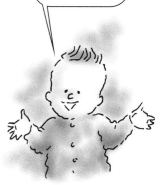

I may cause many physical and mental changes to which my parents must adapt, but I'm worth it!

Physiologic signs of pregnancy

Pregnancy produces several types of physiologic changes that must be evaluated before a definitive diagnosis of pregnancy is made. The changes can be:
• presumptive (subjective)
• probable (objective)
• positive.

Neither presumptive nor probable signs confirm pregnancy because both can be caused by other medical conditions. They simply suggest pregnancy, especially when several are present at the same time. (See *Making sense out of pregnancy signs.*)

Presumptive signs of pregnancy

Presumptive signs of pregnancy are those that can be assumed to indicate pregnancy until more concrete signs develop. These signs include breast changes, nausea and vomiting, amenorrhea, urinary frequency, fatigue, uterine enlargement, quickening, and skin changes. A pregnant patient typically reports some presumptive signs.

Breast changes

Tingling, tender, or swollen breasts can occur as early as a few days after conception. The areola may darken and tiny glands around the nipple, called *Montgomery's tubercles*, may become elevated.

Nausea and vomiting

At least 50% of pregnant women experience nausea and vomiting early in pregnancy (commonly called *morning sickness*). These symptoms are typically the first sensations experienced during pregnancy. The onset of nausea and vomiting usually occurs at 4 to 6 weeks' gestation. These symptoms usually stop at the end of the first trimester, but they may last slightly longer in some patients.

Amenorrhea

Amenorrhea is the cessation of menses. For a woman who has regular menses, this may be the first indication that she's pregnant.

Urinary frequency

A pregnant woman may notice an increase in urinary frequency during the first 3 months of pregnancy. This symptom continues until the uterus rises out of the pelvis and relieves pressure on the bladder.

Memory jogger

To remember the three categories of pregnancy signs, think of the three **P**s:

Presumptive — Think of a presumptive sign as one that suggests, "If I had to guess, I'd say yes!"

Probable — Think of a probable sign as one that means, *most likely this lady is passing on her genes.*

Positive — Think of a positive sign as one that confirms, in about 9 months, this woman is going to give birth

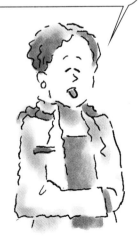

Pregnant patients commonly experience nausea and vomiting early in pregnancy. But tell your patient not to worry because these symptoms usually subside by the end of the first trimester.

Making sense out of pregnancy signs

This chart classifies the signs of pregnancy into three categories: presumptive, probable, and positive.

Sign	Weeks from implantation	Other possible causes
Presumptive		
Breast changes, including feelings of tenderness, fullness, or tingling and enlargement or darkening of areola	2	• Hyperprolactinemia induced by tranquilizers • Infection • Prolactin-secreting pituitary tumor • Pseudocyesis • Premenstrual syndrome
Feeling of nausea or vomiting upon arising	2	• Gastric disorders • Infections • Psychological disorders, such as pseudocyesis and anorexia nervosa
Amenorrhea	2	• Anovulation • Blocked endometrial cavity • Endocrine changes • Medications (phenothiazines) • Metabolic changes
Frequent urination	3	• Emotional stress • Pelvic tumor • Renal disease • Urinary tract infection
Fatigue	12	• Anemia • Chronic illness
Uterine enlargement in which the uterus can be palpated over the symphysis pubis	12	• Ascites • Obesity • Uterine or pelvic tumor
Quickening (fetal movement felt by the woman)	18	• Excessive flatus • Increased peristalsis
Linea nigra (line of dark pigment on the abdomen)	24	• Cardiopulmonary disorders • Estrogen-progestin hormonal contraceptives • Obesity • Pelvic tumor

(continued)

Making sense out of pregnancy signs *(continued)*

Sign	Weeks from implantation	Other possible causes
Presumptive (continued)		
Melasma (dark pigment on the face)	24	• Cardiopulmonary disorders • Estrogen-progestin hormonal contraceptives • Obesity • Pelvic tumor
Striae gravidarum (red streaks on the abdomen)	24	• Cardiopulmonary disorders • Estrogen-progestin hormonal contraceptives • Obesity • Pelvic tumor
Probable		
Serum laboratory tests revealing the presence of human chorionic gonadotropin (hCG) hormone	1	• Cross-reaction of luteinizing hormone (similar to hCG)
Chadwick's sign (vagina changes color from pink to violet)	6	• Hyperemia of cervix, vagina, or vulva
Goodell's sign (cervix softens)	6	• Estrogen-progestin hormonal contraceptives
Hegar's sign (lower uterine segment softens)	6	• Excessively soft uterine walls
Sonographic evidence of gestational sac in which characteristic ring is evident	6	None
Ballottement (fetus can be felt to rise against abdominal wall when lower uterine segment is tapped on during bimanual examination)	16	• Ascites • Uterine tumor or polyps
Braxton Hicks contractions (periodic uterine tightening)	20	• Hematometra • Uterine tumor
Palpation of fetal outline through abdomen	20	• Subserous uterine myoma
Positive		
Sonographic evidence of fetal outline	8	None
Fetal heart audible by Doppler ultrasound	10 to 12	None
Palpation of fetal movement through abdomen	20	None

When lightening strikes

Urinary frequency may return at the end of pregnancy as lightening occurs (the fetal head exerts renewed pressure on the bladder).

Fatigue

A pregnant woman may report that she's often fatigued. During the first trimester, the woman's body works hard to manufacture the placenta and to adjust to the many other physical demands of pregnancy, while she mentally and emotionally prepares for the role of mother. Around 16 weeks' gestation, the body has adjusted to the pregnancy, the placenta's development is complete, and the patient should start to have more energy.

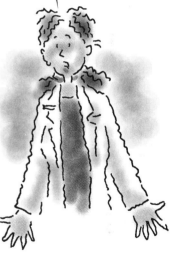

Pregnancy is tiring. Many women experience fatigue during the first trimester.

Uterine enlargement

Softening of the uterus and fetal growth cause the uterus to enlarge and stretch the abdominal wall.

Quickening

Quickening is recognizable movements of the fetus. It can occur anywhere between the 14th and 26th weeks of pregnancy but typically is noticed between weeks 18 and 22.

Flutterflies in the stomach

To the patient, quickening may feel like fluttering movements in her lower abdomen.

Skin changes

Numerous skin changes occur during pregnancy, including those listed here:

• *Linea nigra* refers to a dark line that extends from the umbilicus or above to the mons pubis. In the primigravid patient, this line develops at approximately the third month of pregnancy. In the multigravid patient, linea nigra typically appears before the third month. (See *Skin changes during pregnancy*, page 108.)

• *Melasma*, also known as chloasma or the "mask of pregnancy," are darkened areas that may appear on the face, especially on the cheeks and across the nose. Melasma appears after the 16th week of pregnancy and gradually becomes more pronounced. After childbirth, it typically fades.

• *Striae gravidarum* are red or pinkish streaks that appear on the sides of the abdominal wall and sometimes on the thighs.

Skin changes during pregnancy

Linea nigra and striae gravidarum are two skin changes that occur during pregnancy. Both fade after pregnancy, with striae gravidarum fading to glistening silvery lines.

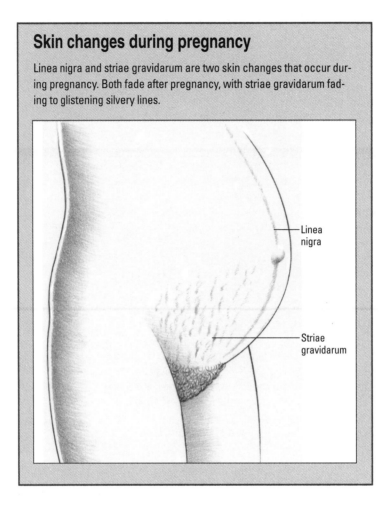

Linea nigra

Striae gravidarum

Probable signs of pregnancy

Probable signs of pregnancy strongly suggest pregnancy. They're more reliable indicators of pregnancy than presumptive signs, but they can also be explained by other medical conditions. Probable signs include positive laboratory tests, such as serum and urine tests; positive results on a home pregnancy test; Chadwick's sign; Goodell's sign; Hegar's sign; sonographic evidence of a gestational sac; ballottement; and Braxton Hicks contractions.

Laboratory tests

Laboratory tests for pregnancy are used to detect the presence of human chorionic gonadotropin (hCG) — a hormone created by the chorionic villi of the placenta—in the urine or blood serum of the woman. Because hCG is produced by trophoblast cells—preplacental cells that wouldn't be present in a nonpregnant woman—detection of hCG is considered a sign of pregnancy. Because laboratory tests for diagnosing pregnancy are accurate only 95% to 98% of the time, positive hCG results are considered probable rather than positive.

Looking for hCG in all the right places

Tests for hCG include radioimmunoassay, enzyme-linked immunosorbent assay, or radioreceptor assay. For these tests, hCG is measured in milli-international units (mIU). In pregnant women, trace amounts of hCG appear in the serum as early as 24 to 48 hours after implantation of the fertilized ovum. They reach a measurable level of about 50 mIU/mL between 7 and 9 days after conception. Levels peak at about 100 mIU/mL between the 60th and 80th days of gestation. After this point, the level declines. At term, hCG is barely detectable in serum or urine.

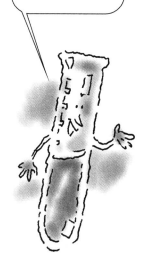

Detection of hCG in a patient's blood or urine is deemed a probable sign of pregnancy.

Home pregnancy tests

Home pregnancy tests, which are available over-the-counter, are 97% accurate when performed correctly. They're convenient and easy to use (they take only 3 to 5 minutes to perform).

Dip stick

Here's how the home pregnancy test works:
• A reagent strip is dipped into the urine stream.
• A color change on the strip denotes pregnancy.
   Most manufacturers suggest that a woman wait until the day of the missed menstrual period to test for pregnancy.

Chadwick's sign

Chadwick's sign is a bluish coloration of the mucous membranes of the cervix, vagina, and vulva. It can be observed at 6 to 8 weeks' gestation by bimanual examination.

Goodell's sign

Goodell's sign is a softening of the cervix that occurs at 6 to 8 weeks' gestation. The cervix of a nonpregnant woman typically has the same consistency as a nose; the cervix of a pregnant woman feels more like an earlobe.

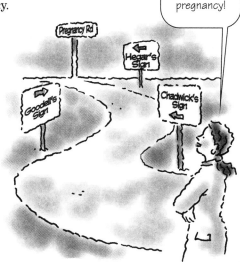

All signs point to pregnancy!

Hegar's sign

Hegar's sign is a softening of the uterine isthmus that can be felt on bimanual examination at 6 to 8 weeks' gestation. As pregnancy advances, the isthmus becomes part of the lower uterine segment. During labor, it expands further.

Ultrasonography

Ultrasonography, or sonographic evaluation, can detect probable and positive signs of pregnancy. At 4 to 6 weeks' gestation, a characteristic ring indicating the gestational sac is visible on sonographic evaluation.

Ballottement

Ballottement is passive movement of the fetus. It can be identified at 16 to 18 weeks' gestation.

Braxton Hicks contractions

Braxton Hicks contractions are uterine contractions that begin early in pregnancy and become more frequent after 28 weeks' gestation. Typically, they result from normal uterine enlargement that occurs to accommodate the growing fetus. Sometimes, however, they may be caused by a uterine tumor.

Positive signs of pregnancy

Positive signs of pregnancy include sonographic evidence of the fetal outline, an audible fetal heart rate, and fetal movement that's felt by the examiner. These signs confirm pregnancy because they can't be attributed to other conditions.

Ultrasonography

Ultrasonography can confirm pregnancy by providing an image of the fetal outline, which can typically be seen by the 8th week. The fetal outline on the ultrasound is so clear that a crown to rump measurement can be made to establish gestational age. Fetal heart movement may be visualized as early as 7 weeks' gestation.

Audible fetal heart rate

Fetal heart rate can be confirmed by auscultation or visualization during an ultrasound. Fetal heart sounds may be heard as early as the 10th to 12th week by Doppler ultrasonography.

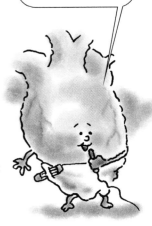

Fetal movement

Even though the pregnant woman can feel fetal movement at a much earlier date (usually around 16 to 20 weeks), other people aren't able to feel fetal movement until the 20th to 24th week. Obese patients may not feel fetal movement until later in pregnancy because of excess adipose tissue.

Physiologic changes in body systems

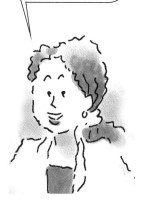

Physiologic changes during pregnancy create a safe and nurturing environment for the fetus.

As the fetus grows and hormones shift during pregnancy, physiologic adaptations occur in every body system to accommodate the fetus. These changes help a pregnant woman to maintain health throughout the pregnancy and to physically prepare for childbirth. Physiologic changes also create a safe and nurturing environment for the fetus. Some of these changes take place even before the woman knows that she's pregnant.

Reproductive system

In addition to the physical changes that initially indicate pregnancy, such as Hegar's sign and Goodell's sign, the reproductive system undergoes significant changes throughout pregnancy.

Out and about

External reproductive structures affected by pregnancy include the labia majora, labia minora, clitoris, and vaginal introitus. These structures enlarge because of increased vascularity. Fat deposits also contribute to the enlargement of the labia majora and labia minora. These structures reduce in size after childbirth, but they may not return to their prepregnant state because of loss of muscle tone or perineal injury (such as an episiotomy or a vaginal tear). For example, in many patients, the labia majora remain separated and gape after childbirth. In addition, varices may be caused by pressure on vessels in the perineal and perianal areas.

The inside story

Internal reproductive structures, including the ovaries, uterus, and other structures, change dramatically to accommodate the developing fetus. These internal structures may not regain their prepregnant states after childbirth.

Ovaries

When fertilization occurs, ovarian follicles cease to mature and ovulation stops. The chorionic villi, which develop from the fertilized ovum, begin to produce hCG to maintain the ovarian corpus luteum. The corpus luteum produces estrogen and progesterone until the placenta is formed and functioning. At 8 to 10 weeks' gestation, the placenta assumes production of these hormones. The corpus luteum, which is no longer needed, then involutes (becomes smaller due to a reduction in cell size).

Uterus

In a nonpregnant woman, the uterus is smaller than the size of a fist, measuring approximately 7.5 cm × 5 cm × 2.5 cm (3″ × 2″ × 1″). It can weigh 60 to 70 g (2 to 2½ oz) in a nulliparous patient (a patient who has never been pregnant) and 100 g (3½ oz) in a parous patient (a patient who has given birth). In a nonpregnant state, a woman's uterus can hold up to 10 ml of fluid. Its walls are composed of several overlapping layers of muscle fibers that adapt to the developing fetus and help in expulsion of the fetus and placenta during labor and childbirth.

Working toward a stronger, more elastic uterus

After conception, the uterus retains the developing fetus for approximately 280 days, or 9 calendar months. During this time, the uterus undergoes progressive changes in size, shape, and position in the abdominal cavity. In the first trimester, the pear-shaped uterus lengthens and enlarges in response to elevated levels of estrogen and progesterone. This hormonal stimulation primarily increases the size of myometrial cells (hypertrophy), although a small increase in cell number (hyperplasia) also occurs. These changes increase the amount of fibrous and elastic tissue to more than 20 times that of the nonpregnant uterus. Uterine walls become stronger and more elastic.

During the first few weeks of pregnancy, the uterine walls remain thick and the fundus rests low in the abdomen. The uterus can't be palpated through the abdominal wall. After 12 weeks of pregnancy, however, the uterus typically reaches the level of the symphysis pubis (the joint at the pubic bone) and then may be palpated through the abdominal wall.

Shape shifters

In the second trimester, the corpus and fundus become globe-shaped. As pregnancy progresses, the uterus lengthens and becomes oval in shape. The uterine walls thin as the muscles stretch; the uterus rises out of the pelvis, shifts to

In the second trimester, the corpus and fundus become globe-shaped.

the right, and rests against the anterior abdominal wall. At 20 weeks' gestation, the uterus is palpable just below the umbilicus and reaches the umbilicus at 22 weeks' gestation. As uterine muscles stretch, Braxton Hicks contractions may occur, helping to move blood more quickly through the intervillous spaces of the placenta.

Final preparations

In the third trimester, the fundus reaches nearly to the xiphoid process (the lower tip of the breast bone). Between weeks 38 and 40, the fetus begins to descend into the pelvis (lightening), which causes fundal height to gradually drop. The uterus remains oval in shape. Its muscular walls become progressively thinner as it enlarges, finally reaching a muscle wall thickness of 5 mm (¼″) or less. At term (40 weeks), the uterus typically weighs approximately 1,100 g (2 lb), holds 5 to 10 L of fluid, and has stretched to approximately 28 cm × 24 cm × 21 cm (11″ × 9½″ × 8¼″). (See *Fundal height throughout pregnancy.*)

Fundal height throughout pregnancy

The illustration below shows approximate fundal heights at various times during pregnancy. The times indicated are in weeks. Note that between weeks 38 and 40, the fetus begins to descend into the pelvis.

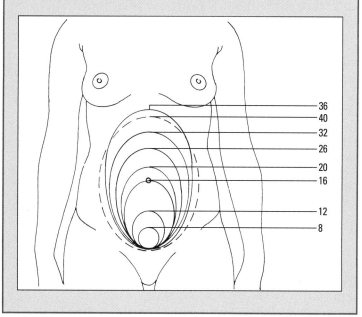

Endometrial development

During the menstrual cycle, progesterone stimulates increased thickening and vascularity of the endometrium, preparing the uterine lining for implantation and nourishment of a fertilized ovum. After implantation, menstruation stops.

The endometrium then becomes the decidua, which is divided into three layers:

✌️ decidua capsularis, which covers the blastocyst (fertilized ovum)

✌️ decidua basalis, which lies directly under the blastocyst and forms part of the placenta

✌️ decidua vera, which lines the rest of the uterus.

Vascular growth

As the fetus grows and the placenta develops, uterine blood vessels and lymphatics increase in number and size. Vessels must enlarge to accommodate the increased blood flow to the uterus and placenta. By the end of pregnancy, an average of 500 ml of blood may flow through the maternal side of the placenta each minute. Maternal arterial pressure, uterine contractions, and maternal position affect uterine blood flow throughout pregnancy.

Because one-sixth of the body's blood supply is circulating through the uterus at any given time, uterine bleeding in pregnancy is always potentially serious and can result in major blood loss. (See *Uterine bleeding*.)

Cervical changes

The cervix consists of connective tissue, elastic fibers, and endocervical folds. This composition allows it to stretch during childbirth. During pregnancy, the cervix softens. It also takes on a bluish color during the second month due to increased vasculature. It becomes edematous and may bleed easily on examination or sexual activity.

Bacteria blocker

During pregnancy, hormonal stimulation causes the glandular cervical tissue to increase in cell number and become hyperactive, secreting thick, tenacious mucus. This mucus thickens into a mucoid weblike structure, eventually forming a mucus plug that blocks the cervical canal. This creates a protective barrier against bacteria and other substances attempting to enter the uterus.

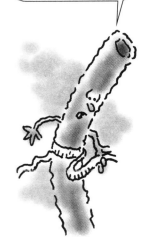

> During pregnancy, it's okay for my waistline to expand a bit, too. I have to be ready to handle increased blood flow to the uterus and placenta.

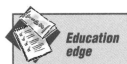

Education edge

Uterine bleeding

Uterine bleeding in a pregnant patient is always potentially serious because it can result in major blood loss. A pregnant woman should be warned that such blood loss poses a major health risk. Advise the pregnant patient to contact her health care provider if uterine bleeding occurs.

Vagina

During pregnancy, estrogen stimulates vascularity, tissue growth, and hypertrophy in the vaginal epithelial tissue. White, thick, odorless, and acidic vaginal secretions increase. The acidity of these secretions helps prevent bacterial infections but, unfortunately, also fosters yeast infections, a common occurrence during pregnancy. (See *Fighting* Candida *infection.*)

Other vaginal changes include:
- development of a bluish color due to increased vascularity
- hypertrophy of the smooth muscles and relaxation of connective tissues, which allow the vagina to stretch during childbirth
- lengthening of the vaginal vault
- possible heightened sexual sensitivity.

Breasts

In addition to the presumptive signs that occur in the breasts during pregnancy (such as tenderness, tingling, darkening of the areola, and appearance of Montgomery's tubercles), the nipples enlarge, become more erectile, and darken in color. The areolae widen from a diameter of less than 3 cm (1½″) to 5 or 6 cm (2″ or 3″) in the primigravid patient.

Rarely, patches of brownish discoloration appear on the skin adjacent to the areolae. These patches, known as *secondary areolae*, may indicate pregnancy if the patient has never breast-fed an infant.

Lactation preparations

The breasts also undergo several changes in preparation for lactation. As blood vessels enlarge, veins beneath the skin of the breasts become more visible and may appear as intertwining patterns over the anterior chest wall. Breasts become fuller and heavier as lactation approaches. They may throb uncomfortably.

Increasing hormones cause the secretion of colostrum (a yellowish, viscous fluid) from the nipples. High in protein, antibodies, and minerals—but low in fat and sugar relative to mature human milk—colostrum may be secreted as early as the 16th week of pregnancy, but it's most common during the last trimester. It continues until 2 to 4 days after delivery and is followed by mature milk production.

More change for first-timers

Breast changes are more pronounced in a primigravida patient than in a multigravida patient. In a multigravida patient, changes are even less significant if the patient has breast-fed an infant within the past year because her areola are still dark and her breasts enlarged. (See *Comparing the nonpregnant and pregnant breast*, page 116.)

Take charge!

Fighting *Candida* infection

Changes in the pH of vaginal secretions during pregnancy favor the growth of *Candida albicans*, a species of yeastlike fungi. This infection can be transmitted to the neonate as he passes through the birth canal during delivery, at which point it's called *thrush* or *oral monila*.

Medication is prescribed to treat and prevent transmission of *Candida* infection if it's properly diagnosed beforehand. Keep on top of possible infections by asking the patient if she has experienced signs and symptoms, such as itching, burning, and a cream cheese–like discharge.

Comparing the nonpregnant and pregnant breast

Subtle changes appear in the breasts of a pregnant patient because of increased estrogen and progestin production.

Nonpregnant breast

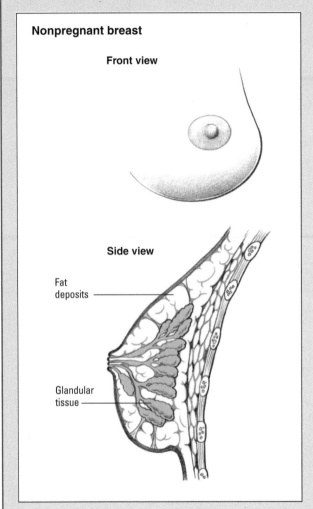

Pregnant breast

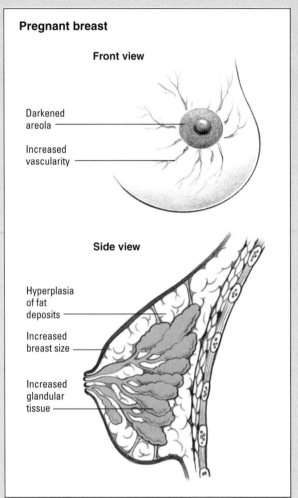

Endocrine system

The endocrine system undergoes many fluctuations during pregnancy. Changes in hormone levels and protein production help support fetal growth and maintain body functions.

Placenta

The most striking change in the endocrine system during pregnancy is the addition of the placenta. The placenta is an endocrine organ that produces large amounts of estrogen, progesterone, hCG, human placental lactogen (hPL), relaxin, and prostaglandins.

The estrogen produced by the placenta causes breast and uterine enlargement as well as palmar erythema (redness in the palm of the hand). Progesterone helps maintain the endometrium by inhibiting uterine contractility. It also prepares the breasts for lactation by stimulating breast tissue development.

Maxin' and relaxin

Relaxin is secreted primarily by the corpus luteum. It helps inhibit uterine activity. It also helps to soften the cervix, which allows for dilation at delivery, and soften the collagen in body joints, which allows for laxness in the lower spine and helps enlarge the birth canal.

How stimulating!

Secreted by the trophoblast cells of the placenta in early pregnancy, hCG stimulates progesterone and estrogen synthesis until the placenta assumes this role.

I predict palmar erythema caused by the estrogen produced by the placenta.

An alternate energy source

Also called *human chorionic somatomammotropin*, the hormone hPL is secreted by the placenta. It promotes fat breakdown (lipolysis), providing the patient with an alternate source of energy so that glucose is available for fetal growth. This hormone, however, has a complicating effect. Along with estrogen, progesterone, and cortisol, hPL inhibits the action of insulin, resulting in an increased insulin need throughout pregnancy.

Prostaglandins

Prostaglandins are found in high concentration in the female reproductive tract and the decidua during pregnancy. They affect smooth muscle contractility to such an extent that they may trigger labor at the pregnancy's term.

Pituitary gland

The pituitary gland undergoes various changes during pregnancy. High estrogen and progesterone levels in the placenta stop the pituitary gland from producing follicle-stimulating hormone and luteinizing hormone. Increased production of growth hormone and melanocyte-stimulating hormone causes skin pigment changes.

Late-breaking developments

Late in pregnancy, the posterior pituitary gland begins to produce oxytocin, which stimulates uterine contractions during labor. Prolactin production also starts late in pregnancy as the breasts prepare for lactation after birth.

Thyroid gland

As early as the second month of pregnancy, the thyroid gland's production of thyroxine-binding protein increases, causing total thyroxine (T_4) levels to rise. Because the amount of unbound T_4 doesn't increase, these thyroid changes don't cause hyperthyroidism; however, they increase basal metabolic rate (BMR), cardiac output, pulse rate, vasodilation, and heat intolerance. BMR increases by about 20% during the second and third trimesters as the growing fetus places additional demands for energy on the woman's system. By term, the woman's BMR may increase by 25%. It returns to the prepregnant level within 1 week after childbirth.

In addition to T_4 level changes, increased estrogen levels augment the circulating amounts of triiodothyronine (T_3). Like the elevation of T_4, the elevation of T_3 levels doesn't lead to a hyperthyroid condition during pregnancy because much of this hormone is bound to proteins and, therefore, nonfunctional.

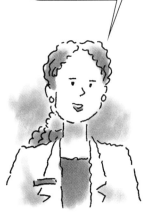

Thyroid changes during pregnancy increase the patient's basal metabolic rate.

Parathyroid gland

As pregnancy progresses, fetal demands for calcium and phosphorus increase. The parathyroid gland responds by increasing hormone production during the third trimester to as much as twice the prepregnancy level.

Adrenal gland

Adrenal gland activity increases during pregnancy as production of corticosteroids and aldosterone escalates.

Corticosteroids deployed

Some researchers believe that increased corticosteroid levels suppress inflammatory reactions and help to reduce the possibility of the woman's body rejecting the foreign protein of the fetus. Corticosteroids also help to regulate glucose metabolism in the woman.

Aldosterone zone

Increased aldosterone levels help to promote sodium reabsorption and maintain the osmolarity of retained fluid. This indirectly helps to safeguard the blood volume and provide adequate perfusion pressure across the placenta.

Pancreas

Although the pancreas itself doesn't change during pregnancy, maternal insulin, glucose, and glucagon production do. In response to the additional glucocorticoids produced by the adrenal glands, the pancreas increases insulin production. Insulin is less effective than normal, however, because estrogen, progesterone, and hPL all act as antagonists to it. Despite insulin's diminished action and increased fetal demands for glucose, maternal glucose levels remain fairly stable because the mother's fat stores are used for energy.

> Although I don't physically change during pregnancy, my production of insulin, glucose, and glucagon does!

Respiratory system

Throughout pregnancy, changes occur in the respiratory system in response to hormonal changes. These changes can be anatomic (biochemical) or functional (mechanical). As pregnancy advances, these respiratory system changes promote gas exchange, providing the woman with more oxygen.

Anatomic changes

The diaphragm rises by approximately 1⅝″ (4 cm) during pregnancy, which prevents the lungs from expanding as much as they normally do on respiration. The diaphragm compensates for this by increasing its excursion ability (its ability to expand outward), allowing more normal lung expansion. In addition, the anteroposterior and transverse diameters of the rib cage increase by approximately ¾″ (2 cm), and the circumference increases by 2″ to 2 ¾″ (5 to 7 cm). This expansion is possible because increased progesterone relaxes the ligaments that join the rib cage. As the uterus enlarges, thoracic breathing replaces abdominal breathing.

All that vascularization

Increased estrogen production leads to increased vascularization of the upper respiratory tract. As a result, the patient may develop respiratory congestion, voice changes, and epistaxis as capillaries become engorged in the nose, pharynx, larynx, trachea, bronchi, and vocal cords. Increased vascularization may also cause the eustachian tubes to swell, leading to such problems as impaired hearing, earaches, and a sense of fullness in the ears. This increased stuffiness in the nose, pharynx, and larynx—combined with the pressure the enlarged uterus places on the patient's diaphragm—may make the patient feel as if she's short of breath.

Education edge

Helping patients breathe easy

Pregnant women commonly experience chronic dyspnea (shortness of breath). Advise the patient that, although her breathing rate is more rapid than normal (18 to 20 breaths per minute), this rate is normal during pregnancy.

To help your patient cope with dyspnea, tell her to try holding her arms above her head. This raises the rib cage and temporarily gives the patient more room to breath. She can also try sleeping on her side with her head elevated by pillows. Show her how to practice slow, deep breathing and tell her to take her time when climbing stairs.

Functional changes

Changes in pulmonary function improve gas exchange in the alveoli and facilitate oxygenation of blood flowing through the lungs. Respiratory rate typically remains unaffected in early pregnancy. By the third trimester, however, increased progesterone may increase the rate by approximately two breaths per minute. (See *Helping patients breathe easy*.)

Rising tide

Tidal volume (the amount of air inhaled and exhaled) rises throughout pregnancy as a result of increased progesterone and increased diaphragmatic excursion. In fact, a pregnant patient breathes 30% to 40% more air during pregnancy than she does when she isn't pregnant. Minute volume (the amount of air expired per minute) increases by approximately 50% by term.

The difference between changes in tidal volume and minute volume creates a slight hyperventilation, which decreases carbon dioxide in the alveoli. The resulting lowered partial pressure of arterial carbon dioxide in maternal blood leads to a greater partial pressure difference of carbon dioxide between fetal and maternal blood, which facilitates diffusion of carbon dioxide from the fetus.

Flux in capacity

An elevated diaphragm decreases functional residual capacity (the volume of air remaining in the lungs after exhalation), which contributes to hyperventilation. Maternal hyperventilation is considered a protective measure that prevents the fetus from being exposed to excessive levels of carbon dioxide. Vital capacity (the largest volume of air that can be expelled voluntarily after

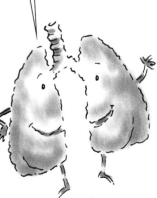

A patient breathes 30% to 40% more air when she's pregnant.

maximum inspiration) increases slightly during pregnancy. These changes, along with increased cardiac output and blood volume, provide adequate blood flow to the placenta.

Assorted aberrations

During the third month of pregnancy, increased progesterone sensitizes respiratory receptors and increases ventilation, leading to a drop in carbon dioxide levels. This increases pH, which might cause mild respiratory alkalosis; however, the decreased level of bicarbonate present in a pregnant woman partially or completely compensates for this tendency.

Cardiovascular system

Pregnancy alters the cardiovascular system so profoundly that, outside of pregnancy, the changes would be considered pathologic and even life-threatening. During pregnancy, however, these changes are vital.

> The vital changes that occur in the cardiovascular system during pregnancy would be considered life-threatening if they occurred at another time.

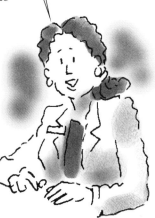

Anatomic changes

The heart enlarges slightly during pregnancy, probably because of increased blood volume and cardiac output. This enlargement isn't marked and reverses after childbirth. As pregnancy advances, the uterus moves up and presses on the diaphragm, displacing the heart upward and rotating it on its long axis. The amount of displacement varies depending on the position and size of the uterus, the firmness of the abdominal muscles, the shape of the abdomen, and other factors.

Auscultatory changes

Changes in blood volume, cardiac output, and the size and position of the heart alter heart sounds during pregnancy. These altered heart sounds would be considered abnormal in a patient who isn't pregnant.

During pregnancy, S_1 tends to exhibit a pronounced splitting, and each component tends to be louder. An occasional S_3 sound may occur after 20 weeks' gestation. Many pregnant patients exhibit a systolic ejection murmur over the pulmonic area.

Break in rhythm

Cardiac rhythm disturbances, such as sinus arrhythmia, premature atrial contractions, and premature ventricular systole, may occur. In the pregnant patient with no underlying heart disease, these arrhythmias don't require therapy and don't indicate the development of myocardial disease.

Hemodynamic changes

Hemodynamically, pregnancy affects heart rate and cardiac output, venous and arterial blood pressures, circulation and coagulation, and blood volume.

Heart rate and cardiac output

During the second trimester, heart rate gradually increases. It may reach 10 to 15 beats/minute above the patient's prepregnancy rate. During the third trimester, heart rate may increase by 15 to 20 beats/minute above the patient's prepregnancy rate. The patient may feel palpitations occasionally throughout pregnancy. In the early months, these palpitations result from sympathetic nervous stimulation.

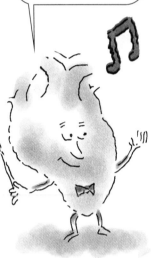

During pregnancy, my rhythm may be slightly off, but it's no reason to worry. I've just got my mind on other things.

All about output

Increased tissue demands for oxygen and increased stroke volume raise cardiac output by up to 50% by the 32nd week of pregnancy. The increase is highest when the patient is lying on her side and lowest when she's lying on her back. The side-lying position reduces pressure on the great vessels, which increases venous return to the heart. Cardiac output peaks during labor, when tissue demands are greatest.

Venous and arterial blood pressure

When the patient lies on her back, femoral venous pressure increases threefold from early pregnancy to term. This occurs because the uterus exerts pressure on the inferior vena cava and pelvic veins, slowing venous return from the legs and feet. The patient may feel light-headed if she rises abruptly after lying on her back. Edema in the legs and varicosities in the legs, rectum, and vulva may occur.

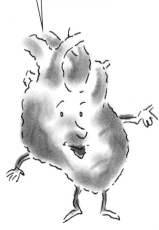

The patient's heart rate increases during the second trimester.

Pressure drop

Early in pregnancy, increased progesterone levels relax smooth muscles and dilate arterioles, resulting in vasodilation. Despite the hypervolemia that occurs during pregnancy, the woman's blood pressure doesn't normally rise because the increased action of the heart enables the body to handle the increased amount of circulating blood. In most women, blood pressure actually decreases slightly during the second trimester because of the lowered peripheral resistance to circulation that occurs as the placenta rapidly expands. Systolic and diastolic pressures may decrease by 5 to 10 mm Hg. The pregnant patient's blood pressure is at its lowest during the second half of the second trimester; it gradually returns to first trimester levels during the third trimester. By term, arterial blood pressure approaches prepregnancy levels.

Position, position, position

Brachial artery pressure is lowest when the pregnant patient lies on her left side because this relieves uterine pressure on the vena cava. Brachial artery pressure is highest when the patient lies on her back (supine). The weight of the growing uterus presses the vena cava against the vertebrae, obstructing blood flow from the lower extremities. This results in a decrease in blood return to the heart and, consequently, immediate decreased cardiac output and hypotension. (See *A look at supine hypotension*, page 124, and *Correcting supine hypotension*, page 125.)

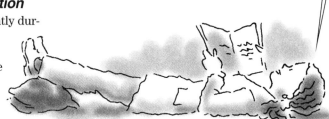

It isn't a problem for me, but a pregnant patient should avoid lying in a supine position. The weight of the uterus on the vena cava when she lays supine could lead to supine hypotension.

Circulation and coagulation

Venous return decreases slightly during the eighth month of pregnancy and, at term, increases to normal levels. Blood is able to clot more easily during pregnancy and the postpartum period because of increased levels of clotting factors VII, IX, and X.

Blood volume

Total intravascular volume increases beginning between 10 and 12 weeks' gestation and peaks with approximately a 40% increase between weeks 32 and 34. This increase can total 5,250 ml in a pregnant patient compared with 4,000 ml in a nonpregnant patient. Volume decreases slightly in the 40th week and returns to normal several weeks after delivery.

Serving a purpose

Increased blood volume, which consists of two-thirds plasma and one-third red blood cells (RBCs), performs several functions. For example:
• it supplies the hypertrophied vascular system of the enlarging uterus
• it provides nutrition for fetal and maternal tissues
• it serves as a reserve for blood loss during childbirth and puerperium.

As the plasma volume first increases, the concentration of hemoglobin and erythrocytes may decline, giving the woman pseudoanemia. The woman's body compensates for this change by producing more RBCs. The body can create nearly normal levels of RBCs by the second trimester.

A look at supine hypotension

When a pregnant woman lays on her back, the weight of the uterus presses on the vena cava and aorta, as shown below left. This obstructs blood flow to and from the legs, resulting in supine hypotension. In a side-lying position, shown below right, pressure on the vessels is relieved, allowing blood to flow freely.

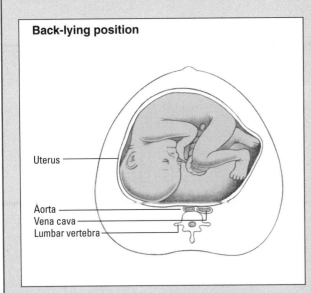

Back-lying position

Uterus

Aorta
Vena cava
Lumbar vertebra

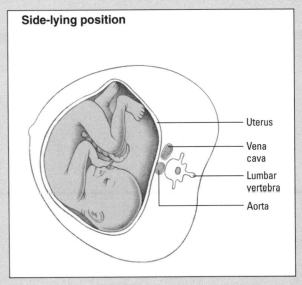

Side-lying position

Uterus

Vena cava

Lumbar vertebra

Aorta

Hematologic changes

Hematologic changes also occur during pregnancy. Pregnancy affects iron demands and absorption as well as RBC, white blood cell (WBC), and fibrinogen levels. In addition, bone marrow becomes more active during pregnancy, producing up to a 30% excess of RBCs.

Ironing out deficiencies

During pregnancy, the body's demand for iron increases. Not only does the developing fetus require approximately 350 to 400 mg of iron per day for healthy growth, but also the mother's iron requirement increases by 400 mg per day. This iron increase is necessary to promote RBC production and accommodate the increased blood volume that occurs during pregnancy. The total daily iron requirements of a woman and her fetus amount to roughly 800 mg. Because the average woman's store of iron is only about 500 mg, a pregnant woman should take iron supplements.

Iron supplements may also be necessary to accommodate for impaired iron absorption. Absorption of iron may be hindered during pregnancy as a result of decreased gastric acidity (iron is absorbed best from an acid medium). In addition, increased plasma volume (from 2,600 ml in a nonpregnant woman to 3,600 ml in a pregnant woman) is disproportionately greater than the increase in RBCs, which lowers the patient's hematocrit (the percentage of RBCs in whole blood) and causes anemia. The hemoglobin level also decreases. A hematocrit below 35% and hemoglobin level below 11.5 g/dl indicate pregnancy-related anemia. Iron supplements are commonly prescribed during pregnancy to reduce the risk of this complication.

Bulking up the blood

The WBC count rises from 7,000 ml before pregnancy to 20,500 ml during pregnancy. The reason for this is unknown. The count may increase to 25,000 ml or more during labor, childbirth, and the early postpartum period.

Fibrin factor

Fibrinogen (a protein in blood plasma) is converted to fibrin by thrombin and is known as coagulation factor I. In a nonpregnant patient, levels average 250 mg/dl. In a pregnant patient, levels average 450 mg/dl, increasing as much as 50% by term. This increase in the coagulation factor plays an important role in preventing maternal hemorrhage during childbirth.

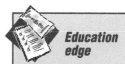

Education edge

Correcting supine hypotension

Supine hypotension can be easily corrected by having the woman turn onto her side (preferably the left side), which enhances blood flow through the vena cava. Teach the pregnant patient to always rest on her left side rather than her back because, even with additional collateral circulation, lying in a supine position can lead to hypotension.

Urinary system

The kidneys, ureters, and bladder undergo profound changes in structure and function during pregnancy.

Anatomic changes

Significant dilation of the renal pelves, calyces, and ureters begins as early as 10 weeks' gestation, probably due to increased estrogen and progesterone levels. As pregnancy advances and the uterus undergoes dextroversion (meaning that it moves more toward the right), the ureters and renal pelves become more dilated above the pelvic brim, particularly on the right side. In addition, the smooth muscle of the ureters undergoes hypertrophy and hyperplasia and muscle tone decreases, primarily because of the muscle-relaxing effects of progesterone. These changes slow the flow of urine through the ureters and result in hydronephrosis and hydroureter (distention of the renal pelves and ureters with urine), predisposing the pregnant patient to urinary tract infections (UTIs). In addition, because of the delay between urine's formation in the kidneys and its arrival in the bladder, inaccuracies may occur during clearance tests.

Maximal capacity, minimal comfort

Hormonal changes cause the bladder to relax during pregnancy, permitting it to distend to hold approximately 1,500 ml of urine. However, hormonal changes and pressure from the growing uterus cause bladder irritation, manifested as urinary frequency and urgency, even if the bladder contains little urine. Bladder vascularity increases and the mucosa bleeds easily.

When the uterus rises out of the pelvis, urinary symptoms reduce. As term approaches, however, the presenting part of the fetus engages in the pelvis, which exerts pressure on the bladder again, causing symptoms to return.

Functional changes

Pregnancy affects fluid retention; renal, bladder, and ureter function; renal tubular resorption; and nutrient and glucose excretion.

Fluid retention

Water is retained during pregnancy to help handle the increase in blood volume and to serve as a ready source of nutrients for the fetus. Because nutrients can only pass to the fetus when dissolved in or carried by fluid, this ready fluid supply is a fetal safeguard. This excess fluid also replenishes the mother's blood volume in case of hemorrhage.

Water, water everywhere

To provide sufficient fluid volume for effective placental exchange, a pregnant woman's total body water increases about 7.5 L from prepregnancy levels of 30 to 40 L. To maintain osmolarity, the body has to increase sodium reabsorption in the tubules. To accomplish this, the body's increased progesterone levels stimulate the angiotensin-renin system in the kidneys to increase aldosterone production. Aldosterone helps with sodium reabsorption. Potassium levels, however, remain adequate despite the increased urine output during pregnancy because progesterone is potassium-sparing and doesn't allow excess potassium to be excreted in the urine.

Renal function

During pregnancy, the kidneys must excrete the waste products of the mother's body as well as those of the growing fetus. Also, the kidneys must be able to break down and excrete additional protein and manage the demands of increased renal blood flow. The kidneys may increase in size, which changes their structure and ultimately affects their function.

A pregnant woman's body retains water to ensure there's a medium in which nutrients can travel to get to the fetus.

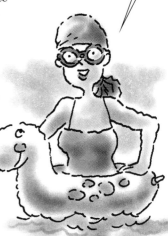

During pregnancy, urine output gradually increases to 60% to 80% more than prepregnancy output (1,500 ml/day). In addition, urine specific gravity decreases. The glomerular filtration rate (GFR) and renal plasma flow (RPF) begin to increase in early pregnancy to meet the increased needs of the circulatory system. By the second trimester, the GFR and RPF have increased by 30% to 50% and remain at this level for the duration of the pregnancy. This rise is consistent with that of the circulatory system increase, peaking at about 24 weeks' gestation. This efficient GFR level leads to lowered blood urea nitrogen and lowered creatinine levels in maternal plasma.

Glucose spill

An increased GFR leads to increased filtration of glucose into the renal tubules. Because reabsorption of glucose by the tubule cells occurs at a fixed rate, glucose sometimes is excreted, or spills, into urine during pregnancy (see *When glucose enters urine*). Lactose, which is being produced by the mammary glands during pregnancy but isn't being used, also spills into the urine.

Ureter and bladder function

During pregnancy, the uterus is pushed slightly toward the right side of the abdomen by the increased bulk of the sigmoid colon. The pressure on the right ureter caused by this movement may lead to urinary stasis and pyelonephritis (inflammation of the kidney cased by bacterial infection). Pressure on the urethra may lead to poor bladder emptying and possible bladder infection,

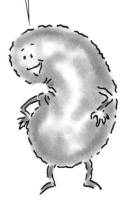

Phew! During pregnancy, I'm working a double shift because I have to excrete maternal and fetal waste.

Take charge!

When glucose enters urine

During each prenatal visit, the woman's urine should be checked for glucose. A finding of more than a trace of glucose in a routine sample of urine from a pregnant woman is considered abnormal until proven otherwise.

Glycosuria on two consecutive occasions that isn't related to carbohydrate intake warrants further investigation. It may indicate gestational diabetes. Such a finding should be reported to the health care provider. In many cases, an oral glucose screening test is ordered. A small percentage of women have glycosuria of pregnancy that isn't diabetes related but is due to a decreased kidney threshold for glucose.

which can become more dangerous if it results in kidney infection. Infection in the kidneys, which serve as the filtering system for toxins in the blood, can be extremely dangerous to the mother. UTIs are also potentially dangerous to the fetus because they're associated with preterm labor.

Renal tubular resorption

To maintain sodium and fluid balance, renal tubular resorption increases by as much as 50% during pregnancy. The patient's sodium requirement increases because she needs more intravascular and extracellular fluid. She may accumulate 6.2 to 8.5 L of water to meet her needs and those of the fetus and placenta. Up to 75% of maternal weight gain is due to increased body water in the extracellular spaces. Amniotic fluid and the placenta account for about one-half of this amount; increased maternal blood volume and enlargement of the breasts and uterus account for the rest.

Posture of elimination

Late in pregnancy, changes in the patient's posture affect sodium and water excretion. For example, the patient excretes less when lying on her back because the enlarged uterus compresses the vena cava and aorta, causing decreased cardiac output. This decreased cardiac output reduces renal blood flow, which in turn decreases kidney function. The patient excretes more when lying on her left side because, in this position, the uterus doesn't compress the great vessels and cardiac output and kidney function remain unchanged.

Nutrient and glucose excretion

A pregnant patient loses increased amounts of some nutrients, such as amino acids, water-soluble vitamins, folic acid, and iodine. Proteinuria (protein in the urine) can occur during pregnancy because the filtered load of amino acids may exceed the tubular reabsorptive capacity. When the renal tubules can't reabsorb the amino acids, protein may be excreted in small amounts in the patient's urine. Values of +1 protein on a urine dipstick aren't considered abnormal until the levels exceed 300 mg/24 hours. Glycosuria (glucose in the urine) may also occur as GFR increases without a corresponding increase in tubular resorptive capacity.

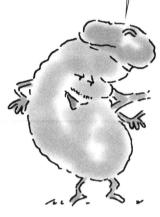

To maintain sodium and fluid balance, renal tubular resorption increases by as much as 50% during pregnancy.

GI system

Changes during pregnancy affect anatomic elements in the GI system and alter certain GI functions. These changes are associated with many of the most commonly discussed discomforts of pregnancy.

Anatomic changes

The mouth, stomach, intestines, gallbladder, and liver are affected during pregnancy. (See *Crowding of abdominal contents*, page 130.)

Mouth

The salivary glands become more active in the pregnant patient, especially in the latter half of pregnancy. The gums become edematous and bleed easily because of increased vascularity.

Stomach and intestines

As progesterone increases during pregnancy, gastric tone and motility decrease, thus slowing the stomach's emptying time and possibly causing regurgitation and reflux of stomach contents. This may cause the patient to complain of heartburn. Progesterone also makes smooth muscle, including that which appears in the intestine, less active.

Make room for the uterus

As the uterus enlarges, it tends to displace the stomach and intestines toward the back and sides of the abdomen. About halfway through the pregnancy, the pressure may be sufficient enough to slow intestinal peristalsis and the emptying time of the stomach, leading to heartburn, constipation, and flatulence. Relaxin may contribute to decreased gastric motility, which may cause a decrease in blood supply to the GI tract as blood is drawn to the uterus.

The enlarged uterus also displaces the large intestine and puts increased pressure on veins below the uterus. This may predispose the patient to hemorrhoids.

Gallbladder and liver

As smooth muscles relax, the gallbladder empties sluggishly. This can lead to reabsorption of bilirubin into the maternal bloodstream, causing generalized itching (subclinical jaundice). A woman who has had previous gallstone formation may have an increased tendency for stone formation during pregnancy as a result of the increased plasma cholesterol level and additional cholesterol incorporated in bile. A patient with a peptic ulcer generally finds her condition improved during pregnancy because the acidity of the stomach decreases.

More work for the liver

The liver doesn't enlarge or undergo major changes during pregnancy. However, hepatic blood flow may increase slightly, causing

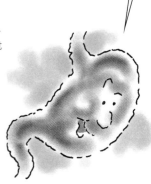

Peptic ulcers tend to improve during pregnancy because the acidity of the stomach decreases.

Crowding of abdominal contents

As the uterus enlarges as a result of the growing fetus, the intestinal contents are pushed upward and to the side. The uterus usually remains midline, although it may shift slightly to the right because of the increased bulk of the sigmoid colon on the left.

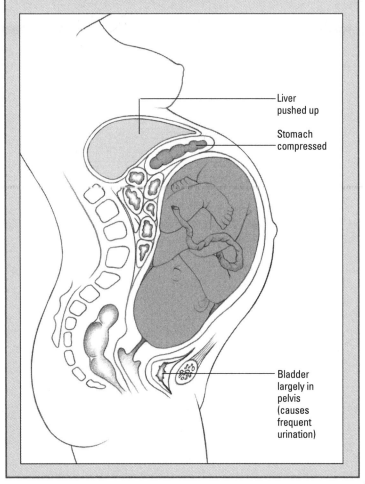

Liver pushed up

Stomach compressed

Bladder largely in pelvis (causes frequent urination)

the liver's workload to increase as BMR increases. Factors within the liver as well as increased estrogen and progesterone decrease bile flow.

Some liver function studies show drastic changes during pregnancy, possibly caused by increased estrogen levels. Test results may show:

- doubled alkaline phosphatase levels, caused in part by increased alkaline phosphatase isoenzymes from the placenta
- decreased serum albumin
- increased plasma globulin levels, causing decreases in albumin globulin ratios
- decreased plasma cholinesterase levels.

These changes would suggest hepatic disease in a nonpregnant patient but are considered normal in the pregnant patient.

Functional changes

Nausea and vomiting during pregnancy may affect appetite and food consumption, even when the patient's energy demand increases.

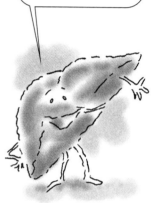

Looks like I'll be putting in some overtime! As BMR increases, the workload of the liver increases.

Appetite and food consumption

A pregnant patient's appetite and food consumption fluctuate. This may be due to several things. For example, the patient may experience nausea and vomiting that decrease her appetite and, therefore, food consumption. These symptoms are more noticeable in the morning when the patient first arises, hence the term *morning sickness*. Nausea and vomiting can also occur when the woman experiences fatigue. If the patient smokes, their occurrence may be more frequent. Nausea and vomiting tend to be noticeable when hCG and progesterone levels begin to rise. These conditions may also be a reaction to decreased glucose levels (because glucose is being used in great quantities by the growing fetus) or increased estrogen levels.

In addition to the reduced appetite caused by nausea and vomiting, increased hCG levels and changes in carbohydrate metabolism may reduce the patient's appetite. When nausea and vomiting stop, the patient's appetite and metabolic needs increase.

Carbohydrate, lipid, and protein metabolism

The patient's carbohydrate needs rise to meet increasing energy demands. The patient needs more glucose, especially during the second half of pregnancy. Plasma lipid levels increase starting in the first trimester, rising at term to 40% to 50% above prepregnancy levels. Cholesterol, triglyceride, and lipoprotein levels increase as well. The total concentration of serum proteins decreases, especially serum albumin and, perhaps, gamma globulin. The primary immunoglobulin transferred to the fetus is lowered in the patient's serum.

Musculoskeletal system

The patient's musculoskeletal system changes in response to hormones, weight gain, and the growing fetus. These changes may affect the patient's gait, posture, and comfort. In addition, increased maternal metabolism creates the need for greater calcium intake. If the patient ingests insufficient calcium, hypocalcemia and muscle cramps may occur.

Skeleton

The enlarging uterus tilts the pelvis forward, shifting the patient's center of gravity. The lumbosacral curve increases, accompanied by a compensatory curvature in the cervicodorsal region. The lumbar and dorsal curves become even more pronounced as breasts enlarge and their weight pulls the shoulders forward, producing a stoop-shouldered stance. Increasing sex hormones (and possibly the hormone relaxin) relax the sacroiliac, sacrococcygeal, and pelvic joints. These changes cause marked alterations in posture and gait. Relaxation of the pelvic joints may also cause the patient's gait to change. Shoe and ring sizes tend to increase because of weight gain, hormonal changes, and dependent edema. Although these changes may persist after childbirth, in most cases, they return to prepregnancy states.

Muscles

In the third trimester, the prominent rectus abdominis muscles (rectus muscles of the abdomen) separate, allowing the abdominal contents to protrude at the midline. Occasionally, the abdominal wall may not be able to stretch enough and the rectus muscles may actually separate, a condition known as *diastasis*. If this happens, a bluish groove appears at the site of separation after pregnancy.

From inny to outty

The umbilicus is stretched by pregnancy to such an extent that, by the 28th week, its depression becomes obliterated and smooth because it has been pushed so far outward. In most women, it may appear as if it has turned inside out, protruding as a round bump at the center of the abdominal wall.

Nerves

In the third trimester, carpal tunnel syndrome may occur when the median nerve of the carpal tunnel of the wrist is compressed by edematous surrounding tissue. The patient may notice tingling

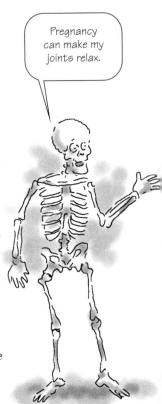

Pregnancy can make my joints relax.

and burning in the dominant hand, possibly radiating to the elbow and upper arm. Numbness or tingling in the hands also may result from pregnancy-related postural changes such as slumped shoulders that pull on the brachial plexus.

Integumentary system

Skin changes vary greatly among pregnant patients. Of those patients who experience skin changes, blacks and whites with brown hair typically show more marked changes.

Because some skin changes may remain after childbirth, they aren't considered an important sign of pregnancy in a patient who has given birth before. The patient may need the nurse's help to integrate these skin changes into her self-concept. Skin changes associated with pregnancy include striae gravidarum, pigment changes, and vascular markings.

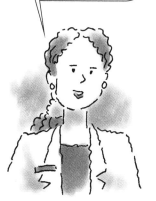

Stretch marks are most common on the skin covering the breasts, abdomen, buttocks, and thighs.

Striae gravidarum

The patient's weight gain and enlarging uterus, combined with the action of adrenocorticosteroids, lead to stretching of the underlying connective tissue of the skin, creating striae gravidarum in the second and third trimesters. Better known as *stretch marks*, striae on light-skinned patients appear as pink or slightly reddish streaks with slight depressions; on dark-skinned patients, they appear lighter than the surrounding skin tone. They develop most commonly on the skin covering the breasts, abdomen, buttocks, and thighs. After labor, they typically grow lighter until they appear silvery white on light-skinned patients and light brown on dark-skinned patients.

Pigment changes

Pigmentation begins to change at approximately the eighth week of pregnancy, partly because of melanocyte-stimulating and adrenocorticotropic hormones and partly because of estrogen and progesterone. These changes are more pronounced in hyperpigmented areas, such as the face, breasts (especially nipples), axillae, abdomen, anal region, inner thighs, and vulva. Specific changes may include linea nigra and melasma.

Vascular markings

Tiny, bright-red angiomas may appear during pregnancy as a result of estrogen release, which increases subcutaneous blood flow. They're called *vascular spiders* because of the branching pattern that extends from each spot. Occurring mostly on the chest, neck, arms, face, and legs, they disappear after childbirth.

Pink-handed

Palmar erythemas, commonly seen along with vascular spiders, are well-delineated, pinkish areas over the palmar surface of the hands. When pregnancy ends and estrogen levels decrease, this condition reverses.

Bubbled gums

Epulides, also known as *gingival granuloma gravidarum*, are raised, red, fleshy areas that appear on the gums as a result of increased estrogen. They may enlarge, cause severe pain, and bleed profusely. An epulis that grows rapidly may require excision.

Other integumentary changes

Nevi (circumscribed, benign proliferations of pigment-producing cells in the skin) may develop on the face, neck, upper chest, or arms during pregnancy. Oily skin and acne from increased estrogen may also occur. Hirsutism (excessive hair growth) may occur, but this reverses when pregnancy ends. By the sixth week of pregnancy, fingernails may soften and break easily — a problem that may be exacerbated by nail polish removers.

Immune system

Immunologic competency naturally decreases during pregnancy, most likely to prevent the woman's body from rejecting the fetus. To the immune system, the fetus is a foreign object. In most cases, the immune system responds to foreign objects by sending defense cells that gang up on the foreign objects and try to destroy them. For certain types of foreign objects, such as a cold virus, this immune response is necessary to protect the body. In a situation such as organ transplantation, however, the patient must be given medications to reduce the immune system response so that the body doesn't attack the transplant.

Make yourself at home

A similar process occurs naturally in a pregnant woman, whereby her immune system response decreases, allowing the fetus to remain. In particular, immunoglobulin G (IgG) production is decreased, which increases the risk of infection during pregnancy. A simultaneous increase in the WBC count may help to counteract the decrease in IgG response.

Neurologic system

Changes in the neurologic system during pregnancy are poorly defined and aren't completely understood. For most patients, neurologic changes are temporary and revert back to normal after pregnancy is over.

Nervous reactions

Functional disturbances called *entrapment neuropathies* occur in the peripheral nervous system as a result of mechanical pressure. In other words, nerves become trapped and pinched by the enlarging uterus and enlarged edematous vessels, making them less functional. For example, the patient may experience meralgia paresthetica, a tingling and numbness in the anterolateral portion of the thigh that results when the lateral femoral cutaneous nerve becomes entrapped in the area of the inguinal ligaments. This feeling is more pronounced in late pregnancy, as the gravid uterus presses on the nerves and as vascular stasis occurs.

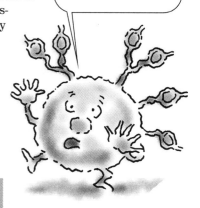

The enlarged uterus and distended vessels trap me, making it difficult for me to do my job. For the patient, this may feel like tingling and numbness.

Psychosocial changes

Pregnancy and childbirth are events that deeply affect the lives of parents, partners, and families. A nurse faces many responsibilities and challenges regarding the expectant family's psychosocial care. Psychological, social, economic, and cultural factors as well as family and individual influences toward sex-specific and family roles affect the parents' response to pregnancy and childbirth. All of these aspects of childbearing affect the health of the parents and their children.

Phases of acceptance

A mother's acceptance of the pregnancy can progress through different phases:
- During the first stage, called *full embodiment*, a woman may become dependent on her partner or significant others and may be introspective and calm. The woman, especially if she's a new mother, may initially feel some ambivalence about finding out that she's pregnant. She may spend the first few weeks imagining how the pregnancy will change her life. As the pregnancy progresses, however, the mother incorporates the fetus into her body image.
- Next comes the developmental stage of *fetal distinction*. In this stage, the woman starts to view her fetus as a separate individual.

She begins to accept her new body image and may even characterize it as being "full of life." She may become closer or more dependent on her mother at this stage.

• The next stage is *role transition*. During this stage, the woman prepares to separate from and give up her attachment to the fetus. She may become anxious about labor and delivery. Discomfort and frustration over the awkwardness of her body may lead the mother to become impatient about the impending delivery. During this stage, the patient also begins to get ready for the baby and to mentally prepare for her role as mother.

> During the role transition stage, the patient begins to prepare for her new role as mother.

Influences affecting acceptance

Such factors as cultural background, family influences, and individual temperaments can affect a mother's acceptance of the pregnancy.

Cultural

A woman's cultural background may strongly influence how she progresses through the stages of acceptance. They may also guide how actively the woman participates in her pregnancy. Certain beliefs and taboos may place restrictions on her behavior and activities. For example, Native Americans may not seek prenatal care as soon as other pregnant women because they view pregnancy as a normal condition.

Family

The home in which a woman was raised can also influence her beliefs about and her acceptance of pregnancy. If a woman was raised in a home in which children were loved and viewed as pleasant additions to a happy family, she'll probably have a more positive attitude toward pregnancy. If she was raised in a home in which children were considered intruders or were blamed for the breakup of a marriage, the woman's view of pregnancy may not be a positive one.

Whence she came

More specifically, the views of the patient's mother commonly influence the patient's attitudes about pregnancy. If her mother hated being pregnant and always reminded her that she was a burden and that children weren't always wanted, she may view her pregnancy in the same way.

Individual

A woman's temperament and ability to cope with or adapt to stress plays a role in how she resolves conflict and adapts to her new life after childbirth. How she accepts her pregnancy depends on her self-image and the support that's given to her. For example, a woman may view pregnancy as a situation that robs her of her career, looks, and freedom.

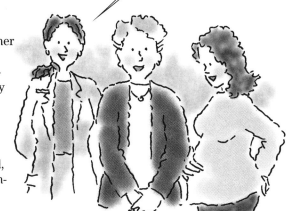

> How a woman views her pregnancy is influenced by her mother's beliefs about pregnancy and motherhood.

Make room for daddy?

A woman's relationship with the child's father also influences her acceptance of the pregnancy. If the father is there to provide emotional support, acceptance of the pregnancy is likely to be easier for the woman than if he isn't a part of the pregnancy. Whether the father of the child is able to accept the pregnancy depends on the same factors that affect the mother: cultural background, past experiences, and relationship with family members.

Promoting acceptance of pregnancy

Pregnancy is a time of profound psychological, social, and biological changes that affect the parents' responsibilities, freedoms, values, priorities, social status, relationships, and self-images. The events of the childbearing year (9 antenatal and 3 postpartum months) also may be unpredictable. Although expectant parents can control some events (for example, obtaining early prenatal care) and adopt positive attitudes, they can't control all that happens during that year.

Supporting change

The nurse must promote family adaptation to the new family member. To achieve these goals, the nurse should take these steps, as expertise allows:
• Promote each family member's self-esteem.
• Elicit questions and concerns from the family and listen to them attentively.
• Discuss the roles and tasks for each family member, affirm their efforts, and inquire about and show concern for each family member's health care needs. Make referrals as needed.
• Involve all family members in prenatal visits, as appropriate.

- Facilitate communication among family members and offer anticipatory guidance about family changes during pregnancy and the postpartum period.
- Help to mobilize the family's resources.
- Offer sexual counseling to the patient and her partner.
- Help the patient maximize her family's positive contributions and minimize negative ones.
- Praise the family's efforts.
- Offer books and other materials that address all family members.
- Promote the family's prenatal bonding (sometimes called *attachment*) with the fetus by sharing information about fetal development and helping the family identify fetal heart tones, position, and movements. Reinforce bonding behaviors, such as patting the abdomen or talking to the fetus, by asking the patient or her partner to note and report fetal movements.

Conquering conflicts

- Facilitate conflict resolution related to pregnancy and childbirth. Help identify underlying conflicts through reflective communication, validation of feelings, and exploration of dreams and fantasies. Promote conflict resolution by teaching such techniques as personal affirmation and dream interpretation and by suggesting literature that helps identify and resolve conflicts. Refer any patient who can't resolve conflicts to counseling.
- Support adaptive coping patterns through realistic patient and family education about pregnancy, childbirth, and the postpartum period. Discuss childbirth and human responses accurately and realistically. Frankly discuss the challenges of parenting.
- Deliver culturally sensitive nursing care. Gather information about the family's customs and beliefs to add to assessment data and to individualize care.
- Identify personal attitudes and feelings about childbearing. Avoid imposing personal values, feelings, and emotional reactions on others. Also avoid making assumptions about the patient and her preferences. Allow her to share her feelings freely.

First trimester

During the first trimester, the family's key psychosocial challenge is to resolve any ambivalence. The mother copes with the common discomforts and changes of the first trimester; the father begins to accept the reality of the pregnancy.

Other psychosocial challenges that the parents face include maternal acceptance of physical changes and paternal acceptance of and preparation for fatherhood.

Ambivalence

The first trimester is known as the *trimester of ambivalence* because parents experience mixed feelings. Many women have unrealistic ideas about maternal instincts, expecting to feel only loving, happy thoughts about the fetus and motherhood. In fact, most women feel some ambivalence about pregnancy and motherhood. Pregnancy involves stressful changes that force women to think and behave differently than they have in the past.

Sharing the joy (and the doubt)

Feelings of ambivalence are inevitable and normal. Encourage the parents to communicate these feelings to each other. Partners who discuss these feelings usually can resolve their grief and fears and enjoy the gratifications of expecting a child. When partners share feelings, they may find they're experiencing similar conflicts.

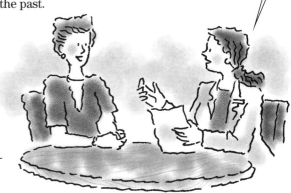

It's okay to have some mixed feelings about your pregnancy at first. Pregnancy and motherhood are major life changes.

Dream a little dream

During this time, both partners may experience vivid dreams about the impending birth. The woman may recall her dreams with greater intensity, however, because she typically is awakened more often at night by heartburn, fetal activity, and a need to urinate. Dreams tend to follow a predictable pattern during pregnancy. By exploring them, expectant parents can better understand themselves and any subconscious conflicts they may have. Dream analysis may be used to help resolve these psychosocial conflicts.

Psychological responses to physical changes

In the early weeks of the first trimester, the woman watches for body changes that confirm her pregnancy. Her body image (her mental image of how her body looks, feels, and moves and how others see her) changes as her breasts enlarge, her menses cease, and she begins to experience nausea, fatigue, waist thickening, and general weight gain. Depending on her acceptance of the pregnancy, the woman may enjoy or dread these changes.

In the mood...or not!

A woman's response to the physical changes her body incurs during pregnancy, as well as other factors, can affect the sexual relationship between her and her partner. A woman's sexual responses during pregnancy vary widely. Some women are too uncomfortable during the first trimester to enjoy sexual intercourse. Others, especially those who have had a past spontaneous abortion, may fear fetal injury. Those who believe sex is only for procreation may feel guilty about sexual activity during pregnancy. Conversely, some patients may feel sexually stimulated by the freedom from contraception, the joy of conception, or the lack of pressure to avoid pregnancy or to have sex on a regular schedule to achieve pregnancy.

A man's sexual response also may change during his partner's pregnancy. Typically, the man worries about how the pregnancy will change his relationship with his partner. He may feel personally rejected when his partner's fatigue, nausea, and other first trimester discomforts diminish her sexual interest. He may also fear causing spontaneous abortion or fetal injury during intercourse. These concerns may increase as the pregnancy advances.

An extra dose of affection

Because of these fears and concerns, both partners may need extra affection from each other, especially during the first trimester. The nurse should encourage them to communicate and share their feelings and preferences about sexual activities.

> Communication is key. Encourage the patient and her partner to discuss their emotions.

Acceptance of and preparation for fatherhood

During the first trimester, the father typically finds the pregnancy unreal and intangible. The idea of the fetus may be abstract to him because he can't observe physical changes in his partner. Accepting the reality of pregnancy is the father's main psychological task in the first trimester.

You've got style

Because he isn't physically pregnant, the father can choose his degree and type of involvement in the pregnancy. There are three fathering styles:

The *observer* style describes a father who's happy about the pregnancy and provides much support to his wife. However, due to personal shyness or cultural values, he doesn't participate in such activities as attending parenting education classes or helping to choose the mode of infant feeding.

The *expressive* style describes a man who shows a strong emotional response to the pregnancy and wishes to be fully involved in it. He demonstrates the same emotional lability and ambivalence as the pregnant woman and may even experience common pregnancy symptoms, such as nausea, vomiting, and fatigue.

In the *instrumental* style of fathering, the man takes on the role of "manager" of the pregnancy. He asks questions and takes pictures throughout the pregnancy, carefully plans for the birthing event, prepares to serve as labor coach, and plans for the infant's arrival home. He's protective and supportive of his wife and feels responsible for the pregnancy outcome.

None of these styles is more competent or mature than another. Although each father becomes more involved as the pregnancy advances, fathering style usually remains consistent. Regardless of fathering style, the man may experience two psychosocial phenomena during the pregnancy: obsession with his role as provider and couvade symptoms.

Show baby the money

Because society values a man's provider role, the expectant father usually ponders the increased financial responsibilities a child brings. Finances remain a major focus throughout pregnancy, and the man may exert tremendous effort to attain financial security. A disproportionate emphasis on finances may reflect deep doubts about his competence as a father. The more secure he feels about his family's economic status, the more open and nurturing he can be with his partner.

Sympathy pains

Couvade syndrome describes physical symptoms—such as backache, nausea, and vomiting—experienced by the man that mimic the symptoms experienced by the pregnant woman. These symptoms commonly result from stress, anxiety, and empathy for the woman. Couvade symptoms aren't associated with the father's attachment to the fetus and aren't limited to first-time fathers. However, they occur most frequently in fathers who are greatly involved in the pregnancy.

Second trimester

During the second trimester, psychosocial tasks include mother-image development, father-image development, coping with body image and sexuality changes, and development of prenatal attachment. Parents may experience various fears. Feeling dependent and vulnerable, the woman may fear for her partner's safety. In touch with mortality, the man may consider how his death would affect his family. He may recall risks he has taken, such as

Let's see... you're experiencing backaches and nausea and your wife is pregnant. I think you're experiencing couvade symptoms.

driving recklessly, and, as a result, he may commit to being more careful to avoid the risk of abandoning his partner and fetus.

Dreams to remember

During the second trimester, the parents' dreams may reflect concerns about the normalcy of the fetus, parental abilities, divided loyalties, and related subjects. To accomplish these tasks, the couple may examine their dreams and fears.

Mother-image development

As the second trimester begins, expectant parents have completed much of the first trimester's grieving. The woman has abandoned old roles and has started to determine what kind of mother she wants to be. Her mother image is a composite of mothering characteristics she has gleaned from role models, readings, and her imagination.

Four aspects of the mother-daughter relationship influence the woman's mother image:

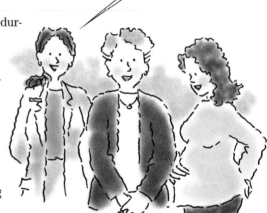

It's all in the family! The development of a pregnant woman's mother image is greatly influenced by what her own mother was like.

her mother's availability in the past and during the pregnancy

her mother's reaction to the pregnancy, her acceptance of the grandchild, and her acknowledgment of her daughter as a mother

her mother's respect for the daughter's autonomy and acceptance of her as a mature adult

her mother's willingness to reminisce about her own childbearing and child-rearing experiences.

Expect introspection

The new mother's preoccupation with forming a mother image causes a period of introspection. As a result, she may show less affection, become more passive, or withdraw from her other children, who react by becoming more demanding. Her partner also may feel neglected during this period.

Father-image development

While the woman develops her mother image, the man begins to form his father image, which is based on his relationship with his father, previous fathering experiences, the fathering styles of friends and family members, and his partner's view of his role in the pregnancy.

Reach out and touch someone

As he starts to develop his father image, the man remembers his relationship with his father and sometimes increases contact with his parents. He may have difficulty viewing his father as a grandfather and coming to terms with his position as a father.

Generally, the woman's expectations about her partner's involvement and the quality of their relationship predict the man's role in delivery and child rearing. Some women desire privacy and modesty during childbirth and don't expect or desire to involve their partners. Others expect their partner's full involvement in tracking fetal movements, attending prenatal visits, and acting as coach, advocate, and primary emotional support during labor. When the patient's expectations about her partner's role doesn't match that of her partner, the couple may need to be referred to counseling.

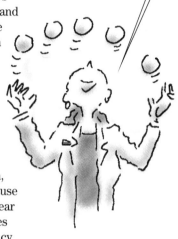

As a new mother juggles with her emotions, she may show less affection for or withdraw from her other children.

Prenatal bonding

A new phase begins at approximately 17 to 20 weeks' gestation, when the woman feels fetal movements for the first time. Because fetal movements are a sign of good health and may dispel the fear of spontaneous abortion, the woman almost always experiences the first flutter of movement positively, even when the pregnancy is unwanted. As a result, she becomes attentive to the type and timing of movements and to fetal responses to environmental factors, such as music, abdominal strokes, and meals.

Yes, sir, that's my baby

The woman may demonstrate bonding behaviors, such as stroking and patting her abdomen, talking to the fetus about eating while she eats, reprimanding the fetus for moving too much, engaging her partner in conversations with the fetus, eating a balanced diet, and engaging in other health promotion behaviors. Bonding is influenced by the woman's health, developmental stage, and culture—not by obstetric complications, general anxiety, or demographic variables such as socioeconomic level.

This prenatal bonding requires positive self-esteem, positive role models, and acceptance of the pregnancy. Social support improves this attachment, which in turn increases the woman's feelings of maternal competence and effectiveness. In general, a woman who displays more bonding behaviors during pregnancy has more positive feelings about the neonate after delivery.

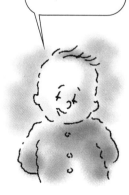

When parents bond with me in utero, they develop positive feelings about their roles as parents.

Third trimester

As the third trimester begins, the woman feels a sense of accomplishment because her fetus has reached the age of viability. She may feel sentimental about the approaching end of her pregnancy, when the mother-child relationship replaces the mother-fetus relationship. At the same time, however, she may look forward to giving birth because the last months of pregnancy involve bulkiness, insomnia, childbirth anxieties, and concern about the neonate's normalcy.

Time to address the special delivery

During the third trimester, the woman and her partner must adapt to activity changes, prepare for parenting, provide partner support, accept body image and sexuality changes, develop birth plans, and prepare for labor. At this time, the woman needs to overcome any fears she may have about the unknown, labor pain, loss of self-esteem, loss of control, and death. The technique of dream and fear examination may help the couple accomplish these tasks.

Adaptation to activity changes

The growing fetus makes daily activities more difficult for the woman and forces her to slow down. This change can affect her emotional state and her family relationships. Decreased social support for the woman on maternity leave can add to anxiety.

Preparation for parenting

Because the pregnant woman is more aware of what's going on in her body, she may begin to prepare for parenting before her partner. As the woman's body grows, however, typically so does the partner's acceptance of the pregnancy and anticipation of fatherhood. To prepare for parenting, the couple may now focus on concrete tasks, such as preparing the nursery, making decisions about childcare, and planning postpartum events.

Partner support and nurture

The couple's ability to support each other through the childbearing cycle is paramount. In many families, husbands and wives get their support from each other.

An easy transition

In relationships in which neither partner is dominant, there may be greater satisfaction and greater closeness during the pregnancy. Relationships that allow flexibility, growth, and risk-taking ease the transition into parenthood.

Acceptance of body image and sexuality changes

A woman's body image can change as the pregnancy progresses and she gains weight. She may begin to feel less attractive. Her body image, as well as her partner's feelings, affects her sexual drive. Poor body image may cause the woman's interest in sex to drop off. Some men also experience diminished sexual interest as pregnancy advances. Couples who desire sexual intimacy in the third trimester must be creative, using new positions and techniques.

Preparation for labor

Childbirth education classes can prepare the woman and her partner for labor and delivery. The partner's attendance at prenatal classes and his participation in all aspects of pregnancy correlate with his degree of relationship satisfaction. Women who feel supported during the pregnancy and delivery experience fewer complications and may make the transition to motherhood more easily.

Development of birth plans

A highly dependent woman may allow the health care provider to make decisions about the birth plans, assuming that the provider's decisions are the wisest. A more independent woman may seek health care that's comfortable to her and that fits with her beliefs and knowledge, thus ensuring that her wishes are honored during labor. A woman who shapes her childbirth experience and who develops realistic expectations of the event has dealt with her fears.

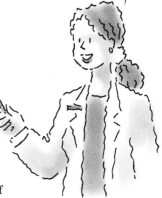

Childbirth education classes can prepare the woman and her partner for labor and delivery.

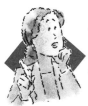

Quick quiz

1. Nausea and vomiting are common because of:
    A.   increased progesterone levels.
    B.   decreased progesterone levels.
    C.   increased estrogen levels.
    D.   decreased estrogen levels.

Answer: C. Nausea and vomiting may occur as a systemic reaction to increased estrogen levels.

2. Which respiratory element doesn't change during pregnancy?

    A.   Vital capacity

    B.   Residual volume

    C.   Tidal volume

    D.   Oxygen consumption

Answer: A. Vital capacity (the maximum volume exhaled following a maximum inspiration) doesn't change during pregnancy.

3. Decreased gastric motility occurring around midpregnancy may occur because of:

    A.   estrogen.

    B.   progesterone.

    C.   relaxin.

    D.   folic acid.

Answer: C. Relaxin (a hormone produced by the ovaries) can contribute to decreased gastric motility, which may cause a decrease in blood supply to the GI tract as blood is drawn into the uterus.

Scoring

☆☆☆ If you answered all three questions correctly, rock on! You're on top of the maternal-neonatal charts.

☆☆ If you answered two questions correctly, kick out the jams! You're adept at the various adaptations to pregnancy.

☆ If you answered only one question correctly, keep on truckin'. You have plenty of chapters to help you get on the road again.

5

Prenatal care

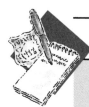

Just the facts

In this chapter, you'll learn:

♦ components of a prenatal patient history

♦ the parts of a prenatal physical assessment

♦ different types of prenatal testing

♦ nutritional needs of the pregnant patient

♦ common discomforts of pregnancy and ways to minimize them.

A close look at prenatal care

Prenatal care is essential to the overall health of the neonate and the mother. Commonly considered elements of prenatal care include assessing the patient, performing prenatal testing, providing nutritional care, and minimizing the discomforts of pregnancy. However, that isn't where prenatal care ends — or, should we say, where it begins.

Long ago...

Believe it or not, prenatal care begins long before pregnancy — it actually begins when the expectant mother herself is still a child! Ideally, to reduce the risk of complications during pregnancy, a woman needs to maintain good health and nutrition throughout her life. For example, adequate calcium and vitamin D intake during the woman's infancy and childhood helps to prevent rickets, which can distort pelvic size, resulting in difficulties during birth. Maintenance of immunizations protects her from viral diseases such as rubella. In addition, such healthy lifestyle practices as eating a nutritious diet, having positive attitudes about sexuality, practicing safer sex, having

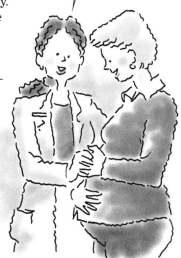

Prenatal care ensures the health of the mother and her neonate. It's essential!

regular pelvic examinations, and receiving prompt treatment for sexually transmitted diseases (STDs) also contribute to the patient's health status throughout pregnancy.

After the fact

Prenatal care after the patient has conceived consists of a thorough assessment, including a health history and physical examination, prenatal testing, nutritional care, and reduction of discomfort. Each of these factors should be addressed at the first prenatal visit.

Occasion for education

The first prenatal visit is also the time when the pregnant woman and her family can receive information on and counseling about what to expect during pregnancy, including necessary care. This promotes the development of healthy behaviors and helps to prevent complications. Keep in mind that the patient education you provide during pregnancy should vary depending on the age and parity of the woman as well as her cultural background. Warn the patient ahead of time that her first visit may be long so that she knows what to expect.

> Developing and maintaining healthy behaviors during pregnancy helps prevent complications.

Assessment

The first prenatal visit is the best time to establish baseline data for the pregnant patient. A thorough assessment of the reproductive system should be included. As with other body systems, this assessment depends on an accurate history (see *Tips for a successful interview*) and a thorough physical examination.

Inform-her

Remember to keep the patient informed about assessment findings. Sharing this information with her may help her to comply with health care recommendations and encourage her to seek additional information about any problems or questions that she has later in the pregnancy.

Health history

Information obtained from the patient's health history helps establish baseline data, which can be used to plan health promotion

Advice from the experts

Tips for a successful interview

Here are some tips that can help you obtain an accurate and thorough patient history.

Location
Pregnancy is too private to be discussed in public areas. Make every effort to interview your patient in a private, quiet setting. Trying to talk to a pregnant woman in a crowded area, such as a busy waiting room in a clinic, is rarely effective. Remember patient confidentially and respect the patient's privacy, especially when discussing intimate topics.

Checklist
To ensure that your history is complete, be sure to ask about:
• the patient's overall patterns of health and illness
• the patient's medical and surgical history
• the patient's history of pregnancy or abortion
• the date of the patient's last menses and whether her menses are regular or irregular
• the patient's sexual history, including number of partners, frequency, current method of birth control, and satisfaction with chosen method of birth control
• the patient's family history
• any allergies the patient has
• health-related habits, such as smoking and alcohol use.

strategies for every subsequent visit as well as identify potential complications. (See *Formidable findings*, page 150.)

The health history you conduct should be extensive. Be sure to include biographic data, information on the patient's nutritional status, a medical history, a family history, a gynecologic history, and an obstetric history.

Biographic data

When obtaining biographic data, assure the patient that the information remains confidential. Topics to discuss include age; cultural considerations, such as race and religion; marital status; occupation; and education.

Age

The patient's age is an important factor in pregnancy because reproductive risks increase among adolescents younger than age 15 and women older than age 35. For example, pregnant adolescents are more likely to have preeclampsia, also known as pregnancy-induced hypertension (PIH). Expectant mothers older than age 35

Formidable findings

When performing your health history and assessment, look for the following findings to determine if a pregnant patient is at risk for complications.

Obstetric history

- History of infertility
- Grandmultiparity
- Incompetent cervix
- Uterine or cervical anomaly
- Previous preterm labor or preterm birth
- Previous cesarean birth
- Previous infant with macrosomia
- Two or more spontaneous or elective abortions
- Previous hydatidiform mole or chorio- carcinoma
- Previous ectopic pregnancy
- Previous stillborn neonate or neonatal death
- Previous multiple gestation
- Previous prolonged labor
- Previous low-birth-weight infant
- Previous midforceps delivery
- Diethylstilbestrol exposure in utero
- Previous infant with neurologic deficit, birth injury, or congenital anomaly
- Less than 1 year since last pregnancy

Medical history

- Cardiac disease
- Metabolic disease
- Renal disease
- Recent urinary tract infection or bac- teriuria
- GI disorders
- Seizure disorders
- Family history of severe inherited dis- orders
- Surgery during pregnancy
- Emotional disorders or mental retarda- tion

- Previous surgeries, particularly those involving the reproductive organs
- Pulmonary disease
- Endocrine disorders
- Hemoglobinopathies
- Sexually transmitted disease (STD)
- Chronic hypertension
- History of abnormal Papanicolaou smear
- Malignancy
- Reproductive tract anomalies

Current obstetric status

- Inadequate prenatal care
- Intrauterine growth restricted fetus
- Large-for-gestational-age fetus
- Pregnancy-induced hypertension (preeclampsia)
- Abnormal fetal surveillance tests
- Polyhydramnios
- Placenta previa
- Abnormal presentation
- Maternal anemia
- Weight gain of less than 10 lb (4.5 kg)
- Weight loss of more than 5 lb (2.3 kg)
- Overweight or underweight status
- Fetal or placenta malformation
- Rh sensitization
- Preterm labor
- Multiple gestation
- Premature rupture of membranes
- Abruptio placentae
- Postdate pregnancy
- Fibroid tumors
- Fetal manipulation
- Cervical cerclage (purse string suture placed around incompetent cervix to

prevent premature opening and subse- quent spontaneous abortion)
- STD
- Maternal infection
- Poor immunization status

Psychosocial factors

- Inadequate finances
- Social problems
- Adolescent
- Poor nutrition
- More than two children at home with no additional support
- Lack of acceptance of pregnancy
- Attempt at or ideation of suicide
- Poor housing
- Lack of involvement of father of baby
- Minority status
- Parental occupation
- Inadequate support systems
- Dysfunctional grieving
- Psychiatric history

Demographic factors

- Maternal age younger than 16 or older than 35
- Less than 11 years of education

Lifestyle

- Smoking (over ten cigarettes per day)
- Substance abuse
- Long commute to work
- Refusal to use seatbelts
- Alcohol consumption
- Heavy lifting or long periods of stand- ing
- Unusual stress
- Lack of smoke detectors in the home

are at risk for other problematic conditions, including placenta previa; hydatidiform mole; and vascular, neoplastic, and degenerative diseases. (See chapter 6, High-risk pregnancy.)

Race and religion

The patient's race and religion, as well as other cultural considerations, may also impact a pregnancy. Obtaining information from your patient about these topics can help you plan patient care. It also gives you greater insight into and an understanding of the patient's behavior, potential problems in health promotion and maintenance, and the patient's ways of coping with illness.

It's important to familiarize yourself with the cultural communities in which you work and to investigate and be familiar with the cultural practices of those communities. (See *Cultural considerations for assessment* and *Southeast Asian views of pregnancy*.)

A race to detect disease

Because some diseases are more common among certain cultural groups, asking the patient about her race can be an important part of your assessment. It may help guide your prenatal testing. For example, a pregnant black woman should be screened for sickle cell trait because this trait primarily occurs in people of African or Mediterranean descent. On the other hand, a Jewish woman of Eastern European ancestry should be screened for Tay-Sachs disease.

Believe it or not

Religious beliefs and practices can also affect the patient's health during pregnancy and can predispose her to complications. For example, Amish women may not be immunized against rubella, putting them at risk. In addition, Seventh-Day Adventists tradition-

Bridging the gap

Cultural considerations for assessment

Encourage the patient to discuss her cultural beliefs regarding health, illness, and health care. Be considerate of the patient's cultural background. Also, be aware that members of many cultures are reluctant to talk about sexual matters and, in some cultures, sexual matters aren't discussed freely with members of the opposite sex.

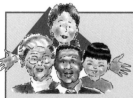

Bridging the gap

Southeast Asian views of pregnancy

Many women from Southeast Asia (Cambodia, Laos, and Vietnam) don't seek care during pregnancy because they don't see it as a time when medical intervention is necessary. In many cases, they're extremely modest and may find pelvic examinations embarrassing. They may rely on herbs and folk remedies to manage common discomforts of pregnancy. In addition, they may hold the belief that blood isn't replaceable, which may prevent them from agreeing to laboratory blood studies. Planning care for these patients may require interpreters, classes in prenatal health, and explanations of how health promotion regimens can fit within their cultural belief systems.

ally exclude dairy products from their diets, and Jehovah's Witnesses refuse blood transfusions. Each of these practices could impact prenatal care and the patient's risk of complications and, thus, you should ask about them when you take the patient's health history.

Marital status

Knowing the patient's marital status may help you identify whether family support systems are available. Marital status can also provide information on the size of the patient's home, her sexual practices, and possible stress factors.

Occupation

Ask about the patient's occupation and work environment to assess possible risk factors. If the patient works in a high-risk environment that exposes her to such hazards as chemicals, inhalants, or radiation, inform her of the dangers of these substances as well as the possible effects on her pregnancy. Knowing the patient's occupation can also help you to identify such risks as working long hours, lifting heavy objects, and standing for prolonged periods.

Several occupational hazards can be harmful to a pregnancy, including heavy lifting.

Education

The patient's formal education and her life experiences may influence several aspects of the pregnancy, including:
- her attitude toward the pregnancy
- her willingness to seek prenatal care
- the adequacy of her at-home prenatal care and nutritional status
- her knowledge of infant care
- her emotional response to childbirth and the responsibilities of parenting.

Obtaining information about the patient's education can help you to plan appropriate patient teaching.

Nutritional status

Adequate nutrition is especially vital during pregnancy. During the prenatal assessment, take a 24-hour diet history (recall). For more information, see the section on nutritional care later in this chapter.

Medical history

When taking a medical history, find out whether the patient is taking any prescription or over-the-counter (OTC) drugs. Also ask about her smoking practices, alcohol use, and use of illegal drugs.

Many drugs—except drugs with molecules that are too large, such as insulin and heparin—are able to cross the placenta and affect the fetus. All of the medications the patient is currently taking should be carefully evaluated, and the benefits of each medication should be weighed against the risk to the fetus.

> Make sure to find out if the patient is taking any prescription or OTC drugs.

> You may need to determine whether certain drugs should be discontinued during pregnancy.

Brushing up on current events

Ask the patient about previous and current medical problems that may jeopardize the pregnancy. For example:
• Diabetes can worsen during pregnancy and harm the mother and fetus. Even a woman who has been successfully managing her diabetes may find it challenging during pregnancy because the glucose-insulin regulatory system changes during pregnancy. Every woman appears to develop insulin resistance during pregnancy. In addition, the fetus uses maternal glucose, which may lead to hypoglycemia in the mother. When glucose regulation is poor, the mother is at risk for PIH and infection, especially monilial infection. The fetus is at risk for asphyxia and stillbirth. Macrosomia (an abnormally large body) may also occur, resulting in an increased risk of birth complications.
• Maternal hypertension, which is more common in women with essential hypertension, renal disease, or diabetes, increases the risk of abruptio placentae.
• Rubella infection during the first trimester can cause malformation in the developing fetus.
• Genital herpes can be transmitted to the neonate during birth. A woman with a history of this disease should have cultures done throughout her pregnancy and may need to deliver by cesarean birth to reduce the risk of transmission.

Other obstacles

Specific problems that you should ask the pregnant patient about include cardiac disorders, respiratory disorders such as tuberculosis; reproductive disorders, such as STDs and endometriosis; phlebitis; epilepsy; and gallbladder disorders. Also, ask the patient if she has a history of urinary tract infections (UTIs), cancer, alcoholism, smoking, drug addiction, or psychiatric problems.

Family history

Knowing the medical histories of the patient's family members can also help you plan care and guide your assessment by identifying complications for which the patient may be at greater risk. For example, if the patient has a family history of varicose veins, she may inherit a weakness in blood vessel walls that becomes evident when she develops varicosities during pregnancy. PIH has also been shown to have a familial tendency, so a history of PIH in the patient's family members means that she's at greater risk for this complication. Be sure to ask whether there's a family history of multiple births, congenital diseases or deformities, or mental disability.

Don't forget the father

When possible, obtain a medical history from the child's father as well. Note that some fetal congenital anomalies may be traced to the father's exposure to environmental hazards.

Gynecologic history

The gynecologic portion of your assessment should include a menstrual history and contraceptive history.

I need to ask you some questions, too, because your family history may also be an important part of prenatal care.

Menstrual history

When obtaining a menstrual history, be sure to ask the patient:
• When did your last menstrual period begin?
• How many days are there between the start of one of your periods and the start of the next?
• Was your last period normal? Was the one before that normal?
• What's the usual amount and duration of your menstrual flow?
• Have you had bleeding or spotting since your last normal menstrual period?

Menarche plays a part

Age of menarche is important when determining pregnancy risks in adolescents. Pregnancy that occurs within 3 years of menarche indicates an increased risk of maternal and fetal mortality; such a pregnancy also places the patient at risk for delivering a neonate who's small for gestational age. Keep in mind that pregnancy can also occur before regular menses are established.

Cramping her style

Ask the patient to describe the intensity of her menstrual cramps. If she indicates that her cramps are very painful, anticipate the need for counseling to help her prepare for labor.

Contraceptive history

To obtain a contraceptive history, ask the patient:
• What form of contraception did you use before your pregnancy?
• How long did you use it?
• Were you satisfied with the method?
• Did you experience any complications while on this type of birth control?

If the patient's method of birth control before becoming pregnant was oral contraceptives, also inquire about how long it was between when the patient ceased taking the pill and when she became pregnant.

Contraceptive catastrophes

A woman whose pregnancy results from contraceptive failure needs special attention to ensure her medical and emotional well-being. Because the pregnancy wasn't planned, the woman may have emotional and financial issues. Offering support and referring her to counselors may help her work through these issues and resolve her ambivalence.

If the patient has an intrauterine device (IUD) in place, be aware of the risk of spontaneous abortion or preterm labor and delivery. If she becomes pregnant with an IUD in place, the device should be removed immediately by her health care provider.

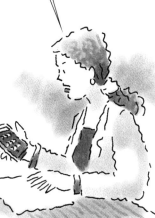

You can use Nägele's rule to calculate the patient's estimated date of delivery.

Calculating estimated date of delivery

Based on information obtained in the patient's menstrual history, you can calculate the patient's estimated date of delivery (EDD) using Nägele's rule: first day of last normal menses, minus 3 months, plus 7 days. Because Nägele's rule is based on a 28-day cycle, you may need to vary the calculation for a woman whose menstrual cycle is irregular, prolonged, or shortened.

Obstetric history

Obtaining an obstetric history is another important part of your assessment. The obstetric history gives important information about the patient's past pregnancies. No matter how old the patient is, don't assume that this is her first pregnancy. (See *Pregnancy classification system*, page 156.)

Getting the details

The obstetric history should include specific details about past pregnancies, including whether the patient had difficult or long labors and whether she experienced complications. Be sure to document each child's sex and the location and date of birth.

Logic says record chronologically

Always record the patient's obstetric history chronologically. For a list of the types of information you should include in a complete obstetric history, see *Taking an obstetric history.*

What's your type?

In addition to asking about pregnancy history, ask the woman if she knows her blood type. If the woman's blood type is Rh-negative, ask if she received $Rh_o(D)$ immune globulin (RhoGAM) after miscarriages, abortions, or previous births so that you'll know whether Rh sensitization occurred. If she didn't receive RhoGAM after any of these situations, her present pregnancy may be at risk for Rh sensitization. Also ask if she's ever had a blood transfusion to establish possible risk of hepatitis B and human immunodeficiency virus (HIV) exposure.

Gravida and para

Two important components of a patient's obstetric history are her gravida and para status. *Gravida* represents the number of times the patient has been pregnant. *Para* refers to the number of children above the age of viability the patient has delivered. The age of viability is the earliest time at which a fetus can survive outside the womb, generally at age 24 weeks or a weight of more than 400 g (14.1 oz). These two pieces of information are important but provide only the most rudimentary information about the patient's obstetric history.

Looking for a little more

A slightly more informative system reflects the gravida and para numbers and includes the number of abortions in the patient's history. For example, G-3, P-2, Ab-1 describes a patient who has been pregnant three times, has had two deliveries after 20 weeks' gestation, and has had one abortion.

TPAL, GTPAL, and GTPALM

In an attempt to provide more detailed information about the patient's obstetric history, many facilities now use one of the following classification systems: TPAL, GTPAL, or GTPALM. These systems involve the assignment of numbers to various aspects of a patient's obstetric past. They offer health care providers a way to

---

Pregnancy classification system

When referring to the obstetric and pregnancy history of a patient, keep these terms in mind:

• A *primigravida* is a woman who's pregnant for the first time.

• A *primipara* is a woman who has delivered one child past the age of viability.

• A *multigravida* is a woman who has been pregnant before but may not necessarily carry to term.

• A *multipara* is a woman who has carried two or more pregnancies to viability.

• A *nulligravida* is a woman who has never been and isn't currently pregnant.

Taking an obstetric history

When taking the pregnant patient's obstetric history, be sure to ask her about:
- genital tract anomalies
- medications used during this pregnancy
- history of hepatitis, pelvic inflammatory disease, acquired immunodeficiency syndrome, blood transfusions, and herpes or other sexually transmitted diseases (STDs)
- partner's history of STDs
- previous abortions
- history of infertility.

Pregnancy particulars

Also ask the patient about past pregnancies. Be sure to note the number of past full-term and preterm pregnancies and obtain the following information about each of the patient's past pregnancies, if applicable:
- Was the pregnancy planned?
- Did any complications — such as spotting, swelling of the hands and feet, surgery, or falls — occur?
- Did the patient receive prenatal care? If so, when did she start?
- Did she take any medications? If so, what were they? How long did she take them? Why?
- What was the duration of the pregnancy?
- How was the pregnancy overall for the patient?

Birth and baby specifics

Also obtain the following information about the birth and postpartum condition of all previous pregnancies:
- What was the duration of labor?
- What type of birth was it?
- What type of anesthesia did the patient have, if any?
- Did the patient experience any complications during pregnancy or labor?
- What were the birthplace, condition, sex, weight, and Rh factor of the neonate?
- Was the labor as she had expected it? Better? Worse?
- Did she have stitches after birth?
- What was the condition of the infant after birth?
- What was the infant's Apgar score?
- Was special care needed for the infant? If so, what?
- Did the neonate experience any problems during the first several days after birth?
- What's the child's present state of health?
- Was the infant discharged from the heath care facility with the mother?
- Did the patient experience any postpartum problems?

quickly obtain fairly comprehensive information about a patient's obstetric history. In particular, these systems offer more detailed information about the patient's para history.

How often, how many, how viable

In TPAL, the most basic of the three systems, the patient is assigned a four-digit number as follows:
- T is the number of full-term infants born (those born at 37 weeks or later).
- P is the number of preterm infants born (those born before 37 weeks).

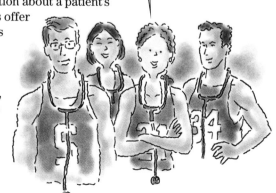

The TPAL, GTPAL, and GTPALM systems are easy ways to share with other members of the health care team information about the patient's obstetric history.

- A is the number of spontaneous or induced abortions.
- L is the number of living children.

Note that the patient's gravida number remains the same, but the TPAL systems allow subclassification of the patient's para status. In most cases, a practitioner includes the patient's gravida status in addition to her TPAL number. Here are some examples:

- A woman who has had two previous pregnancies, has delivered two term children, and is pregnant again, is a gravida 3 and is assigned a TPAL of 2-0-0-2.
- A woman who has had two abortions at 12 weeks (under the age of viability) and is pregnant again is a gravida 3 and is assigned a TPAL of 0-0-2-0.
- A woman who is pregnant for the sixth time, has delivered four term children and one preterm child, and has had one spontaneous abortion and one elective abortion, is a gravida 6 and is assigned a TPAL of 4-1-2-5.

More details, details, details

More comprehensive systems for classifying pregnancy status include the GTPAL and GTPALM systems. In the GTPAL system, the patient's gravida status is incorporated into her TPAL number. In GTPALM, a number is added to the GTPAL to represent the number of multiple pregnancies the patient has experienced (M). Note that a patient who hasn't given birth to multiple pregnancies doesn't receive a number to represent M. These classification tools provide greater detail about the patient's pregnancy history.

Here are some examples:
- If a woman has had two previous pregnancies, has delivered two term children, and is currently pregnant, she's assigned a GTPAL of 3-2-0-0-2.
- If a woman who's pregnant with twins delivers at 35 weeks' gestation and the neonates survive, she's classified as a gravida 1, para 0202 and assigned a GTPAL of 1-0-2-0-2. Using the GTPALM system, the same woman would be identified as 1-0-2-0-2-1.

Preventing history from repeating itself

If the patient is a multigravida, you'll want to know about complications that affected her previous pregnancies. A woman who has delivered one or more large neonates (more than 9 lb [4.1 g]) or who has a history of recurrent *Candida* infections or unexplained unsuccessful pregnancies should be screened for obesity and a family history of diabetes. A history of recurrent second-trimester abortions may indicate an incompetent cervix.

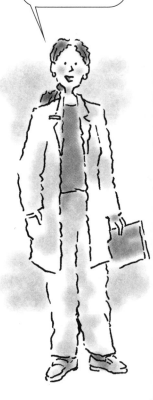

If this isn't your patient's first pregnancy, be sure to ask about previous complications.

Physical assessment

Physical assessment should occur throughout pregnancy, starting with the mother's first prenatal visit and continuing through labor, delivery, and the postpartum period. Physical assessment includes evaluation of maternal and fetal well-being. At each assessment stage, keep in mind the interdependence of the mother and fetus. Changes in the mother's health may affect fetal health, and changes in fetal health may affect the mother's physical and emotional health.

Rounding the baselines

At the first prenatal visit, measurements of height and weight establish baselines for the patient and allow comparison with expected values throughout the pregnancy. Vital signs, including blood pressure, respiratory rate, and pulse rate, are also measured for baseline assessment. (See *Monitoring vital signs.*)

Scheduled surveillance

Prenatal care visits are usually scheduled every 4 weeks for the first 28 weeks of pregnancy, every 2 weeks until the 36th week, and then weekly until delivery, which usually occurs between weeks 38 and 42. Women who have known risk factors for complications and those who develop complications during the pregnancy require more frequent visits.

And now back to our regularly scheduled visit

Regular prenatal visits usually consist of weight measurements, vital signs check, palpation of the abdomen, and fundal height checks. You should also assess the patient for preterm labor symptoms, fetal heart tones, and edema. Also, be sure to ask her

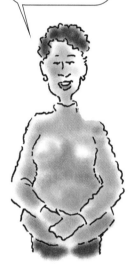

We're in this together! Changes in my health affect my baby and changes in my baby's health affect me.

Advice from the experts

Monitoring vital signs

Monitoring the patient's vital signs, especially blood pressure, during each prenatal visit is an important part of ongoing assessment. A sudden increase in blood pressure is a danger sign of gestational hypertension or pregnancy-induced hypertension. Likewise, a sudden increase in pulse or respiratory rate may suggest bleeding, such as in an early placenta previa or an abruption.

Be sure to report any of these signs or alterations in the patient's vital signs to the health care practitioner for further assessment and evaluation.

if she has felt her baby move. (See *Assessing pregnancy by trimester.*)

Getting started

At the start of a prenatal visit, the woman should undress, put on a gown, and empty her bladder. Emptying the bladder makes the pelvic examination more comfortable for her, allows for easier identification of pelvic organs, and provides a urine specimen for laboratory testing.

Head-to-toe assessment

A thorough physical assessment should include inspection of the patient's general appearance, head and scalp, eyes, nose, ears, mouth, neck, breasts, heart, lungs, back, rectum, extremities, and skin.

General appearance

Inspect the patient's general appearance. This helps form an impression of the woman's overall health and well-being. The manner in which a patient dresses and speaks, in addition to her body posture, can reveal how she feels about herself. Also inspect for signs of spousal abuse. Be sure to document your findings.

Head and scalp

Examine the head and scalp for symmetry, normal contour, and tenderness. Check the hair for distribution, thickness, dryness or oiliness, and use of hair dye. Look for chloasma, an extra pigment on the face that may accompany pregnancy. Dryness or sparseness of hair suggests poor nutrition. Lack of cleanliness suggests fatigue.

Eyes

Be sure to perform a careful inspection of the eyes. Look for edema in the eyelids. Ask the patient if she ever sees spots before her eyes or has diplopia (double vision) or other vision problems. (See *Watching for vision changes*, page 162.) These assessment findings may indicate PIH. In addition, an ophthalmoscopic examination may reveal that the optic disk appears swollen from edema associated with PIH.

Nose

Inspect the nose for nasal congestion and nasal membrane swelling, which may result from increased estrogen levels. If these conditions occur, advise the patient to avoid using topical medicines and nose

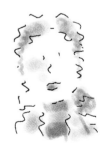

Oh no! Double vision may indicate pregnancy-induced hypertension.

Assessing pregnancy by trimester

Here are some assessment findings you can expect as pregnancy progresses.

Weeks 1 to 4
- Amenorrhea occurs.
- Breasts begin to change.
- Immunologic pregnancy tests become positive: Radioimmunoassay test results are positive a few days after implantation; urine human chorionic gonadotropin test results are positive 10 to 14 days after amenorrhea occurs.
- Nausea and vomiting begin between the 4th and 6th weeks.

Weeks 5 to 8
- Goodell's sign occurs (softening of cervix and vagina).
- Ladin's sign occurs (softening of uterine isthmus).
- Hegar's sign occurs (softening of lower uterine segment).
- Chadwick's sign appears (purple-blue coloration of the vagina, cervix, and vulva).
- McDonald's sign appears (easy flexion of the fundus toward the cervix).
- Braun von Fernwald's sign occurs (irregular softening and enlargement of the uterine fundus at the site of implantation).
- Piskacek's sign may occur (asymmetrical softening and enlargement of the uterus).
- The cervical mucus plug forms.
- Uterus changes from pear shape to globular.
- Urinary frequency and urgency occur.

Weeks 9 to 12
- Fetal heartbeat detected using ultrasonic stethoscope.
- Nausea, vomiting, and urinary frequency and urgency lessen.
- By the 12th week, the uterus is palpable just above the symphysis pubis.

Weeks 13 to 17
- Mother gains 10 to 12 lb (4.5 to 5.5 kg) during the second trimester.
- Uterine soufflé is heard on auscultation.
- Mother's heartbeat increases by about 10 beats/minute between 14 and 30 weeks' gestation. Rate is maintained until 40 weeks' gestation.
- By the 16th week, the mother's thyroid gland enlarges by about 25%, and the uterine fundus is palpable halfway between the symphysis pubis and the umbilicus.
- Maternal recognition of fetal movements, or quickening, occurs between 16 and 20 weeks' gestation.

Weeks 18 to 22
- Uterine fundus is palpable just below the umbilicus.
- Fetal heartbeats are heard with fetoscope at 20 weeks' gestation.
- Fetal rebound or ballottement is possible.

Weeks 23 to 27
- Umbilicus appears to be level with abdominal skin.
- Striae gravidarum are usually apparent.

- Uterine fundus is palpable at the umbilicus.
- Shape of uterus changes from globular to ovoid.
- Braxton Hicks contractions start.

Weeks 28 to 31
- Mother gains 8 to 10 lb (3.5 to 4.5 kg) in third trimester.
- The uterine wall feels soft and yielding.
- The uterine fundus is halfway between the umbilicus and xiphoid process.
- Fetal outline is palpable.
- The fetus is mobile and may be found in any position.

Weeks 32 to 35
- The mother may experience heartburn.
- Striae gravidarum become more evident.
- The uterine fundus is palpable just below the xiphoid process.
- Braxton Hicks contractions increase in frequency and intensity.
- The mother may experience shortness of breath.

Weeks 36 to 40
- The umbilicus protrudes.
- Varicosities, if present, become very pronounced.
- Ankle edema is evident.
- Urinary frequency recurs.
- Engagement, or lightening, occurs.
- The mucus plug is expelled.
- Cervical effacement and dilation begin.

Education edge

Watching for vision changes

Poor vision can be a danger sign of pregnancy, possibly indicating pregnancy-induced hypertension. Instruct the pregnant woman to keep an eye out for symptoms of poor vision, such as spots in the eyes or double vision, and to report them as soon as possible. If she does close desk work on a regular basis, such as computer work or work with small numbers and lists or charts that require tedious and close attention, advise her to take a break every hour so that work-related eye-strain isn't confused with actual danger signs.

sprays for relief without her health care provider's consent. These medications can be absorbed into the bloodstream and may harm the fetus.

Ears

During early pregnancy, nasal stuffiness may lead to blocked eustachian tubes, which can cause a feeling of "fullness" and dampening of sound. This disappears as the body adjusts to the new estrogen level.

Mouth

Examine the inside and outside of the mouth. Cracked corners may reveal a vitamin A deficiency. Pinpoint lesions with an erythematous base on the lips suggest herpes infection. Gingival (gum) hypertrophy may result from estrogen stimulation during pregnancy; the gums may be slightly swollen and tender to the touch. (See *Taking care of the teeth.*)

Neck

Slight thyroid hypertrophy may occur during pregnancy because overall metabolic rate is increased. Lymph nodes normally aren't palpable and, if enlarged, may indicate an infection.

Breasts

During pregnancy, the areola may darken, breast size increases, and breasts become firmer. Blue streaking of veins may occur on the breasts. Colostrum may be expressed as early as 16 weeks' gestation. Montgomery's tubercles may become more prominent.

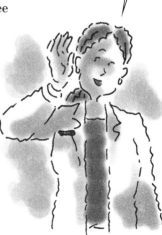

The patient's hearing may be affected early in pregnancy because of blocked eustachian tubes.

Education edge

Taking care of the teeth

Advise the patient that dental hygiene and taking care of dental caries are important during pregnancy. Dental X-rays can be taken during pregnancy as long as the woman reminds her dentist that she's pregnant and needs a lead apron. Extensive dental work requiring anesthesia shouldn't be done during pregnancy without approval from the woman's primary health care provider.

BSE basics

Instruct the patient on how to perform a breast self-examination (BSE), and tell her to perform a BSE monthly. Educate her also on the ongoing changes she'll experience during pregnancy, as appropriate.

Heart

Assess the patient's heart. Heart rate should range from 70 to 80 beats/minute. Occasionally, a benign functional heart murmur that's caused by increased vascular volume may be auscultated. If this occurs, the patient needs further evaluation to ensure that the condition is only a physiologic change related to the pregnancy and not a previously undetected heart condition.

Lungs

Assess respiratory rate and rhythm. Vital capacity (the amount of air that can be exhaled after maximum inspiration) shouldn't be reduced despite the fact that lung tissue assumes a more horizontal appearance as the growing uterus pushes up on the diaphragm. Late in pregnancy, diaphragmatic excursion (diaphragm movement) is reduced because the diaphragm can't descend as fully as usual because of the distended uterus.

Back

When examining the patient's back, be sure to assess for scoliosis. If she has scoliosis, refer her to an orthopedic surgeon to make sure the condition doesn't worsen during pregnancy. Typically, the lumbar curve is accentuated when standing so the patient can maintain body posture in the face of increasing abdominal size. If she has scoliosis, however, the added pressure of the growing fetus on the back may be more bothersome and painful.

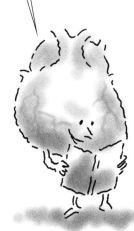

A pregnant patient's heart rate should range from 70 to 80 beats per minute. I can handle that!

Rectum

Assess the rectum for hemorrhoidal tissue, which commonly results from pelvic pressure that prevents venous return.

Extremities and skin

Assess for palmar erythema, an itchy redness in the palms that occurs early in pregnancy as a result of high estrogen levels. Assess for varicose veins and check the filling time of nailbeds. Observe for edema, and assess the patient's gait. The patient should be taught proper posture and walking to prevent musculoskeletal and gait problems later in pregnancy.

Pelvic examination

A pelvic examination provides information on the health of internal and external reproductive organs and is valuable in assessment.

Patient prep

Take the following steps to prepare the patient for the pelvic examination:
• Ask the patient if she has douched within the past 24 hours. Explain that douching can wash away cells and organisms that the examination is designed to evaluate.
• For the patient's comfort, instruct her to empty her bladder before the examination. Provide a urine specimen container, if needed.
• To help the patient relax, which is essential for a thorough pelvic examination, explain what the examination entails and why it's necessary. The patient may desire to have a person in the room with her for support. It may also be beneficial to review some relaxation techniques with the patient such as deep breathing.
• If the patient is scheduled for a Papanicolaou (Pap) test, inform her that she may have to return later for another test if the findings of the first test aren't conclusive. Reassure her that this is done to confirm the results of the first test. If she has never had a Pap test, tell her that the test shouldn't hurt.
• Explain to the patient that a bimanual examination is performed to assess the size and location of the ovaries and uterus.

Shall I compare thee?

During the examination, record the patient's uterine fundal height and fetal heart sounds. Compare the new fundal height findings with the information obtained in the patient's history. In other words, make sure that the information you obtained about the patient's last menstrual period and her estimated date of delivery correlate with the current fundal height.

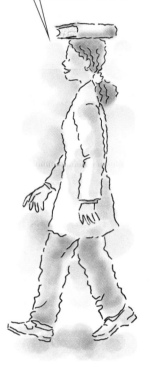

The patient should be taught proper posture and walking to prevent musculoskeletal and gait problems later in pregnancy.

On the move

At about 12 to 14 weeks' gestation, the uterus is palpable over the symphysis pubis as a firm globular sphere. It reaches the umbilicus at 20 to 22 weeks, the xiphoid at 36 weeks, and then, in many cases, returns to about 4 cm below the xiphoid due to lightening at 40 weeks. (See *Measuring fundal height.*)

If the woman is past 12 weeks of pregnancy, palpate fundus location, measure fundal height (from the notch above the symphysis pubis to the superior aspect of the uterine fundus), and plot the height on a graph. This information helps detect variations in fetal growth. If an abnormality is detected, further investigation with ultrasound can be made to determine the cause.

> Checking fundal location and measuring fundal height throughout pregnancy help to detect variations in fetal growth.

Measuring fundal height

Measuring the height of the uterus above the symphysis pubis reflects the progress of fetal growth, provides a gross estimate of the duration of pregnancy, and may indicate intrauterine growth retardation. Excessive increase in fundal height could mean multiple pregnancy or hydramnios (an excess of amniotic fluid).

To measure fundal height, use a pliable (not stretchable) tape measure or pelvimeter to measure from the notch of the symphysis pubis to the top of the fundus, without tipping back the corpus. During the second and third trimesters, make the measurement more precise by using the following calculation, known as McDonald's rule:

$$\text{height of fundus (in centimeters)} \times \tfrac{8}{7}$$
$$= \text{duration of pregnancy in weeks.}$$

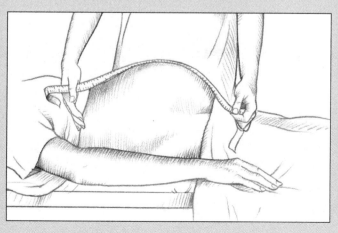

Pelvic shape and potential problems

The shape of a woman's pelvis can affect the delivery of her fetus. Her pelvis may be one of four types.

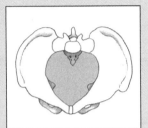 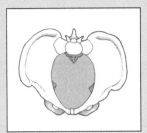 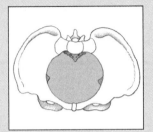 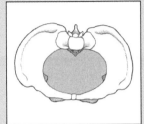

Android pelvis

In an *android* pelvis, the pelvic arch forms an acute triangle, making the lower dimensions of the pelvis extremely narrow. A pelvis of this shape is typically associated with males, but can also occur in women. A pregnant woman with this pelvic shape may experience difficulty delivering the fetus because the narrow shape makes it difficult for the fetus to exit.

Anthropoid pelvis

In an *anthropoid* pelvis, also known as an *apelike pelvis,* the transverse diameter is narrow and the anteroposterior diameter of the inlet is larger than normal. This pelvic shape doesn't accommodate a fetal head as well as a gynecoid pelvis because the transverse diameter is narrow.

Gynecoid pelvis

In a *gynecoid* pelvis, the inlets are well-rounded in both the forward and backward diameters and the pubic arch is wide. This type of pelvis is ideal for childbirth.

Platypelloid pelvis

In a *platypelloid,* or flattened, pelvis, the inlet is oval and smoothly curved but the anteroposterior diameter is shallow. Problems may occur during childbirth for a patient with this pelvic shape if the fetal head is unable to rotate to match the curves of the spine because the anteroposterior diameter is shallow and the pelvis is flat.

After the examination, offer the patient premoistened tissues to clean the vulva.

Estimation of pelvic size

The size and shape of woman's pelvis can affect her ability to deliver her neonate vaginally. It's impossible to predict from a woman's outward appearance if her pelvis is adequate for the passage of a fetus. For example, a woman may look as if she has a wide pelvis, but she may only have a wide iliac crest and a normal, or smaller than normal, internal ring. (See *Pelvic shape and potential problems.*)

Clearly clearance counts

Internal pelvic measurements give actual diameters of the inlet and outlet through which the fetus passes. The internal pelvis must be large enough to allow a patient to give birth vaginally without difficulty. Differences in pelvic contour develop mainly because of heredity factors. However, such diseases as rickets may cause contraction of the pelvis, and pelvic injury may also be responsible for pelvic distortion.

Now or later?

Pelvic measurements can be taken at the initial visit or at a visit later in pregnancy, when the woman's pelvic muscles are more relaxed. If a routine ultrasound is scheduled, estimations of pelvic size may be made through a combination of pelvimetry and fetal ultrasound.

Estimation of pelvic adequacy should be done by the 24th week of pregnancy because, by this time, a danger exists that the fetal head will reach a size that interferes with safe passage and birth if the pelvic measurements are small. In this case, the woman should be advised that she may not be able to deliver her fetus vaginally and may require a cesarean birth. If a woman has already given birth vaginally, her pelvis has proven to be adequate. You don't need to remeasure her pelvis unless trauma occurred to the pelvis after her last vaginal birth.

Diagonal conjugate

The diagonal conjugate is the distance between the anterior surface of the sacral prominence and the anterior surface of the inferior margin of the symphysis pubis. It's the most useful gauge of pelvic size because it indicates the anteroposterior diameter of the pelvic inlet (the narrower diameter). (See *Diagonal conjugate measurement,* page 168.)

Ample room

If the measurement obtained is more than 5″ (12.5 cm), the pelvic inlet is considered adequate for childbirth (the diameter of the fetal head that must pass that point averages 3½″ [9 cm]).

True conjugate

The true conjugate, also known as the *conjugate vera,* is the measurement between the anterior surface of the sacral prominence and the posterior surface of the inferior margin of the symphysis pubis. This measurement can't be made directly but is estimated from the measurement of the diagonal conjugate.

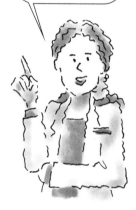

If a woman has previously given birth vaginally, then she's already passed the real test! It isn't necessary to take her pelvic measurements again.

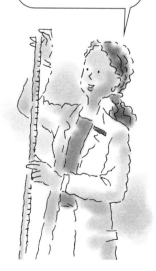

If the diagonal conjugate is more than 5″, the pelvic inlet is big enough for the fetal head to pass through.

Diagonal conjugate measurement

The diagonal conjugate is measured while the woman is in the lithotomy position. Two fingers of the examining hand are placed in the vagina and pressed inward and upward until the middle finger touches the sacral prominence. (The woman may feel the pressure of the examining finger.) The location where the examining hand touches the symphysis pubis is marked by the other hand. After withdrawing the examining hand, the distance between the tip of the middle finger and the marked point is measured with a ruler or a pelvimeter.

If the examining hand is small with short fingers, the fingers may not reach the sacral prominence, making manual pelvic measurements impossible.

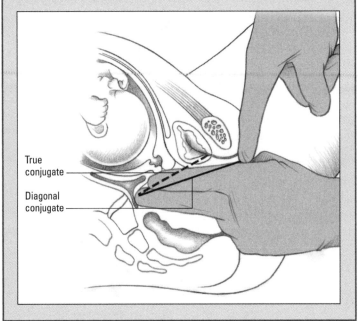

True conjugate

Diagonal conjugate

Tried and true

Here's how it's done:

✍ The usual depth of the symphysis pubis (½″ to ¾″ [1 to 2 cm]) is subtracted from the diagonal conjugate measurement.

✌ The distance remaining is the true conjugate, or the actual diameter of the pelvic inlet through which the fetal head must pass. The average true conjugate diameter is 4″ to 4¼″ (10 to 11 cm).

Ischial tuberosity

The ischial tuberosity is the transverse diameter of the pelvic outlet. This measurement is made at the medial and lowermost aspect of the ischial tuberosities, at the level of the anus. A pelvimeter is generally used to measure the diameter, although it can be measured using a ruler or by comparing it with a known handspan or clenched fist measurement. A diameter of 4¼″ is considered adequate for passage of the fetal head through the outlet.

Prenatal testing

Assess the fetus prenatally by using direct and indirect monitoring techniques. Common tests include fetal heart rate (FHR) monitoring, ultrasonography, fetal activity determination, maternal urinalysis and serum assays, amniocentesis, chorionic villi sampling (CVS), percutaneous umbilical blood sampling (PUBS), fetoscopy, blood studies, prepartum nonstress test (NST), prepartum contraction stress test (CST), and nipple stimulation CST.

Fetal heart rate

You can obtain a FHR by placing a fetoscope or Doppler stethoscope on the mother's abdomen and counting fetal heartbeats. Simultaneously palpating the mother's pulse helps you to avoid confusion between maternal and fetal heartbeats.

With every beat of the heart

A fetoscope can detect fetal heartbeats as early as 20 weeks' gestation. The Doppler ultrasound stethoscope, a more sensitive instrument, can detect fetal heartbeats as early as 10 weeks' gestation and remains a useful tool throughout labor.

To determine the FHR of a fetus who's less than 20 weeks old, place the head of the Doppler stethoscope at the midline of the patient's abdomen above the pubic hairline. After the 20th week of pregnancy, when fetal position can be determined, palpate for the back of the fetal thorax and position the instrument directly over it. Locate the loudest heartbeats and palpate the maternal pulse. Count fetal heartbeats for at least 15 seconds while monitoring maternal pulse. You can use Leopold's maneuvers to determine fetal position, presentation, and attitude. (See *Performing Leopold's maneuvers*, page 170.)

Because FHR usually ranges from 120 to 160 beats/minute, auscultation yields only an average rate at best. It can detect gross (but commonly late) signs of fetal distress, such as tachycardia

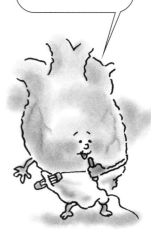

My beat may not be as loud as the beat of my mother's heart. Be sure to palpate the maternal pulse while you're listening for fetal heartbeats to avoid confusion.

Performing Leopold's maneuvers

You can determine fetal position, presentation, and attitude by performing Leopold's maneuvers. Ask the patient to empty her bladder, assist her to a supine position, and expose her abdomen. Then perform the following four maneuvers in order.

First maneuver
Face the patient and warm your hands. Place your hands on the patient's abdomen to determine fetal position in the uterine fundus. Curl your fingers around the fundus. When the fetus is in the vertex position (head first), the buttocks should feel irregularly shaped and firm. When the fetus is in breech position, the head should feel hard, round, and movable.

Second maneuver
Move your hands down the side of the abdomen, applying gentle pressure. If the fetus is in the vertex position, you'll feel a smooth, hard surface on one side—the fetal back. Opposite, you'll feel lumps and knobs—the knees, hands, feet, and elbows. If the fetus is in the breech position, you may not feel the back at all.

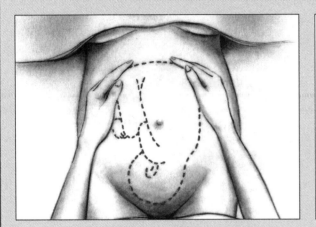

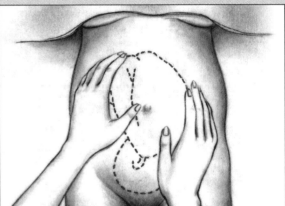

and bradycardia, and is thus recommended only for a patient with an uncomplicated pregnancy. For a patient with a high-risk pregnancy, indirect or direct electronic fetal monitoring provides more accurate information on fetal status. (See *Evaluating FHR*, page 172.)

Ultrasonography

Through the use of sound waves bouncing off of internal structures, ultrasound allows visualization of the fetus without the hazards of X-rays. Ultrasound allows the patient to see her baby and

Third maneuver

Spread apart your thumb and fingers of one hand. Place them just above the patient's symphysis pubis. Bring your fingers together. If the fetus is in the vertex position and hasn't descended, you'll feel the head. If the fetus is in the vertex position and has descended, you'll feel a less distinct mass. If the fetus is in the breech position, you'll also feel a less distinct mass, which could be the feet or knees.

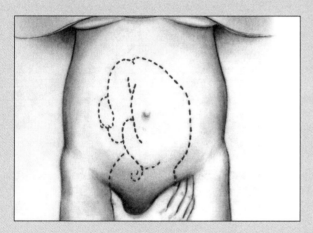

Fourth maneuver

The fourth maneuver can determine flexion or extension of the fetal head and neck. Place your hands on both sides of the lower abdomen. Apply gentle pressure with your fingers as you slide your hands downward, toward the symphysis pubis. If the head is the presenting fetal part (rather than the feet or a shoulder), one of your hands is stopped by the cephalic prominence. The other hand descends unobstructed more deeply. If the fetus is in the vertex position, you'll feel the cephalic prominence on the same side as the small parts; if it's in the face position, on the same side as the back. If the fetus is engaged, you won't be able to feel the cephalic prominence.

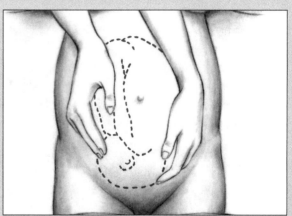

even produces an image (called a *sonogram*) that she can show to friends and family.

How ultra-useful!

Ultrasonography is used to:
- verify the due date and correlate it with the fetus's size
- determine the condition of the fetus when there's a greater than average risk of an abnormality or a greater than average concern
- rule out pregnancy by the seventh week if there has been a suspected false-positive pregnancy test
- determine the cause of bleeding or spotting in early pregnancy
- locate an IUD that was in place at the time of conception

Evaluating FHR

To evaluate fetal heart rate (FHR), position the fetoscope or Doppler ultrasound stethoscope on the patient's abdomen, midway between the umbilicus and symphysis pubis for cephalic presentation, or above or at the level of the umbilicus for breech presentation. Locate the loudest heartbeats, and palpate the maternal pulse. Monitor maternal pulse and count fetal heartbeats for 60 seconds. Notify the health care provider immediately of marked changes in FHR from the baseline.

Fetoscope

A fetoscope is a modified stethoscope attached to a headpiece. A fetoscope can detect fetal heartbeats as early as 20 weeks' gestation.

Doppler stethoscope

A Doppler stethoscope uses ultrasound waves that bounce off the fetal heart to produce echoes or a clicking noise that reflect the rate of the fetal heartbeat. The Doppler stethoscope can detect fetal heartbeats as early as 10 weeks' gestation. The Doppler stethoscope has greater sensitivity than the fetoscope.

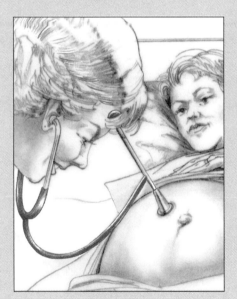

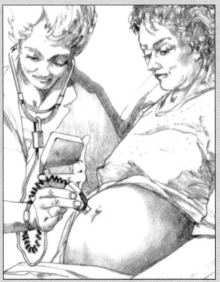

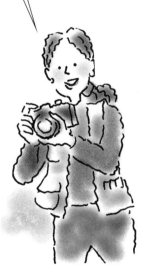

Proud parents like to show off pictures of their baby as soon as possible. A sonogram may be the earliest picture in their collection.

- locate the fetus before amniocentesis and during CVS
- determine the condition of the fetus if no heartbeat has been detected by the 14th week with a Doppler device or if no fetal movement has occurred by the 22nd week
- diagnose the existence of multiple pregnancy, especially if the patient has taken fertility drugs or the uterus is larger than it should be for the expected due date

- determine if abnormally rapid uterine growth is being caused by excessive amniotic fluid
- determine the condition of the placenta when deterioration might be responsible for fetal growth retardation or distress
- evaluate the condition of the fetus through observation of fetal activity, breathing movements, and amniotic fluid volume
- verify presentation and uncommon fetal or cord position before delivery.

Screen debut

Here's how it's usually done. An ultrasonic transducer that's placed on the mother's abdomen transmits high-frequency sound waves through the abdominal wall. These sound waves deflect off the fetus, bounce back to the transducer, and are transformed into a visual image on a monitoring screen.

Filling up with fluid

To prepare a patient for an abdominal ultrasound, have her drink 1 qt (1 L) of fluid 1 to 2 hours before the test. Instruct her not to void before the test because a full bladder serves as a landmark to define other pelvic organs.

A bladder-friendly version

Transvaginal ultrasonography is another type of imaging. It's well tolerated because it eliminates the need for a full bladder and is usually used during the first trimester of pregnancy.

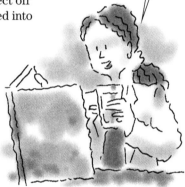

To prepare a patient for an abdominal ultrasound, have her drink 1 qt of fluid approximately 2 hours before the test.

Fetal activity determination

The activity of the fetus (kick counts) determines its condition in utero. Daily evaluation of movement provides an inexpensive, noninvasive way of assessing fetal well-being. Decreased activity in a previously active fetus may reflect a disturbance in placental function.

As early as 7 weeks' gestation, the embryo can produce spontaneous movements; however, these movements don't become apparent to the mother until sometime between the 14th and 26th weeks (but generally between weeks 18 and 22). The first noticeable movement of the fetus by the mother is called *quickening*. The acknowledgment of fetal movements may be delayed if the due date is miscalculated or if the mother doesn't recognize the sensation. A patient who has had a baby before is likely to recognize movement earlier. If the mother hasn't felt any movements by the 22nd week, an ultrasound may be ordered to assess the fetus's condition.

Looking for some fetal action

Fetal movements may be elicited by having the patient lie down for about an hour after having a glass of milk or another snack. The jolt of energy produced by a light snack commonly produces fetal movement. After the 28th week, patients are usually asked to monitor fetal movements twice daily — once in the morning, when activity tends to be sparser, and once in the more-active evening hours. Instruct the patient to check the clock when she's ready to start counting fetal movements. She should count movements of any kind (kicks, flutters, swishes, rolls). After she counts ten movements, she should note the time again.

If the patient doesn't feel 10 movements after 30 minutes, she should eat another snack and then count for another 30 minutes. If the patient feels no movement or less than 10 movements after the second 30-minute period, she should contact her health care provider. The closer the patient is to her due date, the more important regular checking of fetal movements becomes. (See *Monitoring for fetal distress*.)

Maternal urinalysis

During pregnancy, the patient is monitored routinely for potential problems. Some problems may be detected by a simple urine test. The urine specimen should be obtained from the patient during her regularly scheduled visit using a clean-catch technique. The specimen is examined for bacteriuria as well as protein, glucose, and ketones. Urinalysis can detect such problems as infection or diabetes before the patient shows any signs.

Maternal serum assays

Serum assays — including estrogens, human placental lactogen (hPL), and human chorionic gonadotropin (hCG) — are used in addition to urinalysis to monitor the pregnant patient for problems.

Estrogens

Three major estrogens exist: estrone, estradiol, and estriol. Production of estrogens, particularly estriol, increases during pregnancy. During pregnancy, levels of estrone and estradiol increase to about 100 times nonpregnancy levels, whereas estriol levels increase 1,000 times. Estrogen production depends on the interaction of the maternal fetal-placental unit. Estriol is secreted by the placenta into the maternal circulation and eventually excreted in maternal urine.

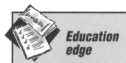

Education edge

Monitoring for fetal distress

If the patient is performing fetal activity determination, make sure that she rests during the counting period. If she's active, such as walking around or otherwise physically moving, she may not feel the movements as much as if she were at rest. If 2 hours go by without ten movements, she should promptly contact her health care provider. Absence of fetal activity doesn't necessarily mean there's a problem but, in some cases, it indicates fetal distress. Immediate action may be needed.

The old estriol test just ain't what it used to be

In the past, a mother's urinary estriol levels were measured regularly to assess fetal and placental well-being. Today, however, estriol levels are measured only as part of the triple screen test. (For more information, see the section on the triple screen test later in this chapter.)

Salivary signs of premature labor

The SalEst test is a salivary test that measures estriol levels. For women at risk, the test is 98% accurate in ruling out premature labor and delivery. The test is performed between 22 and 36 weeks' gestation. Estriol has been found to increase 2 to 3 weeks before the spontaneous onset of labor and delivery. A positive test indicates that the patient is at risk for premature labor. With this knowledge, precautions can be taken to decrease the risk of preterm labor and maintain fetal viability.

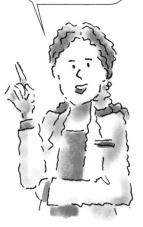

A positive SalEst test indicates that a patient is at risk for premature labor.

Human placental lactogen

Also known as *human chorionic somatomammotropin*, hPL works with prolactin to prepare the breasts for lactation. It also indirectly provides energy for maternal metabolism and fetal nutrition. It facilitates the protein synthesis and mobilization that are essential for fetal growth.

Secretion of hPL is autonomous, beginning around 5 weeks' gestation and declining rapidly after delivery. According to some evidence, however, this hormone may not be essential for a successful pregnancy.

The purpose of hPL testing is to:
• assess placental function and fetal well-being (combined with measurement of estriol levels)
• aid diagnosis of hydatidiform moles and choriocarcinoma
• aid diagnosis and monitor treatment of nontrophoblastic tumors that ectopically secrete hPL.

Serial evaluation

A radioimmunoassay measures plasma hPL levels. The test may be required in high-risk pregnancies, such as those involving diabetes mellitus, hypertension, or suspected placental tissue dysfunction. Because values vary widely during the latter half of pregnancy, serial determinations over several days provide the most reliable test results.

For pregnant women, normal hPL levels slowly increase throughout pregnancy, reaching 7 mg/ml at term. Low hPL concentrations are also characteristically associated with postmaturity syndrome, intrauterine growth retardation, preeclampsia, and eclampsia. However, low hPL concentrations don't confirm fetal distress. Conversely, concentrations over 4 mg/ml after 30 weeks' gestation don't guarantee fetal well-being because elevated levels have been reported after fetal death. An hPL value above 6 mg/ml after 30 weeks' gestation may suggest an unusually large placenta, common in patients with diabetes mellitus, multiple pregnancy, and Rh isoimmunization.

Human chorionic gonadotropin

Although the precise function of hCG (a glycoprotein hormone produced in the placenta) is still unclear, it appears that hCG and progesterone maintain the corpus luteum during early pregnancy. Production of hCG increases steadily during the first trimester, peaking around 10 weeks' gestation. Levels then fall to less than 10% of first-trimester peak levels during the remainder of the pregnancy. About 2 weeks after delivery, the hormone may no longer be detectable.

The serum test for hCG, which is more sensitive (and costlier) than the routine pregnancy test using a urine sample, provides a quantitative analysis. It's used to:
• detect pregnancy
• determine adequacy of hormonal production in high-risk pregnancies
• aid diagnosis of trophoblastic tumors, such as hydatidiform moles and choriocarcinoma
• detect tumors that ectopically secrete hCG
• monitor treatment for induction of ovulation and conception.

Leveling with you

Normal hCG levels are less than 4 IU/L. During pregnancy, hCG levels vary widely, depending partly on the number of days after the last normal menses. Elevated hCG levels indicate pregnancy; significantly higher concentrations are present in a multiple pregnancy. Low hCG levels can occur in ectopic pregnancy or pregnancy of less than 9 days. Unfortunately, hCG levels can't differentiate between pregnancy and tumor recurrence because levels are high in both conditions.

Down and out

In addition, researchers have found that a high level of hCG in a pregnant woman's blood means she's at greater risk for having a baby with Down syndrome. If conception occurs, a specific assay for hCG, commonly called the *beta-subunit assay*, may detect this hormone in the blood as soon as 9 days after ovulation. This interval coincides with the implantation of the

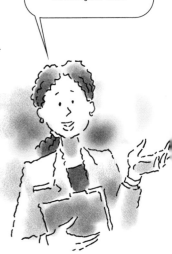

A high level of hCG in a pregnant woman's blood means she's at greater risk for having a baby with Down syndrome.

fertilized ovum into the uterine wall. If hCG levels are indicative of Down syndrome, amniocentesis is used to confirm.

Amniocentesis

Amniocentesis is the sterile needle aspiration of fluid from the amniotic sac for analysis. This procedure is recommended when:
• the mother is older than age 35
• the couple has already had a child with a chromosomal abnormality (such as Down syndrome) or a metabolic disorder (such as Hunter's syndrome)
• the mother is a carrier of an X-linked genetic disorder, such as hemophilia, in which she has a 50% chance of passing the gene on to a son
• a parent is known to have a condition, such as Huntington's chorea, that's passed on by autosomal dominant inheritance, giving the baby a 1 in 2 chance of inheriting the disease
• both parents are carriers of an autosomal recessive inherited disorder, such as Tay-Sachs disease or sickle-cell anemia, and thus have a 1 in 4 chance of bearing an affected child
• results of triple screening tests and ultrasound are abnormal and amniotic fluid evaluation is necessary to determine whether there's a fetal abnormality.

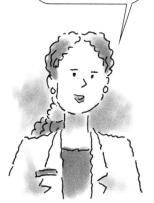

Amniocentesis is recommended to confirm a fetal abnormality when other screening tests detect a possible problem.

Oh, the uses you'll find

Amniocentesis is valuable because it can be used to:
• detect fetal abnormalities, particularly chromosomal and neural tube defects
• detect hemolytic disease of the fetus
• diagnose metabolic disorders, amino acid disorders, and mucopolysaccharidosis
• assess fetal lung maturity (the lungs are the last organs ready to function on their own)
• determine fetal age and maturity, especially fetal lung maturity
• detect the presence of meconium or blood
• measure amniotic levels of estriol and fetal thyroid hormone
• identify fetal gender.

Diagnostic second-trimester amniocentesis is usually performed between the 16th and 18th weeks of pregnancy, although it may be done as early as the 14th week or as late as the 20th week. Most tests require cells to be cultured in the laboratory and take from 24 to 35 days to complete. A few tests — such as those used to detect Tay-Sachs disease, Hunter's syndrome, and neural tube defects — can be performed immediately.

Aspiring toward aspirate

To begin, ask the patient to change into an examination gown and empty her bladder. Then explain that she'll be positioned on the examining table on her back and her body will be draped so that only her abdomen is exposed. During the test, FHR, maternal vital signs, and ultrasound are monitored. The doctor:
- prepares the skin with antiseptic and alcohol
- injects the skin with lidocaine to numb the area
- inserts a 20G spinal needle with a stylet into the amniotic cavity
- aspirates amniotic fluid and places it in an amber or foil-covered test tube (see *Proper handling of amniotic fluid*).

Generally speaking...

Complications of amniocentesis include spontaneous abortion, trauma to the fetus or placenta, bleeding, premature labor, infection, and Rh sensitization from fetal bleeding into the maternal circulation. Because of the potential severity of possible complications, amniocentesis is contraindicated as a general screening test.

Finding meaning in amnio findings

Abnormal test results or failure of the tissue cultures to grow may necessitate repetition of the test. (See *Amniotic fluid analysis findings.*)

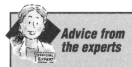

Advice from the experts

Proper handling of amniotic fluid

Aspirated amniotic fluid must be protected from light to prevent the breakdown of pigments such as bilirubin. Properly label all specimen containers or tubes. If the patient is Rh-negative, administer $Rh_0(D)$ immune globulin (RhoGAM), as ordered, to decrease the risk of iso-immunization from the procedure.

Chorionic villi sampling

Performed between 8 and 10 weeks' gestation, CVS involves aspirating chorionic villi from the placenta for prenatal diagnosis of genetic disorders. Chorionic villi are fingerlike projections that surround the embryonic membrane and eventually give rise to the placenta. Cells obtained from the sample are of fetal—rather than maternal—origin and thus can be analyzed for fetal abnormalities. Experts believe that villi in the chorion frondosum reflect fetal chromosome, enzyme, and deoxyribonucleic acid (DNA) content. (See *A close look at CVS*, page 180.)

Two sorts of samples

Either a transcervical or transabdominal approach can be used to obtain a CVS specimen. In transcervical sampling, a sterile catheter is introduced into the cervix using direct visualization with real-time ultrasonography. A small portion of chorionic villi is aspirated through the catheter into a syringe. In transabdominal sampling, the maternal abdomen is cleaned and an 18G to 20G needle is inserted into the chorion frondosum under ultrasound

Advice from the experts

Amniotic fluid analysis findings

Amniotic fluid analysis can provide important information about the condition of the mother, fetus, and placenta. This table shows normal findings and abnormal findings as well as their implications.

Test component	Normal findings	Fetal implications of abnormal findings
Color	Clear, with white flecks of vernix caseosa in a mature fetus	Blood of maternal origin is usually harmless. "Port wine" fluid may indicate abruptio placentae. Fetal blood may indicate damage to the fetal, placental, or umbilical cord vessels.
Bilirubin	Absent at term	High levels indicate hemolytic disease of the neonate in isoimmunized pregnancy.
Meconium	Absent (except in breech presentation)	Presence indicates fetal hypotension or distress.
Creatinine	More than 2 mg/dl in a mature fetus	Decrease may indicate immature fetus (less than 37 weeks).
Lecithin-sphingomyelin ratio	More than 2 generally indicates fetal pulmonary maturity	A ratio of less than 2 indicates pulmonary immaturity and subsequent respiratory distress syndrome.
Phosphatidylglycerol	Present	Absence indicates pulmonary immaturity.
Glucose	Less than 45 mg/dl	Excessive increases at term or near term indicate hypertrophied fetal pancreas and subsequent neonatal hypoglycemia.
Alpha-fetoprotein	Variable, depending on gestation age and laboratory technique; highest concentration (about 18.5 µg/ml) occurs at 13 to 14 weeks	Inappropriate increases indicate neural tube defects, such as spina bifida or anencephaly, impending fetal death, congenital nephrosis, or contamination of fetal blood.
Bacteria	Absent	Presence indicates chorioamnionitis.
Chromosome	Normal karyotype	Abnormal karyotype may indicate fetal sex and chromosome disorders.
Acetylcholinesterase	Absent	Presence may indicate neural tube defects, exomphalos, or other serious malformations.

A close look at CVS

Chorionic villi sampling (CVS) is a prenatal test for quick detection of fetal chromosomal and biochemical disorders that's performed during the first trimester of pregnancy. Preliminary results may be available within 1 hour; complete results, within a few days.

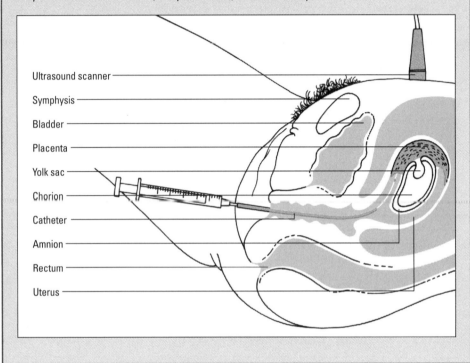

Ultrasound scanner
Symphysis
Bladder
Placenta
Yolk sac
Chorion
Catheter
Amnion
Rectum
Uterus

guidance. The specimen is then aspirated into a syringe. Aspirated villi are placed into a sterile medium for cytogenic analysis.

Painting a picture of the fetus

The cells from the villi normally have the same genetic and biochemical makeup as the embryo. Therefore, examining villi cells provides a complete picture of the genetic makeup of the developing fetus. CVS can detect fetal karyotype, hemoglobinopathies (such as sickle cell anemia, alpha-thalassemias, and some beta-thalassemias), phenylketonuria, alpha antitrypsin$_1$-deficiency, Down syndrome, Duchenne's muscular dystrophy, and factor IX deficiency. The test also identifies sex, allowing early detection of X-linked conditions in male fetuses.

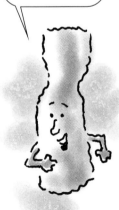

Chorionic villi sampling can provide genetic information about the fetus.

Complicated matters

Test complications include failure to obtain tissue, ruptured membranes or leakage of amniotic fluid, bleeding, intrauterine infection, spontaneous abortion, contamination of the specimen, and possible Rh isoimmunization. If the patient is Rh-negative, administer RhoGAM, as ordered, to cover the risk of Rh sensitization from the procedure. Also, recent research indicates an incidence of limb malformations in neonates whose mothers have undergone CVS. However, this incidence appears to be low when CVS is performed after 10 weeks' gestation.

Many women feel physically and emotionally drained after undergoing this procedure. Advise the patient to have someone drive her home. Tell her not to make other plans for the rest of the day. Instruct her to call her health care provider with any concerns or symptoms of complications, such as fever, vaginal discharge, vaginal bleeding, or cramping.

Percutaneous umbilical blood sampling

PUBS, which is used to obtain blood samples directly from the fetal circulation, is indicated for prenatal diagnosis of inherited blood disorders, detection of fetal infection, and assessment of the acid-base status of a fetus with intrauterine growth retardation. PUBS can be also used to administer blood products or drugs directly to the fetus. Allowing for treatment of the fetus in utero, PUBS reduces the risk of prematurity and mortality for a neonate with erythroblastosis fetalis (hemolytic disease of the newborn due to Rh incompatibility).

Point of origin

In PUBS, a fine needle is passed through the mother's abdomen and uterine wall into a vessel in the umbilical cord. Ultrasonography is used for guidance. The mobility of the cord complicates the procedure. Although the cord is more stable close to the placenta—allowing for a more accurate puncture—maternal intervillous blood lakes occupy this site, creating a risk of contamination with maternal blood. The Betke-Kleihauer procedure, which is used to detect fetal cells in maternal blood, is immediately performed on the blood sample obtained to ensure that it's fetal in origin.

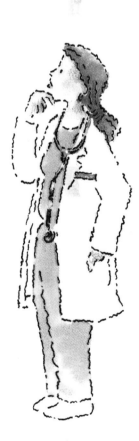

Direct access

Performed anytime after 16 weeks' gestation, PUBS can help diagnose fetal coagulopathies, hemoglobinopathies, hemophilias, and congenital infections. It also provides for rapid fetal karyotyping. Rather than analyzing amniotic fluid to detect abnormalities, PUBS directly assesses fetal blood. This is especially helpful in a patient who may have an isoimmunized pregnancy from Rh disease or another antibody sensitization.

Fetoscopy

Fetoscopy is a procedure in which a fetoscope—a telescope-like instrument with lights and lenses—is inserted into the amniotic sac, where it can view and photograph the fetus. This procedure makes it possible to diagnose, through blood and tissue sampling, several blood and skin diseases that amniocentesis can't detect. Fetoscopy is a relatively risky procedure and, because other safer techniques are becoming available to detect the same disorders, it isn't widely used.

Internal observation

Fetoscopy is typically performed at or after the 16th week of pregnancy. The patient's abdomen is swabbed with antiseptic solution and numbed with a local anesthetic. Tiny incisions are made in the abdomen and uterus. Using ultrasonography to guide the instrument, a fiber-optic endoscope is passed through the incisions and into the uterus. The fetus, placenta, and amniotic fluid are observed and blood samples are taken from the junction of the umbilical cord and the placenta. A small piece of fetal or placental tissue may also be removed for examination.

The procedure carries with it a 3% to 5% chance of fetal loss. Though this risk is greater than that of other diagnostic tests, it's outweighed for some women by the benefit of discovering—and possibly treating or correcting—a defect in the fetus.

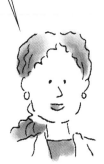

Fetoscopy isn't used much anymore because safer diagnostic techniques are available.

Blood studies

During pregnancy, blood studies are ordered to assess the mother's health, screen for maternal conditions that may endanger the fetus, detect genetic defects, and monitor fetal well-being. Initial studies include blood typing, a complete blood count (CBC) with differential, antibody screening tests, and a serologic test for syphilis and gonorrhea. Other tests may be performed to assess AFP levels, blood glucose, and other chemicals, if indicated.

Blood typing

Blood typing, including Rh factor, is performed to determine the patient's blood type and detect possible blood type incompatibilities. The patient's Rh status is also tested to determine if she's Rh-negative or Rh-positive.

Complete blood count

A CBC includes hemoglobin level, hematocrit, red blood cell (RBC) index, and platelet and white blood cell (WBC) counts. Hemoglobin level and hematocrit help to determine the presence of anemia. The RBC index helps to classify anemia, if present. Platelet count estimates clotting ability. An elevated WBC count may indicate an infection.

Antibody screening tests

The blood studies performed during pregnancy also include antibody screening tests for Rh compatibility (indirect Coombs' test), rubella, and hepatitis B. Antibodies for varicella (chickenpox) may also be assessed.

Indirect Coombs' test

The indirect Coombs' test screens maternal blood for RBC antibodies.

Sorry, but we don't get along

This test should be performed on a patient who's Rh negative because, if her fetus is Rh-positive and its blood mixes with the maternal blood during pregnancy or delivery, the woman's immune system produces antibodies against the fetus's RBCs. This antibody response is called *Rh sensitization*. Rh sensitization usually isn't a problem with the first Rh+ fetus. However, future Rh+ fetuses are in danger of having their RBCs destroyed by the mother's immune system. After sensitization has occurred, the fetus can develop mild to severe problems, such as Rh disease or hemolytic disease of the newborn.

If the patient doesn't show Rh sensitivity, the test is usually repeated at 28 weeks' gestation. If the titers aren't elevated, an Rh-negative woman would receive RhoGAM at this time and after any procedure that might cause placental bleeding (amniocentesis or CVS).

Rubella titer

A rubella (German measles) titer detects antibodies in maternal blood for the virus that causes rubella. If antibodies are found, the woman is immune to rubella. Most women have either had the virus as a child or have received a vaccination for rubella and, therefore, have antibodies in the blood.

Rubella exposure during pregnancy can lead to blindness, deafness, and heart defects in the fetus. If tests reveal that the patient isn't immune, she should avoid anyone who has the infection. She can't receive the vaccination while she's pregnant, but she should get the vaccine after she gives birth to protect future pregnancies.

Hepatitis B

Another antibody screening test, called the *hepatic antibody surface antigen* (HbsAg) test, is used to determine if a patient has hepatitis B. In many cases, the HbsAg test is the only way to tell if a patient has hepatitis B because many people who carry the virus have no symptoms. If the patient is a carrier, she could pass this to her baby during labor or birth.

If the patient tests positive for hepatitis B, the neonate must receive injections of hepatitis B immunoglobulin and hepatitis B vaccine immediately after birth to prevent liver damage. The neonate then receives additional doses of the vaccine at 2 to 4 months and again at 6 to 18 months.

HIV testing

HIV screening may be done for a woman who is at high risk for developing acquired immunodeficiency syndrome. This test uses an enzyme-linked immunosorbent assay on a blood sample to determine the presence of HIV antibodies. If the HIV screening test returns positive results, findings are confirmed by a second test—the Western blot test.

The Centers for Disease Control and Prevention (CDC) recommend that all pregnant women be tested for HIV. However, in some cases, a pregnant woman won't pursue HIV testing because she doesn't want to know if she's infected. This choice should be respected. Screening isn't mandatory in prenatal settings, but is recommended for patients who:
• have a history of I.V. drug use
• have unprotected sex
• have multiple sex partners
• have had a sexual partner who was infected with HIV or was at risk for contracting it (because he was bisexual, an I.V. drug user, or a hemophiliac)
• received a blood transfusion between 1977 and 1985.

> The CDC recommends that all pregnant women be tested for HIV, even if they don't think they're at risk.

Minimizing the damage

A woman who's antibody-positive for HIV may begin therapy with zidovudine (AZT) to decrease the risk of transmitting the disease to her fetus. Alternatively, the patient may choose to terminate the pregnancy to avoid giving birth to a neonate who has a high risk of developing the disease. When discussing test results with a patient, keep in mind that a positive test result or an antibody-positive result indicates that the patient has been exposed to the disease — she doesn't necessarily have the disease.

Purport support

Positive HIV screening results should be presented with tact and compassion. Results are confidential; the information should be reported only to the patient. Extra support needs to be given to the patient who tests positive because there's no known cure for the infection.

VDRL and RPR tests

The Venereal Disease Research Laboratories (VDRL) test and rapid plasma reagin (RPR) test are serologic tests for syphilis. Syphilis needs to be treated early in pregnancy, before fetal damage occurs.

Pregnant women who test positive for syphilis must receive treatment before 16 week' gestation. Untreated syphilis infection during pregnancy can cause miscarriage, premature birth, stillbirth, or birth defects.

Alpha-fetoprotein testing

AFP testing — sometimes called the *MSAFP* test or maternal serum AFP test — is usually used to detect neural tube defects. AFP is a protein that's secreted by the fetal liver and excreted in the mother's blood. When testing by immunoassay, AFP values are less than 15 ng/ml in nonpregnant women.

MOM's levels

The test is considered positive for an increased risk of neural tube defect when the AFP level is greater than 2.5 times the median (midpoint of levels of a group of patients at the same gestational age), or 2.5 MOM (multiples of median).

AFP testing can also indicate:
- abdominal wall defects
- esophageal and duodenal atresia
- renal and urinary tract anomalies
- Turner's syndrome
- low birth weight
- placental complications.

Congenital anomalies, such as Down syndrome, may be associated with low maternal serum AFP concentrations. Elevated maternal serum AFP levels may suggest neural tube defects or other anomalies. Maternal AFP levels rise sharply in the blood of about 90% of women carrying a fetus with anencephaly and in about 50%

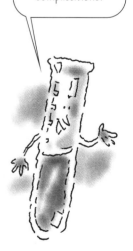

AFP levels can be used to detect neural tube defects, abdominal wall defects, low birth weight, and other complications.

of those carrying a fetus with spina bifida. Definitive diagnosis requires ultrasonography and amniocentesis. High AFP levels can also indicate intrauterine death or other anomalies, such as duodenal atresia, omphalocele, tetralogy of Fallot, and Turner's syndrome.

Glucose tolerance testing

If the patient has a history of previously unexplained fetal loss, has a family history of diabetes, has previously delivered a large-for-gestational age neonate (over 9 lb [4.1 kg]), is obese, or has glycosuria, a 50-g oral 1-hour glucose loading or tolerance test should be scheduled toward the end of the first trimester. This test is performed to rule out or confirm gestational diabetes. It's routinely done between 24 and 28 weeks' gestation to evaluate insulin-antagonistic effects of placental hormones but, in high-risk pregnancies, testing should occur earlier. Fasting plasma glucose levels shouldn't be above 140 mg/dl.

Triple screen

The triple screen is a blood test routinely offered between the 15th and 20th week of pregnancy that measures three chemicals: alpha-fetoprotein (AFP), unconjugated estriol, and hCG.

Picking up on patterns

By detecting chemical patterns, the test predicts if there's an increased risk of bearing a child with a chromosomal abnormality or open tube defect, including:
• Down syndrome — extra chromosome 21 that results in mental retardation
• trisomy 18 — extra chromosome 18 that results in mental retardation that's much more serious than Down syndrome; the neonate usually dies within hours of birth but may live for months or, in rare cases, years
• spina bifida — fetal spine doesn't properly close; size and location of opening determine severity; surgery is required at birth; may cause paralysis
• anencephaly — the most severe type of neural tube defect in which the brain and skull don't form properly; babies are stillborn or die within a few weeks
• omphalocele and gastroschisis — improper closure of the abdominal wall; severity depends on size and location of opening; surgery may correct problem; prognosis depends upon severity.

Suggestive, not definitive

Triple screening doesn't definitively answer whether a fetus has a birth defect. It only suggests that there's a possibility for birth defects. In some cases, results appear to be abnormal because the fetus is younger or older than initially estimated. Suspicions can be confirmed by amniocentesis.

Nonstress testing

Performed by a specially trained nurse, a prepartum NST evaluates fetal well-being by measuring the fetal heart response to fetal movements. Such movements produce transient accelerations in the heart rate of a healthy fetus. Usually ordered during the third trimester of pregnancy, this noninvasive screening test uses indirect electronic monitoring to record FHR and the duration of uterine contractions. It's indicated for suspected fetal distress or placental insufficiency associated with the following maternal conditions:

- diabetes mellitus
- hyperthyroidism
- chronic hypertension or PIH
- collagen disease
- heart disease
- chronic renal disease
- intrauterine growth retardation
- sickle cell disease
- Rh sensitization
- suspected postmaturity (when the woman is suspected of being past her due date)
- history of miscarriage or stillbirth
- abnormal estriol excretion.

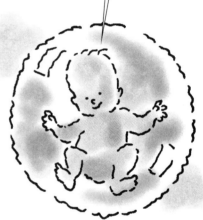

Don't stress over it! Nonstress testing is just used to determine how well I'm doing.

Getting it on the record

To perform the test, the patient is placed in a semi-Fowler or lateral-tilt position with a pillow under one hip. The patient shouldn't be placed in the supine position because pressure on the maternal great vessels from the gravid uterus may cause maternal hypotension and reduced uterine perfusion. Conductive gel is applied to the abdomen and transducers are placed on the patient's abdomen to transmit and record FHR and fetal movement.

Shake it up

The patient is then instructed to depress the monitor's mark or test button when she feels the fetus move. If no spontaneous fetal movement occurs within 20 minutes, apply gentle pressure to the patient's abdomen or shake it to stimulate fetal movement.

A positive reaction

If the monitor records two FHR accelerations that exceed baseline by at least 15 beats/minute, that last longer than 15 seconds, and that occur within a 20-minute period, conclude the test. Such findings, called a *reactive NST,* indicate that an intact fetal autonomic nervous system controls FHR.

Lack of reaction

If reactive results aren't obtained, the fetus should be monitored for an additional 40 minutes. If reactive NST results still aren't obtained, a CST may be performed to more definitively assess fetal status.

Contraction stress test

The prepartum CST evaluates respiratory function of the placenta and indicates whether the fetus will be able to withstand the stress of labor. Performed by a specially trained nurse, this test uses indirect electronic monitoring to measure fetal heart response to spontaneous or oxytocin-induced uterine contractions. The CST is indicated when the NST fails to produce reactive results.

Contraindications to the CST include the following maternal conditions:
- preterm labor or preterm membrane rupture
- multiple pregnancy
- previous vertical cesarean delivery
- abruptio placentae
- placenta previa
- incompetent cervical os
- previous uterine rupture.

If the test must be performed despite the presence of one of these conditions, prepare for emergency delivery.

If I don't respond to an NST, a CST may provide a better indication of how I'm doing.

Places everyone!

To perform the test, the patient is placed in a semi-Fowler or lateral-tilt position with a pillow beneath one hip. As with the NST, the supine position shouldn't be used because pressure on the maternal great vessels from the gravid uterus may cause maternal hypotension and reduced uterine perfusion.

Roll ultrasound...and action!

A tocotransducer and an ultrasound transducer are placed on the abdomen for 20 minutes to record baseline vital signs and baseline measurements of uterine contractions, fetal movements, and

FHR. The contractions cause a temporary decrease in blood and oxygen flow to the fetus, which most fetuses are able to tolerate. Three contractions, each lasting 40 seconds, must occur within a 10-minute period. If the fetus's heart rate stays constant, the test is considered normal.

The lowdown on a slow down

The fetus may experience a decelerated heart rate during the test. If 50% or more of the contractions cause FHR to decrease, the test is stopped and results are considered abnormal. If test results are abnormal, the patient should be observed for 30 minutes after the test to make sure that contractions don't continue. FHR shouldn't drop below baseline at the end of the contraction or after the contraction. This is termed *late deceleration* and can be indicative of fetal hypoxia.

The solution may be a solution

If testing fails to produce spontaneous contractions, an oxytocin solution may be prepared and infused. After three contractions are recorded, the oxytocin drip is stopped. Continue to monitor the patient for 30 minutes or until the contraction rate returns to baseline. Make sure the patient is comfortable while she waits for the results of the test.

If I slow down during a CST for more than 50% of the contractions, stop the test.

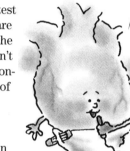

Nipple stimulation contraction stress test

Nipple stimulation can induce the uterine contractions necessary for a prepartum CST by stimulating the body to produce oxytocin itself. This is a natural and practical alternative to I.V. oxytocin administration. However, this test is controversial because it has the potential to cause hyperstimulation and uncontrollable contractions.

The nipple stimulation contraction stress test may cause hyperstimulation and uncontrollable contractions.

A hands-on approach

To stimulate contractions, tell the patient to apply warm washcloths to one of her breasts and then gently roll or tug on one nipple until contractions start. If necessary, she can apply a water-soluble lubricant, such as K-Y jelly, to reduce nipple irritation. If a second contraction doesn't occur within 2 minutes of the first contraction, ask the patient to massage her nipple again. If no contractions occur after 15 minutes of stimulation, the patient may be instructed to stimulate both nipples. The patient should be instructed to discontinue stimulation when three contractions lasting 35 seconds each occur within a 10-minute period.

CAUTION!

Nutritional care

Nutritional needs must also be addressed as a part of prenatal care. A pregnant woman's nutritional intake — including calories, protein, fat, vitamins, minerals, and fluid — needs to be increased to provide sufficient nutrients for her growing fetus. In most cases, the patient doesn't have to increase the quantity of food she eats; she simply needs to increase the quality of the food she eats. (See *RDAs for pregnant women.*)

Let the pyramid be your guide

A pregnant woman's food choices should be based on the Food Guide Pyramid. When discussing nutrition with the patient, refer to servings of food rather than milligrams or percentages. (See *Food guide pyramid.*)

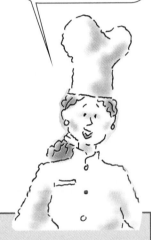

Remember that in most cases pregnant women don't need to increase their intake of food — they just need to increase their intake of nutrients.

RDAs for pregnant women

A pregnant woman's energy and calorie requirements are increased during pregnancy. This increased need is necessary to create new tissue and to meet her increased metabolic needs. Nutrient needs during pregnancy can be met by a diet that provides all of the essential nutrients, fiber, and energy in adequate amounts.

This chart lists the daily recommended dietary allowances (RDAs) for pregnant women, as outlined by the U.S. Department of Agriculture.

Calories	2,500 kcal	**Water-soluble vitamins**		**Minerals**	
Protein	60 g	Ascorbic acid (vitamin C)	75 mg	Calcium	1,200 mg
Fat-soluble vitamins		Folic acid	400 µg	Phosphorus	1,200 mg
Vitamin A	800 µg	Niacin	17 mg	Iodine	175 µg
Vitamin D	10 µg	Riboflavin	1.6 mg	Iron	30 mg
Vitamin E	10 µg	Thiamine	1.5 mg	Zinc	15 mg
		Vitamin B_6	2.2 µg		
		Vitamin B_{12}	2.2 µg		

Food guide pyramid

The food guide pyramid suggests eating a wide variety of foods (with emphasis on fruits, vegetables, and starches) for good health. In this diet, most of the fat comes from the milk-cheese and meat-poultry-eggs groups. Note that this food guide pyramid has been adjusted slightly to accommodate the needs of a pregnant patient.

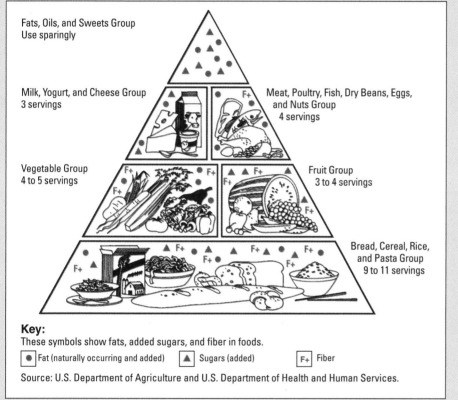

Fats, Oils, and Sweets Group
Use sparingly

Milk, Yogurt, and Cheese Group
3 servings

Meat, Poultry, Fish, Dry Beans, Eggs,
and Nuts Group
4 servings

Vegetable Group
4 to 5 servings

Fruit Group
3 to 4 servings

Bread, Cereal, Rice,
and Pasta Group
9 to 11 servings

Key:
These symbols show fats, added sugars, and fiber in foods.

● Fat (naturally occurring and added)   ▲ Sugars (added)   F+ Fiber

Source: U.S. Department of Agriculture and U.S. Department of Health and Human Services.

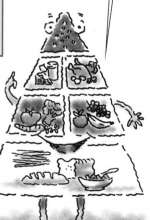

Just because
a patient is
pregnant doesn't
mean that she
can't use me as a
guide for making
healthy food
choices.

Infliction of restriction

Although certain nutritional requirements increase during pregnancy, certain restrictions also become necessary to protect the health of the baby. (See *Foods to avoid during pregnancy*, page 192.)

Education edge

Foods to avoid during pregnancy

Although several nutritional needs increase during pregnancy, other food restrictions become necessary. Tell the patient to avoid the following food products.

Alcohol

A pregnant patient shouldn't drink alcohol because alcohol crosses the placental barrier and can result in fetal alcohol syndrome (FAS). FAS can cause prenatal and postnatal growth failure, microcephaly, facial and musculoskeletal abnormalities, and mental retardation.

Caffeine

Caffeine is a central nervous system stimulant that increases heart rate, urine production in the kidneys, and secretion of acid in the stomach. Sources of caffeine include chocolate, soft drinks, tea, and coffee. A daily caffeine intake of more than 300 mg (about 4 cups of coffee) has been associated with low birth weight. Foods and beverages with caffeine should be avoided or limited. To reduce caffeine intake, suggest that the patient switch to decaffeinated beverages, such as decaffeinated tea or coffee.

Artificial sweeteners and additives

Artificial sweeteners, such as saccharin and aspartame, aren't recommended during pregnancy. According to the results of some animal studies, a large intake of saccharin may be carcinogenic. Some studies also suggest that saccharin may cross the placental barrier. Although no definitive study has been performed that indicates that aspartame crosses the placental barrier, a woman should still be advised to avoid ingesting food products with this substance during pregnancy.

A pregnant patient should also avoid foods that contain food additives because the effects of many of these additives are unknown.

Cholesterol

A pregnant patient should also limit her cholesterol intake. Encourage the patient to eat lean meats, to cook with olive oil instead of lard or butter, and to remove the skin from poultry. Even though such foods as eggs are good sources of protein, a woman who has a family history of high cholesterol shouldn't consume more than one egg per week.

Calories

The recommended daily allowance (RDA) of calories for women of childbearing age is 2,200. To meet the needs of pregnancy, a woman should increase her calorie intake by 300 calories (a total of 2,500 calories daily). These additional calories supply energy for the fetus and placenta as well as accommodate for an increased maternal metabolic rate. Inadequate calorie intake may lead to pro-

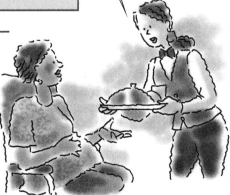

We're only going to increase your calorie intake by 300 calories. That should provide the extra energy that you need.

tein breakdown for energy, depriving the fetus of essential protein and, possibly, resulting in ketoacidosis and neurologic defects.

Meal plan

To help a woman plan for increased calorie intake, consider her lifestyle. Many women skip meals, have erratic eating patterns, and rely on fast or convenient foods. Help the patient plan on adding calories by eating foods rich in protein, iron, and other essential nutrients rather than eating empty-calorie foods, such as pretzels and doughnuts. Suggest such snacks as carrot sticks or cheese and crackers. Encourage the patient to have these snacks on-hand ahead of time to provide needed nutrients.

Ascertain weight gain

The easiest way to determine if your patient's calorie intake is adequate is to assess weight gain. The patient's weight gain pattern is as important as her total weight gain. Even if she surpasses the target weight before the end of the third trimester, encourage her not to restrict her intake—she should continue to gain weight because the fetus is growing rapidly during this time.

Protein

The RDA of protein for pregnant women is 60 g. If protein needs are met, overall nutritional needs are generally met. In many cases, if protein needs are inadequate, iron, B vitamins, calcium, and phosphorus are also inadequate.

You complete me

Good animal sources of protein include meat, poultry, fish, yogurt, eggs, and milk. Because the protein in these forms contains all nine essential amino acids, it's considered *complete protein*. However, lunch meats such as bologna and salami shouldn't be consumed regularly because they're high in fat and aren't typically good sources of protein.

Full of complements

The protein found in nonanimal sources doesn't contain all nine essential amino acids. Vitamin B_{12} is found exclusively in animal proteins. Therefore, a pregnant patient who excludes animal proteins from her diet may have a vitamin B_{12} deficiency. Complete protein can be obtained through nonanimal sources by cooking different protein sources together. For example, eating complementary pro-

You're the best...
No, you're the best...

teins, such as beans and rice, legumes and rice, or beans and wheat together, can provide the patient with all nine essential amino acids.

Got milk?

Milk products are also rich in protein and may be consumed in various forms — buttermilk, yogurt, cheese, custards, eggnogs, and cream soups — to meet daily protein requirements. If the patient is lactose intolerant, lactose supplements may be purchased over the counter. These supplements predigest milk and make it palatable for the patient.

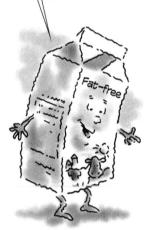

Milk products are great sources of protein, calcium, and vitamin D — which are all necessary nutrients.

Fats

Linoleic acid is an essential fatty acid that's necessary for new cell growth. It isn't manufactured in the body but can be found in such vegetable oils as safflower, corn, olive, peanut, and cottonseed. In addition, these vegetable oils are low in cholesterol compared with animal oils such as lard. They're also recommended for all adults to prevent hypercholesterolemia and atherosclerosis.

Vitamins

Requirements of fat-soluble and water-soluble vitamins increase during pregnancy to support the growth of new fetal cells. A healthy, varied diet with plenty of fruits and vegetables usually allows the pregnant patient to meet these requirements. A specially designed multivitamin supplement is usually also prescribed. The patient should be advised to take these vitamins as directed. The recommended dose shouldn't be exceeded because fat-soluble vitamins can be toxic. In addition, tell the patient not to use mineral oil as a laxative because it can prevent absorption of fat-soluble vitamins from the GI tract.

Source material

A woman who was taking hormonal contraceptives before she became pregnant also needs to include good sources of vitamin A, vitamin B_6, and folic acid in her diet in early pregnancy because hormonal contraceptives may deplete her stores of these vitamins. Vitamin A can be found in milk, eggs, yellow fruits and vegetables, dark green fruits and vegetables, and liver; vitamin B_6, in whole grains, organ meats, brewer's yeast, blackstrap molasses, and wheat germ; folic

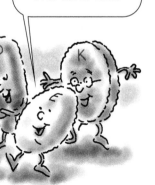

Warn your patient to take us fat-soluble vitamins only as prescribed. Too much of us can be toxic!

acid, in citrus fruits, tomatoes and other vegetables, grain products, and most ready-to-eat cereals (fortified with folic acid).

Too little

Vitamin deficiencies can cause many problems. For example:
• Severe folate deficiency may result in megaloblastic anemia and fetal neural tube defects as well as miscarriages.
• Vitamin D deficiency may result in the breakdown of fetal and maternal mineral bone density (vitamin D is necessary for calcium and phosphorus absorption).

Too much

Likewise, an overdose of vitamins can also cause problems:
• Vitamin A excess can result in fetal malformation and congenital anomalies. Such an excess can occur through the body's absorption of isotretinoin (Accutane), a medication for acne.
• Megadoses of vitamin C may cause withdrawal scurvy in the infant at birth.

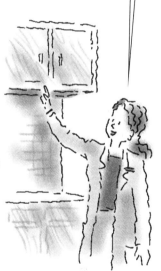

Remind the patient that all vitamins should be kept out of reach of small children because the folic acid and iron in these pills may be poisonous.

Folic acid

Folic acid (folacin) is a water-soluble B-9 vitamin that's necessary for RBC formation. A folic acid deficiency may result in megaloblastic anemia (development of large but ineffective RBCs). If evidence of folic acid deficiency is present at the time of birth, the neonate may be affected as well. Low levels of folic acid in pregnant women have been associated with premature separation of the placenta, spontaneous abortions, and neural tube defects. Good sources of folic acid include fruits and vegetables. Prescribed prenatal vitamins, which contain a folic acid supplement of 0.4 to 1.0 mg, are also essential.

Minerals

Minerals are needed for fetal cell development. They're found in many foods, so most mineral deficiencies in pregnant women are rare. For women whose intake of minerals is below daily requirements, supplements may be necessary.

Calcium and phosphorus

Calcium and phosphorus are vital to the structure of bones and teeth. Between 1,200 and 1,500 mg of calcium and 1,200 mg of phosphorus are recommended per day during pregnancy. In the last trimester of pregnancy, fetal skeletal growth is greatest and the fetus draws calcium directly from the mother's stores. In addition, clinical trials have shown that adequate calcium intake during pregnancy lowers blood pressure and may reduce the incidence of premature births.

Because calcium and phosphorus help with tooth and bone formation in the fetus, a maternal diet high in calcium and vitamin D (a vitamin needed for calcium to enter bones) is necessary. If a woman can't drink milk or eat milk products, such as cheese, a daily calcium supplement may be prescribed. Inadequate calcium intake can result in diminished maternal bone density. The woman should eat foods that are high in protein to ensure adequate phosphorus intake because most foods that are high in protein are also high in phosphorus.

Iodine

The recommended daily requirement of iodine during pregnancy is 175 mg. Iodine is essential for the formation of thyroxine and proper functioning of the thyroid gland. The best sources of this mineral are ocean fish, including cod, haddock, sole, and ocean perch (Atlantic redfish).

If iodine deficiency occurs, it may result in thyroid enlargement (goiter) in the woman or fetus and, in extreme cases, can cause hypothyroidism (cretinism) in the fetus. Thyroid enlargement in the fetus at birth is serious because the increased pressure the enlarged gland places on the airway can result in early respiratory distress. If not discovered at birth, hypothyroidism may lead to cognitive impairment. In areas where water and soil are known to be iodine-deficient, women should use iodized salt and include a serving of seafood in their diet at least once per week.

Iron

The RDA of iron for pregnant women is 30 mg. In most cases, about one-half of this intake comes from supplements because dietary intake alone can't provide sufficient iron. Remember to tell the patient to take iron supplements with orange juice to enhance absorption. Inform her that they may cause her stools to be black and that constipation may develop if she doesn't include enough fluids and fiber in her diet.

Pumping iron

Iron is necessary to build high levels of hemoglobin, which is needed for oxygenation after the baby is born. After the 20th week of pregnancy, the fetus begins to store iron in the liver. These stores need to be adequate to last through the first 3 months of life, when intake consists mainly of milk (which is typically low in

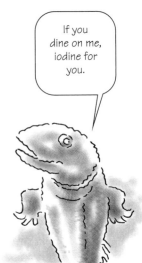

If you dine on me, iodine for you.

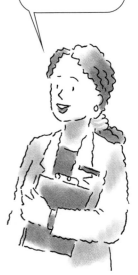

Taking iron supplements with orange juice helps enhance absorption.

iron). The pregnant woman also needs iron to increase her RBC volume and to replace iron lost in blood at delivery.

Because the richest sources of iron are also the most expensive — organ meats, eggs, green leafy vegetables, whole grain, enriched breads, dried fruits — a woman with a low income may have trouble taking in adequate amounts of iron in her diet. Today, many cereals are iron-fortified, but even these foods may not supply the amount of iron that the patient needs.

Fluoride

Fluoride helps to form sound teeth. If the pregnant woman doesn't drink fluoridated water, supplemental fluoride may be recommended. Because large amounts of fluoride stain teeth brown, a woman shouldn't take a supplement if her water contains fluoride and she shouldn't take supplements more often than prescribed.

Sodium

Sodium is a major electrolyte that regulates fluids in the body. It helps with retention of fluid in the maternal circulation to ensure a pressure gradient for optimal exchange across the placenta. It also plays a role in maintaining the acid-base balance of blood and helps nutrients cross cell membranes.

During pregnancy and lactation, a woman's sodium metabolism (utilization) is altered by hormone activity. As a result, sodium needs are slightly higher during these times. However, there's rarely a need for additional sodium intake because a typical diet usually provides adequate amounts. Unless the patient is hypertensive or has heart disease, seasoning foods as usual is recommended during pregnancy. However, extremely salty foods, such as lunch meats and potato chips, should be avoided. Additives, such as monosodium glutamate, should also be avoided. Excessive salt intake could result in fluid retention, which strains the heart.

Excessive salt intake leads to fluid retention, which strains the heart.

Zinc

Zinc is necessary for synthesis of DNA and ribonucleic acid as well as cell division and growth. Zinc deficiency has been associated with preterm birth. The RDA of zinc during pregnancy is 15 mg daily. Meat, liver, eggs, seafood, and prenatal vitamins are good sources of zinc.

Fluid

Because a pregnant woman is excreting not only her own waste products but also those of her fetus, her body requires extra water to promote kidney function. In addition, fluids:

- keep skin soft
- lessen the likelihood of constipation
- rid the body of toxins and waste products
- reduce excessive swelling.

Recommended fluid intake is 2 qt (8 cups) daily. Fluid sources include juices, milk, soups, and carbonated beverages. The patient should avoid excess intake of caffeinated beverages.

Minimizing discomforts of pregnancy

Being aware of patient discomforts during pregnancy allows you to provide information on how to alleviate them. In addition, early monitoring of certain conditions can help reduce their occurrence.

Have them share so you can provide care

A pregnant woman may not mention her concerns or discomforts unless she's specifically asked because she isn't aware of the significance of her problems or she's reluctant to take up a lot of time during a prenatal visit. Encourage the patient to discuss whatever concerns she has at her visits. Although some issues may represent minor common discomforts associated with normal pregnancy, others may be early indicators of potential problems. For example, a problem such as constipation, which the patient may consider a minor discomfort, may result in hemorrhoids that can become a long-term problem if left to progress through the pregnancy.

On the other hand, a woman may see the discomforts of pregnancy as deterrents to good health. The minor discomforts of pregnancy may not seem minor to the patient, especially if they occur daily and make her wonder if she'll ever feel like herself again. You need to provide empathetic and sound advice for relieving discomforts and helping promote the overall health and well-being of a pregnant patient. (See *Dealing with pregnancy discomforts.*)

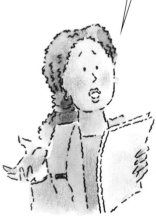

A pregnant patient should be encouraged to discuss the discomforts she's experiencing. Some discomforts can be easily allayed and others may be problematic.

First trimester

Although a pregnant woman may be excited about pregnancy and childbirth, the many discomforts that occur during the first

Education edge

Dealing with pregnancy discomforts

This table lists common discomforts associated with pregnancy and suggestions that you can give to the patient on how to prevent and manage them.

Discomfort	Patient teaching
Urinary frequency	• Void as necessary. • Avoid caffeine. • Perform Kegel exercises.
Fatigue	• Try to get a full night's sleep. • Schedule a daily rest time. • Maintain good nutrition.
Breast tenderness	• Wear a supportive bra.
Vaginal discharge	• Wear cotton underwear. • Avoid tight-fitting pantyhose. • Bathe daily.
Backache	• Avoid standing for long periods. • Apply local heat, such as a heating pad (set on low) or a hot water bottle. Advise the patient to place a towel between the heat source and the skin to prevent burning. • Stoop to lift objects — don't bend.
Round ligament pain	• Slowly rise from a sitting position. • Bend forward to relieve pain. • Avoid twisting motions.
Constipation	• Increase fiber intake in the diet. • Set a regular time for bowel movements. • Drink more fluids, including water and fruit juices (unless contraindicated). Avoid caffeinated drinks.

Discomfort	Patient teaching
Hemorrhoids	• Rest on the left side with the hips and lower extremities elevated to provide better oxygenation to the placenta and fetus. • Avoid constipation. • Apply witch hazel pads to the hemorrhoids. • Keep hemorrhoids reduced by using a well-lubricated gloved finger to push them gently inside the rectum; then tighten the rectal sphincter to support the hemorrhoids and contain them within the rectum. • Take sitz baths with warm water as often as needed to relieve discomfort. • Apply ice packs for reduction of swelling, if preferred over heat.
Varicosities	• Walk regularly. • Rest with the feet elevated daily. • Avoid standing for long periods. • Avoid crossing the legs. • Avoid wearing constrictive knee-high stockings; wear support stockings instead.
Ankle edema	• Avoid standing for long periods. • Rest with the feet elevated. • Avoid wearing garments that constrict the lower extremities.
Headache	• Avoid eyestrain. • Rest with a cold cloth on the forehead.
Leg cramps	• Straighten the leg and dorsiflex the ankle. • Avoid pointing the toes.

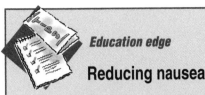

Education edge

Reducing nausea

To help the patient relieve nausea during pregnancy, give her these tips:
• Before getting out of bed in the morning, eat a few dry crackers, toast, or a sour candy.
• Eat small, frequent meals rather than large, infrequent ones.
• Avoid greasy and highly seasoned foods.
• Delay breakfast (or dinner, if experiencing evening nausea) until nausea passes. Make up for missed meals at another time to maintain nutrition.
• Avoid sudden movements and fatigue, which are known to increase nausea.
• If breakfast is usually eaten late in the morning, eat a snack before bedtime to help avoid long periods between meals.
• A wrist acupressure band, available at travel stores, may help to reduce motion sickness.
• Sip carbonated beverages, water, or herbal decaffeinated tea.
• Take a walk outside or take deep breaths through an open window to inhale fresh air.

trimester can take away from the joyful feelings of motherhood. Such discomforts are usually accepted as an expected part of pregnancy. However, there are ways to ease discomforts and prevent further complications. You should pass this information along to your patient as necessary.

Nausea and vomiting

Nausea and vomiting are the most common discomforts during the first trimester. Although these symptoms are commonly referred to as *morning sickness*, they can last all day for some women. Nausea and vomiting rarely interfere with proper nutrition enough to harm the developing fetus.

At least 50% of women experience nausea normally during pregnancy. Medications are rarely prescribed to relieve nausea because they may adversely effect on the fetus.

Cause for queasiness

Although a specific cause of nausea during pregnancy hasn't been determined, it has been suggested that nausea is the body's reaction to the high levels of hCG that occur during the first trimester. Other possible contributors to nausea include the rapid stretching of the woman's uterine muscles, the relative relaxation of the muscle tissue in the digestive tract (making digestion less efficient), excess acid in the stomach, and the woman's enhanced sense of smell. (See *Reducing nausea*.)

Nausea and vomiting are considered abnormal if:
- the patient is losing weight instead of gaining it
- the patient hasn't gained the projected amount of weight for a particular week of pregnancy
- lost meals are unable to be made up for during some time of the day
- signs of dehydration, such as little urine output, are present
- nausea lasts past the 12th week of pregnancy
- the patient vomits more than once daily.

To prevent potential complications, such as hyperemesis gravidarum (severe nausea and vomiting during pregnancy that result in dehydration and loss of at least 10 lb [4.5 kg]), inform the patient's primary health care provider if these signs and symptoms occur. For more information on hyperemesis gravidarum, see the discussion in chapter 6, High-risk pregnancy.

Urinary frequency

Urinary frequency occurs in early pregnancy because of the growing uterus's pressure on the anterior bladder. It may last for about 3 months and disappears in midpregnancy, when the uterus rises above the bladder. It commonly returns again in late pregnancy as the fetal head presses against the bladder.

If a patient reports urinary frequency, ask her if she has experienced burning or pain on urination or if she has noticed blood in her urine — both signs of a UTI. After infection is ruled out, focus on teaching the patient ways to alleviate discomfort. Suggest to the patient that she reduce the amount of caffeine she drinks, if applicable. She can also perform Kegel exercises to help strengthen the pelvic muscles so that the feeling of urgency is less noticeable later in pregnancy. Kegel exercises also help with urinary control.

Breast tenderness

Breast tenderness is commonly noticed early in pregnancy and may be most noticeable when the patient is exposed to cold air. For most women, tenderness is minimal and transient. Many are aware of it but aren't distressed by it.

If breast tenderness is enough to cause the patient discomfort, recommend that she wear a bra with wide shoulder straps for support and she dress warmly to avoid cold drafts (if cold increases symptoms). If actual pain exists, suspect the presence of an underlying condition, such as nipple fissures or mastitis.

Fatigue

Fatigue is common early in pregnancy and may be caused by the body's increased metabolic requirements. Fatigue can also intensify morning sickness. For example, if the patient becomes too tired, she may not eat properly. If she remains on her feet without at least one break during the day, the risk of varicosities and thromboembolitic complications increases.

Putting fatigue to rest

Increasing the amount of rest and sleep may relieve the patient's fatigue. During prenatal visits, ask her whether she manages to take at least one short rest period every day. Modifying her routine to allow rest periods is advised. If the patient has a sedentary job inside or outside of the home, she needs to increase her activity, such as by walking or using a treadmill. By balancing rest and exercise, she can reduce her fatigue.

A modified Sims' position with the top leg forward is a good resting position. This puts the weight of the fetus on the bed, not on the woman, and allows good circulation to the lower extremities.

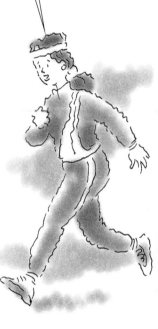

Balancing sedentary activities with physical activities can help reduce fatigue during pregnancy.

Increased vaginal discharge

Leukorrhea is another discomfort of pregnancy. It's a whitish, viscous vaginal discharge or an increase in the amount of normal vaginal secretions. It's caused by the high estrogen levels and increased blood supply to the vaginal epithelium and cervix that occur during pregnancy. A woman who's uncomfortable about discussing this part of her body or who associates vaginal infections with poor hygiene or STDs may be reluctant to mention an irritating vaginal discharge. Be sure to ask every patient at prenatal visits whether they're experiencing this problem.

Deterring discharge

Tell the patient that a daily bath or shower can help wash away accumulated secretions and prevent vulvar excoriation. Warn her not to douche; this is contraindicated throughout pregnancy. She can also use perineal pads to control discharge; she shouldn't use tampons, however, because they promote stasis of secretions, which can lead to infection. Wearing cotton underwear and sleeping without underwear are helpful in reducing moisture and possible excoriation. Tell the patient that she should avoid tight-fitting underwear and pantyhose to prevent yeast infections.

Advise the patient to contact her health care provider if there's a change in the color, odor, or character of the discharge. This could indicate infection. Vulvar pruritus (itching of the vulva) also needs evaluation because this sign also strongly indicates infection. Caution the patient not to self-treat vaginal infections during pregnancy because such preparations as metronidazole (Flagyl) may harm the fetus.

Second and third trimesters

Although the patient may be focused on bonding with the fetus, she must be reminded to report any discomforts she has to ensure that nothing serious is occurring. In addition, at the midpoint of pregnancy, review with the patient precautionary measures that help prevent constipation, varicosities, and hemorrhoids and discuss with her the new symptoms that may occur.

Indigestion

Indigestion may be caused by large amounts of progesterone and estrogen, which tend to relax smooth muscle tissue throughout the body — including the GI tract. This causes food to move through the system more slowly and may result in bloating and indigestion. This slowdown is beneficial because it allows for better absorption of nutrients into the bloodstream and subsequently into the fetus's system.

Feeling the burn

Heartburn results when the cardiac sphincter relaxes, allowing food and digestive juices to back up from the stomach into the esophagus. This irritates the lining, causing a burning sensation. This problem may increase later in pregnancy because of the pressure of the fetus on the mother's internal organs. (See *Relieving heartburn and indigestion*, page 204.)

If measures fail to relieve symptoms, a low-sodium antacid or other OTC medication that's safe to use during pregnancy may be recommended. Sodium or sodium bicarbonate solutions should be avoided because they can exacerbate heartburn.

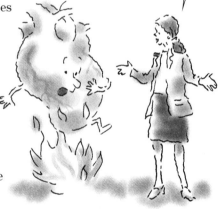

Indigestion and heartburn may result when the relaxation of smooth muscle tissue and the cardiac sphincter causes food processing to slow down.

Ankle edema

Most women experience some swelling of the ankles and feet during late pregnancy, most noticeably at the end of the day. It may result from reduced blood circulation in the lower extremities caused by uterine pressure and general fluid retention. The patient may become aware of it if she takes off her shoes and then can't get them back on again comfortably. As long as proteinuria

Education edge

Relieving heartburn and indigestion

To decrease the incidence of heartburn and indigestion in the pregnant patient, advise her to:
• avoid gaining too much weight (this puts excess pressure on the stomach)
• avoid wearing clothing that's tight around the abdomen and waist
• eat frequent, small meals instead of three large ones
• eat slowly and chew thoroughly
• avoid highly seasoned foods, fried and fatty foods, processed meats, chocolate, coffee, alcohol, carbonated beverages, and spearmint or peppermint
• avoid smoking
• avoid bending at the waist
• sleep with her head elevated about 6″ (15 cm).

and hypertension aren't present, ankle edema is a normal occurrence.

To help relieve edema, tell the patient to rest in a left side-lying position; this increases kidney glomerular filtration rate. Sitting for half an hour in the afternoon and again in the evening with the legs elevated should also help. Tell the patient to avoid constricting panty girdles or knee-high stockings because these garments impede lower-extremity circulation and venous return.

Don't discount a report of lower-extremity edema until you're certain the woman doesn't exhibit signs of proteinuria, edema of other nondependent parts, or sudden weight increase that's indicative of PIH.

Varicose veins

Varicose veins are tortuous veins that commonly appear during pregnancy. They develop because the weight of the distended uterus puts pressure on the veins returning blood from the lower extremities. This causes blood to pool in the vessels, and the veins become engorged, inflamed, and painful. Varicose veins are common in women with a family history and in women who have a large fetus or multiple pregnancies. Sitting for prolonged periods with the legs dependent also promotes venous stasis.

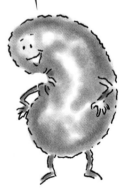

Just lay it out there! Tell your patient to rest in a left side-lying position to increase my glomerular filtration rate. This should help reduce edema.

Simple Sims'

Resting in Sims' position for 15 to 20 minutes twice daily is a good preventive measure against varicose veins. Advise the patient to avoid sitting with her legs crossed or her knees bent and to avoid wearing constrictive knee-high hose or garters. Elastic medical support stockings, such as TEDS, should be used to relieve varicose veins and should be applied before the patient arises in the morning to be most effective. Alternating exercise with rest periods is also effective in alleviating varicose veins. The patient should be advised to break up periods of sitting or standing with a walk at least twice daily. Vitamin C may also be helpful in reducing the size of varicose veins because it's involved in forming collagen and endothelium for blood vessels. Ask at prenatal visits whether fresh fruit is included in the woman's diet.

Surgical removal of varicose veins isn't recommended during pregnancy. In most cases, they improve on their own after delivery, usually by the time prepregnancy weight is reached.

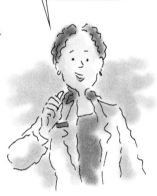

Vitamin C may help reduce the size of varicose veins.

Hemorrhoids

Hemorrhoids are varicosities of the rectal veins. They occur commonly in pregnancy because the bulk of the growing uterus puts pressure on the veins. Measures taken early in pregnancy to prevent their occurrence are key to reducing their incidence as well as severity.

Resting in a modified Sims' position daily helps to reduce the discomfort of hemorrhoids. Tell the patient to assume a knee-chest position at the end of the day to reduce pressure on rectal veins. Because this position can result in light-headedness, advise the patient to start by doing this for only a few minutes and gradually increasing to 10 to 15 minutes. Stool softeners may be recommended as well as application of witch hazel or cold compresses to help relieve pain.

Constipation

As pregnancy progresses, the growing uterus presses against the bowel and slows peristalsis, resulting in constipation and sometimes flatulence. Prescribed oral iron supplements also contribute to constipation. Reinforce the need for the supplements to build fetal iron stores but also help the woman to find a method to relieve or prevent constipation.

Advise the patient not to use home remedies, such as mineral oil and enemas. Mineral oil interferes with the absorption of fat-

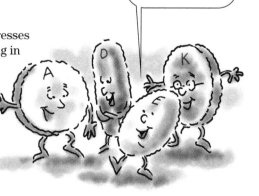

Tell your patient not to fight constipation with mineral oil. Mineral oil can interfere with our absorption.

soluble vitamins (A, D, E, and K), which are necessary for fetal growth. Enemas might initiate labor through their action. OTC laxatives as well as all drugs are contraindicated during pregnancy unless specifically prescribed or authorized by the patient's health care provider. (See *Preventing constipation.*)

If the patient experiences excessive flatulence, recommend that she avoid gas-forming foods, such as cabbage and beans. In addition, if dietary measures and regular bowel evacuation fail, a stool softener (such as docusate sodium [Colace] and evacuation suppositories (such as glycerin) may be prescribed.

Backache

As pregnancy advances, a lumbar lordosis occurs and postural changes necessary to maintain balance may lead to backache. Backache can also be an initial sign of bladder or kidney infection. To determine the cause of the patient's backache, assess the manner in which she walks, determine what type of shoes she wears, and obtain a detailed account of her symptoms.

To help alleviate pain, instruct the patient to wear shoes with low to moderate-height heels. Such shoes reduce the amount of spinal curvature necessary to maintain an upright posture. Advise the patient to walk with her pelvis tilted forward. This helps to alleviate back pain by putting pelvic support under the weight of the uterus. Local heat and a firmer mattress (or a board placed under the mattress) can help to relieve discomfort. Pelvic rocking or tilting can also be beneficial. To avoid back strain, advise the patient to squat—not bend over—to lift objects and to hold objects close to the body when lifting.

Tell the patient not to take muscle relaxants or analgesics (as well as other medications) for back pain without first consulting her health care provider. Generally, acetaminophen (Tylenol) is considered safe and effective for relieving this type of pain during pregnancy.

Leg cramps

Decreased serum calcium, increased serum phosphorus, and interference with circulation commonly cause muscle cramps of the lower extremities during pregnancy. The pain may be extreme and the intensity of the contraction frightening. Make sure to ask the patient at prenatal visits if she's having leg cramps. If leg cramps are a problem, provide her with information on techniques for relieving discomfort.

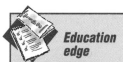

Education edge

Preventing constipation

When teaching the pregnant patient about preventing constipation, include these tips:
• Encourage her to evacuate her bowels regularly.
• Advise her to increase the amount of roughage in her diet by eating raw fruits, bran, and vegetables.
• Instruct her to drink extra amounts of water daily.

Extend and elevate

The best way to relieve symptoms is to have the patient lay on her back momentarily and extend the involved leg while keeping her knee straight and dorsiflexing the foot until the pain is gone. Elevating the lower extremities frequently during the day to improve circulation and avoiding full leg extension, such as stretching with the toes pointed, may also be beneficial.

If the woman is having frequent leg cramps, her doctor may prescribe aluminum hydroxide gel (Amphojel) to bind phosphorus in the intestinal tract, lowering it in the circulation. Lowering milk intake to only a pint daily and supplementing this with calcium lactate may also help to reduce her phosphorus level.

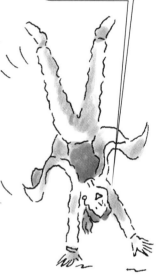

Elevating the lower extremities can help improve circulation during pregnancy.

Light-headedness

Light-headedness in the first trimester may be caused by a blood supply that inadequately fills the rapidly expanding circulatory system. During the second trimester, the pressure of the expanding uterus on maternal blood vessels may cause it. Faintness can occur anytime the patient rises from a sitting or prone position (postural hypotension) because the blood suddenly shifts away from the brain when blood pressure drops rapidly. Advise the patient to get up slowly in these situations.

Light-headedness may also be the result of low glucose levels caused by skipping meals. Carrying fruit or crackers to snack on is helpful to quickly increase glucose levels.

If the patient feels faint, advise her to lie down with her feet elevated or sit down and place her head between her knees until faintness subsides. She should also report to her health care provider any light-headedness because it can be a sign of severe anemia or another illness and should be evaluated.

Shortness of breath

As the expanding uterus puts pressure on the diaphragm, the lungs may compress, causing dyspnea (shortness of breath). This may be more noticeable to the patient on exertion or during the night, when her body is flat.

Sitting upright and allowing the weight of the uterus to fall away from the diaphragm can help relieve the problem. As pregnancy progresses, the patient may require two or more pillows to sleep on at night to avoid dyspnea.

Always question the patient about shortness of breath at prenatal visits to be certain the sensation isn't continuous. Constant shortness of breath may indicate cardiac problems or a respiratory tract infection.

Insomnia

Insomnia is common during pregnancy. It's difficult for a pregnant women to rest physically because her large abdomen makes it difficult to get comfortable, and mentally because she has a lot on her mind. In cases of insomnia, it's helpful to review stress-reduction and relaxation techniques to help the patient get in the frame of mind for a good night's sleep. In addition, a comfortable bed and pillows to support the head, back, and abdomen are helpful. Eating a light snack before bedtime and avoiding caffeine after noontime is also beneficial. If the patient naps during the day, suggest shortening the nap and trying to stay up later to promote better sleep at night. If measures fail, suggest that the patient get out of bed and read, knit, or do a favorite activity until she's drowsy and able to fall asleep.

Abdominal discomfort and Braxton Hicks contractions

A woman may experience uncomfortable feelings of abdominal pressure early in pregnancy. A woman with a multiple pregnancy may notice this throughout pregnancy. The patient can relieve this pressure by putting gentle pressure on the uterine fundus or by standing with her arms crossed in front.

Pain around the round ligaments

When a woman stands up quickly, she may experience a pulling pain in the right or left lower abdomen from tension on the round ligaments. It can be very sharp and frightening and may be prevented by always rising slowly from a lying to a sitting position or from a sitting to a standing position. Keep in mind that round ligament pain may simulate the abrupt pain that occurs with ruptured ectopic pregnancy. The patient's description of the pain needs to be evaluated carefully.

As early as the 12th week of pregnancy, the uterus periodically contracts and relaxes again. These contractions, termed *Braxton Hicks contractions*, usually aren't noticeable early in pregnancy. In middle and late pregnancy, the contractions become stronger, causing the woman to tense and possibly feel minimal pain, similar to a hard menstrual cramp. These feelings are normal and aren't a sign of beginning labor.

Be certain the woman understands that a rhythmic pattern of contractions, characteristic of labor, shouldn't be mistaken for Braxton Hicks contractions.

A rhythmic pattern of contractions is characteristic of labor.

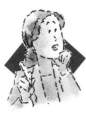

Quick quiz

1. A pregnant patient who is older than age 35 is at greater risk for having:

 A. a low-birth-weight infant.
 B. a preterm infant.
 C. PIH.
 D placenta previa.

Answer: D. Expectant mothers who are older than age 35 are at risk for placenta previa, hydatidiform mole, and vascular, neoplastic, and degenerative diseases. They're also at risk for having fraternal twins or infants with genetic abnormalities, especially Down syndrome.

2. Which familial factor is most likely to cause discomfort during pregnancy?

 A. Anemia
 B. Varicose veins
 C. Cancer
 D. Colitis

Answer: B. Varicose veins are an inherited weakness in blood vessel walls that become evident during pregnancy and can cause the patient discomfort.

3. A patient reports that the first day of her last normal menses was January 7. The calculated EDD is:

 A. October 14.
 B. April 14.
 C. September 31.
 D. April 7.

Answer: A. Based on information obtained in the patient's menstrual history, you can calculate the patient's EDD using Nägele's rule: Take the first day of the last normal menses, minus 3 months, and then add 7 days.

4. Using GTPAL, a patient who has had two previous pregnancies, has had no abortions or miscarriages, delivered two full-term neonates, and is currently pregnant would be considered a:

 A. 3-2-0-2-0.
 B. 3-2-0-0-2.
 C. 2-3-0-0-2.
 D. 3-2-0-2-2.

Answer: B. G is the total number of pregnancies (3). T is the number of full-term neonates born (infants born at 37 weeks' gestation or later), which totals 2. P is the number of preterm infants born (infants born before 37 weeks' gestation), which is 0 for this patient. A is the number of spontaneous or induced abortions, which is 0 for this patient. L is the number of living children.

5. Normal FHR is:
    A.   110 to 150 beats/minute.
    B.   120 to 160 beats/minute.
    C.   130 to 170 beats/minute.
    D.   140 to 180 beats/minute.

Answer: B. Normal FHR usually ranges from 120 to 160 beats/minute.

6. Triple screening combines data from which prenatal tests?
    A.   Ultrasound, amniocentesis, and serum estriol
    B.   Serum hPL, serum estriol, and urinalysis
    C.   Serum hCG, serum estriol, and urinalysis
    D.   MSAFP, serum hCG, and unconjugated estriol

Answer: D. Triple screening combines data from MSAFP, hCG, and unconjugated estriol.

7. A pregnant patient who's fatigued is likely to be more comfortable in which position?
    A.   Modified Sims'
    B.   Supine with legs elevated
    C.   Supine with head elevated
    D.   Sitting upright with legs elevated

Answer: A. A good resting position is a modified Sims' position with the top leg forward. This puts the weight of the fetus on the bed, not on the woman, and allows good circulation in the lower extremities.

Scoring

☆☆☆ If you answered all seven questions correctly, perfecto! You're all that and a bag of chips. (Just recommend a bag of carrots to your patient.)

☆☆ If you answered five or six questions correctly, slammin'! You got game.

☆ If you answered fewer than five questions correctly, stay cool. You're headed in the right direction.

6

High-risk pregnancy

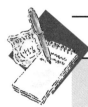

Just the facts

In this chapter, you'll learn:

♦ factors that contribute to high-risk pregnancy

♦ ways to identify high-risk situations based on key assessment findings

♦ appropriate treatments for high-risk pregnancies

♦ relevant nursing interventions for high-risk pregnancies.

A look at high-risk pregnancy

Most women progress through pregnancy without any serious problems. They enter pregnancy in good health and give birth to healthy neonates. However, problems sometimes develop that put a woman and her fetus in jeopardy. These problems may result from a chronic illness in the mother, a complication that developed during the pregnancy, or an external factor that impacts the health and well-being of the mother or the fetus.

Mother + fetus = one

Keep in mind that the health of a woman and her fetus are interdependent. Changes in the woman's health may affect fetal health, and changes in fetal health may affect the mother's physical and emotional health.

Contributing artists

Rarely is just one risk factor responsible for a high-risk pregnancy. Several factors can work together to contribute to a high-risk situation. For example, a pregnant adolescent is considered at higher risk; however, it isn't simply her age that places her in this category. Rather, her age is an indication of other factors that contribute to increased risk.

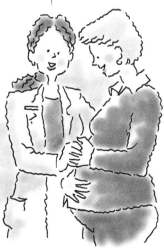

You can depend on it! The health of a woman and her fetus are interdependent.

First, as a pregnant adolescent, she faces a developmental crisis. In addition, adolescents in general tend to lack proper nutrition, adequate support, and knowledge—all contributors to increased risk. Moreover, such conditions as iron deficiency anemia, pregnancy-induced hypertension (PIH), and preterm labor occur more commonly in adolescents.

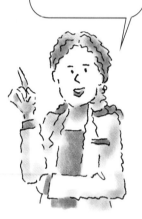

High-risk conditions such as iron deficiency anemia, PIH, and preterm labor are more common in adolescent pregnancies.

Maternal age

Reproductive risks increase among adolescents younger than age 15 and women older than age 35. The adolescent patient faces serious risks, including increased incidence of low-birth-weight and preterm neonates, anemia, labor dysfunction, and cephalopelvic disproportion. Expectant mothers older than age 35 are at risk for placenta previa; hydatidiform mole; and vascular, neoplastic, and degenerative diseases. They're also at risk for having fraternal twins or infants with genetic abnormalities, especially Down syndrome.

Maternal parity

Maternal parity may place a pregnant woman at high risk. For example, a multigravida who has had five or more pregnancies lasting at least 20 weeks is considered high-risk. In addition, if the current pregnancy occurs within 3 months of the last delivery, the pregnancy is considered high-risk.

Maternal obstetric and gynecologic history

Many factors in the mother's obstetric and gynecologic history can place a pregnancy at high risk. These factors may include:
- two or more premature deliveries or spontaneous abortions
- one or more stillbirths at term
- one or more neonates born with gross anomalies
- pelvic inadequacy or abnormal shaping
- cervical incompetency
- uterine incompetency, position, or structural anomalies
- history of multiple pregnancy, placental anomalies, amniotic fluid abnormalities, or poor weight gain
- history of gestational diabetes, PIH, or infection
- history of delivery of postterm neonate
- history of dystocia, precipitous delivery, cervical or vaginal lacerations caused by labor and delivery, cephalopelvic disproportion, hemorrhage during labor and delivery, or retained placenta
- lack of previous prenatal care or preparation for labor or birth.

Uh oh! We could mean double trouble.

History of multiple pregnancy can place a pregnancy at higher risk.

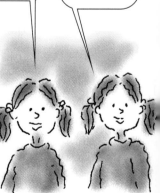

In addition, a pregnancy that occurs within 3 years of menarche indicates an increased risk of maternal mortality and morbidity. Such a pregnancy also places the patient at risk for delivering a neonate who's small for gestational age.

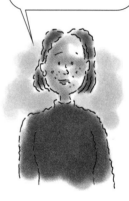

Pregnancy that occurs within 3 years of menarche increases the risk of maternal mortality and morbidity. No thanks!

Maternal medical history

Medical problems can cause complications during pregnancy. For example, abdominal trauma may lead to premature rupture of the membranes or abruptio placentae. Severe cardiac disease can adversely affect placental perfusion, thus jeopardizing fetal nutrition. As a result, the neonate may be born with a low birth weight. PIH, which commonly develops in women with essential hypertension, renal disease, or diabetes, increases the risk of abruptio placentae.

Insulin influx

Diabetes can worsen during pregnancy and harm the mother and fetus. Pregnant women typically develop insulin resistance, requiring increased amounts of insulin. The fetus of a woman with diabetes tends to be large because the increased insulin production needed to counteract the overload of glucose from the mother stimulates fetal growth. This, in turn, can lead to problems of cephalopelvic disproportion and dystocia for the mother.

Gravida aggravations

Stomach displacement by the gravid uterus, along with cardiac sphincter relaxation and decreased GI motility caused by increased progesterone, may aggravate symptoms of peptic ulcer disease such as gastric reflux. Also, the increase in blood volume and cardiac output associated with pregnancy can exhaust a patient with underlying cardiac disease.

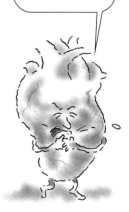

The increase in blood volume and cardiac output associated with pregnancy can be quite taxing on me!

Maternal lifestyle

Lifestyle and occupation can adversely affect a pregnancy. Make the patient aware that what she consumes and what she's exposed to can seriously affect her pregnancy. For example, taking over-the-counter and prescription drugs can be detrimental to the fetus. In addition, cigarette smoking is associated with intrauterine growth retardation and low-birth-weight neonates. Exposure to toxic substances, such as lead, organic solvents, radiation, and carbon monoxide, can also lead to fetal malformations.

Dangerous habits

Substance abuse with illicit drugs or alcohol is another cause of fetal anomalies. After birth, the neonate may experience drug withdrawal. Substance abuse may also interfere with the pregnant woman's ability to obtain adequate nutrition, which can adversely affect fetal growth. Additionally, if the substance abuse involves injection, the pregnant woman is at risk for infection with hepatitis B and human immunodeficiency virus (HIV).

Nourish so baby can flourish

Adequate nutrition is especially vital during pregnancy. Inadequate nutrition can lead to a deficiency of iron, folic acid, or protein. Iron deficiency anemia during pregnancy is associated with low fetal birth weight and preterm birth. Folic acid deficiency is associated with neural tube defects. Protein deficiency can lead to poor development of the fetus and growth restriction.

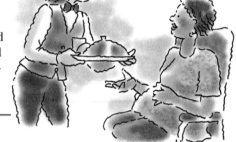

Adequate nutrition is especially vital during pregnancy.

Cultural background

Several genetic disorders are associated with specific cultures. For example, sickle cell anemia occurs primarily in persons of African and Mediterranean descent. Tay-Sachs disease is about 100 times more common in people of Eastern European Jewish (Ashkenazi) ancestry than in the general population.

Faith and the fetus

A woman's religious practices may also affect her health during pregnancy and could predispose her to complications. For example, an Amish woman may not be immunized against rubella. If exposed, the woman's fetus is at risk for congenital anomalies. Seventh-Day Adventists traditionally exclude dairy products from their diets, which may conflict with the woman's need for additional calcium to help fetal bone growth.

Family history

Certain conditions and disorders that contribute to high-risk pregnancy are familial. For example, a family history of multiple births, congenital diseases or deformities, or mental disability may place a pregnancy at higher risk.

Don't forget Dad

Some fetal congenital anomalies may be traced to the father's exposure to environmental hazards. The father's blood type and Rh status are also important because isoimmunization in the fetus may occur if the father is Rh positive, the mother is Rh negative, and the fetus is Rh positive.

On the home front

The family environment is also important in determining whether a pregnancy is high-risk. A history of battering or abuse, lack of support persons, inadequate housing, or lack of adequate finances can increase risk during pregnancy.

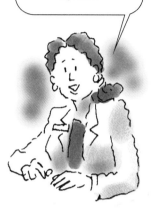

A patient's family history and home environment can put her pregnancy at high risk.

Abruptio placentae

Abruptio placentae — also called *placental abruption* — occurs when the placenta separates from the uterine wall prematurely, usually after the 20th week of gestation, producing hemorrhage. This disorder may be classified according to the degree of placental separation and the severity of maternal and fetal symptoms.

Many births = more risk

Abruptio placentae is most common in multigravidas — usually in women over age 35 — and is a common cause of bleeding during the second half of pregnancy. A confirmed diagnosis of abruptio placentae when there's heavy maternal bleeding generally necessitates termination of the pregnancy. The fetal prognosis depends on its gestational age and the amount of blood lost. The maternal prognosis is good if hemorrhage can be controlled.

What causes it

The cause of abruptio placentae is unknown. Predisposing factors include:
- traumatic injury such as a direct blow to the uterus
- placental site bleeding caused by a needle puncture during amniocentesis
- chronic hypertension or PIH, which raises pressure on the maternal side of the placenta
- multiparity more than 5
- short umbilical cord
- dietary deficiency
- smoking

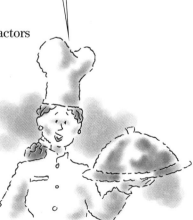

Dietary deficiency is thought to be a predisposing factor in abruptio placentae. So, encourage your patient to eat up!

Understanding abruptio placentae

With abruptio placentae, lack of resiliency or abnormal changes in uterine vasculature cause blood vessels at the placental bed to rupture spontaneously. Hypertension and an enlarged uterus that can't contract sufficiently to seal off the torn blood vessels further complicate the situation. As a result, bleeding continues unchecked, potentially shearing off part or all of the placenta.

External versus internal
About 80% of bleeding is external or marginal, meaning that a peripheral portion of the placenta separates from the uterine wall. The bleeding is internal or concealed if the central portion of the placenta becomes detached and the still-intact peripheral portions trap the blood. This occurs in about 20% of cases.

Effects of bleeding
As blood enters the muscle fibers, detached and still-intact peripheral portions of the placenta trap the blood. Complete relaxation of the uterus becomes impossible. Uterine tone and irritability increase. If bleeding into the muscle fibers is profuse, the uterus turns blue or purple and the accumulated blood prevents its normal contractions after delivery (known as *Couvelaire uterus* or *uteroplacental apoplexy*).

• pressure on the venae cavae from an enlarged uterus. (See *Understanding abruptio placentae.*)

What to look for

Abruptio placentae produces a wide range of signs and symptoms, depending on the extent of placental separation and the amount of blood lost from maternal circulation. In addition to the major complications of abruptio placentae—hemorrhage and shock—it may also cause renal failure, pituitary necrosis (Sheehan's syndrome), disseminated intravascular coagulation (DIC), and maternal and fetal death.

Only three degrees

Three degrees of separation can occur with abruptio placentae:

Mild abruptio placentae (marginal separation) develops gradually and produces mild to moderate bleeding, vague lower abdominal discomfort, mild to moderate abdominal tenderness, and uterine irritability. Fetal heart tones remain strong and regular.

Moderate abruptio placentae (about 50% placental separation) may develop gradually or abruptly and produces continuous abdominal pain, moderate dark red vaginal bleeding, a tender uterus that remains firm between contractions, barely audible or irregular and bradycardic fetal heart tones, and possibly signs of

Placental separation in abruptio placentae

Below are descriptions and illustrations of the three degrees of placental separation in abruptio placentae.

Mild separation

Mild separation begins with small areas of separation and internal bleeding (concealed hemorrhage) between the placenta and uterine wall.

Moderate separation

Moderate separation may develop abruptly or progress from mild to extensive separation with external hemorrhage.

Severe separation

With severe separation, external hemorrhage occurs, along with shock and, possibly, fetal cardiac distress.

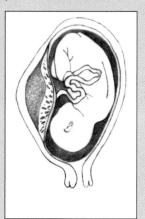

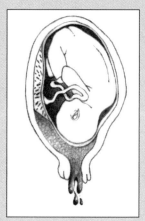

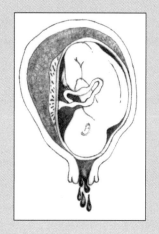

shock. Labor usually starts within 2 hours and usually proceeds rapidly.

Severe abruptio placentae (70% placental separation) develops abruptly and causes agonizing, unremitting uterine pain (described as tearing or knifelike); a boardlike, tender uterus; moderate vaginal bleeding; rapidly progressive shock; and absence of fetal heart tones. (See *Placental separation in abruptio placentae.*)

As abruptio placentae becomes more severe, I'm at greater risk for cardiac distress.

What tests tell you

Pelvic examination (in preparation for emergency cesarean delivery) and ultrasonography are performed to rule out placenta previa. Decreased hemoglobin levels and platelet counts support the diagnosis. Periodic assays for fibrin split products aid in monitoring the progression of abruptio placentae and in detecting DIC.

Differential diagnosis excludes placenta previa, ovarian cysts, appendicitis, and degeneration of leiomyomas.

How it's treated

Treatment of abruptio placentae focuses on assessing, controlling, and restoring the amount of blood lost; delivering a viable neonate; and preventing coagulation disorders.

Top priorities

Immediate measures for abruptio placentae include:
• starting an I.V. infusion (through a large-bore catheter) of lactated Ringer's solution to combat hypovolemia
• placing a central venous pressure (CVP) line and urinary catheter to monitor fluid status
• drawing blood for hemoglobin level, hematocrit, coagulation studies, and typing and crossmatching
• external electronic fetal monitoring and monitoring of maternal vital signs and vaginal bleeding.

Delivery details

After the severity of abruption has been determined and fluid and blood has been replaced, prompt cesarean delivery is necessary if the fetus is in distress. If the fetus isn't in distress, monitoring continues; delivery (vaginal or cesarean) is usually performed at the first sign of fetal distress.

Because of possible fetal blood loss through the placenta, a pediatric team should be ready at delivery to assess and treat the neonate for shock, blood loss, and hypoxia. If placental separation is severe and no signs of fetal life are present, vaginal delivery may be performed unless uncontrolled hemorrhage or other complications contraindicate it.

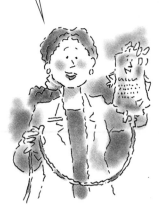

One of the top priorities for treating abruptio placentae is to start an I.V. infusion of lactated Ringer's solution.

What to do

• Assess the patient's extent of bleeding and monitor fundal height every 30 minutes for changes. Count the number of perineal pads used by the patient, weighing them as needed to determine the amount of blood loss.
• Monitor maternal blood pressure, pulse rate, respirations, CVP, intake and output, and amount of vaginal bleeding every 10 to 15 minutes.
• Begin electronic fetal monitoring to assess fetal heart rate (FHR) continuously.

• Have equipment for emergency cesarean delivery readily available.

• If vaginal delivery is elected, provide emotional support during labor. Because of the neonate's prematurity, the mother may not receive analgesics during labor and may experience intense pain. Reassure the patient of her progress through labor, and keep her informed of the fetus's condition.

• Prepare the patient and her family for the possibility of an emergency cesarean delivery of a premature neonate and the changes to expect in the postpartum period. Offer emotional support and an honest assessment of the situation.

• Tactfully discuss the possibility of neonatal death. Tell the mother that the neonate's survival depends primarily on gestational age, the amount of blood lost, and associated hypertensive disorders. Assure her that frequent monitoring and prompt management greatly reduce the risk of death.

• Encourage the patient and her family to verbalize their feelings.

• Help the patient and her family develop effective coping strategies. Refer them for counseling if necessary.

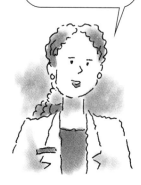

Provide emotional support to the mother during a vaginal delivery, and keep her informed of the fetus's condition.

Cardiac disease

The pregnant woman with preexisting cardiac disease is considered high-risk. Despite improvements in early identification and management of cardiac problems, these disorders contribute to complications in approximately 1% of pregnancies.

Rating the risk

The type and extent of the woman's cardiac disease determines whether she can successfully complete a pregnancy. Guidelines developed by the New York Heart Association are commonly used to predict a pregnancy's outcome. These guidelines categorize pregnancy based on the degree of compromise. (See *Cardiac disease classification*, page 220.)

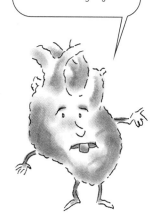

Because more women are becoming pregnant at an older age, incidence of cardiac disease in pregnancy is increasing. Oy.

What causes it

The most common underlying cause of cardiac disease in pregnancy involves congenital anomalies, such as atrial septal defect and coarctation of the aorta that hasn't been corrected. Valvular disease caused by rheumatic fever or Kawasaki disease may also be an underlying problem. Moreover, with an increase in the number of women becoming pregnant at an older age, the incidences

Cardiac disease classification

Below are the New York Heart Association's guidelines for classifying the degree of compromise in a pregnant woman with cardiac disease. Typically, a woman with Class I or II cardiac disease can complete a pregnancy and delivery without major complications. A woman with Class III cardiac disease usually must maintain complete bed rest during the pregnancy. A woman with Class IV cardiac disease is a poor candidate for pregnancy and should be strongly urged to avoid becoming pregnant.

Class	Description
I	*Uncompromised*—The woman has unrestricted physical activity. Ordinary physical activity causes no discomfort, cardiac insufficiency, or anginal pain.
II	*Slightly compromised*—The woman has a slight limitation on physical activity. Ordinary activity causes excess fatigue, palpitations, dyspnea, or anginal pain.
III	*Markedly compromised*—The woman has a moderate or marked limitation on physical activity. With less than ordinary activity, she experiences excessive fatigue, palpitations, dyspnea, or anginal pain.
IV	*Severely compromised*—The woman can't engage in any physical activity without experiencing discomfort. Cardiac insufficiency or anginal pain occurs even at rest.

Adapted with permission from Criteria Committee of the New York Heart Association. *Nomenclature and Criteria for Diagnosis of Diseases of the Heart and Great Vessels*, 9th ed. Boston, Mass: Little, Brown, & Co., 1994:253-256.

of ischemic cardiac disease and myocardial infarction are increasing.

On rare occasion

Peripartal cardiomyopathy (cardiac disease that manifests primarily with pregnancy) is rare. Although the exact cause is unknown, it's believed to result from the effects of pregnancy on the circulatory system. In many cases, previously undiagnosed cardiac disease is the cause.

What to look for

Signs and symptoms of cardiac disease in a pregnant woman depend on the type and severity of the underlying disease. Primarily, these signs and symptoms are those associated with heart failure. (See *The weaker weeks*.) Fetal signs of maternal cardiac disease

> ## The weaker weeks
>
> The most dangerous time for a pregnant woman with cardiac disease and her fetus is between 28 and 32 weeks' gestation. During this time, blood volume peaks and the woman's heart may be unable to compensate adequately for the increase. As a result, cardiac decompensation can occur, causing the woman's cardiac output to drop, possibly to such an extent that perfusion to vital organs, including the placenta, is significantly affected. Consequently, oxygen and nutrients aren't delivered in adequate amounts to the cells, including those of the fetus.

are nonspecific, such as abnormally low FHR and fetal growth retardation, so diagnosis depends mainly on maternal signs and symptoms.

Failure to the left

Left-sided heart failure occurs with such conditions as mitral valve disorder and congenital coarctation of the aorta. Common signs and symptoms are those associated with pulmonary hypertension and pulmonary edema and may include:
- decreased systemic blood pressure
- productive cough with blood-streaked sputum
- tachypnea
- dyspnea on exertion, progressing to dyspnea at rest
- tachycardia
- orthopnea
- paroxysmal nocturnal dyspnea
- edema.

Failure to the right

Right-sided heart failure can occur in a woman with a congenital heart defect, such as atrial and ventricular septal defect and pulmonary valve stenosis. Signs and symptoms may include:
- hypotension
- jugular vein distention
- liver and spleen enlargement
- ascites
- dyspnea and pain.

My, oh, myocardial failure

For the woman with peripartal cardiac disease, signs and symptoms typically reflect myocardial failure. Shortness of breath, chest pain, and edema are common. Cardiomegaly also may occur.

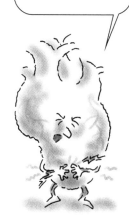

I've got coarctation to the left of me, defects to the right. Here I am, stuck in the middle.

What tests tell you

An electrocardiogram (ECG) may show cardiac changes in the mother but may be less accurate later in pregnancy as the enlarged uterus pushes the diaphragm upward and displaces the heart. Echocardiography shows cardiomegaly. If the mother's cardiac decompensation has reached the point of placental insufficiency and incompetency, late decelerations during fetal monitoring may indicate fetal distress. Ultrasonography may show growth retardation.

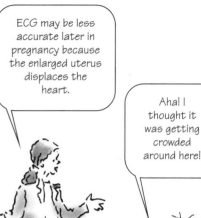

How it's treated

Treatment focuses on ensuring the health and safety of the mother and fetus. Commonly, more frequent prenatal visits are scheduled, such as every 2 weeks and then every week during the last month, to achieve this goal.

Minor adjustments

If the woman was taking cardiac medications before becoming pregnant, the medications are typically continued during pregnancy. However, maintenance doses may need to be increased to aid in compensating for the increased blood volume associated with pregnancy.

The deal with other drugs

If the patient required digoxin before her pregnancy, she can continue use during pregnancy without risk. Even if she wasn't taking digoxin before her pregnancy, she may require it to help increase or strengthen her cardiac output as her pregnancy advances. The effects on pregnancy of propranolol (Inderal), a beta-adrenergic blocker commonly used for cardiac arrhythmias, aren't known; however, the drug doesn't appear to cause fetal abnormalities. The effects of nitroglycerin, a compound commonly prescribed for angina, are also unknown; however, the drug appears to be safe. A woman who's taking heparin for venous thromboembolitic disease shouldn't take any after labor begins. If the woman has had a valve replacement and is receiving warfarin (Coumadin) therapy, warfarin — which is associated with an increase in fetal anomalies — is discontinued and heparin is used instead.

Prophylactic tactics

For women with valvular or congenital cardiac disease, some doctors may begin prophylactic antibiotic therapy near to the patient's expected due date to prevent the development of possible subacute bacterial endocarditis secondary to bacterial invasion from the placental site into the bloodstream. If the woman was taking prophylactic antibiotics to prevent a recurrence of rheumatic fever before becoming pregnant, they're continued during pregnancy.

Rest for the weary

Another key area of treatment is rest. A pregnant woman with cardiac disease requires more rest than the average pregnant woman. In addition, doctors commonly recommend complete bed rest for the woman after gestational week 30 to ensure that the woman carries the fetus to term or to at least week 36, thus helping to ensure that the fetus is mature.

> Doctors recommend complete bed rest after week 30 for a pregnant woman with cardiac disease.

Sustaining the heart

Maintaining good nutrition is an important component of ensuring a healthy mother and fetus. Weight gain must be balanced to ensure that the nutritional needs of the mother and fetus are met, while also ensuring that the mother's heart isn't overburdened. As a general practice, salt intake may be limited; however, it shouldn't be severely restricted because sodium is needed for fluid volume. Prenatal vitamins are essential to help ensure adequate iron intake and avoid anemia, which reduces the blood's capacity to carry oxygen. The pregnant woman with cardiac disease and her fetus need as much oxygen as possible, so anemia must be avoided.

> Maintaining good nutrition helps make my job a little easier!

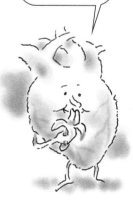

What to do

- Assess maternal vital signs and cardiopulmonary status closely for changes; question the patient about increased shortness of breath, palpitations, or edema; monitor FHR for changes.
- Monitor weight gain throughout pregnancy. Assess for edema and note any pitting.
- Explain signs and symptoms of worsening disease and tell the patient to report them immediately.
- Reinforce use of prescribed medications to control cardiac disease. Explain possible adverse reactions to these medications and instruct the patient to report these reactions immediately.
- Anticipate the need for increased doses of maintenance medications; explain to the patient the rationale for this increase.

• Assess nutritional pattern. Work with the patient to develop a feasible meal plan. Stress the need for prenatal vitamins.
• Assess FHR and ultrasound results to monitor fetal growth.
• Encourage frequent rest periods throughout the day. Discuss measures for pacing activities and conserving energy.
• Advise the woman to immediately report signs and symptoms of infection, such as upper respiratory or urinary tract infection (UTI), to prevent overtaxing the heart.
• Advise the woman to rest in the left lateral recumbent position to prevent supine hypotension and provide the best possible oxygen exchange to the fetus; if necessary, use semi-Fowler's position to relieve dyspnea.
• Prepare the woman for labor, anticipating the use of epidural anesthesia to avoid overtaxing the patient's heart.
• Monitor FHR, uterine contractions, and maternal vital signs closely for changes during labor.
• Assess vital signs closely after delivery. Anticipate anticoagulant and cardiac glycoside therapy immediately after delivery for the woman with severe heart failure.
• Encourage ambulation, as ordered, as soon as possible after delivery.
• Anticipate administration of prophylactic antibiotics, if not already ordered, after delivery to prevent subacute bacterial endocarditis.

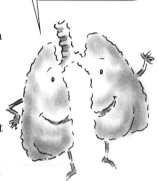

Tell the pregnant woman with cardiac disease to immediately report signs of upper respiratory tract infection or other infection.

Diabetes mellitus

Diabetes mellitus is a metabolic disorder characterized by hyperglycemia (elevated serum glucose level) resulting from lack of insulin, lack of insulin effect, or both. It's a disorder of carbohydrate, protein, and fat metabolism.

Three general classifications are recognized:

Type 1 diabetes (absolute insulin insufficiency) usually occurs before age 30, although it may occur at any age. The patient is typically thin and requires exogenous insulin and dietary management to achieve control.

Type 2 diabetes (insulin resistance with varying degrees of insulin secretory defects) usually occurs in obese adults after age 40. It's treated with diet and exercise in combination with various antidiabetic drugs, although treatment may also include insulin therapy.

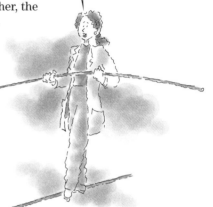

Mom and baby can be adversely affected by poor glucose control. The key is to maintain balance between glucose levels and insulin.

 Gestational diabetes (diabetes that emerges during pregnancy) typically develops during the middle of the pregnancy when insulin resistance is most apparent.

Losing balance

Diabetes affects approximately 2% to 5% of all pregnancies. The overall problem associated with diabetes and pregnancy is controlling the balance between glucose levels and insulin requirements. Poor glucose control can adversely affect the mother, the fetus, or both. The risk of PIH and infection (most commonly candidal infections) is higher in pregnant women with diabetes. Moreover, continued fetal consumption of glucose may lead to maternal hypoglycemia, especially between meals and during the night. Additionally, polyhydramnios (increased amount of amniotic fluid) may occur because of increased fetal urine production caused by fetal hyperglycemia.

Neonates who are born to mothers with poorly controlled diabetes typically are large, possibly more than 10 lb (4.5 kg). This large size may complicate labor and delivery, necessitating a cesarean birth. The risks of congenital anomalies, spontaneous abortions, and stillbirths also increase in women with poorly controlled or uncontrolled diabetes.

What causes it

Evidence indicates that diabetes mellitus has various causes, including:
- heredity
- environment (infection, diet, exposure to toxins and stress)
- lifestyle in genetically susceptible persons.

Deficient

Although the cause of type 1 diabetes isn't known, scientists believe that the tendency to develop diabetes may be inherited and related to viruses. In persons with a supposed genetic predisposition to type 1 diabetes, a triggering event (possibly infection with a virus) spurs the production of autoantibodies that destroy the pancreas's beta cells. The destruction of beta cells causes insulin secretion to decrease or ultimately stop. When more than 90% of the beta cells have been destroyed, the subsequent insulin deficiency leads to hyperglycemia, enhanced lipolysis (decomposition of fat), and protein catabolism.

Resistant

Type 2 diabetes is a chronic disease caused by one or more of these factors:
- impaired insulin production
- inappropriate hepatic glucose production
- peripheral insulin receptor insensitivity
- history of gestational diabetes
- stress.

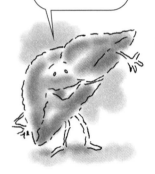

Inappropriate glucose production can cause type 2 diabetes. Oops!

Intolerant

Gestational diabetes occurs when a woman who hasn't been previously diagnosed with diabetes shows glucose intolerance during pregnancy. Of those women who don't have diabetes when they become pregnant, approximately 3% develop gestational diabetes. It isn't known whether gestational diabetes results from inadequate insulin response to carbohydrates, excessive insulin resistance, or both. Identifiable risk factors include:
- obesity
- history of delivering large neonates (usually more than 10 lb [4.5 kg]), unexplained fetal or perinatal loss, or evidence of congenital anomalies in previous pregnancies
- age older than 25
- family history of diabetes.

What to look for

The signs and symptoms noted in the pregnant woman with diabetes are the same as those for any person with diabetes. Common signs and symptoms include hyperglycemia, glycosuria, and polyuria. Dizziness and confusion may be related to hyperglycemia. In addition, the woman may experience an increased incidence of monilial infections. Hydramnios may be present along with poor FHR and variability arising from inadequate tissue (placental) perfusion.

The woman with type 1 or 2 diabetes may also exhibit signs and symptoms related to microvascular and macrovascular changes, such as peripheral vascular disease, retinopathy, nephropathy, and neuropathy.

What tests tell you

All women are screened for gestational diabetes during pregnancy. Testing typically occurs between weeks 24 and 28 and may be repeated at week 32 if the woman is obese or older than age 40. If the woman has risk factors for gestational diabetes, this screening

Glucose challenge values in pregnancy

Below are normal values for pregnant patients taking the oral glucose challenge test to determine risk of diabetes. These values are determined after a 100-g glucose load. Normal blood glucose levels should remain between 90 and 120 mg/dl. If a pregnant woman's plasma glucose value exceeds these levels, she should be treated as a potential diabetic.

Test type	Pregnancy glucose level (mg/dl)
Fasting	95
1 hour	180
2 hour	155
3 hour	140

takes place at the first prenatal visit and again between weeks 24 and 28.

The glucose challenge

Screening involves an oral glucose challenge test (a test that obtains a fasting plasma glucose level) using 100-g glucose load. One hour after ingestion, a venous blood sample is obtained. If the glucose level is greater than 180 mg/dl, the woman is scheduled for a 3-hour glucose tolerance test using a 100-g glucose load. Two abnormal levels or a fasting glucose level greater than 95 mg/dl confirms a diagnosis of gestational diabetes. (See *Glucose challenge values in pregnancy*.)

If the woman is known to have diabetes, serial blood glucose monitoring and measurement of glycosylated hemoglobin levels are used to determine the degree of glucose control.

How it's treated

Any woman with diabetes, whether preexisting or gestational, requires more frequent prenatal visits to ensure optimal control of glucose levels, minimizing the risks to the woman and her fetus. Additionally, treatment focuses on balancing rest with exercise and maintaining adequate nutrition for fetal growth and control of blood glucose levels.

Ideally, the woman with preexisting diabetes should consult with her doctor before becoming pregnant to ensure the best possible health for herself and her fetus. At that time, blood glucose levels can be assessed closely and medication adjustments can be made to ensure optimal regulation before she becomes pregnant.

Diet right

Nutritional therapy is crucial in the treatment of women with diabetes. Typically, an 1,800- to 2,200-calorie diet is prescribed for the pregnant woman with diabetes. Alternatively, caloric requirements may be calculated at 35 kcal/kg of ideal body weight. The caloric requirement is usually divided among three meals and three snacks, allowing the calories to be distributed throughout the day in an attempt to maintain constant glucose levels.

Additional dietary recommendations include reduced saturated fat and cholesterol and increased dietary fiber. Carbohydrates should make up more than half of daily caloric intake, with protein and fat supplying the remainder. The goal is to allow a weight gain of approximately 25 to 30 lb (11.3 to 13.6 kg) so that the neonate doesn't grow too large and vaginal delivery remains a possibility.

Slight modifications

For the woman with preexisting diabetes, insulin adjustments are necessary. Early in pregnancy, insulin may be reduced because of the increased utilization of glucose by the fetus for growth. However, later in pregnancy, an increase in insulin typically occurs because of an increase in the woman's metabolism. Insulin therapy dosages and types are highly individualized. A continuous subcutaneous insulin infusion via a pump may be ordered to maintain constant blood glucose levels. The woman with gestational diabetes may require insulin if diet therapy doesn't adequately control blood glucose levels.

Check 1: Glucose levels

To assist with blood glucose control, fingerstick blood glucose monitoring is important. For the woman with preexisting diabetes, typically this monitoring is performed daily, possibly as often as four times per day. For women with gestational diabetes, however, blood glucose monitoring may be performed only weekly. Regardless of monitoring frequency, the goal is to obtain fasting blood glucose levels below 95 mg/dl and 2-hour postprandial values below 120 mg/dl.

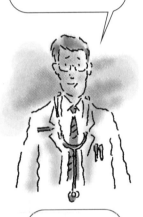

A woman with preexisting diabetes should consult with her doctor before becoming pregnant.

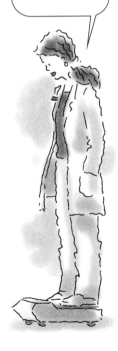

Pregnant patients with diabetes should allow for a weight gain of about 25 to 30 lb.

Check 2: Eyes and urinary tract

Throughout the pregnancy, follow-up monitoring is performed. A urine culture may be done each trimester to detect UTIs that produce no symptoms. Ophthalmic examination is done at each trimester for the woman with preexisting diabetes and at least once during the pregnancy for the woman with gestational diabetes. Retinal changes may develop or progress during pregnancy.

Check 3: The fetus

Because the risk of fetal complications is high, fetal monitoring is crucial. A serum alpha-fetoprotein level may be done at 15 to 17 weeks' gestation to assess for neural tube defects. Ultrasonography may be done at 18 to 20 weeks to detect gross abnormalities, and then be repeated at 28 weeks and again at 36 to 38 weeks to determine fetal growth, amniotic fluid volume, placental location, and biparietal diameter. At 36 weeks, the woman may undergo an amniocentesis to assess the lecithin-sphingomyelin ratio, an indicator of fetal maturity.

Delivery time

In the past, delivery occurred at approximately 37 weeks' gestation via cesarean birth. More recently, however, vaginal delivery has become the preferred route of delivery. During labor, uterine contractions and FHR are monitored continuously. The mother's glucose level is regulated with I.V. infusions of regular insulin based on blood glucose levels that are obtained hourly.

What to do

- Carefully monitor the woman's weight gain, blood glucose levels, and nutritional intake as well as fetal growth parameters throughout pregnancy.
- Review results of fingerstick blood glucose monitoring; assess for signs and symptoms of hypoglycemia and hyperglycemia.
- Assist with scheduling of follow-up laboratory studies, including glycosylated hemoglobin levels and urine studies as necessary.
- Encourage the patient to maintain a consistent exercise program and explain the benefits of eating certain snacks before exercise. (See *Preventing hypoglycemia during exercise.*)
- Instruct the woman in all aspects of managing diabetes, including insulin administration techniques, self-monitoring, nutrition, and danger signs and symptoms. (See *Teaching topics for pregnant patients with diabetes*, page 230.)
- Assist with preparations for labor, including explanations about possible labor induction and required monitoring.

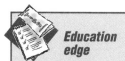

Education edge

Preventing hypoglycemia during exercise

Hypoglycemia during exercise is a common problem for patients with diabetes but one that has an easy solution, if the patient is careful.

The problem

During exercise, the muscles increase their uptake of glucose, causing blood glucose levels to decrease. This effect can last up to 12 hours after exercise. In addition, if the woman injects insulin into the extremity involved in exercise, the insulin is released more quickly. As a result, blood glucose levels decrease even more dramatically, causing hypoglycemia.

The solution

To prevent hypoglycemia, encourage the patient with diabetes to eat a snack consisting of a protein or a complex carbohydrate before she exercises and to maintain a consistent exercise pattern each day.

Education edge

Teaching topics for pregnant patients with diabetes

Be sure to cover the following topics when teaching a pregnant patient with diabetes:
• insulin type and dosage
• insulin syringe preparation and injection technique or insulin pump use and care
• sites to use (Most women prefer not to use the abdomen as an injection site.)
• site rotation (Insulin is absorbed more slowly from the thigh than from the upper arm.)
• blood glucose monitoring technique, including frequency of monitoring and desired glucose levels
• nutritional plan, including suggestions for ap-

propriate foods to include and avoid
• consistent exercise regimen
• signs and symptoms of urinary tract and monilial infections, including the need to report one immediately
• signs and symptoms of hypoglycemia and hyperglycemia
• measures to prevent and manage hypoglycemia and hyperglycemia
• fetal monitoring methods, including fetal movement count and follow-up testing
• preparations for labor and delivery
• care after delivery.

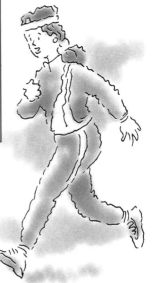

Encourage the pregnant patient with diabetes to maintain a consistent exercise program.

• Closely assess the woman in the postpartum period for changes in blood glucose levels and insulin requirements. Typically the woman with preexisting diabetes will require no insulin in the immediate postpartum period (because insulin resistance is gone), and won't return to her prepregnancy insulin requirements for several days. The woman with gestational diabetes usually exhibits normal blood glucose levels within 24 hours after delivery, requiring no further insulin or diet therapy.
• Encourage the patient with gestational diabetes to keep all follow-up appointments so that glucose testing can be performed to detect possible type 2 diabetes.

Ectopic pregnancy

Ectopic pregnancy is the implantation of a fertilized ovum outside the uterine cavity. It most commonly occurs in the fallopian tube but may occur in other sites as well. (See *Sites of ectopic pregnancy.*)

Ectopic pregnancy occurs in 1 of every 200 white women and about 1 of every 120 nonwhite women. The prognosis for the patient is good with prompt diagnosis, appropriate surgical intervention, and control of bleeding. Rarely, in cases of abdominal implantation, the fetus may survive to term. Usually, only 1 in 3

Sites of ectopic pregnancy

In most women with ectopic pregnancy, the ovum implants in the fallopian tube, either in the fimbria, ampulla, or isthmus. Other possible sites of implantation include the interstitium, tubo-ovarian ligament, ovary, abdominal viscera, and internal cervical os.

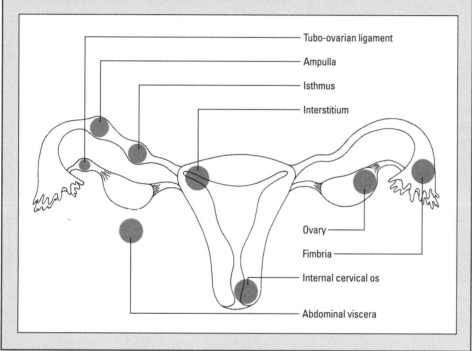

- Tubo-ovarian ligament
- Ampulla
- Isthmus
- Interstitium
- Ovary
- Fimbria
- Internal cervical os
- Abdominal viscera

Prognosis for the patient with ectopic pregnancy is good with prompt diagnosis and appropriate intervention.

women who experience an ectopic pregnancy give birth to a live neonate in a subsequent pregnancy. Rupture of the tube causes life-threatening complications, including hemorrhage, shock, and peritonitis. Infertility results if the uterus, both fallopian tubes, or both ovaries are removed.

What causes it

Conditions that prevent or slow the fertilized ovum's passage through the fallopian tube into the uterine cavity include:
- endosalpingitis, an inflammatory reaction that causes folds of the tubal mucosa to agglutinate, narrowing the tube
- diverticula (blind pouches that cause tubal abnormalities)
- tumors pressing against the tube
- previous surgery, such as tubal ligation or resection, or adhesions from previous abdominal or pelvic surgery

• transmigration of the ovum from one ovary to the opposite tube resulting in delayed implantation.

Ectopic pregnancy may also result from congenital defects in the reproductive tract or ectopic endometrial implants in the tubal mucosa. Additional factors include sexually transmitted tubal infections as well as intrauterine devices that cause irritation of the cellular lining of the uterus and the fallopian tubes.

What to look for

Symptoms of ectopic pregnancy are sometimes similar to those of a normal pregnancy, making diagnosis difficult. Mild abdominal pain may occur, especially in cases of abdominal pregnancy. Typically, the patient reports amenorrhea or abnormal menses (in cases of fallopian tube implantation), followed by slight vaginal bleeding and unilateral pelvic pain over the mass. During a pelvic examination, the patient may report extreme pain when the cervix is moved and the adnexa is palpated. The uterus feels boggy and is tender. The patient may complain of lower abdominal pain precipitated by activities that increase abdominal pressure, such as a bowel movement.

No time to waste

If the tube ruptures, the patient may complain of sharp lower abdominal pain, possibly radiating to the shoulders and neck. This condition is an emergent situation that requires immediate transport to a clinic or hospital.

Complaints of sharp lower abdominal pain indicate tube rupture, a medical emergency!

CAUTION!

What tests tell you

Differential diagnosis is necessary to rule out intrauterine pregnancy, ovarian cyst or tumor, pelvic inflammatory disease (PID), appendicitis, and spontaneous abortion. The following tests confirm ectopic pregnancy:
• Serum pregnancy test results show an abnormally low level of human chorionic gonadotropin (hCG) that remains lower than that in a normal intrauterine pregnancy when the test is repeated in 48 hours.
• Real-time ultrasonography performed after a positive serum pregnancy test detects intrauterine pregnancy or ovarian cyst.
• Culdocentesis (aspiration of fluid from the vaginal cul-de-sac) detects free blood in the peritoneum. This test is performed if ultrasonography detects the absence of a gestational sac in the uterus.

• Laparoscopy, performed if culdocentesis is positive, may reveal pregnancy outside the uterus.

How it's treated

If culdocentesis shows blood in the peritoneum, laparotomy and salpingectomy (excision of the fallopian tube) are indicated, possibly preceded by laparoscopy to remove the affected fallopian tube and control bleeding. Patients who wish to have children can undergo microsurgical repair of the fallopian tube. The ovary is saved, if possible; however, ovarian pregnancy requires oophorectomy. Interstitial pregnancy may require hysterectomy. Abdominal pregnancy requires a laparotomy to remove the fetus, except in rare cases, when the fetus survives to term or calcifies undetected in the abdominal cavity.

See ya, cells

Nonsurgical management of ectopic pregnancy involves oral administration of methotrexate (Folex), a chemotherapeutic drug and folic acid inhibitor that stops cell reproduction. The drug destroys remaining trophoblastic tissue, thus avoiding the need for laparotomy.

Methotrexate stops cell reproduction in ectopic pregnancy.

Support, in short

Supportive treatment includes whole blood or packed red blood cells (RBCs) to replace excessive blood loss, broad-spectrum I.V. antibiotics for sepsis, supplemental iron (either oral or I.M.), and a high-protein diet. Grief counseling for the loss of a wanted child is also recommended.

What to do

• Ask the patient the date of her last menses, and obtain serum hCG levels as ordered.
• Assess vital signs, and monitor vaginal bleeding for extent of fluid loss.
• Check the amount, color, and odor of vaginal bleeding; monitor perineal pad count.
• Withhold food and fluid orally in anticipation of possible surgery. Prepare the patient for surgery as indicated.
• Assess for signs and symptoms of hypovolemic shock secondary to blood loss from tubal rupture. Monitor closely for decreased urine output, which suggests fluid volume deficit.
• Administer blood transfusions, as ordered, and provide emotional support.

• Record the location and character of the pain, and administer analgesics as ordered.

• Determine if the patient is Rh-negative. If she is, administer $Rh_o(D)$ immune globulin (human), also known as RhoGAM, as ordered after treatment or surgery.

• Provide a quiet, relaxing environment and encourage the patient and her partner to express their feelings of fear, loss, and grief. Help the patient to develop effective coping strategies. Refer her to a mental health professional for additional counseling if necessary.

• To prevent recurrent ectopic pregnancy from diseases of the fallopian tube, urge the patient to get prompt treatment of pelvic infections.

• Inform patients who have undergone surgery involving the fallopian tubes or those with confirmed PID that they're at increased risk for another ectopic pregnancy.

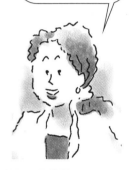

Providing a relaxing environment helps the patient and her partner express feelings of fear, loss, and grief.

Folic acid deficiency anemia

Folic acid deficiency anemia is a common, slowly progressive, megaloblastic (involving enlarged RBCs) anemia. Folic acid, or folacin, is a B vitamin needed for RBC formation and deoxyribonucleic acid (DNA) synthesis. It's also thought to play a role in preventing neural tube defects in the developing fetus.

Where it acts

Folic acid is found in most body tissues. It acts as a coenzyme in metabolic processes. Although its body stores are relatively small, folic acid can be found in most well-balanced diets. Even so, folic acid is water soluble and is affected by heat, so it's easily destroyed by cooking. Moreover, about 20% of folic acid intake is excreted unabsorbed. Insufficient intake—typically less than 50 mcg/day—usually results in folic acid deficiency anemia within 4 months.

Folic acid deficiency anemia is a risk factor in approximately 1% to 5% of pregnancies, becoming most apparent during the second trimester. It's believed to be a risk factor contributing to early spontaneous abortion and abruptio placentae.

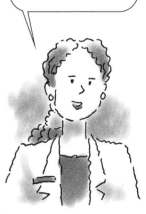

Folic acid deficiency anemia is believed to be a risk factor contributing to spontaneous abortion and abruptio placentae.

What causes it

Alcohol abuse, which suppresses the metabolic effects of folic acid, is probably the most common cause of folic acid deficiency anemia. During pregnancy, folic acid deficiency anemia occurs most commonly in women with multiple pregnancy, probably because of the increased fetal demand for folic acid. Folic acid deficiency anemia is also seen in women who have underlying hemolytic illness that results in rapid destruction and production of RBCs. In addition, certain drugs—such as phenytoin (Dilantin), an anticonvulsant agent that interferes with folate absorption, and hormonal contraceptives—have a role in folic acid deficiency anemia.

What to look for

The main symptom of folic acid deficiency anemia is a history of severe, progressive fatigue. Associated findings include shortness of breath, palpitations, diarrhea, nausea, anorexia, headaches, forgetfulness, and irritability. The impaired oxygen-carrying capacity of the blood from lowered hemoglobin levels may produce complaints of weakness and light-headedness.

Assessment may reveal generalized pallor and jaundice. The patient may also appear wasted. Cheilosis and glossitis may be present. Neurologic impairment is present only if the folic acid deficiency anemia is associated with a vitamin B_{12} deficiency.

What tests tell you

Typically, blood studies reveal:
- macrocytic RBCs
- decreased reticulocyte count
- increase mean corpuscular volume
- abnormal platelet count
- decreased serum folate levels (below 4 mg/ml).

How it's treated

During pregnancy, treatment consists primarily of folic acid supplements. Supplements may be given orally or parenterally (for patients who are severely ill, have malabsorption, or can't take oral medication). In addition, a diet high in folic acid is urged. Many patients respond favorably to a well-balanced diet.

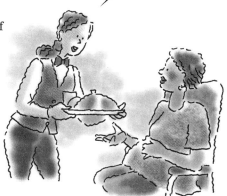

Many patients with folic acid deficiency anemia respond favorably to a well-balanced diet.

Education edge

Foods high in folic acid

If your patient is planning to become pregnant or is pregnant, encourage her to eat these foods high in folic acid to help prevent folic acid deficiency anemia:

- asparagus
- beef liver
- broccoli
- green leafy vegetables such as collards
- mushrooms
- oatmeal
- peanut butter
- red beans
- wheat germ
- whole wheat bread.

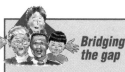

Bridging the gap

Supplement use

Prenatal vitamins are prescribed to prevent folic acid deficiency because over-the-counter (OTC) multivitamins generally don't contain adequate amounts of folic acid for pregnancy. Compliance may be an issue if the patient doesn't have the money to pay for the prescription supplements or lacks understanding of their role in preventing folic acid deficiency. Patients may substitute OTC vitamins, thinking they're just as effective as prescription vitamins. At prenatal visits, be sure to ask if the patient is taking her prescribed vitamin, and stress the importance of using prescription supplements during pregnancy.

What to do

- Strongly urge women trying to become pregnant to take a vitamin supplement or be conscious about eating foods rich in folic acid. (See *Foods high in folic acid.*)
- Assist with planning a well-balanced diet that includes meals and snacks that are high in folic acid.
- Encourage the woman to eat or drink a rich source of vitamin C at each meal to enhance absorption of folic acid.
- Administer a folic acid supplement as ordered throughout pregnancy, and assess for patient compliance. (See *Supplement use.*)
- If the patient has severe anemia and requires hospitalization, plan activities, rest periods, and diagnostic tests to conserve energy. Monitor pulse rate often. If tachycardia occurs, the patient's activities are too strenuous.
- Monitor the patient's complete blood count (CBC), platelet count, and serum folate levels as ordered.
- Assess maternal vital signs and FHR as indicated.
- Instruct the pregnant woman in the use of prescribed folic acid supplements and the need to continue taking them throughout pregnancy.

Gestational trophoblastic disease

Gestational trophoblastic disease, also called *hydatidiform mole* or *molar pregnancy*, is the rapid deterioration of trophoblastic villi cells. Trophoblast cells are located in the outer ring of the blastocyst (the structure that develops around the third or fourth day after fertilization) and eventually become part of the structure that forms the placenta and fetal membranes. As trophoblast cells begin to deteriorate, they fill with fluid. The cells become edematous, appearing as grapelike clusters of vesicles. As a result of these cell abnormalities, the embryo fails to develop past the early stages.

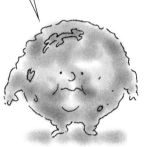

As trophoblast cells deteriorate, they fill with fluid. I'm pretty full already!

Leading to bleeding

Gestational trophoblastic disease is a major cause of second trimester bleeding. It's also associated with choriocarcinoma (a fast-growing, highly invasive malignant tumor that develops in the uterus), which is why early detection is important.

All or some

Chromosomal analysis helps classify gestational trophoblastic disease as a complete or partial mole. A complete mole is characterized by swelling and cystic formation of all trophoblastic cells. No fetal blood is present. If an embryo does develop, it's most likely only 1 to 2 mm in size and will probably die early in development. This form is associated with the development of choriocarcinoma.

A partial mole is characterized by edema of some of the trophoblastic villi with some of the normal villi. Fetal blood may be present in the villi, and an embryo up to the size of 9 weeks' gestation may be present. Typically, a partial mole has 69 chromosomes in which there are 3 chromosomes for every one pair.

Gestational trophoblastic disease is associated with the development of choriocarcinoma.

Hard to recognize

Gestational trophoblastic disease is reported to occur in about 1 in every 2,000 pregnancies. Recent research indicates that the incidence would be much higher if all cases of the disorder were identified. Some cases aren't recognized because the pregnancy is aborted early and the products of conception aren't available for analysis. The incidence is higher in women from low socioeconomic groups, older women, and multiparous women. The incidence is highest in Asian women, especially those from Southeast Asia.

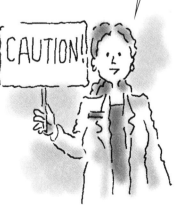

CAUTION!

What causes it

The cause of gestational trophoblastic disease is unknown. Several unconfirmed theories relate gestational trophoblastic disease to chromosomal abnormalities, hormonal imbalances, or deficiencies in protein and folic acid. About one-half of patients with choriocarcinoma have had a preceding molar pregnancy. In the remaining one-half of patients, the disease is usually preceded by a spontaneous or induced abortion, an ectopic pregnancy, or a normal pregnancy.

What to look for

A patient with gestational trophoblastic disease may report vaginal bleeding, ranging from brownish red spotting to bright red hemorrhage. She may report passing tissue that resembles grape clusters. Her history may also include hyperemesis, lower abdominal cramps (such as those that accompany spontaneous abortion), and signs and symptoms of preeclampsia.

On inspection, a uterus that's exceptionally large for the patient's gestational date is detected. Pelvic examination may reveal grapelike vesicles in the vagina. Palpation may detect ovarian enlargement caused by cysts. Auscultation of the uterus may reveal the absence of fetal heart tones that had been noted at a previous visit.

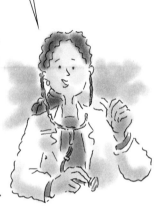

Hmmm...an exceptionally large uterus, presence of grapelike vesicles, and absence of fetal heart tones. Sounds like gestational trophoblastic disease.

What tests tell you

Differential diagnosis is necessary to rule out normal pregnancy, imminent spontaneous abortion, uterine leiomyomas, multiple pregnancy, and incorrect gestational date. The following diagnostic test results suggest the presence of gestational trophoblastic disease:
• Radioimmunoassay detects extremely elevated hCG levels for early pregnancy.
• Histologic examination confirms presence of vesicles.
• Ultrasonography performed after the 3rd month shows grapelike clusters instead of a fetus.
• Amniography (a procedure that introduces a water-soluble dye into the uterus) reveals the absence of a fetus. (This test is done only when the diagnosis is in question.)
• Doppler ultrasonography shows the absence of fetal heart tones.

• Hemoglobin level and hematocrit, RBC count, prothrombin time, partial thromboplastin time, fibrinogen levels, and hepatic and renal function findings are abnormal.
• White blood cell (WBC) count and erythrocyte sedimentation rate (ESR) are increased.

How it's treated

Gestational trophoblastic disease necessitates uterine evacuation by dilatation and suction curettage. Labor induction with oxytocin or prostaglandins is contraindicated because of the increased risk of hemorrhage.

Postoperative treatment varies, depending on the amount of blood lost and complications. If no complications develop, hospitalization is usually brief and normal activities can be resumed quickly as tolerated.

Monitoring for malignancy

Because of the possibility that choriocarcinoma will develop following gestational trophoblastic disease, scrupulous follow-up care is essential. Such care includes monitoring hCG levels once weekly until titers are negative for 3 consecutive weeks, then once monthly for 6 months, then every 2 months for 6 months.

Follow-up also includes chest X-rays to check for lung metastasis once monthly until hCG titers are negative, then once every 2 months for 1 year. Contraceptive methods are used to prevent another pregnancy until at least 1 year after all titers and X-ray findings are negative.

The role of chemo

Prophylactic chemotherapy with methotrexate or actinomycin-D (Cosmegen) after evacuation of the uterus has been successful in preventing malignant gestational trophoblastic disease. Chemotherapy and irradiation are used for metastatic choriocarcinoma.

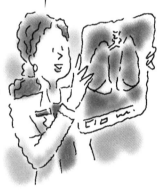

There's no sign of lung metastasis and hCG levels are negative. This patient hasn't developed choriocarcinoma.

What to do

• Assess the patient's vital signs to obtain a baseline for future comparison.
• Preoperatively, observe for signs of complications, such as hemorrhage and uterine infection, and vaginal passage of vesicles. Save any expelled tissue for laboratory analysis.
• Prepare the patient for surgery.
• Postoperatively monitor vital signs and fluid intake and output, and check for signs of hemorrhage.

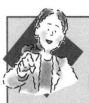

Take charge!

Monitoring hCG levels

When evaluating serum human chorionic gonadotropin (hCG) levels in a woman previously diagnosed with gestational trophoblastic disease, gradually declining levels suggest no further disease. However, if hCG levels plateau three times or increase at any time during the monitoring period, suspect the development of a malignancy.

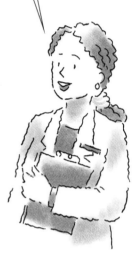

Explain to the patient the importance of reporting new symptoms promptly.

• Encourage the patient and her family to express their feelings about the disorder. Offer emotional support and help them through the grieving process.
• Help the patient and her family develop effective coping strategies. Refer them to a mental health professional for additional counseling if needed.
• Assist with obtaining baseline information—including a pelvic examination, chest X-ray, and serum hCG levels—and with ongoing monitoring. (See *Monitoring hCG levels*.)
• Stress the need for regular monitoring (hCG levels and chest X-rays) to detect malignant changes.
• Instruct the patient to report new symptoms promptly (for example, hemoptysis, cough, suspected pregnancy, nausea, vomiting, and vaginal bleeding).
• Explain to the patient that she must use contraceptives to prevent pregnancy for at least 1 year after hCG levels return to normal and her body reestablishes regular ovulation and menstrual cycles.

HELLP syndrome

HELLP is an acronym that stands for **h**emolysis, **e**levated **l**iver enzymes, and **l**ow **p**latelets. HELLP syndrome is a category of PIH that involves changes in blood components and liver function.

Temporary HELLP

HELLP syndrome develops in 12% of women with PIH. It can occur in primigravidas and multigravidas. When it occurs, maternal and infant mortality is high; approximately one-fourth of women and one-third of infants die from this disorder. However, after

Memory jogger

HELLP is an acronym that helps identify the underlying signs associated with the syndrome.

H – Hemolysis

E, L – Elevated Liver enzymes

L, P – Low Platelets

birth, laboratory results return to normal usually within 1 week and the mother experiences no further problems.

What causes it

Although the exact cause of HELLP is unknown, theories have been proposed about the development of its signs and symptoms. Hemolysis is believed to result because RBCs are damaged by their travel through small, impaired blood vessels. Elevated liver enzymes are believed to result from obstruction in liver flow by fibrin deposits. Low platelets are believed to be the result of vascular damage secondary to vasospasm. Women with severe preeclampsia are at high risk for developing HELLP syndrome.

HELLP! I've been damaged by a blood vessel!

What to look for

Typically, the patient complains of pain, most commonly in the right upper quadrant, epigastric area, or lower chest. Additional signs and symptoms include nausea, vomiting, general malaise, and severe edema. The right upper quadrant may be tender on palpation because of a distended liver. In addition, the woman exhibits signs and symptoms of preeclampsia.

What tests tell you

Laboratory studies reveal:
• hemolysis of RBCs (appearing fragmented and irregular on a peripheral blood smear)
• thrombocytopenia (a platelet count below 100,000/µl)
• elevated levels of alanine aminotransferase and serum aspartate aminotransferase.

How it's treated

Treatment involves intensive care management for the woman and her fetus. Drug therapy, such as magnesium sulfate, is instituted to reduce blood pressure and prevent seizures. Transfusions of fresh frozen plasma or platelets may be used to reverse thrombocytopenia. When the fetus has matured enough, delivery may occur vaginally or by cesarean birth.

What to do

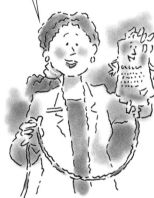

Expect to administer dextrose I.V. if hypoglycemia develops.

• Assess maternal vital signs and FHR frequently; be alert for signs and symptoms of complications, including hemorrhage, hypoglycemia, hyponatremia, subcapsular liver hematoma, and renal failure.
• Maintain a quiet, calm, dimly lit environment to reduce the risk of seizures; institute seizure precautions.
• Avoid palpating the abdomen because this increases intra-abdominal pressure, which could lead to rupture of a subcapsular liver hematoma.
• Limit visitation to maintain a quiet environment.
• Institute bleeding precautions, and monitor the patient for signs and symptoms of bleeding. Administer blood transfusions and medications as ordered.
• If the patient develops hypoglycemia, expect to administer I.V. dextrose solutions.
• Prepare the patient for delivery; explain all events and procedures being done; assist with evaluations for fetal maturity.
• Be aware that because of the increased risk of bleeding due to thrombocytopenia the woman may not be a candidate for epidural anesthesia.
• Assess the patient carefully throughout labor and delivery for possible hemorrhage.

HIV infection

HIV is the organism that causes acquired immunodeficiency syndrome (AIDS). Considered a sexually transmitted disease (STD), HIV infection can have serious implications for the pregnant woman and her fetus.

Women on the rise

Currently, women are the fastest growing segment of the population infected with HIV. Research also shows that women are diagnosed with HIV infection later in the course of the disease than men are. HIV infection and AIDS are considered the third leading cause of death in women between ages 25 and 45. Approximately 2 out of every 100 women giving birth are HIV-positive.

Still hope

Nevertheless, studies demonstrate that pregnancy doesn't accelerate progression of the infection in the mother. In addition, women who stay healthy during pregnancy reduce the risk of transmitting the virus to their fetus because the placenta provides a barrier to disease transmission. Even so, if HIV infection occurred concurrently or close to the time of conception or the mother suffers from disorders that affect placental health, such as infections unrelated to HIV or complications of advanced HIV infection (malnutrition), the placenta may not be an effective barrier.

Suspending transmission

Before advances in drug therapy, the risk of a neonate becoming infected via maternal virus transmission ranged from 25% to 35%. However, with appropriate antiviral drug therapy during and after pregnancy, the rate of possible infection has dropped to nearly 5%. Unfortunately, if infection occurs in the fetus or neonate, it progresses more quickly than in an adult.

What causes it

HIV infection is caused by a retrovirus that targets helper T-cells containing the CD4+ antigen (cells that regulate normal immune response). The virus integrates itself into the cells' genetic make-up, causing cellular dysfunction that disrupts immune response. This makes patients vulnerable to opportunistic infections.

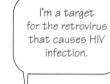

I'm a target for the retrovirus that causes HIV infection.

HIV is transmitted in several ways:
• through sexual intercourse
• through contact with infected blood
• across the placenta to the fetus during pregnancy (in cases of active disease, medication noncompliance, and placental inflammation)
• through contact during labor and delivery
• through breast milk.

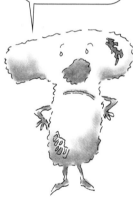

For women, heterosexual contact and injection drug use are the two major modes of HIV transmission. Other risk factors for contracting HIV include:
• history of multiple sexual partners (either in the patient or her partner)
• having bisexual partners
• use of injection drugs by the patient's partner
• blood transfusions (rare).

What to look for

Signs and symptoms of HIV infection include lymphadenopathy, bacterial pneumonia, fevers, night sweats, weight loss, dermatologic problems, thrush, thrombocytopenia, and diarrhea. In addition, women commonly experience severe vaginal yeast infections that are difficult to treat.

Other manifestations specific to women may include:

• abnormal Papanicolaou tests
• frequent human papilloma virus infections
• frequent and recurrent bacterial vaginosis, trichomonas, and genital herpes infections
• severe PID.

Pneumocystis carinii pneumonia is the most common opportunistic infection associated with female HIV infection. Cervical cancer ranks second in prevalence. Kaposi's sarcoma may also occur in women, although it's rare.

What tests tell you

In some cases, a woman doesn't know that she's HIV-positive until it's discovered at a prenatal visit, after pregnancy has begun. Positive results from two enzyme-linked immunosorbent assays that are then further confirmed by the Western Blot test classify a woman as HIV-positive. Positive status means that the woman has developed antibodies to the virus after having been exposed. In addition, CD4+ T-cell count less than 200 cells/µl and presence of one or more opportunistic infections confirms diagnosis.

Load up on viral load

Viral load testing measures the level of HIV in the blood. Although blood levels don't reflect all possible areas of HIV infection, research suggests that these levels effectively demonstrate virus levels throughout the body. This testing relies on the detection of ribonucleic acid (RNA) in HIV molecules. This RNA is responsible for replication of the virus. Scientists have a good idea of what some parts of HIV RNA look like. With this image, they can find HIV RNA in the blood of a potentially infected person. Two techniques are used to detect HIV RNA strands in a blood sample:

• Branched-chain DNA sets off a chemical reaction in the HIV RNA so it gives out light and measures the amount of light to determine the levels of HIV RNA in a sample.
• Quantitative polymerase chain reaction encourages the HIV RNA to replicate in a test tube. This replication makes it easier to measure the amount of HIV RNA that was originally in the blood sample.

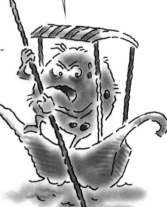

Viral load measures HIV levels in the bloodstream, which effectively indicates levels throughout the body.

How it's treated

The Centers for Disease Control and Prevention recommend treating the pregnant woman who's HIV-positive with combination antiretroviral therapy. This treatment attempts to reduce the mother's viral load and minimize the risk of transmitting the infection to the fetus.

Risky delivery

Cesarean delivery provides the lowest risk of HIV transmission from mother to fetus — lowest if performed before labor begins or membranes are ruptured. If vaginal delivery is unavoidable, episiotomy is contraindicated as well as amniocentesis and fetal monitoring via scalp electrodes. For every hour of labor after membranes rupture, the risk of transmission from mother to fetus increases by 2%.

When breast isn't best

Risk of transmission during breast-feeding depends on the mother's health, including her nutritional and immune status and viral load, as well as the length of time the child nurses at each feeding and whether the mother breast-feeds exclusively. In addition, the duration of breast-feeding impacts the likelihood of transmission. About 15% of infected mothers who breast-feed for 24 months or more transmit the infection to their neonates.

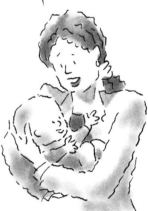

Although breast-feeding is best if the mother is healthy, mothers with HIV who breast-feed increase the risk of transmission to their infants.

Shutting the door on opportunity

Zidovudine (AZT) and didanosine (Videx) are used to slow progression of opportunistic infections such as *P. carinii* pneumonia, the most common. These drugs are given orally during pregnancy, I.V. during labor, and then to the neonate in syrup form. Co-trimoxazole (Bactrim) is also used but may be teratogenic in early pregnancy. Additionally, sulfamethoxazole may cause increased bilirubin levels in the neonate if administered late in pregnancy.

What to do

• Institute standard precautions when caring for the mother throughout the pregnancy, after delivery, and when caring for the neonate.
• Teach the pregnant woman measures to minimize the risk of virus transmission.
• Provide emotional support and guidance for the woman who's HIV-positive and considering pregnancy.

- Allow the pregnant woman who's HIV-positive to verbalize feelings and provide her with support.
- Monitor CD4+ T-cell counts and viral loads as indicated.
- Assess the patient for signs and symptoms of opportunistic infections, such as *P. carinii* pneumonia (fever, dry cough, chest discomfort, fatigue, shortness of breath on exertion and later at rest) and Kaposi's sarcoma (slightly raised, painless lesions on the skin or oral mucous membranes that are reddish or purple in fair-skinned patients and bluish or brown in dark-skinned patients; painful swelling, especially in the lower legs; nausea, vomiting, and bleeding if GI tract is involved; difficulty breathing if lungs are involved).
- Encourage the patient to keep prenatal follow-up appointments to evaluate the status of her pregnancy.
- Administer antiretroviral therapy as ordered, and instruct the patient about this regimen. Assist with scheduling medications, and evaluate for compliance on return visits.
- Institute measures during labor and delivery to minimize the fetus's risk of exposure to maternal blood or body fluids. Avoid the use of internal fetal monitors, scalp blood sampling, forceps, and vacuum extraction to prevent the creation of an open lesion on the fetal scalp.
- Advise the mother that breast-feeding isn't recommended because of the risk of transmitting the virus.
- Withhold blood sampling and injections of the neonate until maternal blood has been removed with the first bath.
- Educate the mother about the mode of HIV transmission and safer sex practices.

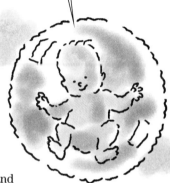

Special precautions must be taken during pregnancy to reduce my risk of contracting HIV.

Hyperemesis gravidarum

Unlike the transient nausea and vomiting that's normally experienced until about the 12th week of pregnancy, hyperemesis gravidarum is severe and unremitting nausea and vomiting that persists after the 1st trimester. It usually occurs with the first pregnancy and commonly affects pregnant women with conditions that produce high levels of hCG, such as gestational trophoblastic disease or multiple pregnancy.

This disorder occurs in about 7 out of 1,000 pregnancies in blacks and in about 16 out of 1,000 pregnancies in whites. The prognosis is usually good. However, if untreated, hyperemesis gravidarum produces substantial weight loss, starvation with ketosis and acetonuria, dehydration with subsequent fluid and electrolyte imbalance (hypokalemia), and acid-base disturbances (acidosis and alkalosis). Retinal, neurologic, and renal damage may also occur.

What causes it

The specific cause of hyperemesis gravidarum is unknown. Possible causes include pancreatitis (elevated serum amylase levels are common), biliary tract disease, decreased secretion of free hydrochloric acid in the stomach, decreased gastric motility, drug toxicity, inflammatory obstructive bowel disease, and vitamin deficiency (especially B_6). In some patients, this disorder may be related to psychological factors.

What to look for

The patient typically complains of unremitting nausea and vomiting. The vomitus initially contains undigested food, mucus, and small amounts of bile. Later, it contains only bile and mucus. Finally, the vomitus includes blood and material that resembles coffee grounds.

The body's other responses

The patient may report thirst, hiccups, oliguria, vertigo, and headache as well as substantial weight loss and eventual emaciation caused by persistent vomiting. She may appear confused or delirious. Lassitude, stupor and, possibly, coma may occur. Additional findings may include:
- pale, dry, waxy and, possibly, jaundiced skin with decreased skin turgor
- dry, coated tongue
- subnormal or elevated temperature
- rapid pulse
- fetid, fruity breath (from acidosis).

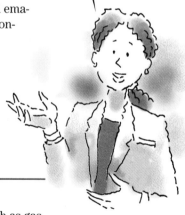

In cases of suspected hyperemesis gravidarum, diagnostic tests are used to rule out other disorders that produce similar effects.

What tests tell you

Diagnostic tests are used to rule out other disorders, such as gastroenteritis, cholecystitis, and peptic ulcer, which produce similar clinical effects. Differential diagnosis also rules out gestational trophoblastic disease, hepatitis, inner ear infection, food poisoning, emotional problems, and eating disorders.

Urine test results show ketonuria and slight proteinuria. The following results of serum analysis support a diagnosis of hyperemesis gravidarum:
- decreased protein, chloride, sodium, and potassium levels

- increased blood urea nitrogen levels
- elevated hemoglobin levels
- elevated WBC count.

How it's treated

Other possible causes, such as gastroenteritis, gall bladder disease, and pancreatic or liver disorders, must be ruled out before the diagnosis of hyperemesis gravidarum is confirmed. The patient with hyperemesis gravidarum may require hospitalization to correct electrolyte imbalances and prevent starvation. I.V. infusions are used to maintain nutrition until she can tolerate oral feedings.

Infuse while you snooze — and snack

An infusion of 3,000 ml of I.V. fluid over 24 hours will usually cause a reduction in symptoms. Oral fluids and food are usually withheld until there's no vomiting for 24 hours. Then clear liquids can be initiated. Metoclopramide (Reglan) may be administered to control vomiting. This infusion can be performed at the mother's home in the presence of a visiting nurse. She progresses slowly to a clear liquid diet, then a full liquid diet, and finally, small, frequent meals of high-protein solid foods. A midnight snack helps stabilize blood glucose levels. Parenteral vitamin supplements and potassium replacements are used to help correct deficiencies.

Stop the ride

If persistent vomiting jeopardizes the patient's health, antiemetic medications may be prescribed. Note, however, that no drug has been approved by the FDA for the treatment of nausea and vomiting during pregnancy. Therefore, any antiemetic must be prescribed with caution and the benefits must outweigh the risks to the patient and her fetus. Meclizine (Antivert) and diphenhydramine (Benadryl) may be prescribed.

More commonly, however, a continuous I.V. infusion of metoclopramide (Reglan) is administered through a portable I.V. pump worn under the patient's clothes. The latter treatment is highly successful. After vomiting stops and the patient's electrolyte balance has been restored, the pregnancy usually continues without recurrence of hyperemesis gravidarum. Most patients feel better as they begin to regain normal weight, but some continue to vomit throughout the pregnancy, requiring extended treatment. If appropriate, some patients may benefit from consultations with clinical nurse specialists, psychologists, or psychiatrists.

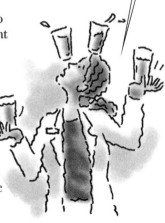

When a patient with hyperemesis gravidarum can tolerate oral feedings, she'll start with a clear liquid diet.

What to do

- Administer I.V. fluids as ordered until the patient can tolerate oral feedings.
- Monitor fluid intake and output, vital signs, skin turgor, daily weight, serum electrolyte levels, and urine for ketones; anticipate the need for electrolyte replacement therapy.
- Provide frequent mouth care.
- Consult a dietitian to provide a diet high in dry, complex carbohydrates. Suggest decreased liquid intake during meals. Company and diversionary conversation at mealtime may be beneficial.
- Instruct the patient to remain upright for 45 minutes after eating to decrease reflux.
- Suggest that the patient eat two or three dry crackers before getting out of bed in the morning to alleviate nausea.
- Provide reassurance and a calm, restful atmosphere. Encourage the patient to discuss her feelings about her pregnancy and the disorder.
- Help the patient develop effective coping strategies. Refer her to a mental health professional for additional counseling if necessary. Refer her to the social service department for help in caring for other children at home if appropriate.
- Teach the patient protective measures to conserve energy and promote rest. Include relaxation techniques, fresh air and moderate exercise (if tolerated), and activities scheduled appropriately to prevent fatigue.

Iron deficiency anemia

Iron deficiency anemia is a disorder in which hemoglobin synthesis is deficient and the body's capacity to transport oxygen is impaired. A common disease worldwide, iron deficiency anemia affects 10% to 30% of the adult population of the United States. It's the most common anemia during pregnancy, affecting up to one-fourth of all pregnancies. Iron deficiency anemia during pregnancy is associated with low fetal birth weight and preterm birth.

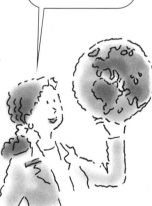

Iron deficiency anemia is common worldwide.

What causes it

During pregnancy, maternal iron stores are used for fetal RBC production, thus causing an iron deficiency in the mother. In addition, many women have deficient iron stores when they enter pregnancy because of factors such as a diet low in iron (inadequate intake), heavy menses (blood loss), or misguided weight-reduction programs. Iron stores also tend to be low in

women who have fewer than 2 years in between pregnancies and in those from low socioeconomic communities. Other possible causes of iron deficiency anemia may include:
- iron malabsorption
- intravascular-hemolysis-induced hemoglobinuria or paroxysmal nocturnal hemoglobinuria
- mechanical trauma to RBCs caused by a prosthetic heart valve or vena caval filter.

No iron, no hemoglobin, no oxygen

Iron deficiency anemia is considered a microcytic, hypochromic anemia, meaning that inadequate iron intake results in smaller RBCs that contain less hemoglobin. Cells that aren't as large and rich in hemoglobin as they should be affect the proper transport of oxygen.

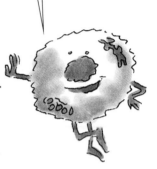

Adequate iron intake helps me grow rich with hemoglobin so I can properly transport oxygen.

What to look for

Typically, the signs and symptoms exhibited by the pregnant woman with iron deficiency anemia are the same as those for any patient with this disorder. They tend to develop gradually and may include fatigue, listlessness, pallor, and exercise intolerance. Some women develop pica (eating of substances such as ice or starch) in response to the body's need for increased nutrients. If the anemia is severe or prolonged, other signs and symptoms may include:
- dyspnea on exertion
- inability to concentrate
- susceptibility to infection
- tachycardia
- coarsely ridged, spoon-shaped, brittle, thin nails
- sore, red, burning tongue
- sore, dry skin in the corners of the mouth.

What tests tell you

Diagnosis of iron deficiency anemia must not precede exclusion of other causes of anemia, such as thalassemia minor, cancer, and chronic inflammatory, hepatic, or renal disease. Blood studies (serum iron, total iron-binding capacity, ferritin levels) and iron stores in bone marrow may confirm iron deficiency anemia. However, the results of these tests can be misleading because of complicating factors, such as infection, blood transfusion, or iron supplements. Characteristic blood test results for women include:
- low hemoglobin (less than 10 g/dl)
- low hematocrit (less than 33%)

- low serum iron (less than 30 µg/dl) with high binding capacity (over 400 µg/dl)
- low serum ferritin (less than 100 mg/dl)
- low RBC count with microcytic and hypochromic cells (in early stages, RBC count may be normal)
- decreased mean corpuscular hemoglobin (less than 30 g/dl) in severe anemia
- depleted or absent iron stores (identified by specific staining) and hyperplasia of normal precursor cells (identified by bone marrow studies).

How it's treated

Preventing iron deficiency anemia with prescription prenatal vitamins is the primary goal. However, if iron deficiency anemia does develop, an iron supplement, such as ferrous sulfate and ferrous gluconate, is prescribed. Additionally, patients should be advised to eat a well-balanced diet that includes foods high in vitamins and iron.

Fe via I.V.

If the woman's anemia is severe or she can't comply with the prescribed oral therapy, parenteral iron may be prescribed. Because total-dose I.V. infusion of supplemental iron is painless and requires fewer injections, it's usually preferred to I.M. administration. In pregnant patients with severe anemia, total-dose infusion of iron dextran in normal saline solution is given over 1 to 8 hours. A test dose of 0.5 ml I.V. is given first to help minimize the risk of allergic reaction.

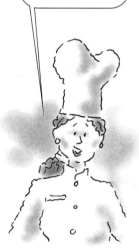

Don't let your patient skimp on foods high in vitamins and iron if you want to treat her iron deficiency anemia!

What to do

- Instruct the patient to use prenatal vitamins as prescribed.
- If the patient is hospitalized, administer oral iron with an acid, such as orange juice, to enhance absorption; for outpatients, advise women to take prescribed iron supplements with orange juice or a vitamin C supplement.
- Monitor the patient's CBC and serum iron and ferritin levels regularly.
- Assess the family's dietary habits for iron intake, noting the influence of childhood eating patterns, cultural food preferences, and family income on adequate nutrition.
- Monitor the woman's vital signs, especially heart rate, noting any tachycardia, which suggests that her activities are too strenuous.
- Evaluate for signs and symptoms of decreased perfusion to vital organs (such as dyspnea, chest pain, and dizziness) and symptoms of neuropathy (such as tingling in the extremities).

Advice from the experts

Z-track injection for iron

When administering iron using the I.M. route, use the Z-track injection method to displace the skin. This technique blocks the needle pathway after an injection, thereby preventing discomfort and tissue irritation secondary to drug leakage into subcutaneous tissue. To perform a Z-track injection, follow these steps:

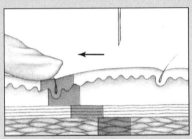

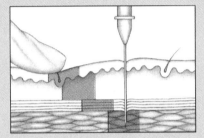

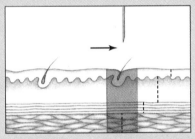

• Place your finger on the skin surface, and pull the skin and subcutaneous layers out of alignment with the underlying muscle. You should move the skin approximately ½″ (1 cm).

• Insert the needle at a 90-degree angle at the site where you initially placed your finger.
• Aspirate for blood return; if none appears, inject the drug slowly.
• Wait 10 seconds and then withdraw the needle slowly.
• Remove your finger from the skin surface, letting the layers return to normal, thus sealing the needle track. The needle track (as shown by the dotted line in the illustration above right) is now broken at the junction of each tissue layer, trapping the drug in the muscle.

• Don't massage the site or allow the patient to wear a tight fitting garment over the site because doing so could force medication into the subcutaneous tissue.
• Encourage the patient to walk or move about in bed to facilitate drug absorption from the injection site.

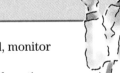

• Assess FHR at each visit; if the patient is hospitalized, monitor FHR at least every 4 hours.
• Provide frequent rest periods to decrease physical exhaustion. Assist the patient with planning activities so that she has sufficient rest between them.
• If the anemia is severe, expect to administer oxygen, as ordered, to help prevent and reduce hypoxia.
• Administer iron supplements as ordered. Use the Z-track injection method when administering iron I.M. to prevent skin discoloration, scarring, and irritating iron deposits in the skin. (See *Z-track injection for iron*.)

Education edge

Teaching topics on iron supplements

Be sure to cover the following topics when teaching your pregnant patient about iron supplements:
• reinforcement of the doctor's explanation of the anemia
• prescribed treatments and possible complications
• need for continuing therapy—even if the patient feels better—because replacement of iron stores takes time
• foods that interfere with absorption, such as milk and antacids
• foods that enhance absorption, such as citrus juices and foods containing vitamin C
• administration guidelines, including using a straw when taking liquid form to prevent staining the teeth and taking iron on an empty stomach (if possible) with a vitamin C food or taking with food if gastric irritation occurs
• need to report adverse effects of iron therapy, such as nausea, vomiting, diarrhea, and constipation, because dosage adjustment or supplemental stool softeners may be necessary
• change in stool appearance
• components of a nutritionally balanced diet, including red meats, green vegetables, eggs, whole wheat, iron-fortified bread, and milk
• intake of high-fiber foods to prevent constipation
• infection prevention measures
• need to report signs and symptoms of infection, such as fever and chills
• need for regular checkups and compliance with prescribed treatments.

• If the patient receives iron I.V., monitor the infusion rate carefully. Stop the infusion and begin supportive treatment immediately if the patient shows signs of an allergic reaction. Also, watch for dizziness and headache and for thrombophlebitis around the I.V. site.
• Assist with planning a well-balanced diet with an increased intake of foods high in vitamins and iron. Consult a nutrition therapist as indicated.
• Provide patient teaching about therapy. (See *Teaching topics on iron supplements.*) Offer suggestions for high-fiber foods to prevent possible constipation from iron therapy; also warn the patient that the medication may cause stools to appear black and tarry.

Isoimmunization

Isoimmunization, also called *Rh incompatibility*, refers to a condition in which the pregnant woman is Rh-negative but her fetus is Rh-positive. This condition, if left untreated, can lead to hemolytic disease in the neonate. Isoimmunization develops in about 7% of all pregnancies in the United States. Before the development of RhoGAM, this condition was a major cause of kernicterus (nerve cell deterioration) and neonatal death.

What causes it

During her first pregnancy, an Rh-negative woman may become sensitized to Rh antigens by:
• being exposed to Rh-positive fetal blood antigens inherited from the father
• receiving alien Rh antigens from a blood transfusion, causing agglutinins to develop
• receiving inadequate doses of $Rh_o(D)$ or failing to receive $Rh_o(D)$ after significant fetal-maternal leakage from abruptio placentae.

Subsequent pregnancy with an Rh-positive fetus provokes increasing amounts of maternal agglutinating antibodies to cross the placental barrier, attach to Rh-positive cells in the fetus, and cause hemolysis and anemia. To compensate for this, the fetus steps up the production of RBCs, and erythroblasts (immature RBCs) appear in the fetal circulation. Extensive hemolysis results in the release of large amounts of unconjugated bilirubin, which the liver can't conjugate and excrete, causing hyperbilirubinemia and hemolytic anemia. (See *Pathogenesis of Rh isoimmunization*.)

What to look for

Typically, the pregnant woman doesn't exhibit any signs or symptoms of this disorder. The fetus and subsequently the neonate are affected. Bilirubin levels in amniotic fluid are monitored for early delivery intervention or intrauterine fetal transfusion if needed. Repeated transfusions may be needed in the neonate.

What tests tell you

At the first pregnancy visit, an anti-D antibody titer should be performed on all women with Rh-negative blood. If the results are normal (titer is 0) or the titer is minimal (a ratio below 1:8), the test will be repeated at week 28. No therapy is needed at this time.

Sensitive blood

An anti-D antibody titer of 1:16 or greater indicates Rh sensitization. Continued titer monitoring will occur every 2 weeks for the remainder of the pregnancy. Amniocentesis will be performed approximately every 2 weeks to evaluate the status of the fetus.

Pathogenesis of Rh isoimmunization

Rh isoimmunization spans pregnancies in Rh-negative mothers who give birth to an Rh-positive neonate. The illustrations below outline the process of isoimmunization.

Before pregnancy, the woman has Rh-negative blood.

She becomes pregnant with an Rh-positive fetus. Normal antibodies appear.

Placental separation occurs.

After delivery, the mother develops anti–Rh-positive antibodies.

With the next Rh-positive fetus, antibodies enter fetal circulation, causing hemolysis.

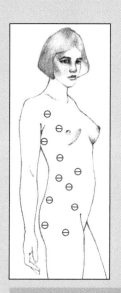
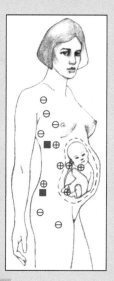
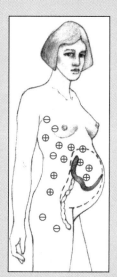
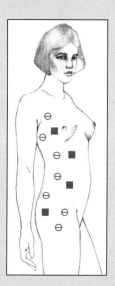
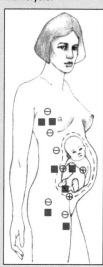

Rh- blood ⊖
Rh+ blood ⊕
Normal antibodies ■

During amniocentesis, the fluid density of the amniotic fluid is determined using spectrophotometry. The results are plotted on a graph and correlated with gestational age to determine the extent of involvement and the amount of bilirubin present.

Also, amniotic fluid analysis may show increased bilirubin levels (indicating possible hemolysis) and increased anti-Rh titers. Radiologic studies may show edema and, in those with hydrops fetalis (edema of the fetus), the halo sign (edematous, elevated, subcutaneous fat layers).

How it's treated

Treatment focuses on preventing Rh isoimmunization by administering RhoGAM to any unsensitized Rh-negative woman as soon as possible after the birth of an Rh-positive neonate or after spontaneous or elective abortion. In addition, screening for Rh isoimmunization or irregular antibodies is indicated for the following patients:
• Rh-negative mothers during their first prenatal visit and at 24, 28, 32, and 36 weeks' gestation
• Rh-positive mothers with a history of transfusion, a neonate with jaundice, stillbirth, cesarean birth, induced abortion, placenta previa, or abruptio placentae.

Towering titer

If the mother's Rh antibody titer is high, she may be given high doses of gamma globulin to help reduce fetal involvement, hoping to interfere with the rapid destruction of fetal RBCs. The fetus may receive a blood transfusion in utero via an injection of RBCs directly into a vessel in the fetal cord or instillation in the fetal abdomen via amniocentesis. After birth, the neonate may receive an exchange transfusion to remove hemolyzed RBCs and replace them with healthy blood cells.

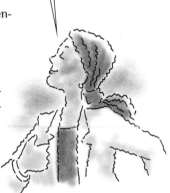

I'm positive! RhoGAM should be administered to an unsensitized Rh-negative woman as soon as possible after delivery of an Rh-positive neonate to prevent isoimmunization.

What to do

• Assess all pregnant women for possible Rh incompatibility.
• Expect to administer $Rh_0(D)$ I.M., as ordered, to Rh-negative women after transfusion reaction, ectopic pregnancy, spontaneous or induced abortion, or during the second and third trimesters to patients with abruptio placentae, placentae previa, or amniocentesis. (See *Administering RhoGAM.*)
• Administer RhoGAM to Rh-negative women at 28 weeks' gestation as ordered.
• Assist with intrauterine transfusion as indicated; before intrauterine transfusion, obtain a baseline FHR through electronic monitoring. Afterward, carefully observe the mother for uterine contractions and fluid leakage from the puncture site. Monitor FHR for tachycardia or bradycardia.
• Prepare the woman for a planned delivery, usually 2 to 4 weeks before term date, depending on maternal history, serologic tests, and amniocentesis.
• Assist with labor induction if indicated from the 34th to 38th week of gestation. During labor, monitor the fetus electronically; obtain capillary blood scalp sampling to determine acid-base bal-

Advice from the experts

Administering RhoGAM

$Rh_0(D)$ immune globulin (human), also known as RhoGAM, is a concentrated solution of immune globulin containing $Rh_0(D)$ antibodies. I.M. injection of RhoGAM keeps the Rh-negative mother from producing active antibody responses and forming anti-$Rh_0(D)$ to Rh-positive fetal blood cells and endangering future Rh-positive fetuses.

RhoGAM is administered to the Rh-negative mother after abortion, ectopic pregnancy, delivery of a neonate having $Rh_0(D)$-positive blood and cord blood that's direct Coombs' negative, accidental transfusion of Rh-positive blood, amniocentesis, abruptio placentae, or abdominal trauma. It's given within 72 hours to prevent future maternal sensitization. Administration at approximately 28 weeks' gestation can also protect the fetus of the Rh-negative mother.

RhoGAM is given I.M. into the gluteal site. When administering RhoGAM, the same steps are followed as for any I.M. injection. However, be sure to include the following:
• Check the vial's identification numbers with another nurse, and sign the triplicate form that comes with the RhoGAM.
• Attach the top copy to the patient's chart.
• Send the remaining two copies along with the empty RhoGAM vial to the laboratory or blood bank.
• Give the woman a card indicating her Rh-negative status, and instruct her to carry it with her or keep it in a convenient location.

ance. An indication of fetal distress necessitates immediate cesarean delivery.
• Administer RhoGAM within 72 hours of delivery to prevent complications in subsequent pregnancies.
• Provide emotional support to the patient and her family.
• Encourage the patient and her family to express their fears concerning possible complications of treatment.
• Before intrauterine transfusion, explain the procedure and its purpose.

Multiple pregnancy

Multiple pregnancy, or *multiple gestation*, refers to a pregnancy involving more than one fetus. It's considered a complication of pregnancy because the woman's body must adjust to the effects of carrying multiple fetuses.

Baby boom

The increased use of fertility drugs has lead to a more than 50% rise in the incidence of multiple pregnancy. For example, births of triplets (or greater) is 100 times more common now than in 1978. Twins — monozygotic (identical) or dizygotic (fraternal) — occurred about 68,000 times in 1978 and increased to about 104,000 births in 1997. (See *Types of twins*.)

Multiple pregnancies may be single-ovum conceptions (monozygotic twins) or multiple-ova conceptions (dizygotic twins and greater). Naturally occurring multiple pregnancies are more common in nonwhites than in whites. The higher a woman's parity and age, the more likely she is to have a multiple pregnancy. Inheritance, based on the mother's family pattern, also appears to play a role in natural dizygotic twinning.

Double, triple, or quadruple the risks

The risks of such complications as PIH, hydramnios, placenta previa, preterm labor, and anemia are higher in women with multiple pregnancy. Additionally, postpartum bleeding is more common because the uterus is stretched more. Multiple pregnancies also tend to end before normal term, meaning that the fetuses are at risk for premature birth.

It's a twin thing

With twins, the risk of congenital anomalies, such as spinal cord defect, is higher. The incidence of velamatous cord insertion (the cord inserted into the fetal membranes) is also higher and increases the risk of bleeding during delivery due to a torn cord. With monozygotic twins, fetuses share the placenta, which may lead to a condition known as twin-to-twin transfusion. In this condition, one fetus overgrows while the other undergrows. Additionally, if a single amnion is present, the umbilical cords can become knotted or twisted, leading to fetal distress or difficulty with birth.

Best to be first

In addition, the second fetus (twin B) is at more risk for birth-related complications, such as umbilical cord prolapse, malpresentation, and abruptio placentae.

What causes it

Multiple pregnancy is the result of the fertilization of one ova forming one zygote that divides into two identical zygotes or the simultaneous fertilization of two or more ova. The increasing use of fertility drugs has led to a rise in the number of multiple preg-

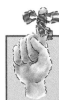

Memory jogger

To remember the difference between monozygotic (identical) and dizygotic (fraternal) twins, picture the "i" in "identical" as the Roman numeral one (I). One egg fertilized by one spermatozoan makes an Identical twin.

Types of twins

There are two types of twins: monozygotic and dizygotic.

 Monozygotic

Monozygotic (identical) twins begin with one ovum and one spermatozoan. In the process of fusion, or in one of the first cell divisions, the zygote divides into two identical individuals. Single-ovum twins usually have one placenta, one chorion, two amnions, and two umbilical cords. The twins are always the same sex.

 Dizygotic

Dizygotic, (fraternal) twins are the result of the fertilization of two separate ova by two separate spermatozoa. Double-ova twins have two placentas, two chorions, two amnions, and two umbilical cords. The twins may be of the same or different sex.

nancies because these drugs stimulate the ovaries to release multiple ova to increase chances of fertilization.

What to look for

When the uterus begins to grow at a rate faster than usual, a multiple pregnancy is suspected. In addition, the woman may report that with quickening she feels fluttering actions at different areas of her abdomen rather than at one specific and consistent spot. She also may report an increased amount of fetal activity than expected for the date. Auscultation may reveal multiple sets of fetal heart sounds.

The woman may report an increase in fatigue and backache. Resting or sleeping may be difficult because of the increased discomfort and fetal activity level. Appetite and intake may decrease because the enlarging uterus is compressing her stomach.

What tests tell you

Diagnostic test results that help determine multiple pregnancy may include:
- elevated alpha-fetoprotein levels
- evidence of multiple gestational sacs on ultrasound and, possibly, evidence of multiple amniotic sacs early in pregnancy.

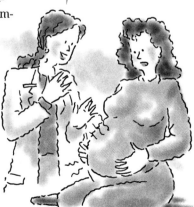

If you're experiencing this much fetal activity at this stage of your pregnancy, you may be expecting more than one baby.

How it's treated

Multiple gestation pregnancies put the mother at risk for developing many complications of pregnancy, such as preterm labor, intrauterine growth retardation, premature rupture of membranes, PIH, and abruptio placentae. Treatment centers on any of these complications that may arise. In addition, the patient may be ordered to go on complete bed rest for a period of her pregnancy to prevent such complications as preterm labor. Depending on the number of fetuses, their gestational age, and their position, the manner of delivery will vary. Vaginal delivery is possible for a mature twin gestation at term when both twins are in the head down, or *vertex*, position. If the first, or *presenting*, twin is vertex and the second is breech, it's possible to proceed with a vaginal birth; however, because this situation is more complicated, a cesarean delivery would most probably be the method of choice.

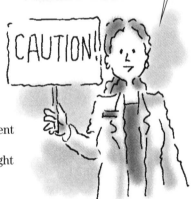

A multiple gestation pregnancy puts the patient at risk for preterm labor and premature rupture of membranes.

What to do

Other than more frequent monitoring, nursing care for the woman with multiple pregnancy is similar to that for any pregnancy:
• Assist the woman with understanding her current condition and the need for close, frequent follow-up.
• Encourage frequent rest periods throughout the day to help relieve fatigue.
• Urge the woman to rest in the side-lying position to prevent supine hypotension syndrome.
• Monitor maternal vital signs, weight gain, and fundal height at every visit.
• Assess FHR and position at every visit.
• Arrange for follow-up testing, such as ultrasounds and non-stress-test monitoring, as well as 24-hour fetal monitoring if the patient is on complete bed rest for the 3rd trimester of her pregnancy.
• Urge the woman to comply with prenatal vitamins and eat a well-balanced diet high in vitamins and iron.
• Explain danger signs and symptoms to report immediately, especially those related to preterm labor.
• Provide emotional support to the woman and her family; allow the pregnant woman to verbalize her fears and anxieties about the pregnancy and fetuses. Correct any misconceptions that the woman verbalizes.
• During labor, provide separate electronic fetal monitoring for each fetus.

- Maintain the patient in the side-lying position to aid breathing during labor.
- Be alert for hypotonic labor, which might necessitate labor augmentation or cesarean delivery.
- At delivery, have on hand all medication for each neonate.
- Usually an anesthesiologist and a pediatrician or a neonatal nurse practitioner should be present in anticipation of maternal or neonatal problems.
- During delivery, one nurse should be available for each neonate and one for the mother.

Placenta previa

Placenta previa occurs when the placenta implants in the lower uterine segment, obstructing the internal cervical os and failing to provide as much nourishment as the fundus. The placenta tends to spread out, seeking the blood supply it needs, and it becomes larger and thinner than normal. Eccentric insertion of the umbilical cord commonly develops, for unknown reasons. Hemorrhage occurs as the internal cervical os effaces and dilates, tearing the uterine vessels. One of the most common causes of bleeding during the second half of pregnancy, this disorder occurs in about 1 in 200 pregnancies and more commonly in multigravidas than primigravidas. If the patient has heavy maternal bleeding and is then diagnosed with placenta previa, the pregnancy must be terminated.

Partial or complete coverage

The placenta may cover all or part of the internal cervical os, or it may gradually overlap the os as the cervix dilates. Complete obstruction is known as total, complete, or central placenta previa. Partial obstruction is known as incomplete or partial placenta previa. Obstruction that occurs as the cervix dilates is caused by marginal implantation or a low-lying placenta. The apparent degree of placenta previa may depend largely on the extent of cervical dilation at the time of examination. Maternal prognosis is good if hemorrhage can be controlled. Fetal prognosis depends on gestational age and the amount of blood lost. (See *Three types of placenta previa*, page 262.)

What causes it

The specific cause of placenta previa is unknown. Factors that may affect the site of the placenta's attachment to the uterine wall include:

Three types of placenta previa

Placenta previa has three basic types: low marginal, partial, and complete.

Low marginal
In low marginal placenta previa, a small placental edge can be felt through the maternal os.

Partial
In partial placenta previa, the placenta partially caps the internal os.

Complete
In complete placenta previa, the placenta completely covers the internal os.

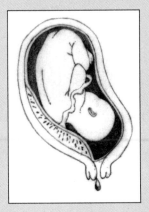
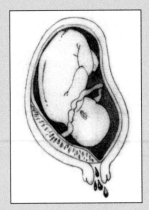
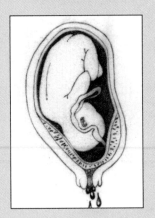

- defective vascularization of the decidua
- multiple pregnancy (the placenta requires a larger surface for attachment)
- previous uterine surgery
- multiparity
- advanced maternal age.

What to look for

Typically, a patient with placenta previa reports the onset of painless, bright red, vaginal bleeding after the 20th week of pregnancy. Such bleeding, beginning before the onset of labor, tends to be episodic; it starts without warning, stops spontaneously, and resumes later.

About 7% of patients with placenta previa are asymptomatic. In these women, ultrasound examination reveals the disorder incidentally.

Palpation may reveal a soft, nontender uterus. Abdominal examination using Leopold's maneuvers reveals various malpresentations because the placenta's abnormal location has interfered with descent of the fetal head. Minimal descent of the fetal presenting part may indicate placenta previa. The fetus remains active, however, with good heart tones audible on auscultation.

What tests tell you

A differential diagnosis is necessary to exclude genital lacerations, excessive bloody show, abruptio placentae, and cervical lesions. Laboratory studies may reveal decreased maternal hemoglobin levels (due to blood loss).

Ultrasound is most sound

Transvaginal ultrasound scanning is used to determine placental position. Radiologic tests, such as femoral arteriography, retrograde catheterization, or radioisotope scanning or localization, may be done to locate the placenta. However, these tests have limited value, are risky, and are usually performed only when ultrasound is unavailable.

Only just before

Pelvic examination should be performed only in a surgical suite or a birthing room that's equipped for cesarean birth in the event that hemorrhage necessitates immediate delivery.

How it's treated

Treatment of placenta previa focuses on assessing, controlling, and restoring blood loss; delivering a viable neonate; and preventing coagulation disorders. Immediate therapy includes:
- starting an I.V. infusion using a large-bore catheter
- drawing blood for hemoglobin and hematocrit levels, typing, and crossmatching
- initiating external electronic fetal monitoring
- monitoring maternal blood pressure, pulse rate, and respirations
- assessing the amount of vaginal bleeding.

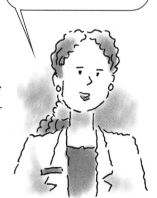

Treatment of placenta previa focuses on controlling and restoring blood loss, delivering the neonate, and preventing coagulation disorders.

When the bun's not done

If the fetus is premature (following determination of the degree of placenta previa and necessary fluid and blood replacement), treatment consists of careful observation to allow the fetus more time to mature. If clinical evaluation confirms complete placenta previa, the patient is usually hospitalized because of the increased risk of hemorrhage. As soon as the fetus is sufficiently mature, or in cases of severe hemorrhage, immediate cesarean delivery may be necessary. Vaginal delivery is considered only when the bleeding is minimal and the placenta previa is marginal or when the labor is rapid.

Have hands on hand

Because of possible fetal blood loss through the placenta, a pediatric team should be on hand during such a delivery to immediately assess and treat neonatal shock, blood loss, and hypoxia.

What to do

• If the patient with placenta previa shows active bleeding, continuously monitor her blood pressure, pulse rate, respirations, central venous pressure, intake and output, and amount of vaginal bleeding as well as the fetus's heart rate and rhythm.

• Anticipate the need for electronic fetal monitoring, and assist with application as indicated.

• Have oxygen readily available in case fetal distress occurs. (Many facilities will administer oxygen continuously in labor and delivery to increase the oxygen amount delivered to the fetus). Evidence of fetal distress includes bradycardia, tachycardia, or late or variable decelerations.

• If the patient is Rh-negative, administer RhoGAM after every bleeding episode.

• Institute complete bed rest.

• Prepare the patient and her family for a possible cesarean delivery and the birth of a preterm neonate. Thoroughly explain postpartum care so the patient and her family know which measures to expect.

• If the fetus isn't mature, expect to administer an initial dose of betamethasone (Celestone) I.M. to aid in promoting fetal lung maturity. Explain that additional doses may be given again in 24 hours and, possibly, 1 to 2 weeks.

• Provide emotional support during labor. Because of the fetus's prematurity, the patient may not be given analgesics, so labor pain may be intense. Reassure her of her progress throughout labor, and keep her informed of the fetus's condition.

• If the patient's bleeding ceases and she's to return home on bed rest, anticipate the need for a referral for home care.

• Assess for signs of infection (fever, chills). The patient is at increased risk for infection because of the proximity of vaginal organisms to the placenta and the susceptibility of the placental environment to the growth of microorganisms.

• Teach the patient to identify and report signs of placenta previa (bleeding, cramping) immediately.

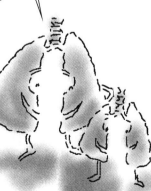

I.M. betamethasone will help you grow big and strong.

• During the postpartum period, monitor the patient for signs of hemorrhage and shock caused by the uterus's diminished ability to contract.

• Tactfully discuss the possibility of neonatal death. Tell the mother that the neonate's survival depends primarily on gestational age, the amount of blood lost, and associated hypertensive disorders. Assure her that frequent monitoring and prompt management greatly reduce the risk of death.

• Encourage the patient and her family to verbalize their feelings, and help them develop effective coping strategies. Refer them for counseling if necessary.

Pregnancy-induced hypertension

PIH, also called *hypertension of pregnancy*, is a potentially life-threatening disorder that usually develops after the 20th week of pregnancy. It occurs most commonly in nulliparous women. Currently, PIH and its complications are the most common cause of maternal and fetal death in developed countries.

With or without seizure

PIH is typically classified as preeclampsia or eclampsia. Preeclampsia, the nonconvulsive form of the disorder, is marked by the onset of hypertension after 20 weeks' gestation. It develops in about 7% of pregnancies and may be mild or severe. The incidence is significantly higher in patients from low socioeconomic groups. Eclampsia, the convulsive form, occurs between 24 weeks' gestation and the end of the first postpartum week. The incidence increases among women who are pregnant for the first time, have multiple fetuses, and have a history of vascular disease.

About 5% of women with preeclampsia develop eclampsia; of these, about 15% die of eclampsia or its complications. Fetal mortality is high because of the increased incidence of premature delivery.

Complicating the situation

Generalized arteriolar vasoconstriction associated with PIH is thought to produce decreased blood flow through the placenta and maternal organs. This can result in intrauterine growth retardation (or restriction), placental infarcts, and abruptio placentae. Hemolysis, elevated liver enzyme levels, and a low platelet count (HELLP syndrome) are associated with severe preeclampsia. Other possible complications include stillbirth of the neonate, seizures, coma, premature labor, renal failure, and hepatic damage in the mother.

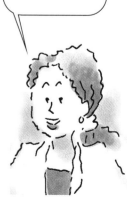

Preexisting vascular disease may contribute to PIH.

What causes it

Although the exact cause of PIH is unknown, systemic peripheral vasospasm occurs that affects every organ system. (See *Changes associated with PIH*.) Geographic, ethnic, racial, nutritional, immunologic, and familial factors may contribute to preexisting vascular disease which, in turn, may contribute to its occurrence. Age is also a factor. Adolescents and primiparas older than age 35 are at higher risk for preeclampsia.

Other possible causes include potential toxic sources (such as autolysis of placental infarcts), autointoxication, uremia, maternal sensitization to total proteins, and pyelonephritis.

What to look for

A patient with mild preeclampsia typically reports a sudden weight gain of more than 3 lb (1.4 kg) per week in the second trimester or more than 1 lb (0.5 kg) per week during the third trimester. The patient's history reveals hypertension, as evidenced by high blood pressure readings (140 mm Hg or more systolic, or an increase of 30 mm Hg or more above the patient's normal systolic pressure, measured on two occasions, 6 hours apart; and 90 mm Hg or more diastolic, or an increase of 15 mm Hg or more above the patient's normal diastolic pressure, measured on two occasions, 6 hours apart). Further examination may reveal generalized edema, especially of the face. Palpation may reveal pitting edema of the legs and feet. Deep tendon reflexes may indicate hyperreflexia.

As preeclampsia worsens, the patient may demonstrate oliguria (urine output of 400 ml/day or less), blurred vision caused by retinal arteriolar spasms, epigastric pain or heartburn, irritability, and emotional tension. She may also complain of a severe frontal headache.

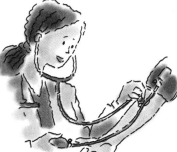

Two or more high blood pressure readings obtained 6 hours apart while the patient is on bed rest may indicate preeclampsia.

Pressure, spasm, hemorrhage — oh my!

In severe preeclampsia, blood pressure readings increase to 160/110 mm Hg or higher on two occasions, 6 hours apart, during bed rest. Ophthalmoscopic examination may reveal vascular spasm, papilledema, retinal edema or detachment, and arteriovenous nicking or hemorrhage.

Pre no more

The onset of seizures signifies eclampsia. The patient with eclampsia may appear to cease breathing, then suddenly take a deep, gasping breath and resume breathing. The patient may then lapse into a coma, lasting a few minutes to several hours. When waking from the coma, the patient may have no memory of the

Changes associated with PIH

The following flowchart illustrates the physiologic affects of pregnancy-induced hypertension (PIH) on the body.

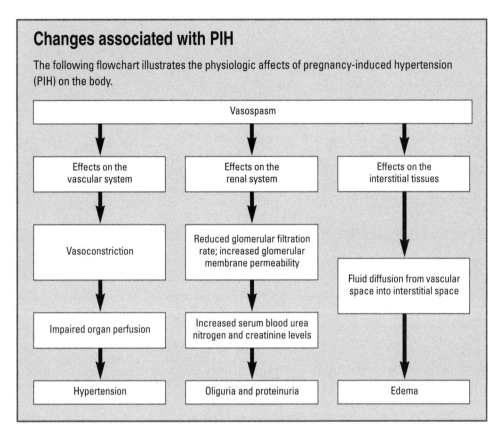

seizure. Mild eclampsia may involve more than one seizure; severe eclampsia up to 20 seizures.

Kicked up a notch

In eclampsia, physical examination findings are similar to those in preeclampsia but more severe. Systolic blood pressure may increase to 180 mm Hg or even to 200 mm Hg. Marked edema may be present; some patients, however, don't show visible signs of edema.

What tests tell you

A differential diagnosis is used to distinguish the disorder from viral hepatitis, idiopathic thrombocytopenia, cholecystitis, hemolytic uremic syndrome, peptic ulcer, neuroangiopathic syndrome, appendicitis, renal calculi, pyelonephritis, and gastroenteritis. Laboratory test findings reveal proteinuria (more than 300 mg/24 hours [1+] with preeclampsia, and 5 g/24 hours [5+] or more with severe eclampsia). Test results may also suggest HELLP syndrome. Additionally, ultrasonography, stress and nonstress tests, and biophysical profiles evaluate fetal well-being.

How it's treated

Adequate nutrition, good prenatal care, and control of preexisting hypertension during pregnancy help decrease the incidence and severity of preeclampsia. However, if preeclampsia does develop, early recognition and prompt treatment can prevent progression to eclampsia.

Suppress the progress

Therapy for patients with preeclampsia is intended to stop the disorder's progression and ensure fetal survival. Some doctors advocate the prompt inducement of labor, especially if the patient is near term; others follow a more conservative approach. Therapy may include:
• complete bed rest in the preferred left lateral lying position to enhance venous return
• administration of antihypertensive drugs, such as methyldopa and hydralazine
• if the patient's blood pressure fails to respond to bed rest and antihypertensives and persistently rises above 160/100 mm Hg or central nervous system irritability increases, administration of magnesium to promote diuresis, reduce blood pressure, and prevent seizures.

> Treatment of preeclampsia may include complete bed rest to enhance venous return.

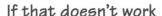

If that doesn't work

If these measures fail to improve the patient's condition, or if fetal life is endangered (as determined by stress or nonstress tests and biophysical profiles), cesarean delivery or labor induction with oxytocin may be required. If the woman develops seizures, emergency treatment consists of immediate I.V. administration of magnesium, oxygen therapy, and electronic fetal monitoring. After the patient's condition stabilizes, cesarean delivery may be indicated.

What to do

• Monitor the patient regularly for changes in blood pressure, pulse rate, respiratory rate, FHR, vision, level of consciousness, and deep tendon reflexes as well as headache unrelieved by medication. Report changes immediately. Assess these signs and symptoms before administering medications. (See *Emergency interventions for PIH.*)

• If the woman is receiving I.V. magnesium, administer the loading dose over 15 to 30 minutes and then maintain the infusion at a rate of 1 to 2 g/hour. (See *Administering magnesium safely,* page 270.)

• Monitor the extent and location of edema. Elevate affected extremities to promote venous return. Avoid constricting pantyhose, slippers, or bed linens.

• Assess fluid balance by measuring intake and output and checking daily weight. Insert an indwelling urinary catheter, if necessary, to provide a more accurate measurement of output.

• Provide a quiet, darkened room, limit visitation by friends and family members until the patient's condition stabilizes, and enforce complete bed rest.

• Provide emotional support for the patient and her family. Encourage them to verbalize their feelings. If the patient's condition requires premature delivery, point out that infants of mothers with PIH are usually small for gestational age but sometimes fare better than other premature babies of the same weight, possibly because they have developed adaptive responses to stress in utero.

• Encourage the patient to eat a well-balanced, high-protein diet; limit high-sodium foods, include high-fiber foods, and drink at least eight 8-oz glasses of noncaffeinated drinks each day.

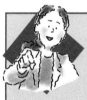

Take charge!

Emergency interventions for PIH

When caring for a patient with pregnancy-induced hypertension (PIH), be prepared to perform these nursing interventions:

• Observe for signs of fetal distress by closely monitoring the results of stress and nonstress tests.

• Keep emergency resuscitative equipment and anticonvulsant drugs readily available in case of seizures and cardiac or respiratory arrest.

• Maintain a patent airway and have oxygen readily available.

• Carefully monitor the I.V. infusion of magnesium sulfate, observing for signs and symptoms of toxicity, such as absence of patellar reflexes, flushing, muscle flaccidity, decreased urine output, a significant drop in blood pressure (more than 15 mm Hg), and respiratory rate less than 12 breaths/minute.

• Keep calcium gluconate readily available at the bedside to counteract the toxic effects of magnesium sulfate.

• Prepare for emergency cesarean delivery if indicated.

• Maintain seizure precautions to protect the patient from injury. Never leave an unstable patient unattended.

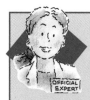

Advice from the experts

Administering magnesium safely

If your patient requires I.V. magnesium therapy, use caution when administering the drug because magnesium toxicity may occur. Follow these guidelines to ensure the patient's safety during administration:

• Always administer the drug as a piggyback infusion so that it can be discontinued immediately if the patient develops signs and symptoms of toxicity.

• Obtain a baseline serum magnesium level before initiating therapy and monitor levels frequently thereafter.

• Keep in mind that for I.V. magnesium to be effective as an anticonvulsant, serum magnesium levels should be between 5 and 8 mg/dl. Levels above 8 mg/dl indicate toxicity and place the patient at risk for respiratory depression, cardiac arrhythmias, and cardiac arrest.

• Assess the patient's patellar reflex. If the patient has received epidural anesthesia, test the biceps or triceps reflex. Diminished or hypoactive reflexes suggest magnesium toxicity.

• Assess for ankle clonus (alternating contractions and relaxations of the muscles) by rapidly dorsiflexing the patient's ankle three times, then removing your hand and observing the foot's movement. If no further motion is noted, ankle clonus is absent; if the foot continues to move involuntarily, clonus is present. Moderate (3 to 5 movements) or severe (6 or more movements) suggests possible magnesium toxicity.

• Have calcium gluconate readily available at the patient's bedside. Anticipate administering this antidote for magnesium I.V.

• Teach the patient to report signs and symptoms that indicate a worsening of PIH which include headache, visual disturbances (blurring, flashes of light, "spots" before the eyes); GI symptoms (nausea, pain); worsening edema, especially of the face and fingers; noticeable decrease in urine output.

• Teach the woman the importance of keeping her prenatal appointments, which will be more frequent because she has PIH.

• Help the patient and her family develop effective coping strategies.

Premature labor

Premature labor, also known as *preterm labor*, is the onset of rhythmic uterine contractions that produce cervical changes after fetal viability but before fetal maturity. It usually occurs between the 20th and 37th weeks of gestation. Between 5% and 10% of pregnancies end prematurely; about 75% of neonatal deaths result from this disorder.

Weighing in

Fetal prognosis depends on birth weight and length of gestation. Fetuses born at less than 26 weeks' gestation and weighing less than 737 g (1 lb, 10 oz) have a survival rate of about 10%. Fetuses born at 27 to 28 weeks' gestation and weighing between 737 g and 992 g (1 lb, 10 oz and 2 lb, 3 oz) have a survival rate of more than 50%. Those born at more than 28 weeks' gestation and weighing 992 g to 1,219 g (2 lb, 3 oz to 2 lb, 11 oz) have a 70% to 90% survival rate.

What causes it

Causes of premature labor include premature rupture of membranes, (in 30% to 50% of cases), PIH, chronic hypertensive vascular disease, hydramnios, multiple pregnancy, placenta previa, abruptio placentae, incompetent cervix, abdominal surgery, trauma, structural anomalies of the uterus, infections (such as group B streptococci), and fetal death.

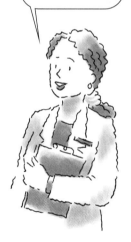

In premature labor, fetal prognosis depends on birth weight and length of gestation.

What to look for

The patient reports the onset of rhythmic uterine contractions, possible rupture of membranes, passage of the cervical mucus plug, and a bloody discharge. Her history indicates that she's in the 20th to 37th week of pregnancy. Vaginal examination shows cervical effacement and dilation.

What tests tell you

Premature labor is confirmed by the combined results of prenatal history, physical examination, presenting signs and symptoms, and ultrasonography (if available) showing the position of the fetus in relation to the mother's pelvis.

How it's treated

Treatment is designed to suppress preterm labor when tests show immature fetal pulmonary development, cervical dilation of less than 4 cm, and the absence of factors that contraindicate continuation of pregnancy. Such treatment consists of bed rest and, when necessary, tocolytic drug therapy.

Prevention first

Taking steps to prevent premature labor is important. This requires good prenatal care, adequate nutrition, and proper rest. Inserting a purse-string suture (cerclage) to reinforce an incompetent cervix at 14 to 18 weeks' gestation may prevent premature labor in a patient with a history of this disorder.

Some patients have prevented premature labor by receiving tocolytic drugs at home (either orally or through an I.V. infusion pump). Women at risk who are treated at home can have their contractions monitored via telephone hookup to a center, such as Health-Dyne or Tokos.

Slow to a stop

Several types of drug therapy may be used to stop the patient's contractions. Magnesium sulfate is typically the first drug of choice. It acts as a central nervous system (CNS) depressant, resulting in the slowing and cessation of contractions. A beta-adrenergic agent such as terbutaline (Brethine) is used to stimulate beta-2 receptors, thus inhibiting the contractility of uterine smooth muscle. Terbutaline is the most widely used drug for tocolysis.

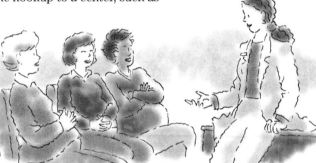

> Good prenatal care, adequate nutrition, and proper rest can help prevent premature labor.

Indomethacin (Indocin), a prostaglandin synthesis inhibitor, may be given, but its use has been associated with premature closure of ductus arteriosus if given after 34 weeks' gestation.

Coming to terms with preterm delivery

Sometimes preterm delivery is the lesser risk if maternal factors, such as intrauterine infection, abruptio placentae, placental insufficiency, and severe preeclampsia, jeopardize the fetus. Fetal problems, particularly isoimmunization and congenital anomalies, can become more perilous as pregnancy nears term and may require preterm delivery.

In an ideal world

Ideally, treatment of active premature labor should take place in a perinatal intensive care center, where the staff is specially trained to handle this situation. In such settings, the infant can remain close to his parents. (Community hospitals commonly lack the facilities for special neonatal care and transfer the neonate alone to a perinatal center.)

Treatment and delivery require intensive team effort. The fetus's health requires continuous assessment through fetal monitoring. Sedatives and narcotics, which may harm the fetus, shouldn't be used. Although morphine (Duramorph) and meperidine (Demerol) have little effect on uterine contractions, they depress CNS function and may cause fetal respiratory depression; therefore, they should be administered in the smallest doses possible and only when absolutely necessary.

Amniotomy is avoided, if possible, to prevent cord prolapse or damage to the fetus's tender skull. Adequate hydration is maintained with I.V. fluids.

Whoa there, contractions!

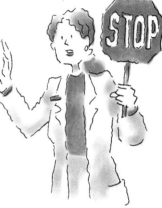

What to do

- Closely observe the patient in premature labor for signs of fetal or maternal distress and provide comprehensive supportive care.
- During attempts to suppress premature labor, make sure the patient maintains bed rest.
- Encourage the mother to stay in the left side-lying position to ensure better placental blood flow to the fetus.
- Administer medications as ordered. (See *Administering terbutaline*, page 274.)
- Give sedatives and analgesics sparingly because they may be harmful to the fetus. Minimize the need for these drugs by providing comfort measures, such as frequent repositioning and good perineal and back care.
- Monitor blood pressure, pulse rate, respirations, FHR, and uterine contraction pattern when administering a beta-adrenergic stimulant, sedative, or narcotic. Minimize adverse reactions by keeping the patient in a side-lying position as much as possible to ensure adequate placental perfusion.
- Administer fluids as ordered to ensure adequate hydration.
- Assess deep tendon reflexes frequently when administering magnesium sulfate. Monitor the neonate for signs of magnesium toxicity, including neuromuscular and respiratory depression.
- During active premature labor, remember that the preterm fetus has a lower tolerance for the stress of labor and is more likely to become hypoxic than a full-term fetus. If necessary, administer oxygen to the patient through a nasal cannula. Encourage the patient to lie on her left side or sit up during labor; this position prevents vena caval compression, which can cause supine hypotension and subsequent fetal hypoxia.
- Observe fetal response to labor through continuous monitoring. Prevent maternal hyperventilation; use a rebreathing bag as necessary. Continually reassure the patient throughout labor to help reduce her anxiety.

Advice from the experts

Administering terbutaline

I.V. terbutaline may be ordered for a woman in premature labor. When administering this drug, follow these steps:
• Obtain baseline maternal vital signs, fetal heart rate (FHR), and laboratory studies, including hematocrit, and serum glucose and electrolyte levels.
• Institute external monitoring of uterine contractions and FHR.
• Prepare the drug with lactated Ringer's solution instead of dextrose in water to prevent additional glucose load and hyperglycemia.
• Administer the drug as an I.V. piggyback infusion into a main I.V. solution so that the drug can be discontinued immediately if adverse effects occur.
• Use microdrip tubing and an infusion pump to ensure an accurate flow rate.
• Expect to adjust infusion flow rate every 10 minutes until contractions cease or adverse effects become problematic.
• Monitor maternal vital signs every 15 minutes while the infusion rate is increased, then every 30 minutes thereafter until contractions cease; monitor FHR every 15 to 30 minutes.
• Auscultate breath sounds for evidence of crackles or changes; be alert for complaints of dyspnea and chest pain.
• Monitor for maternal pulse rate greater than 120 beats/minute, blood pressure less than 90/60 mm Hg, or persistent tachycardia or tachypnea, chest pain, dyspnea, or abnormal breath sounds, which can indicate developing pulmonary edema. Notify the doctor immediately.
• Watch for fetal tachycardia or late or variable decelerations in FHR pattern because these could indicate possible uterine bleeding or fetal distress necessitating an emergency birth.
• Monitor intake and output closely, every hour during the infusion and then every 4 hours after.
• Expect to continue the infusion for 12 to 24 hours after contractions have ceased and then to switch to oral therapy.
• Administer the first dose of oral therapy 30 minutes before discontinuing the I.V. infusion.
• Instruct the patient in how to take the oral therapy, continuing therapy until 37 weeks' gestation or fetal lung maturity has been confirmed by amniocentesis; alternatively, if the patient is prescribed subcutaneous terbutaline therapy via a continuous pump, teach the patient how to use the pump.
• Teach the woman how to measure her pulse rate before each dose of oral terbutaline, or at the recommended times with subcutaneous therapy; instruct the patient to call the doctor if her pulse rate is over 120 beats/minute or if she experiences palpitations or severe nervousness.

• Help the patient proceed through labor with as little analgesic and anesthetic as possible. To minimize fetal CNS depression, avoid administering an analgesic when delivery seems imminent. Monitor fetal and maternal response to local and regional anesthetics.

Premature rupture of membranes

PROM occurs in about 10% of pregnancies of more than 20 weeks' gestation.

Premature rupture of membranes (PROM) is a spontaneous break or tear in the amniotic sac before onset of regular contractions that results in progressive cervical dilation. This common abnormality of parturition occurs in nearly 10% of all pregnancies over 20 weeks' gestation, and labor usually starts within 24 hours; more than 80% of these infants are mature.

In labor limbo

The latent period (between membrane rupture and labor onset) is generally brief when membranes rupture near term. When the neonate is premature, the latent period is prolonged, which increases the risk of mortality from maternal infection (amnionitis, endometritis), fetal infection (pneumonia, septicemia), and prematurity.

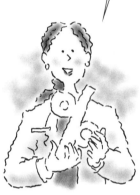

If membranes rupture when the fetus isn't near term, the neonate is then at increased risk for mortality from maternal infection (amnionitis, endometritis), fetal infection (pneumonia, septicemia), and prematurity.

PROM problems for mom

Maternal complications associated with PROM include:
- endometritis
- amnionitis
- septic shock and death if amnionitis goes untreated.

Baby's PROM predicament

Neonatal complications of PROM include:
- increased risk of respiratory distress syndrome
- asphyxia
- pulmonary hypoplasia
- congenital anomalies
- malpresentation
- cord prolapse
- severe fetal distress that can result in neonatal death.

What causes it

Although the cause of PROM is unknown, malpresentation and a contracted pelvis commonly accompany the rupture.

PROM suspects

Predisposing factors include:
- lack of proper prenatal care

- poor nutrition and hygiene
- maternal smoking
- incompetent cervix
- increased intrauterine tension from hydramnios or multiple gestation
- reduced amniotic membrane tensile strength
- uterine infection.

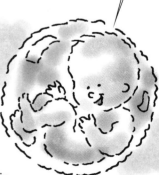

Poor nutrition may play a part in PROM. We sure don't want that!

What to look for

Typically, PROM causes blood-tinged amniotic fluid containing vernix caseosa particles to gush or leak from the vagina. Maternal fever, fetal tachycardia, and foul-smelling vaginal discharge indicate infection.

What tests tell you

Differential diagnosis is used to exclude urinary incontinence or vaginal infection as the underlying cause. Passage of amniotic fluid confirms the rupture. Slight fundal pressure or Valsalva's maneuver may expel fluid through the cervical os. Physical examination identifies if multiple pregnancy is involved. Abdominal palpation (Leopold's maneuvers) determines fetal presentation and size. Patient history and physical examination findings determine gestational age.

Diagnosis of PROM is confirmed by the following test results:
- Alkaline pH of fluid collected from the posterior fornix turns Nitrazine paper deep blue. (The presence of blood can give a false-positive result.) Staining the fluid with Nile blue sulfate reveals two categories of cell bodies. Blue-stained bodies represent sheath fetal epithelial cells; orange stained bodies originate in sebaceous glands. Incidence of prematurity is low when more than 20% of cells stain orange.
- If fluid is amniotic, a smear of the fluid placed on a slide and allowed to dry takes on a fernlike pattern (because of the high sodium and protein content of amniotic fluid). Verification of amniotic fluid leak confirms PROM.
- Vaginal probe ultrasonography allows visualization of the amniotic sac to detect tears or ruptures.

Treatment of PROM depends on fetal age and the risk of infection.

How it's treated

Treatment of PROM depends on fetal age and the risk of infection. In a term pregnancy, if spontaneous labor and vaginal delivery don't result within a relatively short time (usually within

24 hours after the membranes rupture), induction of labor with oxytocin usually follows, and then, if induction fails, cesarean delivery is performed. Cesarean hysterectomy may be recommended with gross uterine infection.

Before 34

Management of a preterm pregnancy of less than 34 weeks is controversial. However, with advances in technology, a conservative approach to PROM has been effective. Treatment of preterm pregnancy between 28 and 34 weeks includes hospitalization and observation for signs of infection (such as maternal leukocytosis or fever and fetal tachycardia) while the fetus matures.

Suspect infect, induce to reduce

If the presence of infection is suspected, baseline cultures and sensitivity tests are appropriate. If these tests confirm infection, labor must be induced, followed by I.V. administration of an antibiotic. A culture of gastric aspirate or a swabbing from the neonate's ear may also be done, as antibiotic therapy may be indicated for him as well. During such a delivery, resuscitative equipment must be readily available to treat neonatal distress.

What to do

• Prepare the patient for a vaginal examination. Before physically examining a patient who's suspected of having PROM, explain all diagnostic tests and clarify any misunderstandings she may have.
• During the exam, stay with the patient and offer reassurance.
• Provide sterile gloves and sterile lubricating jelly. Don't use iodophor antiseptic solution because it discolors Nitrazine paper and makes pH determination impossible.
• After the examination, provide proper perineal care.
• Send fluid specimens to the laboratory promptly because bacteriologic studies require immediate evaluation.
• Anticipate administering prophylactic antibiotics to the woman who's positive for streptococcal B infection to reduce the risk of this infection in the neonate.
• If labor starts, observe the mother's contractions and monitor vital signs every 2 hours.
• Watch for signs and symptoms of maternal infection (fever, abdominal tenderness, changes in amniotic fluid, such as purulence and foul odor) and fetal tachycardia. Fetal tachycardia may precede maternal fever. Report such signs and symptoms immediately.
• Perform patient teaching. (See *Teaching about PROM.*)
• Encourage the patient and her family to express their feelings and concerns for the fetus's health and survival.

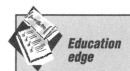

Education edge

Teaching about PROM

Here are some guidelines to follow when teaching a patient about premature rupture of membranes (PROM):
• Inform the patient about PROM, including its signs and symptoms, during the early stages of pregnancy.
• Make sure the patient understands that amniotic fluid doesn't always gush; it sometimes leaks slowly in PROM.
• Stress the importance of immediately reporting PROM (prompt treatment may prevent dangerous infection).
• Warn the patient not to engage in sexual intercourse, douche, or take a tub bath after her membranes rupture.
• Advise the patient to refrain from orgasm and breast stimulation, which can stimulate uterine contractions.
• Tell the patient to report to the health care provider a temperature above 100.4° F (38° C), which may indicate the onset of infection.

• Tell the patient to record fetal kick counts and to report fewer than 10 kicks in a 12-hour period. A decrease in fetal kick counts may indicate fetal distress.

• Tell the patient to report uterine contractions, reduced fetal activity, or signs of infection (fever, chills, foul-smelling discharge).

Sickle cell anemia

Sickle cell anemia is a congenital hematologic disease that causes impaired circulation, chronic ill health, and premature death. It results from an inherited mutation in the formation of hemoglobin, the blood component that carries oxygen to body tissues. Patients who suffer from this disease inherit the sickling gene from both parents, although some parents may be only carriers and don't experience symptoms. If both parents are carriers, chances are that one in four of their children will be affected. (See *Sickle cell anemia and race.*)

A threat in the blood

The sickle cell trait doesn't appear to influence the course of pregnancy; however, women with the trait tend to experience bacteriuria (which commonly produces no symptoms), which leads to pyelonephritis. Sickle cell anemia can threaten the woman's life if such vital blood vessels as those to the liver, kidneys, heart, lungs, or brain become blocked. During pregnancy, placental circulation may become blocked, causing low fetal birth weight and, possibly, fetal death.

What causes it

Sickle cell anemia results from homozygous inheritance of an autosomal recessive gene that produces a defective hemoglobin molecule (hemoglobin S). The defect is caused by a structural change in the gene that encodes the beta chain of hemoglobin. The amino acid valine is substituted for glutamic acid in the sixth position of the beta chain, causing the hemoglobin's structure to change.

Hemoglobin S causes RBCs to become sickle-shaped. The sickle cells start to build up in the capillaries and smaller blood vessels, making the blood more viscous. Normal circulation is impaired, causing pain, tissue infarctions, and swelling. The level of oxygen deficiency in sickle cell anemia and the factors that trigger a sickle cell crisis differ in each patient. (See *Sickle cell crisis.*)

Sickle cell trait, which results from heterozygous inheritance of this gene, causes few or no symptoms. However, people with this trait are carriers who may pass the gene to their offspring.

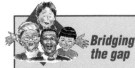
Bridging the gap

Sickle cell anemia and race

Sickle cell anemia is an inherited disease that's most common in people of African or Mediterranean descent. About 1 in 10 blacks carries the abnormal gene, and 1 in every 400 to 600 black children has sickle cell anemia.

Sickle cell crisis

Infection, exposure to cold, high altitudes, overexertion or other situations that cause cellular oxygen deprivation may trigger a sickle cell crisis. The deoxygenated, sickle-shaped red blood cells stick to the capillary wall and each other, blocking blood flow and causing cellular hypoxia. The crisis worsens as tissue hypoxia and acidic waste products cause more sickling and cell damage. With each new crisis, organs and tissues, especially the kidney and spleen, are slowly destroyed.

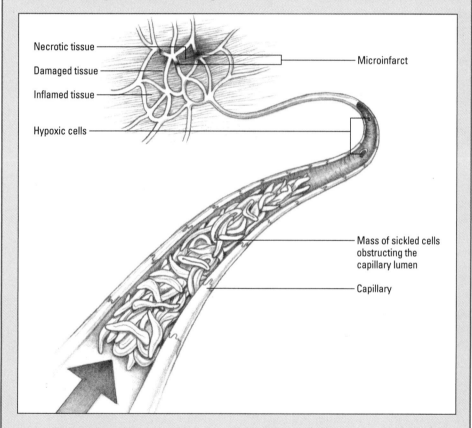

Necrotic tissue

Damaged tissue

Inflamed tissue

Hypoxic cells

Microinfarct

Mass of sickled cells obstructing the capillary lumen

Capillary

What to look for

The disease begins to manifest in the later part of the first year of life. Signs and symptoms include unusual swelling of the fingers and toes, chronic anemia, pallor, fatigue, and decreased appetite. Signs and symptoms of sickle cell crisis include severe abdominal pain, muscle spasms, leg pains, painful and swollen joints, fever, vomiting, hematuria, seizures, stiff neck, coma, and paralysis.

What tests tell you

Diagnosis of sickle cell anemia is based on:
- positive family history and presence of typical clinical features
- hemoglobin electrophoresis revealing hemoglobin S
- stained blood smear showing sickled cells
- hemoglobin level of 6 to 8 mg/dl or less, possibly decreasing to as low as 5 to 6 mg/dl during a crisis
- decreased RBC count and ESR
- increased indirect bilirubin level (during a crisis)
- clean-catch urine specimen positive for bacteria.

How it's treated

Although sickle cell anemia can't be cured, treatments can alleviate symptoms and prevent painful crises. Any pregnant woman who's considered at risk for this disease but hasn't been tested should be screened for sickle cell anemia at the first prenatal visit.

Drugs for bugs

Anti-infectives such as low-dose oral penicillin and certain vaccines, such as polyvalent pneumococcal vaccine and *Haemophilus influenzae* B vaccine, can minimize complications of sickle cell disease and transfusion therapy. Analgesics may be used to relieve pain of crisis.

Some supplements

For pregnant women, it's crucial to maintain adequate fluid intake and administer folic acid supplements. Iron supplements typically aren't prescribed because the woman's cells can't absorb iron in the usual manner; taking supplements can lead to iron overload.

Sickle stock exchange

Periodic exchange transfusions throughout the pregnancy may be used to replace sickle cells with normal cells. This procedure also helps reduce the high levels of bilirubin produced from the breakdown of RBCs.

What to do

- Monitor the patient's CBC regularly.
- Assess the patient's hydration status. Monitor her intake and output, and check for signs of dehydration.

• Urge the woman to drink at least eight 8-oz glasses of fluid each day.
• Monitor the patient's vital signs and FHR as indicated. Monitor weight gain, and assess fundal height for changes indicating adequate fetal growth.
• Assess the patient for signs and symptoms of sickle cell crisis and chronic complications. Administer analgesics and I.V. fluids as ordered if crisis develops.
• Expect to administer hypotonic saline solution I.V. for fluid replacement because the woman's kidneys have difficulty concentrating urine to remove large amounts of fluid.
• Obtain clean-catch urine specimen for culture to assess for possible bacteriuria.
• Assess lower extremities for venous pooling. Encourage the woman to avoid standing for long periods and to rest in a chair with her legs elevated or in a side-lying position to promote venous return to the heart.
• Prepare the patient for ultrasound at 16 to 24 weeks' gestation and weekly nonstress tests beginning at approximately 30 weeks' gestation.
• Be aware that blood flow velocity tests may be ordered to evaluate blood flow through the uterus and placenta. Reduced blood flow may suggest intrauterine growth retardation.
• Anticipate the patient's desire to determine if the fetus has the disease. Assist with percutaneous umbilical blood sampling to obtain a sample for RBC electrophoresis.
• Watch for signs and symptoms of infection, such as fever, chills, and purulent drainage.
• Assess the patient's respiratory status. Perform regular respiratory assessments, including auscultation of breath sounds. Expect to administer oxygen if sickle cell crisis develops.
• Provide comfort and emotional support to the patient and her family.
• Assist with measures to maintain hydration during labor and delivery.

Sexually transmitted diseases

STDs are those conditions spread through sexual contact with an infected partner. Although all STDs can be serious, certain STDs place the pregnant woman at greater risk for problems because of their potential effect on the pregnancy, fetus, or neonate. (See *Selected STDs and pregnancy*, pages 283 to 286.)

What causes it

STDs can be caused by infection with various organisms, including:
- fungi
- bacteria
- protozoa
- parasites
- viruses.

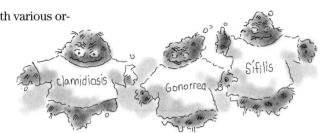

What to look for

The signs and symptoms exhibited by the patient with an STD typically involve some type of vaginal discharge or lesion. Vulvar or vaginal irritation, such as itching and pruritus, commonly accompany the discharge or lesion.

How it's treated

Treatment focuses on the underlying causative organism. Typically, antimicrobial or antifungal agents are prescribed.

Preventing the spread

In addition, education about the mode of transmission and safer sex practices are important to prevent the spread of infection.

What to do

- Explain the mode of transmission of the STD, and instruct the patient in measures to reduce the risk of transmission.
- Administer drug therapy, as ordered, and instruct the patient in drug therapy regimen. Advise the patient to comply with therapy, completing the entire course of medication even if she feels better.
- Urge the patient to refrain from sexual intercourse until the active infection is completely gone.
- Instruct the patient to have her partner arrange to be examined so that treatment can be initiated, thus preventing the risk of reinfection.
- Provide comfort measures for the client to reduce vulvar and vaginal irritation; encourage the woman to keep the vulvar area clean and dry and to avoid using strong soaps, creams, or ointments unless prescribed.
- Suggest the use of cool or tepid sitz baths to relieve itching.
- Encourage the woman to wear cotton underwear and avoid tight-fitting clothing as much as possible.

(Text continues on page 287.)

Selected STDs and pregnancy

The chart below lists several sexually transmitted diseases (STDs) along with their causative organisms and assessment findings as well as appropriate treatment for pregnant patients.

STD	Causative organism	Assessment findings	Treatment	Special considerations
Candidiasis	*Candida* fungal infection	• Thick, cheesylike vaginal discharge • Intense pruritus • Vaginal redness and irritation • Wet mount slide positive for organism	• Antifungal agent, such as miconazole cream (Monistat) or oral fluconazole (Diflucan)	• Common during pregnancy because increased estrogen levels cause changes in vaginal pH • Most commonly occurs in women receiving antibiotic therapy for another infection and women with gestational diabetes or human immunodeficiency virus infection • Possible neonatal infection if infection is present at the time of delivery
Trichomoniasis	Single-cell protozoan infection	• Yellow-gray, frothy, odorous vaginal discharge • Vulvar itching, edema, and redness • Vaginal secretions on a wet slide treated with potassium hydroxide positive for organism	• Topical clotrimazole (Gyne-Lotrimin) instead of metronidazole (Flagyl) because of its possible teratogenic effects if used during the first trimester of pregnancy	• Possibly associated with preterm labor, premature rupture of membranes, and postcesarean infection • Treatment of partner required, even if asymptomatic
Bacterial vaginosis	*Gardnerella vaginalis* infection (most commonly)	• Thin, gray vaginal discharge with a fishlike odor • Intense pruritus • Wet mount slide positive for clue cells (epithelial cells with numerous bacilli clinging to the cells' surface)	• Topical vaginal metronidazole after the first trimester, usually late in pregnancy	• Rapid growth and multiplication of organisms, replacing the normal lactobacilli organisms that are found in the healthy woman's vagina • Treatment goal of reestablishing the normal balance of vaginal flora • Untreated infections associated with amniotic fluid infections and, possibly, preterm labor and premature rupture of membranes

(continued)

Selected STDs and pregnancy *(continued)*

STD	Causative organism	Assessment findings	Treatment	Special considerations
Chlamydia	*Chlamydia trachomatis*	• Commonly produces no symptoms; suspicion raised if partner treated for nongonococcal urethritis • Heavy, gray-white vaginal discharge • Painful urination • Positive vaginal culture using special chlamydial test kit	• Amoxicillin (Amoxil)	• Screening for infection at first prenatal visit because it's one of the most common types of vaginal infection seen during pregnancy • Repeated screening in the 3rd trimester if the woman has multiple sexual partners • Doxycycline (Vibramycin)— drug of choice for treatment if the woman isn't pregnant—contraindicated during pregnancy due to association with fetal long bone deformities • Concomitant testing for gonorrhea due to high incidence of concurrent infection • Possible premature rupture of the membranes, preterm labor, and endometritis in the postpartum period resulting from infection • Possible development of conjunctivitis or pneumonia in neonate born to mother with infection present in the vagina
Syphilis	*Treponema pallidum*	• Painless ulcer on vulva or vagina (primary syphilis) • Hepatic and splenic enlargement, headache, anorexia, and maculopapular rash on the palms of the hands and soles of the feet (secondary syphilis; occurring about 2 months after initial infection)	• Penicillin G benzathine (Bicillin L-A) I.M. (single dose)	• Possible transmission across placenta after approximately 18 weeks' gestation, leading to spontaneous miscarriage, preterm labor, stillbirth, or congenital anomalies in the neonate • Standard screening for syphilis at the first prenatal visit, screening at 36 weeks' gestation for women with multiple partners, and possible rescreening at beginning of labor, with neonates tested for congenital syphilis using a sample of cord blood

Selected STDs and pregnancy (continued)

STD	Causative organism	Assessment findings	Treatment	Special considerations
Syphilis *(continued)*		• Cardiac, vascular, and central nervous system changes (tertiary syphilis; occurring after an undetermined latent phase) • Positive Venereal Disease Research Laboratory (VDRL) serum test; confirmed with positive rapid plasma reagin and fluorescent treponemal antibody absorption tests • Dark-field microscopy positive for spirochete		• Jarisch-Herxheimer reaction (sudden hypotension, fever, tachycardia, and muscle aches) after medication administration, lasting for about 24 hours, and then fading because spirochetes are destroyed
Genital herpes	Herpes simplex virus, type 2	• Painful, small vesicles with erythematous base on vulva or vagina rupturing within 1 to 7 days to form ulcers • Low-grade fever • Dyspareunia • Positive viral culture of vesicular fluid • Positive enzyme linked immunosorbent assay	• Acyclovir (Zovirax) orally or in ointment form	• Reduction or suppression of symptoms, shedding, or recurrent episodes only with drug therapy, not a cure for infection • Abstinence urged until vesicles completely heal • Primary infection transmission possible across the placenta, resulting in congenital infection in the neonate • Transmission to neonate possible if active lesions are present in the vagina or on the vulva at birth, which can be fatal • Cesarean delivery recommended if patient has active lesions
Gonorrhea	*Neisseria gonorrhoeae*	• May not produce symptoms • Yellow-green vaginal discharge	• Cefixime (Suprax) as a one-time I.M. injection	• Associated with spontaneous miscarriage, preterm birth, and endometritis in the postpartum period

(continued)

Selected STDs and pregnancy (continued)

STD	Causative organism	Assessment findings	Treatment	Special considerations
Gonorrhea *(continued)*		• Male partner who experiences severe pain on urination and purulent yellow penile discharge • Positive culture of vaginal, rectal, or urethral secretions		• Treatment of sexual partners required to prevent reinfection • Major cause of pelvic infectious disease and infertility • Severe eye infection leading to blindness in the neonate (ophthalmia neonatorum) if infection present at birth
Condyloma acuminata	Human papillomavirus	• Discrete papillary structures that spread, enlarge, and coalesce to form large lesions; increasing in size during pregnancy • Possible secondary ulceration and infection with foul odor	• Topical application of trichloroacetic acid or bichloroacetic acid to lesions • Lesion removal with laser therapy, cryocautery, or knife excision	• Serious infections associated with the development of cervical cancer later in life • Lesions left in place during pregnancy unless bothersome and removed during the postpartum period
Group B streptococci infection	Spirochete	• Usually no symptoms	• Broad-spectrum penicillin such as ampicillin	• Occurs in as many as 15% to 35% of pregnant women • May lead to urinary tract infection, intra-amniotic infection leading to preterm birth, and postpartum endometritis • Screening for all pregnant women recommended by The Centers for Disease Control and Prevention at 35 to 38 weeks' gestation • Approximately 40% to 70% infection rate in neonates of actively infected mothers due to placental transfer or direct contact with the organisms at birth, possibly leading to severe pneumonia, sepsis, respiratory distress syndrome, or meningitis in the neonate

- Instruct the patient in safer sex practices, including the use of condoms and spermicides such as nonoxynol 9.
- Encourage follow-up to ensure complete resolution of the infection (if possible).

Spontaneous abortion

Abortion refers to the spontaneous or therapeutically induced expulsion of the products of conception from the uterus before fetal viability (fetal weight of less than 496.1 g [17½ oz] and gestation of less than 20 weeks). Up to 15% of all pregnancies and about 30% of first pregnancies end in spontaneous abortion (miscarriage). At least 75% of spontaneous abortions occur during the first trimester. (See *Types of spontaneous abortion*, page 288.)

What causes it

Spontaneous abortion may result from abnormal fetal, placental, or maternal factors.

Small flaws

Fetal factors usually cause spontaneous abortions at 6 to 10 weeks' gestation. Such factors include defective embryologic development from abnormal chromosome division (the most common cause of fetal death), faulty implantation of the fertilized ovum, and failure of the endometrium to accept the fertilized ovum.

Poor placenta performance

Placental factors usually cause spontaneous abortion around the 14th week, when the placenta takes over the hormone production needed to maintain the pregnancy. Placental factors include premature separation of the normally implanted placenta, abnormal placental implantation, and abnormal platelet function.

Maternal mechanical difficulties

Maternal factors usually cause abortion between 11 and 19 weeks and include maternal infection, severe malnutrition, and abnormalities of the reproductive organs (especially incompetent cervix, in which the cervix dilates painlessly and without blood in the second trimester). Other maternal factors include endocrine

Types of spontaneous abortion

Spontaneous abortions occur without medical intervention and in various ways:

• In *complete abortion,* the uterus passes all products of conception. Minimal bleeding usually accompanies complete abortion because the uterus contracts and compresses the maternal blood vessels that feed the placenta.

• Spontaneous loss of three or more consecutive pregnancies constitutes habitual abortion.

• In *incomplete abortion,* the uterus retains part or all of the placenta. Before 10 weeks' gestation, the fetus and placenta are usually expelled together; after the 10th week, they're expelled separately. Because part of the placenta may adhere to the uterine wall, bleeding continues. Hemorrhage is possible because the uterus doesn't contract and seal the large vessels that feed the placenta.

• In *inevitable abortion,* the membranes rupture and the cervix dilates. As labor continues, the uterus expels the products of conception.

• In *missed abortion,* the uterus retains the products of conception for 2 months or more after the fetus has died. Uterine growth ceases; uterine size may even seem to decrease. Prolonged retention of the dead products of conception may cause coagulation defects such as disseminated intravascular coagulation.

• In *septic abortion,* infection accompanies abortion. This may occur with spontaneous abortion but usually results from a lapse in sterile technique during therapeutic abortion.

• In *threatened abortion,* bloody vaginal discharge occurs during the first half of pregnancy. About 20% of pregnant women have vaginal spotting or actual bleeding early in pregnancy. Of these, about 50% abort.

---

problems (such as thyroid dysfunction and lowered estriol secretion), trauma (including any type of surgery that requires manipulation of the pelvic organs), ABO blood group incompatibility and Rh isoimmunization, and drug ingestion.

What to look for

Prodromal symptoms of spontaneous abortion include a pink discharge for several days or a scant brown discharge for several weeks before the onset of cramps and increased vaginal bleeding. For a few hours, the cramps intensify and occur more frequently; then, the cervix dilates for expulsion of uterine contents. If the entire contents are expelled, cramps and bleeding subside. However, if contents remain, cramps and bleeding continue.

What tests tell you

Diagnosis of spontaneous abortion is based on evidence of expulsion of uterine contents, pelvic examination, and laboratory studies. If the blood or urine contains hCG, pregnancy is confirmed; decreased hCG levels suggest spontaneous abortion. Pelvic examination determines the size of the uterus and whether the size is consistent with the stage of the pregnancy. Expelled tissue cytology provides evidence of products of conception. Laboratory tests reflect decreased hemoglobin levels and hematocrit from blood loss. Ultrasonography confirms presence or absence of fetal heartbeats or an empty amniotic sac.

> Decreased hCG levels suggest spontaneous abortion.

How it's treated

An accurate evaluation of uterine contents is necessary before planning treatment. Spontaneous abortion can't be stopped, except in those cases attributed to an incompetent cervix. Control of severe hemorrhage requires hospitalization. Severe bleeding requires transfusion with packed RBCs or whole blood. Initially, I.V. administration of oxytocin stimulates uterine contractions. If there are remnants in the uterus, dilatation and vacuum extraction or dilatation and curettage should be performed.

RhoGAM guarantee

After an abortion, an Rh-negative female with a negative indirect Coombs' test should receive RhoGAM to prevent future Rh isoimmunization.

Employing reinforcements

Habitual abortion can result from an incompetent cervix. Treatment involves surgical reinforcement of the cervix (cerclage) about 14 to 16 weeks after the patient's last menses. A few weeks before the estimated delivery date, the sutures are removed and the patient waits for the onset of labor. An alternative procedure — particularly used for cases in which the woman wants to have more children — is to leave the sutures in place and to deliver the neonate by cesarean birth.

What to do

- Don't allow bathroom privileges because the patient may expel uterine contents without knowing it. After she uses the bedpan, inspect the contents carefully for intrauterine material.
- Note the amount, color, and odor of vaginal bleeding. Save all pads the patient uses for evaluation.
- Place the patient's bed in Trendelenburg's position as ordered.
- Administer analgesics and oxytocin as ordered.

Education edge

After spontaneous abortion

If your patient experiences a spontaneous abortion, be sure to include these instructions in your teaching plan:

• Expect vaginal bleeding or spotting to continue for several days.

• Immediately report bleeding that lasts longer than 8 to 10 days, or bleeding that's excessive or appears as bright red blood.

• Watch for signs of infection, such as a temperature higher than 100° F (37.8° C) and foul-smelling vaginal discharge.

• Gradually increase daily activities to include whatever tasks are comfortable to perform, as long as the activities don't increase vaginal bleeding or cause fatigue.

• Abstain from sexual intercourse for approximately 2 weeks.

• Use a contraceptive when you and your partner resume intercourse.

• Avoid the use of tampons for 1 to 2 weeks.

• Schedule a follow-up visit with the doctor in 2 to 4 weeks.

• Assess vital signs every 4 hours for 24 hours (or more frequently depending on the extent of bleeding).

• Monitor urine output closely.

• Provide good perineal care by keeping the perineal area clean and dry.

• Check the patient's blood type and administer RhoGAM as ordered.

• Provide emotional support and counseling during the grieving process.

• Encourage the patient and her partner to express their feelings. Some couples may want to talk to a member of the clergy or, depending on their religion, may wish to have the fetus baptized.

• Help the patient and her partner develop effective coping strategies.

• Explain all procedures and treatments to the patient and provide teaching about aftercare and follow-up. (See *After spontaneous abortion.*)

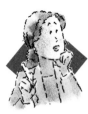

Quick quiz

1. The risks for a pregnant woman with cardiac disease and her fetus are greatest between:
- A. weeks 8 and 12.
- B. weeks 16 and 24.
- C. weeks 28 and 32.
- D. weeks 36 and 40.

Answer: C. Although the risks for the pregnant woman with cardiac disease and her fetus are always present, the most dangerous time is between weeks 28 and 32, when blood volume peaks and the woman's heart may be unable to compensate adequately for this change.

2. Screening for gestational diabetes in women is usually performed at:
- A. 4 to 8 weeks' gestation.
- B. 12 to 16 weeks' gestation.
- C. 24 to 28 weeks' gestation.
- D. 32 to 36 weeks' gestation.

Answer: C. All women are typically screened for gestational diabetes at 24 to 28 weeks' gestation.

3. The ovum of an ectopic pregnancy most commonly lodges in the:
- A. fallopian tube.
- B. abdominal viscera.
- C. ovary.
- D. cervical os.

Answer: A. The most common site of an ectopic pregnancy is the fallopian tube, either in the fimbria, ampulla, or isthmus.

4. After a spontaneous abortion, a woman who's Rh-negative would be given:
- A. magnesium sulfate.
- B. RhoGAM.
- C. terbutaline.
- D. betamethasone.

Answer: B. A woman who's Rh-negative would receive RhoGAM after a spontaneous abortion to reduce the risk of possible isoimmunization of the fetus in a future pregnancy.

5.   A major factor contributing to the increased incidence of multiple pregnancy is:
>   A.   increased use of fertility drugs.
>   B.   women becoming pregnant at a younger age.
>   C.   previous pregnancy.
>   D.   underlying iron deficiency anemia.

Answer: A. The increased use of fertility drugs has led to a doubling of the incidence of multiple pregnancy.

6.   Assessment of a woman with placenta previa would most likely reveal:
>   A.   absence of fetal heart tones.
>   B.   boardlike abdomen.
>   C.   painless, bright red vaginal bleeding.
>   D.   signs of shock.

Answer: C. A patient with placenta previa would most likely report the onset of painless, bright red vaginal bleeding after the 20th week of gestation.

7.   The drug of choice for a treating a pregnant woman with chlamydia is:
>   A.   doxycycline (Vibramycin).
>   B.   azithromycin (Zithromax).
>   C.   acyclovir (Zovirax).
>   D.   miconazole (Monistat).

Answer: B. Chlamydia infection in the pregnant woman is treated with azithromycin or amoxicillin.

Scoring

☆☆☆   If you answered all seven questions correctly, way to go! You know the in's and out's of high-risk pregnancy.

☆☆   If you answered five or six questions correctly, good going! You're maternal-neonatal nursing instincts are kicking in.

☆   If you answered fewer than five questions correctly, don't rupture your membranes. Allowing the material to gestate a little more will deliver positive results.

Labor and birth

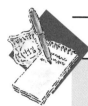

Just the facts

In this chapter, you'll learn:

♦ types of fetal presentations and positions

♦ ways in which labor can be stimulated

♦ signs and symptoms of labor

♦ stages and cardinal movements of labor

♦ nursing responsibilities during labor and birth, including ways to provide comfort and support.

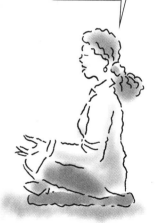

Ohm...Ohm. Providing measures to promote relaxation is key during labor and birth.

A look at labor and birth

Labor and birth is physically and emotionally straining for a woman. As the patient's body undergoes physical changes to help the fetus pass through the cervix, she may also feel discomfort, pain, panic, irritability, and loss of control. To ensure the safest outcome for the mother and child, you must fully understand the stages of labor as well as the factors affecting its length and difficulty. With an understanding of the labor and birth process, you'll be better able to provide supportive measures that promote relaxation and help increase the patient's sense of control.

Fetal presentation

Fetal presentation is the relationship of the fetus to the cervix. It can be assessed through vaginal examination, abdominal inspection and palpation, sonography, or auscultation of fetal heart tones. By knowing the fetal presentation, you can anticipate which part of the fetus will first pass through the cervix during delivery.

How long and how hard

Fetal presentation can affect the length and difficulty of labor as well as how the fetus is delivered. For example, if the fetus is in a breech presentation (the fetus's soft buttocks are presenting first), the force exerted against the cervix by uterine contractions is less than it would be if the fetus's firm head presented first. The decreased force against the cervix decreases the effectiveness of the uterine contractions that help open the cervix and push the fetus through the birth canal.

Presenting difficulties

Sometimes, the fetus's presenting part is too large to pass through the mother's pelvis or the fetus is in a position that's undeliverable. In such cases, cesarean birth may be necessary. In addition to the usual risks associated with surgery, an abnormal fetal presentation increases the risk of complications for the mother and fetus.

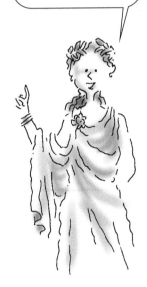

By Julius! When the fetus's presenting part is too large to pass through the mother's pelvis, cesarean birth may be necessary.

Factors determining fetal presentation

The primary factors that determine fetal presentation during birth are attitude, lie, and position.

Fetal attitude

Fetal attitude (degree of flexion) is the relationship of the fetal body parts to one another. It indicates whether the presenting parts of the fetus are in flexion or extension.

Complete flexion

The most common fetal attitude is *complete flexion*. This attitude results in a vertex (top of the head) presentation of the fetus through the birth canal. Commonly called "the fetal position," complete flexion is the traditional attitude referred to when describing a fetus in utero.

Tucked, folded, and crossed

In complete flexion, the head of the fetus is tucked down onto the chest, with the chin touching the sternum. The fetus's arms are folded over the chest with the elbows flexed. The lower legs are crossed, and the thighs are drawn up onto the abdomen. The calf of each leg is pressed against the thigh of the opposite leg.

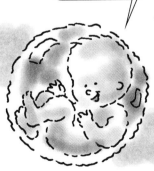

I may look uncomfortable, but I have a good attitude!

The award for best attitude goes to...

Complete flexion is the ideal attitude for gestation and birth because the fetus occupies as little space as possible in the uterus. Birth of a fetus in complete flexion is easier because the smallest anteroposterior diameter of the fetal skull is presented to pass through the pelvis first.

Moderate flexion

Moderate flexion (military position) is the second most common fetal attitude. It tends to result in a sinciput (forehead) presentation through the birth canal. Many fetuses assume this attitude early in labor but convert to complete flexion as labor progresses.

Ten-hut!

In moderate flexion, the head of the fetus is slightly flexed but held straighter than in complete flexion. The chin doesn't touch the chest. This attitude is commonly called the *military position* because the straightness of the head makes the fetus appear to be at attention.

Low rank of difficulty

The birth of a fetus in moderate flexion usually isn't difficult because the second smallest anteroposterior diameter of the skull is presented through the pelvis first.

Partial extension

Partial extension is an uncommon fetal attitude that results in a brow presentation through the birth canal. The head of the fetus is extended, with the head pushed slightly backward so that the brow becomes the first part of the fetus to pass through the pelvis during birth. Partial extension of the fetus can make birth difficult because the anteroposterior diameter of the skull may be the same size as or larger than the opening in the woman's pelvis.

Complete extension

Complete extension is a relatively rare and abnormal fetal attitude that results in a face presentation through the birth canal. This attitude occurs in an average of 1 in 500 births.

Extended and arched

In complete extension, the head and neck of the fetus are hyperextended and the occiput touches the fetus's upper back. The back is usually arched, which increases the degree of hyperextension. The occipitomental diameter of the head presents first to pass through the pelvis. Commonly, this skull diameter is too large

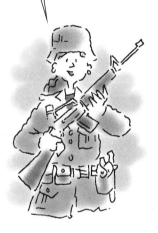

Moderate flexion is also known as the military position because the fetal head looks as if it's at attention.

to pass through the pelvis. About 12% to 20% of patients with a fetus in complete extension require cesarean birth.

Complete extension may be caused by:

- oligohydramnios (less than normal amniotic fluid)
- neurologic abnormalities
- multiparity
- a large abdomen with decreased uterine tone
- a nuchal cord with multiple coils around the fetus's neck
- fetal malformation (found in up to 60% of cases).

Fetal lie

The relationship of the fetal spine to the maternal spine is referred to as *fetal lie*. Fetal lie can be described as longitudinal, transverse, or oblique.

Longitudinal lie

When the fetal spine is parallel to the maternal spine, the fetus is in a longitudinal lie. This means that the fetus is lying vertically (top to bottom) in the uterus. Approximately 99% of fetuses are in longitudinal lie at the onset of labor.

Heads or tails?

Longitudinal lie can be further classified as *cephalic* or *breech*. In cephalic longitudinal lie, an area of the fetal head—determined by attitude and position—is the presenting part. In a breech longitudinal lie, the fetal buttocks or foot (possibly feet) is the presenting part.

Transverse lie

When the fetal spine and the maternal spine are at 90-degree angles to each other, the fetus is in transverse lie. This means that the fetus is lying horizontally (side to side) in the uterus. Transverse lie is considered abnormal, and it occurs in less than 1% of deliveries. If labor progresses while the fetus is in transverse lie, the presenting part may be a shoulder, iliac crest, hand, or elbow.

Oblique lie

When the fetal spine and the maternal spine are at 45-degree angles to each other—midway between the transverse and the longitudinal lies—the fetus is in an oblique lie. This lie is rare and is considered abnormal if the fetus remains in this position after the onset of labor.

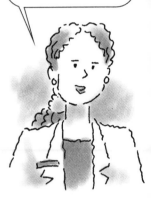

A cesarean birth may be necessary if the fetus is in complete extension because occipitomental skull diameter makes it impossible for the fetus to pass through the pelvis.

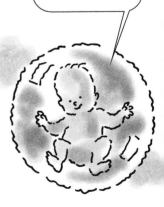

It's no lie! When I'm in line with my mom's spine, I'm in longitudinal lie.

Fetal position abbreviations

Here's a list of abbreviations, organized according to variations in presentation, that are used when documenting fetal position.

Vertex presentations (occiput)

LOA, left occipitoanterior
LOP, left occipitoposterior
LOT, left occipitotransverse
ROA, right occipitoanterior
ROP, right occipitoposterior
ROT, right occipitotransverse

Breech presentations (sacrum)

LSaA, left sacroanterior
LSaP, left sacroposterior
LSaT, left sacrotransverse
RSaA, right sacroanterior
RSaP, right sacroposterior
RSaT, right sacrotransverse

Face presentations (mentum)

LMA, left mentoanterior
LMP, left mentoposterior
LMT, left mentotransverse
RMA, right mentoanterior
RMP, right mentoposterior
RMT, right mentotransverse

Shoulder presentations (acromion process)

LAA, left scapuloanterior
LAP, left scapuloposterior
RAA, right scapuloanterior
RAP, right scapuloposterior

Fetal position

Fetal position is the relationship of the presenting part of the fetus to a specific quadrant of the mother's pelvis. It's important to define fetal position because it influences the progression of labor and whether surgical intervention is needed.

Spelling it out

Fetal position is defined using three letters. The first letter designates whether the presenting part is facing the woman's right (R) or left (L) side. The second letter or letters refer to the presenting part of the fetus: the occiput (O), mentum (M), sacrum (Sa), or scapula or acromion process (A). The third letter designates whether the presenting part is pointing to the anterior (A), posterior (P), or transverse (T) section of the mother's pelvis. The occiput typically presents first when the fetus is in the vertex fetal presentation; the mentum, in face presentation; the sacrum, in breech presentation; and the scapula or acromion process, in shoulder presentation.

The most common fetal positions are left occiput anterior (LOA) and right occiput anterior (ROA). (See *Fetal position abbreviations*.)

Duration determinant

Commonly, the duration of labor and birth is shortest when the fetus is in the LOA or ROA position. When the fetal position is posterior, such as left occiput posterior (LOP), labor tends to be longer and more painful for the woman because the fetal head puts pressure on her sacral nerves. (See *Determining fetal position*, page 298.)

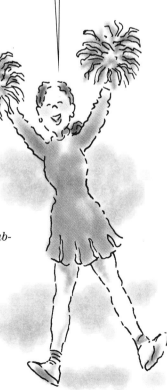

Give me an L! Give me an O! Give me an A! What does that spell? An ideal fetal position!

Determining fetal position

Fetal position is determined by the relationship of a specific presenting part (occiput, sacrum, mentum [chin], or sinciput [deflected vertex]) to the four quadrants (anterior, posterior, right, or left) of the maternal pelvis. For example, a fetus whose occiput (O) is the presenting part and who is located in the right (R) and anterior (A) quadrant of the maternal pelvis is identified as ROA.

The illustrations below show the possible positions of a fetus in vertex presentation.

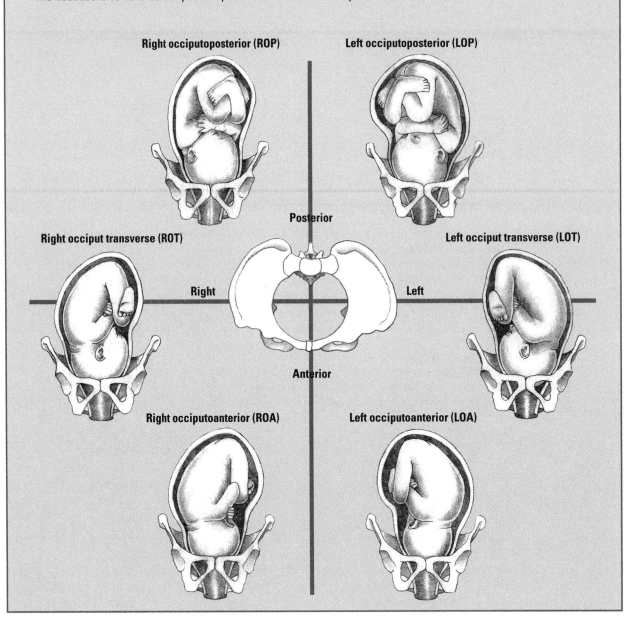

Right occiputoposterior (ROP)

Left occiputoposterior (LOP)

Posterior

Right occiput transverse (ROT)

Left occiput transverse (LOT)

Right

Left

Right occiputoanterior (ROA)

Left occiputoanterior (LOA)

Anterior

Types of fetal presentation

Fetal presentation refers to the part of the fetus that presents into the birth canal first. It's determined by fetal attitude, lie, and position. Fetal presentation should be determined in the early stages of labor in case an abnormal presentation endangers the mother and the fetus. (See *Classifying fetal presentation*, pages 300 and 301.)

The four main types of fetal presentation are:

 cephalic

 breech

 shoulder

 compound.

Cephalic presentation

When the fetus is in cephalic presentation, the head is the first part to contact the cervix and expel from the uterus during delivery. About 95% of all fetuses are in cephalic presentation at birth.

The four types of cephalic presentation are vertex, brow, face, and mentum (chin).

Vertex

In the vertex cephalic presentation, the most common presentation overall, the fetus is in a longitudinal lie with an attitude of complete flexion. The parietal bones (between the two fontanels) are the presenting part of the fetus. This presentation is considered optimal for fetal descent through the pelvis.

Brow

In brow presentation, the fetus's brow or forehead is the presenting part. The fetus is in a longitudinal lie and exhibits an attitude of moderate flexion. Although this isn't the optimal presentation for a fetus, few suffer serious complications from the delivery. In fact, many brow presentations convert to vertex presentations during descent through the pelvis.

Face

The face type of cephalic presentation is unfavorable for the mother and the fetus. In this presentation, the fetus is in a longitudinal lie and exhibits an attitude of partial extension. Because the face is the presenting part of the fetal head, severe edema and facial distortion may occur from the pressure of uterine contractions during labor.

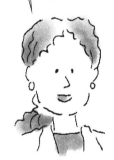

Vertex presentation is considered optimal for delivery.

Classifying fetal presentation

Fetal presentation may be broadly classified as cephalic, shoulder, compound, or breech. Almost all births are cephalic presentations. Breech births are the second most common type.

Cephalic
In the cephalic, or head-down, presentation, the position of the fetus may be further classified by the presenting skull landmark, such as vertex, brow, sinciput, or mentum (chin).

Shoulder
Although a fetus may adopt one of several shoulder presentations, examination can't differentiate among them; thus, all transverse lies are considered shoulder presentations.

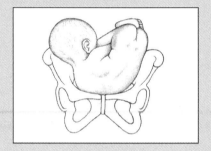

Compound
In compound presentation, an extremity prolapses alongside the major presenting part so that two presenting parts appear in the pelvis at the same time.

Vertex	Brow
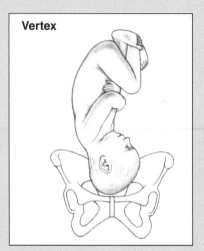	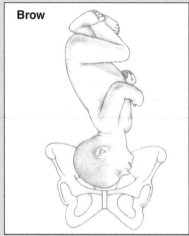

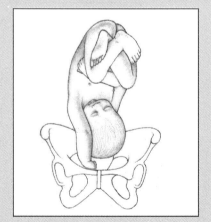

Sinciput	Mentum
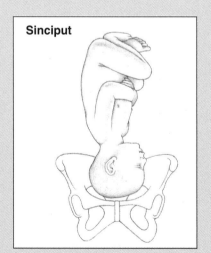	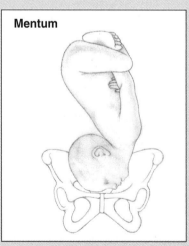

Classifying fetal presentation *(continued)*

Breech

In the breech, or head-up, presentation, the position of the fetus may be further classified as *complete,* where the knees and hips are flexed; *frank,* where the hips are flexed and knees remain straight; *kneeling,* where the knees are flexed and the hips remain extended; and *incomplete,* where one or both hips remain extended and one or both feet or knees lie below the breech.

Frank

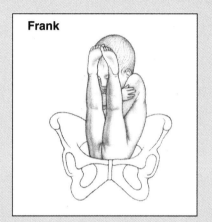

Complete

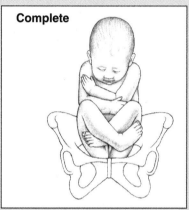

Footling

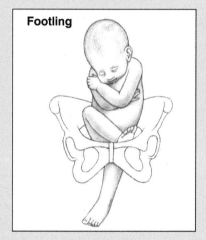

Kneeling

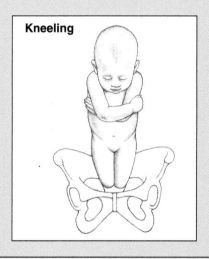

Incomplete

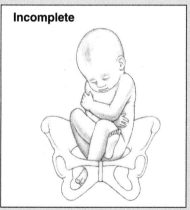

Faced with potential complications

If labor is allowed to progress, careful monitoring of both the fetus and the mother is necessary to reduce the risk of compromise. Labor may be prolonged and ineffective in some instances, and vaginal birth may not be possible because the presenting part has a larger diameter than the pelvic outlet. Attempts to manually convert the face presentation to a more favorable position are rarely successful and are associated with high perinatal mortality and maternal morbidity.

Mentum

The mentum, or chin, type of cephalic presentation is also unfavorable for the mother and the fetus. In this presentation, the fetus is in a longitudinal lie with an attitude of complete extension. The presenting part of the fetus is the chin, which may lead to severe edema and facial distortion from the pressure of the uterine contractions during labor. The widest diameter of the fetal head is presenting through the pelvis because of the extreme extension of the head. If labor is allowed to progress, careful monitoring of both the fetus and the mother is necessary to reduce the risk of compromise. Labor is usually prolonged and ineffective. Vaginal delivery is usually impossible because the fetus can't pass through the ischial spines.

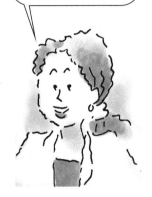

For fetuses in the mentum cephalic presentation, pressure from uterine contractions may cause severe edema and facial distortion.

Breech presentation

Although 25% of all fetuses are in breech presentation at week 30 of gestation, most turn spontaneously at 32 to 34 weeks' gestation. However, breech presentation occurs at term in about 3% of births. Labor is usually prolonged with breech presentation because of ineffective cervical dilation caused by decreased pressure on the cervix and delayed descent of the fetus.

It gets complicated

In addition to prolonging labor, the breech presentation increases the risk of complications. In the fetus, cord prolapse; anoxia; intracranial hemorrhage caused by rapid molding of the head; neck trauma; and shoulder, arm, hip, and leg dislocations or fractures may occur. Complications that may occur in the mother include perineal tears and cervical lacerations during delivery and infection from premature rupture of the membranes.

How will I know?

A breech presentation can be identified by abdominal and cervical examination. The signs of breech presentation include:
• fetal head is felt at the uterine fundus during an abdominal examination
• fetal heart tones are heard above the umbilicus
• soft buttocks or feet are palpated during a cervical examination.

Once, twice, three types more

The three types of breech presentation are complete, frank, and incomplete.

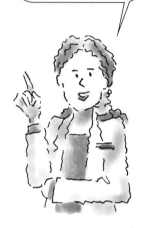

Presented with the buttocks and the feet? That means the breech is complete.

Complete breech

In a complete breech presentation, the fetus's buttocks and the feet are the presenting parts. The fetus is in a longitudinal lie and is in complete flexion. The fetus is sitting crossed-legged and both legs are drawn up (hips flexed) with the anterior of the thighs pressed tightly against the abdomen; the lower legs are crossed with the calves pressed against the posterior of the thighs; and the feet are tightly flexed against the outer aspect of the posterior thighs. Although considered an abnormal fetal presentation, complete breech is the least difficult of the breech presentations.

Frank breech

In a frank breech presentation, the fetus's buttocks are the presenting part. The fetus is in a longitudinal lie and is in moderate flexion. Both legs are drawn up (hips flexed) with the anterior of the thighs pressed against the body; the knees are fully extended and resting on the upper body with the lower legs stretched upward; the arms may be flexed over or under the legs; the feet are resting against the head. The attitude is moderate.

Incomplete breech

In an incomplete breech presentation, also called a *footling breech*, one or both of the knees or legs are the presenting parts. If one leg is extended, it's called a *single-footling breech* (the other leg may be flexed in the normal attitude); if both legs are extended, it's called a *double-footling breech.* The fetus is in a longitudinal lie. At least one of the thighs and one of the lower legs are extended with little or no hip flexion.

Perhaps expect prolapse

A footling breech is the most difficult of the breech deliveries. Cord prolapse is common in a footling breech because of the space created by the extended leg. A cesarean birth may be necessary to reduce the risk of fetal or maternal mortality.

Shoulder presentation

Although common in multiple pregnancies, the shoulder presentation of the fetus is an abnormal presentation that occurs in less than 1% of deliveries. In this presentation, the shoulder, iliac crest, hand, or elbow is the presenting part. The fetus is in a transverse lie, and the attitude may range from complete flexion to complete extension.

Lacking space and support

In the multiparous woman, shoulder presentation may be caused by the relaxation of the abdominal walls. If the abdominal walls are relaxed, the unsupported uterus falls forward, causing the fetus to turn horizontally. Other causes of shoulder presentation may include pelvic contraction (the vertical space in the pelvis is smaller than the horizontal space) or placenta previa (the low-lying placenta decreases the vertical space in the uterus).

Early identification and intervention are critical when the fetus is in a shoulder presentation. Abdominal and cervical examination and sonography are used to confirm if the mother's abdomen has an abnormal or distorted shape. Attempts to turn the fetus may be unsuccessful unless the fetus is small or preterm. A cesarean delivery may be necessary to reduce the risk of fetal or maternal death.

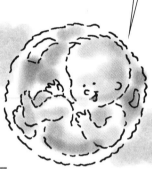

A compound presentation compounds the difficulty of birth because an extremity presents with the major presenting part.

Compound presentation

In a compound presentation, an extremity presents with another major presenting part, usually the head. In this type of presentation, the extremity prolapses alongside the major presenting part so that they present simultaneously.

Engagement

Engagement is when the presenting part of the fetus passes into the pelvis to the point where, in cephalic presentation, the biparietal diameter of the fetal head is at the level of the mid-pelvis (or at the level of the ischial spines). Vaginal and cervical examinations are used to assess the degree of engagement before and during labor.

A good sign

Because the ischial spines are usually the narrowest area of the female pelvis, an engagement indicates that the pelvic inlet is large enough for the fetus to pass through (because the widest part of the fetus has already passed through the narrowest part of the pelvis).

Floating away

In the primipara, nonengagement of the presenting part at the onset of labor may indicate a complication, such as cephalopelvic disproportion, abnormal presentation or position, or an abnormality of the fetal head. The nonengaged presenting part is described as "floating." In the multipara, nonengagement is common at the onset of labor; however, the presenting part quickly becomes engaged as labor progresses.

Station

Station is the relationship of the presenting part of the fetus to the mother's ischial spines. If the fetus is at station 0, the fetus is considered to be at the level of the ischial spines. The fetus is considered engaged when it reaches station 0.

Grand central stations

Fetal station is measured in centimeters. The measurement is called "minus" when it's above the level of the ischial spines and "plus" when it's below that level. Station measurements range from −1 to −3 cm (minus station) and +1 to +4 cm (plus station).

A crowning achievement

When the station is measured at +4 cm, the presenting part of the fetus is at the perineum—commonly known as "crowning." (See *Assessing fetal engagement and station.*)

Advice from the experts

Assessing fetal engagement and station

During a vaginal examination, you'll assess the extent of the fetal presenting part into the pelvis. This is referred to as *fetal engagement.*

After you have determined fetal engagement, palpate the presenting part and grade the fetal station (where the presenting part lies in relation to the ischial spines of the maternal pelvis). If the presenting part isn't fully engaged into the pelvis, you won't be able to assess station.

Station grades range from −3 (3 cm above the maternal ischial spines) to +4 (4 cm below the maternal ischial spines, causing the perineum to bulge). A zero grade indicates that the presenting part lies level with the ischial spines.

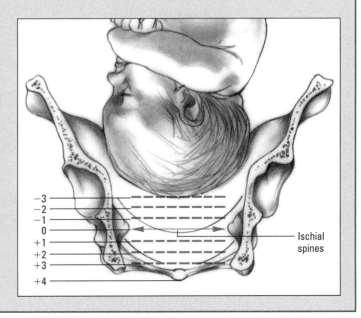

A look at labor stimulation

For some patients, it's necessary to stimulate labor. The stimulation of labor may involve induction (artificially starting labor) or augmentation (assisting a labor that started spontaneously).

Although induction and augmentation involve the same methods and risks, they're performed for different reasons. Many high-risk pregnancies must be induced because the safety of the mother or fetus is in jeopardy. Medical problems that justify induction of labor include preeclampsia, eclampsia, severe hypertension, diabetes, Rh sensitization, prolonged rupture of the membranes (over 24 hours), and a postmature fetus (a fetus that's 42 weeks' gestation or older). Augmentation of labor may be necessary if the contractions are too weak or infrequent to be effective.

Conditions for labor stimulation

Before stimulating labor, the fetus must be:
- mature
- in longitudinal lie
- engaged
- in cephalopelvic proportion (the fetal head can pass through the pelvis).

The ripe type for induction

In addition to the above fetal criteria, the mother must have a ripe cervix before labor is induced. A ripe cervix is soft and supple to the touch rather than firm. Softening of the cervix allows for cervical effacement, dilation, and effective coordination of contractions. Using Bishop's scale, you can determine whether a cervix is ripe enough for induction. (See *Bishop's scale*.)

When it isn't so great to stimulate

Stimulation of labor should be done with caution in women age 35 and older and in those with grand parity or uterine scars.

Labor shouldn't be stimulated if:
- vaginal birth is too risky.
- stimulation of the uterus increases the risk of such complications as placenta previa, abruptio placenta, uterine rupture, and decreased fetal blood supply caused by the increased intensity or duration of contractions.
- multiple pregnancy is involved.
- the woman has an active genital herpes infection.
- evidence of fetal distress exists.

A ripe cervix allows for effacement and dilation.

Bishop's scale

Bishop's scale is a tool that you can use to assess whether a woman is ready for labor. A score ranging from 0 to 3 is given for each of five factors: cervical dilation, length (effacement), consistency, position, and station.

If the woman's score exceeds 8, the cervix is considered suitable for induction.

Factor	Score
Cervical dilation	
• Cervix dilated < 1 cm	0
• Cervix dilated 1 to 2 cm	1
• Cervix dilated 2 to 4 cm	3
• Cervix dilated > 4 cm	2
Cervical length (effacement)	
• Cervical length > 4 cm (0% effaced)	0
• Cervical length 2 to 4 cm (0% to 50% effaced)	1
• Cervical length 1 to 2 cm (50% to 75% effaced)	2
• Cervical length < 1 cm (> 75% effaced)	3
Cervical consistency	
• Firm cervical consistency	0
• Average cervical consistency	1
• Soft cervical consistency	2
Cervical position	
• Posterior cervical position	0
• Middle or anterior cervical position	1
Zero station notation (presenting part level)	
• Presenting part at ischial spines −3 cm	0
• Presenting part at ischial spines −1 cm	1
• Presenting part at ischial spines +1 cm	3
• Presenting part at ischial spines +2 cm	2

Modifiers

Add 1 point to score for:
• Preeclampsia
• Each prior vaginal delivery

Subtract 1 point from score for:
• Postdates pregnancy
• Nulliparity
• Premature or prolonged rupture of membranes

Adapted with permission from Bishop, E.H. "Pelvic Scoring for Elective Induction," *Obstetrics and Gynecology* 24:266-68, 1964.

• the fetus is in an unusual presentation (such as a footling breech presentation).
• the uterus is unusually large (which increases the risk of uterine rupture).

Methods of labor stimulation

If labor is to be induced or augmented, one method or a combination of methods may be used. Methods of labor stimulation include breast stimulation, amniotomy, oxytocin administration, and ripening agent application.

Breast stimulation

In breast stimulation, the nipples are massaged to induce labor. Stimulation results in the release of oxytocin, which causes contractions that sometimes result in labor.

The patient or her partner can help with breast stimulation by:
• applying a water-soluble lubricant to the nipple area (to prevent irritation)
• gently rolling the nipple through the patient's clothing.

Too much, too soon?

One drawback of breast stimulation is that the amount of oxytocin being released by the woman's body can't be controlled. In some cases (rarely), too much oxytocin leads to excessive uterine stimulation (hyperstimulation, or tetanic contractions), which impairs fetal or placental blood flow, causing fetal distress.

Amniotomy

Amniotomy (artificial rupturing of the membranes) is performed to augment or induce labor when the membranes haven't ruptured spontaneously. This procedure allows the fetal head to contact the cervix more directly, thus increasing the efficiency of contractions. Amniotomy is virtually painless for both the mother and the fetus because the membranes don't have nerve endings.

System requirements

To perform amniotomy, the fetus must be in the vertex presentation with the fetal head at −2 station or lower. In addition, the mother must have a Bishop's score of at least 8 and her cervix must be dilated at least 3 cm.

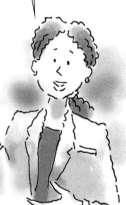

Amniotomy helps increase the efficiency of contractions.

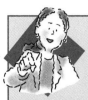

Take charge!

Complications of amniotomy

Umbilical cord prolapse—a life-threatening complication of amniotomy—is an emergency that requires immediate cesarean birth to prevent fetal death. It occurs when amniotic fluid, gushing from the ruptured sac, sweeps the cord down through the cervix. Prolapse risk is higher if the fetal head isn't engaged in the pelvis before rupture occurs.

Cord prolapse can lead to cord compression as the fetal presenting part presses the cord against the pelvic brim. Immediate action must be taken to relieve the pressure and prevent fetal anoxia and fetal distress. Here are some options:

• Insert a gloved hand into the vagina and gently push the fetal presenting part away from the cord.
• Place the woman in Trendelenburg position to tilt the presenting part backward into the pelvis and relieve pressure on the cord.
• Administer oxygen to the mother by face mask to improve oxygen flow to the fetus.

If the cord has prolapsed to the point that it's visible outside the vagina, don't attempt to push the cord back in. This can add to the compression and may cause kinking. Cover the exposed portion with a compress soaked with sterile saline solution to prevent drying, which could result in atrophy of the umbilical vessels.

Let it flow, let it flow, let it flow

During amniotomy, the woman is placed in a dorsal recumbent position. An amniohook (a long, thin instrument similar to a crochet hook) is inserted into the vagina to puncture the membranes. If puncture is properly performed, amniotic fluid gushes out.

Persevere if it isn't clear

Normal amniotic fluid is clear. Bloody or meconium-stained amniotic fluid is considered abnormal and requires careful, continuous monitoring of the mother and fetus. Bloody amniotic fluid may indicate a bleeding problem. Meconium-stained amniotic fluid may indicate fetal distress. If the fluid is meconium stained, note whether the staining is thin, moderate, or dark.

Prolapse potential

Amniotomy increases the risk to the fetus because there's a possibility that a portion of the umbilical cord will prolapse with the amniotic fluid. Fetal heart rate (FHR) should be monitored during and after the procedure to make sure that umbilical cord prolapse didn't occur. (See *Complications of amniotomy*.)

Oxytocin administration

Synthetic oxytocin (Pitocin) is used to induce or augment labor. It may be used in patients with pregnancy-induced hypertension (PIH), prolonged gestation, maternal diabetes, Rh sensitization, premature or prolonged rupture of membranes, and incomplete or inevitable abortion. Oxytocin is also used to evaluate for fetal distress after 31 weeks' gestation and to control bleeding and enhance uterine contractions after the placenta is delivered.

Oxytocin is always administered I.V. with an infusion pump. Throughout administration, FHR and uterine contractions should be assessed and monitored to ensure that they're occurring in a 20-minute span.

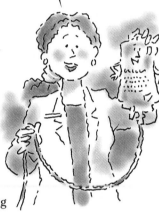

Oxytocin is always administered I.V. with an infusion pump.

Nursing interventions

Here's how to administer oxytocin:
• Start a primary I.V. line.

For starters

• Insert the tubing of the administration set through the infusion pump, and set the drip rate to administer the oxytocin at a starting infusion rate of 0.5 to 1.0 mU/minute. The maximum dosage of oxytocin is 20 to 40 mU/minute. Typically, the recommended labor-starting dosage is 10 units of oxytocin in 100 ml isotonic solution to run at 0.5 to 1.0 mU/minute, with the maximum dosage being 20 to 40 mU.

Piggyback ride

• The oxytocin solution is then piggybacked to the primary I.V. line.
• If a problem occurs, such as decelerations of FHR or fetal distress, stop the piggyback infusion immediately and resume the primary line.

Immediate action

• Because oxytocin begins acting immediately, be prepared to start monitoring uterine contractions.
• Increase the oxytocin dosage as ordered — but never increase the dose more than 1 to 2 mU/minute once every 15 to 60 minutes. Typically, the dosage continues at a rate that maintains activity closest to normal labor.

If more is in store

• Before each increase, be sure to assess contractions, maternal vital signs, and fetal heart rhythm and rate. If you're using an external fetal monitor, the uterine activity strip or grid should show

contractions occurring every 2 to 3 minutes. The contractions should last for about 60 seconds and be followed by uterine relaxation. If you're using an internal fetal monitor, look for an optimal baseline value ranging from 5 to 15 mm Hg. Your goal is to verify uterine relaxation between contractions.
• Assist with comfort measures, such as repositioning the patient on her other side, as needed.

Following through

• Continue assessing maternal and fetal responses to the oxytocin.
• Review the infusion rate to prevent uterine hyperstimulation. To manage hyperstimulation, discontinue the infusion and administer oxygen. (See *Complications of oxytocin administration*, page 312.)
• To reduce uterine irritability, try to increase uterine blood flow. Do this by changing the patient's position and increasing the infusion rate of the primary I.V. line. After hyperstimulation resolves, resume the oxytocin infusion per your facility's policy.

Ripening agent application

If a woman's cervix isn't soft and supple, a ripening agent may be applied to the cervix to stimulate labor. Drugs containing prostaglandin E_2—such as dinoprostone (Cervidil, Prepidil, Prostin E2)—are commonly used to ripen the cervix. These drugs initiate the breakdown of the collagen that keeps the cervix tightly closed.

The ripening agent can be:
• applied to the interior surface of the cervix with a catheter or suppository.
• applied to a diaphragm that's then placed against the cervix.
• inserted vaginally.

Additional doses may be applied every 6 hours; however, two or three doses are usually enough to cause ripening. The woman should remain flat after application to prevent leakage of the medication.

Success half the time

The success of this labor stimulation method varies with the agent used. After just a single application of a ripening agent, about 50% of women go into labor spontaneously and deliver within 24 hours. Those women who don't go into labor require a different method of labor stimulation.

Not to be mixed

A prostaglandin cervical ripening product should be removed from the cervix before oxytocin administration because

Take charge!

Complications of oxytocin administration

Oxytocin can cause uterine hyperstimulation. This, in turn, may progress to tetanic contractions, which last longer than 2 minutes. Signs of hyperstimulation include contractions that are less than 2 minutes apart and last 90 seconds or longer, uterine pressure that doesn't return to baseline between contractions, and intrauterine pressure that rises over 75 mm Hg.

What else to watch for
Other potential complications include fetal distress, abruptio placentae, uterine rupture, and water intoxication. Water intoxication, which can cause maternal seizures or coma, can result because the antidiuretic effect of oxytocin causes decreased urine flow.

Stop signs
Watch for the following signs of oxytocin administration complications. If any indication of any potential complications exists, stop the oxytocin administration, administer oxygen via face mask, and notify the doctor immediately.

Fetal distress
Signs of fetal distress include:
• late decelerations
• bradycardia.

Abruptio placentae
Signs of abruptio placentae include:
• sharp, stabbing uterine pain
• pain over and above the uterine contraction pain
• heavy bleeding
• hard, boardlike uterus.

Also watch for signs of shock, including rapid, weak pulse; falling blood pressure; cold and clammy skin; and dilation of the nostrils.

Uterine rupture
Signs of uterine rupture include:
• sudden, severe pain during a uterine contractions
• tearing sensation
• absent fetal heart sounds.
    Also watch for signs of shock, including rapid, weak pulse; falling blood pressure; cold and clammy skin; and dilation of the nostrils.

Water intoxication
Signs and symptoms of water intoxication include:
• headache and vomiting (usually seen first)
• hypertension
• peripheral edema
• shallow or labored breathing
• dyspnea
• tachypnea
• lethargy
• confusion
• change in level of consciousness.

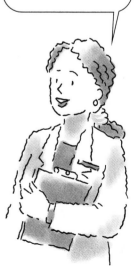

Prostaglandin application may cause uterine hyperstimulation. Monitor the patient's uterine activity.

prostaglandin potentiates the effect of oxytocin. Oxytocin induction can be started 6 to 12 hours after the last application of prostaglandin. If oxytocin is started earlier, hyperstimulation of the uterus may occur.

Prostaglandin should also be removed before amniotomy. Use this drug with caution in women with asthma, glaucoma, and renal or cardiac disease.

Not to be ignored

While the ripening agent is applied, carefully monitor the patient's uterine activity. If uterine hyperstimulation occurs or if labor begins, the prostaglandin agent should be removed. The patient should also be monitored for adverse effects of prostaglandin application, including headache, vomiting, fever, diarrhea, and hypertension. FHR should be monitored continuously for at least 30 minutes after each application and up to 2 hours after vaginal insertion.

Onset of labor

True labor begins when the woman has bloody show, her membranes rupture, and she has painful contractions of the uterus that cause effacement and dilation of the cervix. The actual mechanism that triggers this process is unknown.

Before the onset of true labor, preliminary signs appear that indicate the beginning of the birthing process. Although not considered to be a true stage of labor, these signs signify that true labor isn't far away.

Preliminary signs and symptoms of labor

Preliminary signs and symptoms of labor include lightening, increased level of activity, Braxton Hicks contractions, and ripening of the cervix. Subjective signs, such as restlessness, anxiety, and sleeplessness, may also occur. (See *Labor: True or false?* page 314.)

Lightening

Lightening is the descent of the fetal head into the pelvis. The uterus lowers and moves into a more anterior position, and the contour of the abdomen changes. In primiparas, these changes commonly occur about 2 weeks before birth. In multiparas, these changes can occur on the day labor begins or after labor starts.

More pressure here, less pressure there

Lightening increases pressure on the bladder, which may cause urinary frequency. In addition, leg pain may occur if the shifting of the fetus and uterus increases pressure on the sciatic nerve. The mother may also notice an increase in vaginal

I said lightening — not lightning!

Advice from the experts

Labor: True or false?

Use this chart to help differentiate between the signs and symptoms of true labor and those of false labor.

Signs and symptoms	True labor	False labor
Cervical changes	Cervix softens and dilates	No cervical dilation or effacement
Level of discomfort	Intense	Mild
Location of contractions	Start in the back and spread to the abdomen	Abdomen or groin
Uterine consistency when palpated	Hard as a board; can't be indented	Easily indented with a finger
Regularity of contractions	Regular with increasing frequency and duration	Irregular; no discernable pattern
Frequency and duration of contractions affected by position or activity	No	Yes
Ruptured membranes	Possible	No

discharge because of the pressure of the fetus on the cervix. Breathing, however, becomes easier for the woman after lightening because pressure on the diaphragm is decreased.

Increased level of activity

After having endured increased fatigue for most of the third trimester, it's common for a woman to experience a sudden increase in energy before true labor starts. This phenomenon is sometimes referred to as "nesting" because, in many cases, the woman directs this energy toward last-minute activities, such as organizing the baby's room, cleaning and straightening her home, and preparing other children in the household for the new arrival.

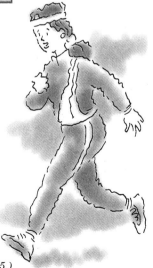

A pregnant woman won't be running marathons before she goes into labor, but she may experience an increase in her energy level.

(Text continues on page 315.)

Female pelvic organs

The female pelvis includes reproductive, urinary, and GI structures. Reproductive structures include the internal and external genitalia. Hormonal influences determine the development and function of these structures and affect fertility and childbearing.

Most of the structures of the female reproductive system are internal, housed within the pelvic cavity.

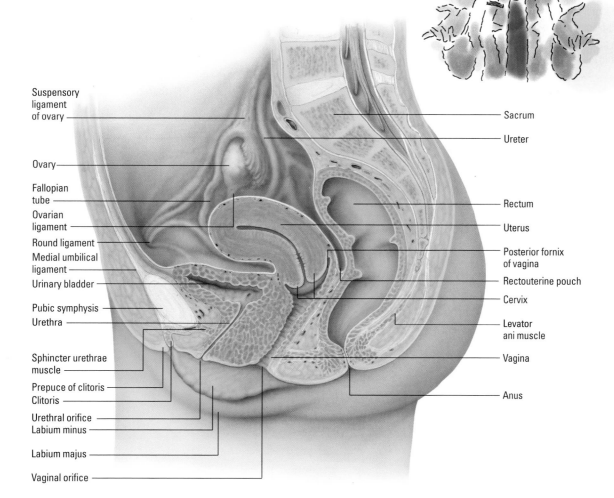

Suspensory ligament of ovary

Ovary

Fallopian tube

Ovarian ligament

Round ligament

Medial umbilical ligament

Urinary bladder

Pubic symphysis

Urethra

Sphincter urethrae muscle

Prepuce of clitoris

Clitoris

Urethral orifice

Labium minus

Labium majus

Vaginal orifice

Sacrum

Ureter

Rectum

Uterus

Posterior fornix of vagina

Rectouterine pouch

Cervix

Levator ani muscle

Vagina

Anus

Ovarian and uterine changes during the menstrual cycle

The hypothalamus, ovaries, and pituitary gland secrete hormones that effect the buildup and shedding of the endometrium during the menstrual cycle. The menstrual cycle normally occurs over 28 days, although it may range from 22 to 34 days. The cycle is regulated by fluctuating hormone levels that, in turn, are regulated by negative and positive feedback mechanisms involving the hypothalamus, pituitary glands, and ovaries.

The hormonal changes of the menstrual cycle trigger a series of changes in the uterine endometrium as follows:
- menstrual (preovulatory) phase—endometrium exfoliates and sheds
- proliferative (follicular) phase and ovulation—endometrium proliferates
- luteal (secretory) phase—endometrium becomes thick and secretory to prepare for the implantation of a fertilized ovum
- premenstrual phase—in absence of fertilization, estrogen and progesterone levels drop and the endometrium sheds.

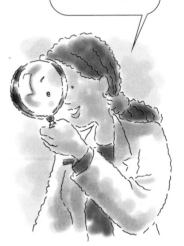

These illustrations show the relationship between ovarian changes and uterine changes during the menstrual cycle.

Ovary

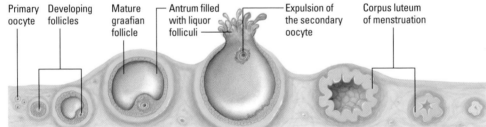

Primary oocyte · Developing follicles · Mature graafian follicle · Antrum filled with liquor folliculi · Expulsion of the secondary oocyte · Corpus luteum of menstruation

Uterus

Ovulation

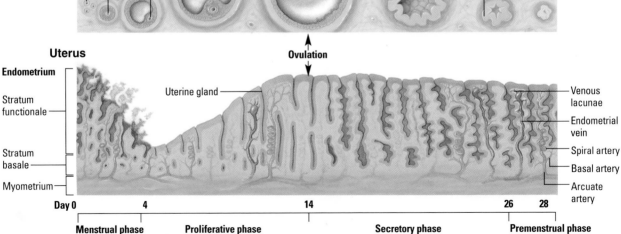

Endometrium · Stratum functionale · Stratum basale · Myometrium · Uterine gland · Venous lacunae · Endometrial vein · Spiral artery · Basal artery · Arcuate artery

Day 0 · 4 · 14 · 26 · 28

Menstrual phase · Proliferative phase · Secretory phase · Premenstrual phase

Fertilization and implantation

During monthly ovulation, an ovum is released from the ovary into the fallopian tube, where it travels toward the uterus. If present, sperm from the male move through the fallopian tube, where they meet the ovum.

If a sperm penetrates the ovum, fertilization occurs and the ovum is called a *zygote*. The zygote continues to travel toward the uterus, dividing many times until it becomes a blastocyst. When the blastocyst reaches the uterus, it implants in the uterine wall and continues to develop over the next nine months.

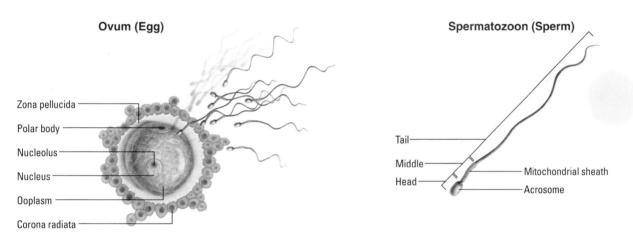

Ovum (Egg)

- Zona pellucida
- Polar body
- Nucleolus
- Nucleus
- Ooplasm
- Corona radiata

Spermatozoon (Sperm)

- Tail
- Middle
- Head
- Mitochondrial sheath
- Acrosome

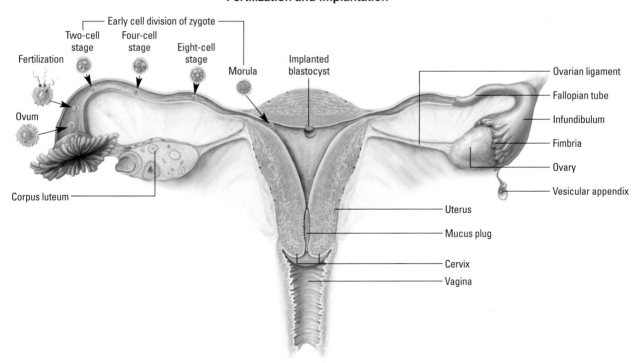

Fertilization and implantation

Early cell division of zygote

- Two-cell stage
- Four-cell stage
- Eight-cell stage
- Fertilization
- Ovum
- Morula
- Implanted blastocyst
- Corpus luteum
- Ovarian ligament
- Fallopian tube
- Infundibulum
- Fimbria
- Ovary
- Vesicular appendix
- Uterus
- Mucus plug
- Cervix
- Vagina

Male pelvic structures

In the male, pelvic structures include GI, reproductive, and urinary organs. These structures are illustrated below.

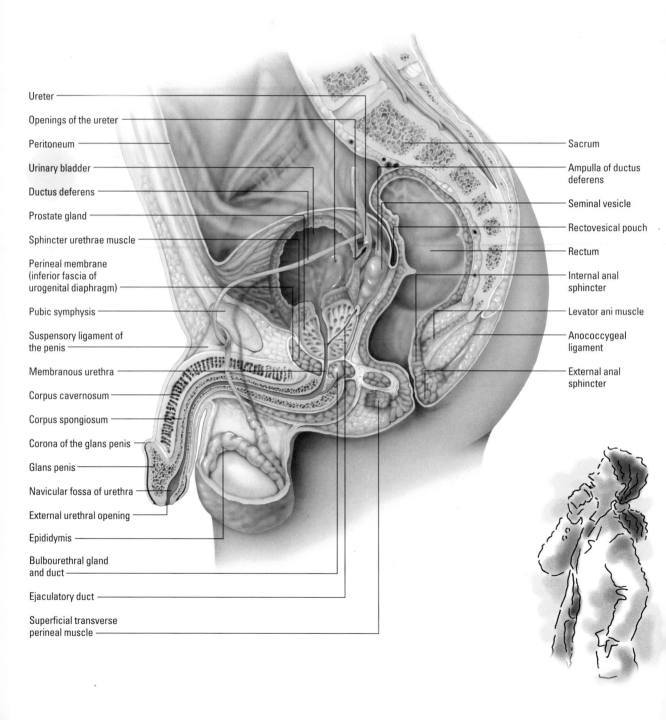

Ureter

Openings of the ureter

Peritoneum

Urinary bladder

Ductus deferens

Prostate gland

Sphincter urethrae muscle

Perineal membrane
(inferior fascia of
urogenital diaphragm)

Pubic symphysis

Suspensory ligament of
the penis

Membranous urethra

Corpus cavernosum

Corpus spongiosum

Corona of the glans penis

Glans penis

Navicular fossa of urethra

External urethral opening

Epididymis

Bulbourethral gland
and duct

Ejaculatory duct

Superficial transverse
perineal muscle

Sacrum

Ampulla of ductus
deferens

Seminal vesicle

Rectovesical pouch

Rectum

Internal anal
sphincter

Levator ani muscle

Anococcygeal
ligament

External anal
sphincter

A built-in energy source

The woman's increase in activity may be caused by a decrease in placental progesterone production (which may also be partly responsible for the onset of labor) that results in an increase in the release of epinephrine. This epinephrine increase gives the woman extra energy for labor.

Braxton Hicks contractions

Braxton Hicks contractions are mild contractions of the uterus that occur throughout pregnancy. They may become extremely strong a few days to a month before labor begins, which may cause some women, especially a primipara, to misinterpret them as true labor. Several characteristics, however, distinguish Braxton Hicks contractions from labor contractions.

> Eating can help calm Braxton Hicks contractions.

Patternless

Braxton Hicks contractions are irregular. There's no pattern to the length of time between them and they vary widely in their strength. They gradually increase in frequency and intensity throughout the pregnancy, but they maintain an irregular pattern. In addition, Braxton Hicks contractions can be diminished by increasing activity or by eating, drinking, or changing position. Labor contractions can't be diminished by these activities.

Painless

Braxton Hicks contractions are commonly painless—especially early in pregnancy. Many women feel only a tightening of the abdomen in the first or second trimester. If the woman does feel pain from these contractions, it's felt only in the abdomen and the groin—usually not in the back. This is a major difference from the contractions of labor.

No softening or stretching

Probably the most important differentiation between Braxton Hicks contractions and true labor contractions is that Braxton Hicks contractions don't cause progressive effacement or dilation of the cervix. The uterus can still be indented with a finger during a contraction, which indicates that the contractions aren't efficient enough for effacement or dilation to occur.

Ripening of the cervix

Ripening of the cervix refers to the process in which the cervix softens to prepare for dilation and effacement. It's thought to be the result of hormone-mediated biochemical events that initiate breakdown of the collagen in the cervix, thus causing it to soften and become flexible. As the cervix ripens, it also changes position by tipping forward in the vagina.

Ripening of the cervix doesn't produce outwardly observable signs or symptoms. The ripeness of the cervix is determined during a pelvic examination, usually in the last weeks of the third trimester.

Signs of true labor

Signs of true labor include uterine contractions, show, and spontaneous rupture of membranes.

Uterine contractions

The involuntary uterine contractions of true labor help effacement and dilation of the uterus and push the fetus through the birth canal. Although uterine contractions are irregular when they begin, as labor progresses they become regular with a predictable pattern.

Early contractions occur anywhere from 5 to 30 minutes apart and last about 30 to 45 seconds. The interval between the contractions allows blood flow to resume to the placenta, which supplies oxygen to the fetus and removes waste products. As labor progresses, the contractions increase in frequency, duration, and intensity. During the transition phase of the first stage of labor — when contractions reach their maximum intensity, frequency, and duration — they each last 60 to 90 seconds and recur every 2 to 3 minutes.

Sweeping waves

Uterine contractions are painful and wavelike — they build and recede — beginning in the lower back and moving around to the abdomen and, possibly, the legs. They're stronger in the upper uterus than in the lower uterus so they can push the fetus downward and allow for dilation. These contractions cause a palpable hardening of the uterus that can't be indented with a finger.

Efface it!

Most important, the uterine contractions of labor cause progressive effacement and dilation of the cervix. As labor progresses, a visible bulging of intact membranes can be observed.

Cowabunga! Uterine contractions are wavelike.

Show

Bloody show occurs as the cervix thins and begins to dilate, allowing passage of the mucus plug that seals the cervical canal during pregnancy. Mucus from the plug mixes with blood from the cervical capillaries due to the pressure of the fetus on the canal and other changes in the cervix. Because of this, show may appear pinkish, blood-tinged, or brownish. Occasionally, in primiparas it may be passed up to 2 weeks before labor begins.

Spontaneous rupture of membranes

Twenty-five percent of all labors begin with spontaneous rupture of the membranes. The membranes — consisting of the amniotic and chorionic membranes — cover the fetal surface of the placenta and form a sac that contains and supports the fetus and the amniotic fluid. This fluid, produced by the amniotic membrane, acts as a cushion throughout gestation, protects the fetus from temperature changes, protects the umbilical cord from pressure, and is believed to aid in fetal muscular development by allowing the fetus to move freely.

Fluid facts

Spontaneous rupture of the membranes may occur as a sudden gush of fluid, or as a steady or intermittent, slow leakage of fluid. Rupture isn't painful because the membranes don't have a nerve supply. Even though much of the amniotic fluid is lost when the membranes rupture, the fetus is still protected. The amniotic membrane continues to produce more fluid that surrounds and protects the fetus until it's delivered.

Color-coded

The amniotic fluid that's lost after the rupture of the membranes should be odorless and clear or milky. Colored fluid usually indicates a problem. Yellow fluid indicates that the amniotic fluid is bilirubin-stained from the breakdown of red blood cells, which may be caused by blood incompatibility. Green fluid indicates meconium-staining, possibly from a breech presentation or fetal anoxia, and needs immediate evaluation.

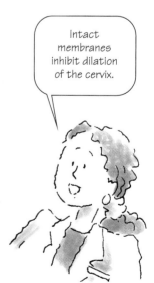

Intact membranes inhibit dilation of the cervix.

Rupture or be ruptured

If a woman's membranes haven't ruptured spontaneously before the transition phase of the first stage of labor, they may rupture when the cervix becomes fully dilated at 10 cm or amniotomy may be performed. Membrane rupture shortens the duration of labor and aids in the dilation of the cervix. Membranes that remain intact delay full dilation and lengthen the duration of labor because the amniotic fluid cushions the pressure of the fetal head against the cervix, preventing the contractions from exerting their full impact.

A little premature

Premature rupture of membranes (rupture that occurs more than 24 hours before labor begins) is associated with a risk of infection and umbilical cord prolapse.

Stages of labor

Labor is typically divided into four stages:

The first stage, when effacement and dilation occur, begins with the onset of true uterine contractions and ends when the cervix is fully dilated.

The second stage, which encompasses the actual birth, begins when the cervix is fully dilated and ends with the delivery of the fetus.

The third stage, also called the *placental stage*, begins immediately after the neonate is delivered and ends when the placenta is delivered.

The fourth stage begins after delivery of the placenta. During this stage, homeostasis is reestablished.

First stage

The first stage of labor begins with the onset of contractions and ends when the cervix is dilated to 10 cm (full dilation). It's divided into three phases: latent, active, and transition.

Latent phase

The latent phase of labor begins with the onset of regular contractions. Usually, the contractions during this phase are mild. They last about 20 to 40 seconds and recur every 5 to 30 minutes. Initially, the contractions may vary in intensity and duration, but they become consistent within a few hours.

Waiting for dilation

The latent phase lasts about 6 hours in the primipara and 4½ hours in the multipara and ends when rapid cervical dilation begins. During this phase, the cervix dilates from 0 cm to 3 cm and becomes fully effaced; however, there's minimal fetal descent through the pelvis. The contractions usually cause little discomfort if the woman remains relaxed and continues to walk around.

Lasting longer than expected?

Premature analgesia administration, poor fetal position, cephalopelvic disproportion, and a cervix that hasn't softened sufficiently may increase the duration of the latent phase.

Keep her calm, moving, or voiding

Nursing care during the latent phase is mainly supportive. Provide the woman with a calm environment and psychological support for the conflicting emotions — such as excitement, anxiety and, possibly, depression — that she's experiencing. Give a clear liquid diet or ice chips as tolerated, and encourage the woman to move and empty her bladder frequently. Be sure to involve the woman's partner or support person in her care as much as possible.

Technical stuff

Obtain the required blood sample and urine specimen, monitor the woman's vital signs, monitor FHR, and explain and initiate electronic monitoring as ordered.

It's all about timing and intensity

During the latent phase, start timing the frequency and length of the contractions and assessing their intensity. To time the frequency of contractions, gently rest a hand on the woman's abdomen at the fundus of the uterus. Count from the beginning of one contraction to the beginning of the next. Begin timing at the start of the gradual tensing and upward rising of the fundus (initially, these sensations may not be felt by the woman); end timing when the uterus has fully relaxed.

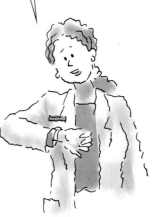

> During the latent phase, start timing the frequency and length of contractions.

Do you feel a nose, a chin, or a forehead?

The intensity of contractions can be determined by assessing the uterus. With mild contractions, the uterus is minimally tense. It may be easily indented with a fingertip, and feel similar to pressing on the tip of the nose. With moderate contractions, the uterus feels firmer. It can't be indented with a finger and it feels similar to pressing on the chin. With strong contractions, the uterus feels extremely hard. It can't be indented — even with firm pressure — and it feels similar to pressing on the forehead.

Active phase

During the active phase of labor, the release of show increases and the membranes may rupture spontaneously. The contractions are stronger, each lasting about 40 to 60 seconds and recurring about every 3 to 5 minutes. The increased strength of the contractions commonly causes pain. Cervical dilation occurs more rapidly, increasing from about 3 cm to 7 cm, and the fetus begins to descend through the pelvis at an increased rate.

Whole lot of changing going on

The active phase is an emotionally charged time for the woman. She may be feeling excitement as well as fear. The woman also undergoes many systemic changes. (See *Systemic changes in the active phase of labor*.)

How long must this go on?

The active phase of labor lasts about 3 hours in a primipara and 2 hours in a multipara. If analgesics are given at this time, they won't slow labor. Poor fetal position and a full bladder may prolong this phase.

Shower her with comfort and support

Nursing care during the active phase focuses on the psychological status of the woman as well as her physical care. Expect the woman to have mood swings and difficulty coping. Offer support and encourage the woman to use proper breathing techniques. In addition, continue to involve the woman's partner or labor support person in her care. Placing the woman in an upright or side-lying position may provide additional comfort.

Other nursing measures that may be necessary include:
• monitoring I.V. fluids as ordered to maintain fluid balance
• monitoring intake and output
• monitoring vital signs and FHR
• performing perineal care frequently to reduce the risk of infection, especially after each voiding and bowel movement.

Transition phase

During the transition phase, contractions reach maximum intensity. They each last 60 to 90 seconds and they occur every 2 to 3 minutes. The cervix dilates from about 7 cm to 10 cm to become fully dilated and effaced. If the membranes aren't already ruptured, they usually rupture when the woman is 10 cm dilated, and the remainder of the mucus plug is expelled from the cervix.

The transition phase peaks when cervical dilation slows slightly at 9 cm. This slowdown signifies the end of the first stage of labor. For multiparas, birth may be imminent at this time.

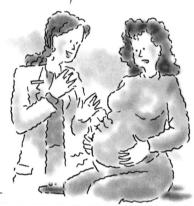

In the active phase, the strength of contractions increases.

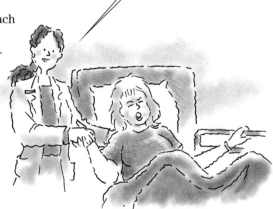

Contractions reach maximum intensity during the transition phase of labor.

Systemic changes in the active phase of labor

This chart shows the systemic changes that occur during the active phase of labor.

System	Change
Cardiovascular	• Increased blood pressure • Increased cardiac output • Supine hypotension
Respiratory	• Increased oxygen consumption • Increased rate • Possible hyperventilation leading to respiratory alkalosis, hypoxia, and hypercapnia (if breathing isn't controlled)
Renal	• Difficulty voiding • Proteinuria (1+ normal)
Musculoskeletal	• Diaphoresis • Fatigue • Backache • Joint pain • Leg cramps
Neurologic	• Increased pain threshold and sedation caused by endogenous endorphins • Anesthetized perineal tissues caused by constant intense pressure on nerve endings
GI	• Dehydration • Decreased motility • Slow absorption of solid food • Nausea • Diarrhea
Endocrine	• Decreased progesterone level • Increased estrogen level • Increased prostaglandin level • Increased oxytocin level • Increased metabolism • Decreased blood glucose

What she's feeling

When in the transition phase, the woman may experience intense pain or discomfort as well as nausea and vomiting. She may also experience intense mood swings and feelings of anxiety, panic, irritability, and loss of control because of the intensity and duration of contractions.

What you're doing

Nursing care during the transition phase includes monitoring vital signs and FHR, encouraging proper breathing techniques, and administering medications as ordered. Arrange for a nurse to be with the woman at all times because there's a possibility that birth is imminent. In addition, expect the patient to experience irritability, mood swings, and difficulty coping. Make sure to provide emotional support to the woman and her partner or support person during this time.

Second stage

The second stage of labor starts with full dilation and effacement of the cervix and ends with the delivery of the neonate. It lasts about 1 to 3 hours for the primipara and 30 to 60 minutes for the multipara. During the second stage, the frequency of the contractions slows to about one every 3 to 4 minutes; however, they continue to last 60 to 90 seconds and are accompanied by the uncontrollable urge to push or bear down. The decreased frequency of the contractions gives the woman a chance to rest.

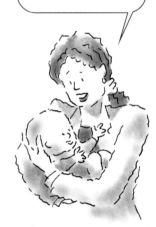

Although the second stage of labor ends with delivery of the neonate, the work isn't done yet. There are still two stages of labor to go!

Movin' out

Whereas the previous stage of labor primarily involved thinning and opening of the uterus, the second stage involves moving the fetus through the birth canal and out of the body.

As the uterine contractions work to accomplish this movement, the fetus pushes on the internal side of the perineum, causing the perineum to bulge and become tense. The fetal scalp becomes visible at the opening to the vagina (called *crowning*). The vaginal opening changes from a slit to an oval and then to a circle. The circular opening then gradually increases in size to allow the fetus's head to emerge. The combination of involuntary uterine contractions and the mother pushing with her abdominal muscles helps the fetus proceed through the cardinal movements of labor and expel from the body.

The physiologic changes that began in the first stage of labor continue throughout the second stage. In addition, the mother's oxytocin level increases, which helps to intensify the contractions.

Cardinal movements of labor

The cardinal movements of labor are fetal position changes that occur during the second stage of labor. They help the fetus pass through the birth canal. These movements are necessary because of the size of the fetal head in relation to the irregularly-shaped pelvis. Specific, deliberate, and precise, the various movements allow the smallest diameter of the fetus to pass through the corresponding diameter of the woman's pelvis. (See *Cardinal movements of labor*, page 324.)

Descent

Descent, the first of the cardinal movements, is the downward movement of the fetus. It's determined when the biparietal diameter of the head passes the ischial spines and moves into the pelvic inlet.

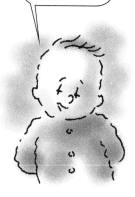

I had some smooth cardinal moves back when I was born.

May the forces be with you

Descent progresses intermittently with contractions and occurs because of several forces:
- direct pressure on the fetus by the contracting uterine fundus
- pressure of the amniotic fluid
- contraction of the abdominal muscles (fetal pressure on the mother's sacral nerves causes her to experience an uncontrollable need to push)
- extension and straightening of the fetal body.

Making contact

Full descent is accomplished when the fetal head passes beyond the dilated cervix and contacts the posterior vaginal floor.

Flexion

Flexion, the second of the cardinal movements, occurs during descent. It's caused by the resistance of the fetal head against the pelvic floor. The combined pressure from this resistance and uterine and abdominal muscle contractions forces the head of the fetus to bend forward so that the chin is pressed to the chest. This allows the smallest diameter of the fetal head to descend through the pelvis.

A different angle

Flexion causes the presenting diameter to change from occipitofrontal (nasal bridge to the posterior fontanel) to suboccipitobregmatic (posterior fontanel to subocciput) in an occiput anterior position. If the fetus is an occiput posterior position, flexion is

Cardinal movements of labor

These illustrations show the fetal movements that occur during the cardinal movements of labor.

Descent

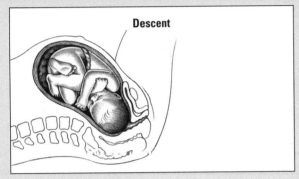

Internal rotation

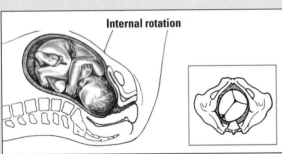

Extension beginning (rotation complete)

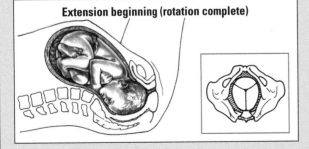

Extension complete

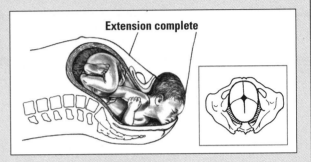

External rotation (restitution)

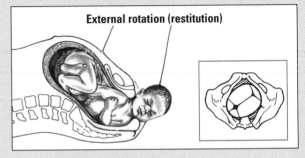

External rotation (shoulder rotation)

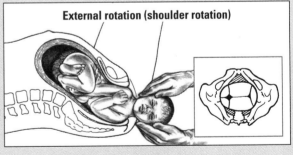

Expulsion

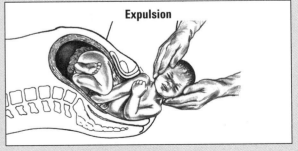

incomplete and the fetus has a larger presenting diameter, which can prolong labor.

Internal rotation

The fetal head typically enters the pelvis with its anteroposterior head diameter in a transverse (right to left) position. This position is beneficial when entering the pelvis because the diameter at the pelvic inlet is widest from right to left. However, if the head remains in the transverse position, the shoulders are in a position where they're too wide to pass through the pelvic inlet.

Shifting toward the same plane

To allow the shoulders to pass through the pelvic inlet, the fetal head rotates about 45 degrees as it meets the resistance of the pelvic floor. With the head rotated, the anteroposterior diameter of the head is in the anteroposterior plane of the pelvis (front to back), which places the widest part of the shoulders in line with the widest part of the pelvic inlet and outlet. At this point, the face of the fetus is usually against the woman's back and the back of the fetal head is against the front of the woman's pelvis.

Extension

Extension occurs after the internal rotation is complete. As the head passes through the pelvis, the occiput emerges from the vagina, and the back of the neck stops under the symphysis pubis (pubic arch). Further descent is temporarily halted because the fetus's shoulders are too wide to pass through the pelvis or under the pubic arch.

Pivotal movements

With the back of the fetal neck resting against the pubic arch, the arch acts as a pivot. The upward resistance from the pelvic floor causes the head to extend. As this occurs, the brow, nose, mouth, and chin are born.

External rotation

External rotation (also called *restitution*) is necessary because the shoulders, which previously turned to fit through the pelvic inlet, must now turn again to fit through the pelvic outlet and under the pubic arch.

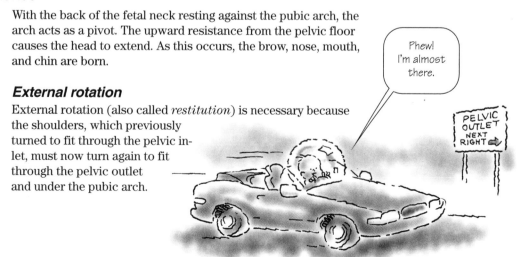

Phew! I'm almost there.

PELVIC OUTLET NEXT RIGHT

Return the fetus to the transverse position...

After the head is born, the face, which is facing down after the completion of extension, is turned to face one of the mother's inner thighs. The head rotates about 45 degrees, returning the anteroposterior head diameter to the transverse (right to left) position assumed during descent.

...and prepare for shoulder delivery

The anterior shoulder (closest to the front of the mother) is delivered first with the possible assistance of downward flexion on the head. After the anterior shoulder is delivered, a slight upward flexion may be necessary to deliver the posterior shoulder.

Weighing in

During external rotation, a neonate who weighs more than 9.9 lb (4.5 kg) has a greater likelihood of experiencing shoulder dystocia than one who weighs less. Shoulder dystocia occurs when lack of room for passage causes the shoulders to stop at the pelvic outlet. Commonly, shoulder dystocia is resolved by sharply flexing the maternal thighs against the maternal abdomen (McRobert's technique). This movement reduces the angle between the sacrum and the spine and allows the shoulders to pass through; however, the neonate may sustain some injury to the brachial plexus.

Expulsion

After delivery of the shoulders, the remainder of the body is delivered quickly and easily. Termed *expulsion*, this step signifies the end of the second stage of labor.

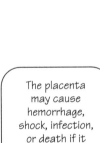

Unlike in school, expulsion during labor is a good thing.

Third stage

The third stage of labor, also called the *placental stage,* occurs after delivery of the neonate and ends with the delivery of the placenta. It consists of two phases: placental separation and placental expulsion. This stage of labor is important because a placenta that remains in place may cause hemorrhage, shock, infection, or even death.

From round to discoid

After the neonate has been delivered, uterine contractions commonly stop for several minutes. During this time, the uterus is a round mass located below the level of the umbilicus that feels firm to the touch. When contractions resume, the uterus takes on a discoid shape until the placenta has separated from the uterus.

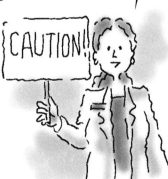

The placenta may cause hemorrhage, shock, infection, or death if it isn't delivered.

Delivery in 30 minutes or less

The duration of the third stage varies widely. It may last from several minutes to up to 30 minutes.

Placental separation

Separation of the placenta from the uterus occurs after the uterus resumes contractions. Uterine contractions continue to occur in the wavelike pattern that they assumed throughout the other stages of labor; however, in the other stages, the fetus exerted pressure on the placenta during contractions, which prevented the placenta from separating prematurely. When the fetus is no longer in the uterus, the uterine walls contract on an almost empty space. Nothing exerts reverse pressure on the placenta. As a result, the placenta folds and begins to separate from the uterine wall. This separation causes bleeding that further pushes the placenta away from the uterine wall, ultimately causing the placenta to fall to the upper vagina or lower uterine segment.

Ready to roll

Signs that the placenta has separated and is ready to be delivered include:
- absence of cord pulse
- lengthening of the umbilical cord
- sudden gush of vaginal blood
- change in the shape of the uterus.

Separating from the center...

Approximately 80% of all separated placentas are *Schultze placentas*. A Schultze placenta starts to separate at the center and folds onto itself. It delivers with the fetal surface exposed and appears shiny and glistening from the fetal membranes.

...or the edge

A *Duncan placenta* separates at the edges, then slides down the surface of the uterus and delivers with the maternal surface exposed. It appears red, raw, and irregular because of the ridges that separate the blood collection spaces.

Placental expulsion

Natural bearing down by the mother or gentle pressure on the fundus of the contracting uterus (Credé's maneuver) aids in the delivery of the placenta. To avoid possible eversion (turning inside out) of the uterus, which can result in gross hemorrhage, never exert pressure on the uterus when it isn't contracted. Manual removal of the placenta may be indicated if it doesn't deliver spontaneously.

Memory jogger

To help remember which type of placenta is which, think "Shiny Schultze" and "Dirty Duncan." The Schultze placenta is shiny from the fetal membrane. The Duncan placenta exposes the maternal side and appears red and dirty with an irregular surface.

Check it out

After delivery, examine the placenta to make sure it's intact and normal in appearance and weight. This helps determine whether any has been retained in the uterus. The placenta is usually one-sixth the weight of the infant.

Additional layers

An outer area of decidua (the lining of the uterus) is expelled at the same time as the placenta. The remainder of the decidua separates into two layers:

☞ the superficial layer that's shed in the lochia during the postpartum period

✌ the basal layer that remains in the uterus to regenerate new endothelium.

Blood volume matters

Normal bleeding occurs until the uterus contracts with enough force to seal the blood collection spaces. A blood loss of 300 to 500 ml should be expected. Blood loss exceeding 500 ml may indicate a cervical tear or a problem at the episiotomy site. It may also indicate that the uterus isn't contracting properly due to retained placenta or a full bladder.

Commonly, after the placenta is delivered, the mother is given I.V. oxytocin (Pitocin) or I.M. methylergonovine (Methergine) to increase uterine contractions and minimize bleeding; however, these drugs shouldn't be given if the mother's blood pressure is increased because they cause vasoconstriction and hypertension.

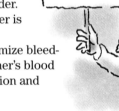

Neither Pitocin nor Methergine should be administered if the mother's blood pressure is increased because they can cause vasodilation and hypertension.

Fourth stage

The fourth stage of labor occurs immediately after the delivery of the placenta. It usually lasts for about 1 to 4 hours, and it initiates the postpartum period. During this stage, the woman should be monitored closely because her body has just undergone many changes.

Risks associated with the fourth stage of labor include hemorrhage, bladder distention, and venous thrombosis. Oxygen, type O-negative blood or blood tested for compatibility, and I.V. fluids must be available for 2 to 3 hours after delivery.

Inspect and repair

Initially, the cervix and vagina are inspected to check for and repair lacerations that may have occurred during birth. If an episiotomy was performed, the incision is sutured. Keep in mind that a woman who delivered without the aid of an anesthetic requires a local anesthetic for this procedure; a woman who received regional or local anesthesia during the birth probably won't need additional medication. When suturing is complete, the woman's legs should be lowered from the stirrups. Make sure the legs are lowered simultaneously to prevent back injury.

Monitoring mommy

Monitor the woman's vital signs every 15 minutes for a minimum of 1 hour, then as ordered. Expect the woman's pulse, respirations, and blood pressure to be slightly increased at this time because of the birth process, excitement, and oxytocin administration. In addition, the woman may experience a normal chill and shaking sensation shortly after the birth. This is common and may be caused by excess epinephrine production during labor or the sudden release of pressure on the pelvic nerves.

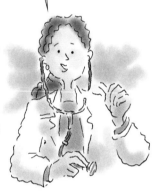

After delivery, the woman's pulse, respirations, and blood pressure will be slightly increased.

The incredible shrinking uterus

After delivery, the uterus gradually decreases in size and descends into its prepregnancy position in the pelvis — a process known as *involution*. To evaluate this process, palpate the uterine fundus and determine uterine size, degree of firmness, and rate of descent (which is measured in fingerbreadths above or below the umbilicus). Involution normally begins immediately after delivery, when the firmly contracted uterus lies almost at the umbilicus. If the woman is breast-feeding, the release of natural oxytocics should help to maintain or stimulate contraction of the uterus. If it doesn't remain contracted, gently massage the uterus or administer medications as ordered.

Void to avoid interference

Encourage the woman to void because a full bladder interferes with uterine contractions that work to compress the open blood vessels at the placental site. If these blood vessels are allowed to bleed freely, hemorrhage may occur. Observe the amount, color, and consistency of the lochia and watch for its absence, which may indicate that a clot is blocking the cervical os. Sudden heavy bleeding could result if a change of position dislodges the clot.

Clot watch

Pregnant and postpartum women have higher fibrinogen levels, which increase the possibility of clot formation. A woman has an additional risk of clot formation if she has varicose veins or a history of thrombophlebitis or if she had a cesarean delivery. Monitor closely for signs of venous thrombosis, especially if the duration of labor was abnormally long or if the woman was confined to bed for an extended period.

Ongoing support

Be sure to take the following steps as well:
• Offer emotional support as needed to the mother and her partner or labor support person.
• Perform perineal care and apply a clean perineal pad as needed.
• Offer a regular diet as soon as the patient requests food (sometimes this request is made shortly after delivery).
• Encourage full ambulation as soon as possible.
• Provide comfort measures, such as a clean gown and a warmed blanket.

Nursing procedures

Nursing procedures performed during labor and delivery include uterine contraction palpation, external electronic monitoring, internal electronic monitoring, and vaginal examination.

Uterine contraction palpation

External uterine palpation can tell you the frequency, duration, and intensity of contractions and the relaxation time between them. The character of contractions varies with the stage of labor and the body's response to labor-inducing drugs, if administered. As labor advances, contractions become more intense, occur more often, and last longer. In some patients, labor progresses rapidly, preventing the patient from entering a health care facility.

To palpate uterine contractions:
• Review the patient's admission history to determine the onset, frequency, duration, and intensity of contractions. Also, note where contractions feel strongest or exert the most pressure.
• Describe the procedure to the patient.
• Assist the patient into a comfortable side-lying position.
• Drape the patient with a sheet.
• Place the palmar surface of your fingers on the uterine fundus, and palpate lightly to assess contractions. Each contraction has three phases: increment (rising), acme (peak), and decrement (letting down or ebbing).

How fast?

• To assess *frequency*, time the interval between the beginning of one contraction and the beginning of the next.

Take charge!

Contraction without relaxation

If any contraction lasts longer than 90 seconds and isn't followed by uterine muscle relaxation, or if the relaxation period is less than 1 minute between contractions, notify the doctor. This may indicate hyperstimulation of the uterus or tetanic contractions. When the uterus doesn't relax, or the relaxation period is less than 1 minute, uteroplacental blood flow is interrupted, which can lead to fetal hypoxia and fetal distress.

If you determine that the patient's contractions last longer than 90 seconds or if the re-

laxation period is less than 1 minute, follow these steps:
• Discontinue the oxytocin infusion to stop uterine stimulations (if the patient is receiving oxytocin).
• Make sure that the patient is lying on her left side; this increases uteroplacental perfusion.
• Administer oxygen via face mask to increase fetal oxygenation.
• Notify the doctor or nurse-midwife immediately.

How long?

• To assess *duration*, time the period from when the uterus begins tightening until it begins relaxing.

How hard?

• To assess intensity, press your fingertips into the uterine fundus when the uterus tightens. During mild contractions, the fundus indents easily; during moderate contractions, the fundus indents less easily; during strong contractions, the fundus resists indenting.
• Determine how the patient copes with discomfort by assessing her breathing and relaxation techniques.
• Assess contractions in low-risk patients every 30 minutes in the latent phase, every 15 to 30 minutes in the active phase, and every 15 minutes in the transition phase. More frequent assessments are required for high-risk patients. High-risk fetal status assessments should also occur every 30 minutes during the latent phase, every 15 minutes during the active phase, and every 5 minutes in the second stage. (See *Contraction without relaxation*.)

External electronic monitoring

External electronic monitoring is an indirect, noninvasive procedure. Two devices, an ultrasound transducer and a tocotransducer, are placed on the mother's abdomen to evaluate fetal well-being and uterine contractions during labor. These devices are held in place with an elastic stockinette or by using plastic or soft straps.

Two readings, one printout

The ultrasound transducer transmits high-frequency sound waves aimed at the fetal heart. The tocotransducer, in turn, responds to the pressure exerted by uterine contractions and simultaneously records the duration and frequency of the contractions. (See *Applying external monitoring devices.*) The monitoring apparatus traces FHR and uterine contraction data onto the same printout paper.

External fetal monitoring is used for most women, especially those with a high-risk pregnancy or oxytocin-induced labor.

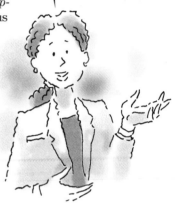

External fetal monitoring is a noninvasive way to assess contractions and fetal heart rate.

Monitoring FHR and uterine contractions

Here are the steps you should take when monitoring the FHR and uterine contractions:
• Explain the procedure to the patient and make sure that she has signed a consent form, if required by your facility.

Who and when?

• Label the monitoring strip with, or enter into the computer, the patient's identification number or birth date, her name, the date, maternal vital signs and position, the paper speed, and the number of the strip paper.
• Assist the patient to the semi-Fowler or left-lateral position with her abdomen exposed, and palpate the abdomen to locate the fundus—the area of greatest muscle density in the uterus.

Buckle up and get tracing

• Using transducer straps or a stockinette binder, secure the tocotransducer over the fundus.
• Adjust the pen set tracer controls so that the baseline values read between 5 and 15 mm Hg on the monitor strip or as indicated by the model.

Goo for good contact

• Apply conduction gel to the ultrasound transducer, and use Leopold's maneuvers to palpate the fetal back, through which fetal heart tones resound most audibly.
• Start the monitor, and apply the ultrasound transducer directly over the site having the strongest heart tones.
• Activate the control that begins the printout.

Advice from the experts

Applying external monitoring devices

To ensure clear tracings that define fetal status and labor progress, be sure to precisely position external monitoring devices. These devices include an ultrasound transducer and a tocotransducer.

Fetal heart monitor

Palpate the uterus to locate the fetus's back and place the ultrasound transducer, which reads the fetal heart rate, over the site where the fetal heartbeat sounds the loudest. Then tighten the belt. Use the fetal heart tracing on the monitor strip to confirm the transducer's position.

Tocotransducer

A tocotransducer records uterine motion during contractions. Place the tocotransducer over the uterine fundus where it contracts, either midline or slightly to one side. Place your hand on the fundus, and palpate a contraction to verify proper placement. Secure the tocotransducer's belt; then adjust the pen set so that the baseline values read between 5 and 15 mm Hg on the monitor strip.

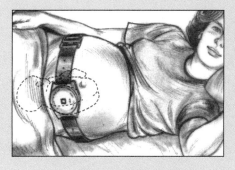

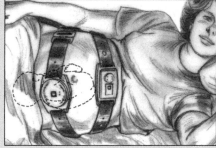

• Observe the tracings to identify the frequency and duration of uterine contractions, but palpate the uterus to determine intensity of contractions.

Compare and contract

• Note the baseline FHR, and assess periodic accelerations or decelerations from the baseline. Compare the FHR patterns with those of the uterine contractions.

• Move the tocotransducer and the ultrasound transducer to accommodate changes in maternal or fetal position. Readjust both transducers every hour, and assess the patient's skin for reddened areas caused by the pressure of the monitoring device.

• Clean the ultrasound transducer periodically with a damp cloth to remove dried conduction gel, and apply fresh gel as necessary.

- If the patient reports discomfort in the position that provides the clearest signal, try to obtain a satisfactory 5- or 10-minute tracing with the patient in this position before assisting her to a more comfortable position.

Internal electronic monitoring

Internal monitoring, also called *direct monitoring*, is an invasive procedure that uses a spiral electrode attached to the presenting fetal part (usually the scalp). This electrode detects the fetal heartbeat and transmits it to the monitor, which converts the signals to a fetal electrocardiogram (ECG) waveform. This helps assess fetal response to uterine contractions, measures intrauterine pressure, tracks labor progress, and allows evaluation of short- and long-term FHR variability.

Without a tracing

Internal monitoring is indicated for high risk pregnancies. However, it can only be performed if the amniotic sac has ruptured, the cervix is dilated at least 2 cm, and the presenting part of the fetus is at least at the –1 station. Maternal complications of internal fetal monitoring may include uterine perforation and intrauterine infections. Fetal complications may include abscess, hematoma, and infection.

An intrauterine pressure catheter may be used if external uterine monitoring doesn't provide satisfactory information. It may also be necessary in high-risk pregnancies or if the patient is obese.

Monitoring uterine contractions

Follow these steps when monitoring uterine contractions:
- Make sure that the patient understands the procedure and that she signs a consent form, if required by your facility.
- Label the printout paper with the patient's identification number or name, her birth date, the date, the paper speed, and the number on the monitor strip.
- Help the patient into a lithotomy position.

Cable connection

- Attach the connection cable to the uterine activity outlet on the monitor, and zero the catheter with a gauge on the distal end of the catheter.
- Cover the patient's perineum with a sterile drape, and clean the perineum with antiseptic solution, according to your facility's policy.
- The doctor will perform a vaginal examination, insert the catheter into the uterine cavity until it advances to the black line,

and secure the catheter with hypoallergenic tape to the patient's inner thigh.

Strip tips

• You'll need to observe the monitoring strip to verify proper placement and a clear tracing. Periodically evaluate the strip to determine the amount of pressure exerted with each contraction. Note all such data on the strip and the patient's medical record. (See *Applying an internal electronic fetal monitor.*)

Monitoring fetal heart rate

Follow these steps when monitoring FHR:
• Help the patient into the lithotomy position so the doctor can perform a vaginal examination.

Advice from the experts

Applying an internal electronic fetal monitor

During internal electronic fetal monitoring, a spiral electrode monitors the fetal heart rate (FHR) and an internal catheter monitors uterine contractions.

Monitoring FHR
The spiral electrode is inserted after a vaginal examination that determines the position of the fetus. As shown at right, the electrode is attached to the presenting fetal part, usually the scalp or buttocks.

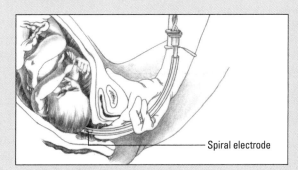

Spiral electrode

Monitoring uterine contractions
The intrauterine catheter is inserted up to a premarked level on the tubing and then connected to a monitor that interprets uterine contraction pressures.

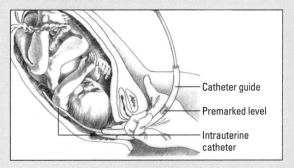

Catheter guide

Premarked level

Intrauterine catheter

- After identifying the presenting fetal part and level of descent, the doctor applies a fetal scalp electrode to the fetal scalp.
- Attach the internal fetal scalp electrode to a cable from the monitor. Then secure the electrode to the mother's body.
- Finally, observe the FHR.

Check and compare

- Check the baseline FHR, and assess periodic accelerations or decelerations from the baseline. Compare the FHR pattern with the uterine contraction pattern. Note the interval between the onset of deceleration and uterine contractions, the interval between the lowest level of an FHR deceleration and the peak of a uterine contraction, and the range of FHR deceleration. (See *Reading a fetal monitor strip.*)
- Check for FHR variability, which is a measure of fetal oxygen reserve and neurologic integrity and stability.
- Interpret FHR and uterine contractions at regular intervals. Guidelines of the Association of Women's Health, Obstetric, and Neonatal Nurses specify that high-risk patients need continuous FHR monitoring, whereas low-risk patients should have FHR auscultated every 30 minutes after a contraction during the first stage and every 15 minutes after a contraction during the second stage. First, determine the baseline FHR within 10 beats/minute; then assess the degree of baseline variability. Identify changes such as decelerations (early late, variable, or mixed) and nonperiodic changes such as a sinusoidal pattern. (See *Identifying baseline FHR irregularities*, pages 338 to 340.) If vaginal delivery isn't imminent (within 30 minutes) and fetal distress patterns are identified, cesarean birth is necessary.

Vaginal examination

During first-stage labor, a vaginal examination may be done to assess cervical dilation and effacement; membrane status; and fetal presentation, position, and engagement. If the patient has excessive vaginal bleeding, which may signal placenta previa, vaginal examination is contraindicated.

Only specially trained nurses can perform vaginal examinations. In early labor, perform the vaginal examination between contractions, focusing on the extent of cervical dilation and effacement. At the end of first-stage labor, perform the examination during a contraction to focus on assessing fetal descent.

Get into position

Follow these steps during vaginal examination:
- Explain the procedure to the patient.

Advice from the experts

Reading a fetal monitor strip

Presented in two parallel recordings, the fetal monitor strip records the fetal heart rate (FHR) in beats per minute in the top recording and uterine activity (UA) in millimeters of mercury (mm Hg) in the bottom recording. You can obtain information on fetal status and labor progress by reading the strips horizontally and vertically.

Reading horizontally on the FHR or the UA strip, each small block represents 10 seconds. Six consecutive small blocks, separated by a dark vertical line, represent 1 minute. Reading

vertically on the FHR strip, each block represents an amplitude of 10 beats/minute. Reading vertically on the UA strip, each block represents 5 mm Hg of pressure.

Assess the baseline FHR (the "resting" heart rate) between uterine contractions when fetal movement diminishes. This baseline FHR (normal range: 120 to 160 beats/minute) pattern serves as a reference for subsequent FHR tracings produced during contractions.

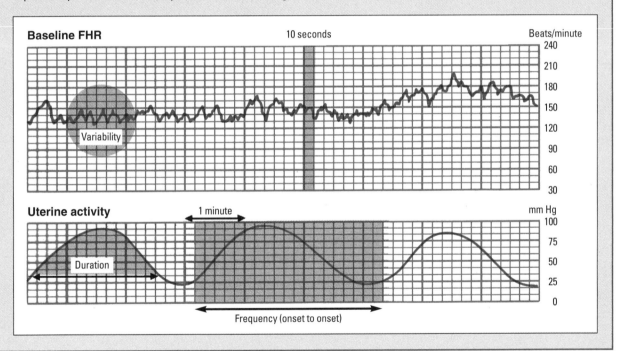

- Ask the patient to empty her bladder.
- Use Leopold's maneuvers to identify the fetal presenting part and position.
- Help the patient into a lithotomy position. Place a linen-saver pad under the patient's buttocks.
- Put on sterile gloves, and lubricate the index and middle fingers of your examining hand with sterile water or sterile water-soluble

(Text continues on page 340.)

Advice from the experts

Identifying baseline FHR irregularities

When monitoring fetal heart rate (FHR), you need to be familiar with irregularities that may occur, the possible causes, and nursing interventions to take. Here's a guide to these irregularities.

Irregularity	Possible causes	Clinical significance	Nursing interventions
Baseline tachycardia beats/minute 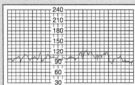	• Early fetal hypoxia • Maternal fever • Parasympathetic agents, such as atropine and scopolamine • Beta-adrenergics, such as ritodrine and terbutaline • Amnionitis (inflammation of inner layer of fetal membrane, or amnion) • Maternal hyperthyroidism • Fetal anemia • Fetal heart failure • Fetal arrhythmias	Persistent tachycardia without periodic changes doesn't usually adversely affect fetal well-being, especially when associated with maternal fever. However, tachycardia is an ominous sign when associated with late decelerations, severe variable decelerations, or lack of variability.	• Intervene to alleviate the cause of fetal distress, and provide supplemental oxygen as ordered. Also administer I.V. fluids as prescribed. • Discontinue oxytocin infusion to reduce uterine activity. • Turn the patient onto her left side and elevate her legs. • Continue to observe FHR. • Document interventions and outcomes. • Notify the doctor; further medical intervention may be necessary.
Baseline bradycardia beats/minute	• Late fetal hypoxia • Beta-adrenergic blockers, such as propranolol, and anesthetics • Maternal hypotension • Prolonged umbilical cord compression • Fetal congenital heart block	Bradycardia with good variability and no periodic changes doesn't signal fetal distress if FHR remains higher than 80 beats/minute. However, bradycardia caused by hypoxia and acidosis is an ominous sign when associated with loss of variability and late decelerations.	• Intervene to correct the cause of fetal distress. Administer supplemental oxygen as ordered. Start an I.V. line and administer fluids as prescribed. • Discontinue oxytocin infusion to reduce uterine activity. • Turn the patient onto her left side, and elevate her legs. • Continue observing FHR. • Document interventions and outcomes. • Notify the doctor; further medical intervention may be necessary.

Identifying baseline FHR irregularities *(continued)*

Irregularity	Possible causes	Clinical significance	Nursing interventions
Early decelerations beats/minute 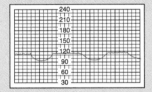 mm Hg 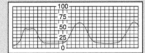	• Fetal head compression	Early decelerations are benign, indicating fetal head compression at dilation of 4 to 7 cm.	• Reassure the patient that the fetus isn't at risk. • Observe FHR. • Document the frequency of decelerations.
Late decelerations beats/minute mm Hg	• Uteroplacental circulatory insufficiency (placental hypoperfusion) caused by decreased intervillous blood flow during contractions or a structural placental defect such as abruptio placentae • Uterine hyperactivity caused by excessive oxytocin infusion • Maternal hypotension • Maternal supine hypotension	Late decelerations indicate uteroplacental circulatory insufficiency and may lead to fetal hypoxia and acidosis if the underlying cause isn't corrected.	• Turn the patient onto her left side to increase placental perfusion and decrease contraction frequency. • Increase the I.V. fluid rate to boost intravascular volume and placental perfusion, as prescribed. • Administer oxygen by mask to increase fetal oxygenation as ordered. • Assess for signs of the underlying cause, such as hypotension or uterine tachysystole. • Take other appropriate measures such as discontinuing oxytocin as prescribed. • Document interventions and outcomes. • Notify the doctor; further medical intervention may be necessary.

(continued)

Identifying baseline FHR irregularities (continued)

Irregularity	Possible causes	Clinical significance	Nursing interventions
Variable decelerations beats/minute mm Hg	• Umbilical cord compression causing decreased fetal oxygen perfusion	Variable decelerations are the most common deceleration pattern in labor because of contractions and fetal movement.	• Help the patient change position. No other intervention is necessary unless you detect fetal distress. • Assure the patient that the fetus tolerates cord compression well. Explain that cord compression affects the fetus the same way that breath-holding affects her. • Assess the deceleration pattern for reassuring signs: a baseline FHR that isn't increasing, short-term variability that isn't decreasing, abruptly beginning and ending decelerations, and decelerations lasting less than 50 seconds. If assessment doesn't reveal reassuring signs, notify the doctor. • Start I.V. fluids and administer oxygen by mask at 10 to 12 L/minute, as prescribed. • Document interventions and outcomes. • Discontinue oxytocin infusion to decrease uterine activity.

lubricant. If the membranes are ruptured, use an antiseptic solution.

Breathe and release

- Ask the patient to relax by taking several deep breaths and slowly releasing the air.
- Insert your lubricated fingers (palmar surface down) into the vagina. Keep your uninserted fingers flexed to avoid the rectum.
- Palpate the cervix, noting its consistency. The cervix gradually softens throughout pregnancy, reaching a buttery consistency before labor begins. (See *Cervical effacement and dilation*.)

Cervical effacement and dilation

As labor advances, so do cervical effacement and dilation, promoting delivery. During effacement, the cervix shortens and its walls become thin, progressing from 0% effacement (palpable and thick) to 100% effacement (fully indistinct, or effaced, and paper thin). Full effacement obliterates the constrictive uterine neck to create a smooth, unobstructed passageway for the fetus.

At the same time, dilation occurs. This progressive widening of the cervical canal—from the upper internal cervical os to the lower external cervical os—advances from 0 to 10 cm. As the cervical canal opens, resistance decreases. This further eases fetal descent.

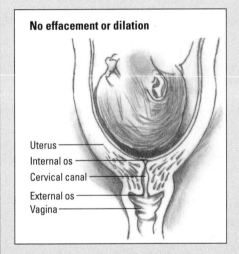

No effacement or dilation

Uterus
Internal os
Cervical canal
External os
Vagina

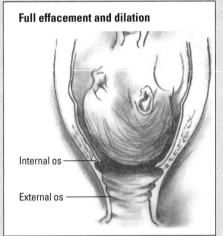

Full effacement and dilation

Internal os

External os

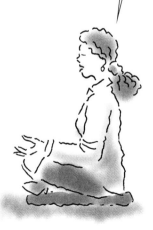

A vaginal exam works best when the patient is relaxed. Take a moment to help her breathe deeply.

• After identifying the presenting fetal part and position and evaluating dilation, effacement, engagement, station, and membrane status, gently withdraw your fingers.
• Help the patient clean her perineum, and change the linen-saver pad, as necessary.

Flood zone

If the amniotic membrane ruptures during the examination, record FHR and time, and describe the color, odor, and approximate amount of fluid. If FHR becomes unstable, determine fetal station and check for umbilical cord prolapse. After the membranes rupture, perform the vaginal examination only when labor changes significantly to minimize the risk of introducing intrauterine infection.

Comfort and support issues

Labor and birth usually involve a significant amount of discomfort and can be emotionally draining for the woman. Comfort and support measures, such as prenatal education, planning, and the presence of a birthing partner or coach, can promote relaxation and decrease or eliminate the need for analgesia or anesthesia during labor and birth.

Expect the unexpected

Although it's helpful for the woman to make decisions about the issue of pain relief during labor before the actual event, advise the woman to keep an open mind. She should be aware of the other acceptable pain relief options available in case the situation changes during labor and birth. Sometimes, it may be necessary to take the decision regarding pain relief out of the woman's hands—for example, in cases of cesarean birth. No matter what method of pain relief is used, the woman should feel comfortable with it and it should be medically safe.

To provide comfort and support to the woman during labor and birth, the nurse must understand:
• sources of pain
• pain perception and how it affects the woman's response to relief measures
• cultural and familial influences on responses to pain
• different approaches to relieving pain.

By using appropriate comfort and support measures, you can decrease the need for analgesia or anesthesia during labor and birth.

Sources of pain

The pain experienced during labor and birth comes from several sources.

Uterine contractions

The contraction of the uterine muscles is a prominent source of pain during labor and birth. Like the heart, stomach, and intestine, the uterus is part of an involuntary muscle group. Although most muscles of this type don't cause pain when they contract, uterine contractions do. During a contraction, the blood vessels constrict, which reduces the blood supply to the uterine and cervical cells, causing temporary hypoxia or anoxia and pain. As labor progresses and contractions increase in intensity and duration, the blood supply to the cells decreases further, thus increasing the pain.

Dilation

Dilation and stretching of the cervix and lower uterine segment also cause pain during labor. Similar to the intestinal pain caused by accumulated gas in the bowel, this pain increases as the dilation increases.

Distention

Distention of the vagina and perineum to accommodate passage of the fetal head also causes pain during labor. As the fetal head is delivered, an episiotomy or possible tearing of the perineum intensifies this pain.

Pressure on adjacent organs

Another source of pain during labor is the pressure of the presenting part on the adjacent organs, such as the bladder, urethra, or lower colon. This varies depending on the position of the fetus.

Tension

Tension also contributes to pain during labor and birth. The woman's anticipation of pain and her inability to relax commonly cause tension or constriction of the voluntary muscles, including the muscles of the abdominal wall. Tense abdominal muscles increase the pressure on the uterus by preventing the uterus from rising with the contractions.

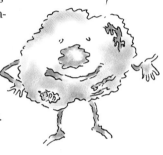

Ack! When contractions increase in intensity and duration, the blood supply to cells decreases.

Pain perception

Pain is a subjective symptom that's unique to each individual who experiences it. What may be slight discomfort to one person may be intense, unbearable pain to another. Only the woman who is experiencing the pain can describe it or know its extent. When assessing the woman in labor, watch for signs of pain, such as increased respiratory and pulse rates, clenched fists, facial tenseness, and flushed or pale areas of the skin.

Under the influence of endorphins

Many factors influence how pain is perceived. A woman's pain threshold (the amount of pain perceived at a given time) may be influenced by her level of endorphins, the opiate-like substances that are produced by the body in response to pain.

If you expect it, pain will come

Expectations of pain can also affect how pain is perceived. A woman who expects the pain of labor to be the most horrible pain she has ever experienced commonly becomes increasingly tense with each contraction and episode of pain, which can intensify her overall perception of the pain.

Too tired and weak for distractions

Fatigue, nutritional status, and sleep deprivation can also affect pain perception. A tired or malnourished individual has less energy than a rested one and can't focus on distraction strategies.

Mind games

Psychological factors, including fear, anxiety, body image, self-concept, and feelings of having no control over the situation, also affect a woman's pain perception. In addition, memories of previous childbirth experiences affect how the labor pains of the current pregnancy are perceived.

More pieces to the pain puzzle

Other factors that influence pain perception during labor include the intensity of labor, pelvic size and shape, and the interventions of caregivers (which can be a positive or negative influence on pain perception).

> Pain is subjective. Each patient's experience during labor and birth will be unique, just like her!

Cultural influences on pain

Individuals tend to react to pain in ways that are acceptable to their culture and family. Commonly learned through previous experience and conditioning, some women react to pain by becoming silent and avoiding interaction with other individuals; others may scream, verbalize their feelings of distress, or become verbally abusive to other individuals. Make sure that you determine the level of comfort each woman desires to receive and the manner in which she chooses to express her discomfort. (See *How certain cultures handle pain.*)

Nonpharmacologic pain relief

Most nonpharmacologic pain relief methods are based on the gate control theory of pain, which poses that local physical stimulation can interfere with pain stimuli by closing a hypothetical gate in the spinal cord, thus blocking pain signals from reaching the

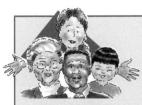

Bridging the gap

How certain cultures handle pain

Cultural and familial influences play a role in how a woman expresses, or represses, pain as well as whether she uses pharmacologic methods of pain relief. If her family views childbirth as a natural process or function for the female in the family unit, the woman is less likely to outwardly react to labor pains and she's less likely to require pharmacologic methods of pain relief. For example:

• Middle Eastern women are verbally expressive during labor and often cry out and scream loudly; in addition, many refuse pain medication.

• Samoan women believe they shouldn't express any pain verbally because they believe the pain must simply be endured. They may also refuse pain medication.

• Filipino women lie quietly during labor.

• Guatemalan women express pain verbally.

• Vietnamese, Laotian, and other women of Southeast Asian descent believe that crying out during labor is shameful and that pain during labor must be endured.

• Hispanic women are taught by *parteras* (midwives) to endure pain and to keep their mouths closed during labor because to cry out would cause the uterus to rise and retard labor.

brain. Nonpharmacologic pain relief methods may be used as the only method of pain management during labor and delivery, or they may be used in conjunction with pharmacologic interventions. Be flexible when a woman chooses an alternative method of pain relief, and provide support and reassurance if she finds that the method she has chosen isn't working effectively.

Nonpharmacologic pain relief methods include various relaxation techniques, breathing techniques, heat and cold application, counterpressure, transcutaneous electrical nerve stimulation (TENS), hypnosis, acupuncture and acupressure, and yoga.

Relaxation techniques

Most childbirth education classes teach relaxation techniques to their students. Relaxation turns the woman's focus away from the pain, which reduces tension. The reduced tension leads to a perceived decrease in pain, which then further reduces tension, thus breaking the pain cycle.

Let the sound take you away...

Relaxation techniques include positioning, focusing and imagery, therapeutic touch and massage, music therapy, and the support of a birthing partner or

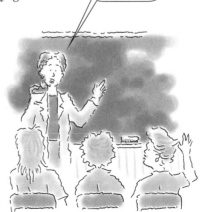

Relaxation techniques take focus away from the pain.

coach. Many women find these techniques helpful in the early stages of labor, even if they later decide that they need supplemental analgesia or anesthesia. Usually, the amount of pharmacologic assistance that's needed is reduced when used in conjunction with relaxation techniques.

Positioning

Part of the relaxation process involves positioning. The woman should be taught to shift her position during labor until she finds the one that's most comfortable for her. Commonly, the position of the fetus and its presenting part determines the most comfortable position for the mother. For example, a woman with a fetus in an occiput posterior position usually experiences intense back pain during labor. A change from a back- or side-lying position to one on her hands and knees with her head lower than her hips usually helps to ease this pain. Left side-lying position provides the greatest perfusion of blood to the mother's organs and to the placenta, so it's the position of choice no matter what the fetal position is.

Focusing and imagery

Focusing is a relaxation technique that's used to keep the sensory input perceived during the contraction from reaching the pain center in the cortex of the brain. During contractions, the woman concentrates intently on an object that has special meaning or appeal to her, such as a photograph.

When using imagery, the woman mentally places herself in a relaxing environment.

Picture this

In imagery (also known as *visualization*), the woman concentrates on a mental image of a person, place, or thing. The woman may picture herself on a beach with the waves crashing on shore, in a forest or meadow with the sound of rustling leaves or singing birds, or near a stream or river with the sound of the water flowing by.

Stop, hey, what's that sound?

The sounds the woman hears during this process are an important part of effective imagery because they help her stay concentrated on the image. She may want to use an item such as a music box playing her favorite tune to help her visualize her image. If a person participating in the delivery is included in the woman's visualization, the individual should speak softly and offer words of comfort. The person could also sing or read a favorite poem to the woman.

Education edge

Using imagery during contractions

Teach your patient about using imaging techniques by telling her to follow these steps:
- Begin with a deep cleansing breath.
- Close your eyes.
- Relax every part of your body: head and neck, shoulders, arms, hands, fingers, chest, back, stomach, hips, bottom, legs, feet, and toes.
- Picture a place in your mind where you feel warm and safe. The place could be your home, a place you remember from your childhood, or a place that reminds you of peacefulness, such as a warm sandy beach or a quiet meadow. Keep these details in your mind so that when a contraction gets closer, you can focus on this image and have all the details in place.
- Slowly breathe with the contraction.
- When the contraction ends, take a deep cleansing breath and return to reality.
- Open your eyes.

Zip the lip

You shouldn't talk to the woman or ask her questions when she's using focusing or imagery techniques because the dialogue could break her concentration and allow the painful stimuli to cross into the brain. An exception should be made if a coach or other support person is assisting her in maintaining her concentration by providing verbal cues. (See *Using imagery during contractions*.)

Therapeutic touch and massage

Therapeutic touch is based on the premises that the body contains energy fields that lead to either good or ill health and that the hands can be used to redirect the energy fields that lead to pain. Touching and massage actually offer a distraction that directs the woman's focus from the pain to the action of the hands. Although not well documented, it's also believed that touch and massage cause the release of endorphins that block the perception of pain.

Music therapy

As an adjunct to relaxation, focusing, and imagery, it's usually helpful for the woman to have her favorite music available during labor and delivery. Listening to her favorite tunes usually helps the woman throughout the focusing or imagery process. It also acts as a form of diversion. Although it's recommended that the music be soft and soothing, many women find greater distraction from dance or rock and roll rhythms. It may also be used in conjunction with breathing exercises; however, de-

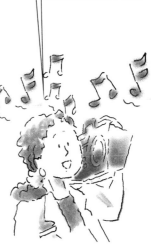

Turn on the tunes! Music can help with focusing or imagery and divert attention from the pain of labor and delivery.

pending on the rhythm, music may serve to disrupt an established breathing pattern, rather than support it.

Birthing partner or coach

Having a capable birthing partner or coach to provide support during labor and deliver is one of the most important factors in making the birth experience a positive one. The presence of a birthing partner can alleviate the woman's anxiety and increase her self-esteem and feelings of control over the experience, which can effectively reduce the pain or at least increase her ability to deal with it. The birthing partner or coach may be the woman's husband, partner, parent, sibling, or friend. The most important factor in choosing a support person is determining who will provide the most effective coaching and support without being influenced on an emotional level.

> A birthing partner helps alleviate anxiety during labor and delivery, which can help decrease the amount of pain and discomfort the woman feels.

Doula on duty

Sometimes, a woman doesn't have someone close to her who can take on birthing partner responsibilities. In such cases, the woman may use a *doula*, an independent contractor without formal medical training who provides support during labor and delivery. As effective as a traditional support person, the doula can help increase the woman's self-esteem and decrease the use of pharmacologic pain relief. Using a doula as a birthing partner or coach doesn't prevent the woman's partner or the baby's father from being present, providing emotional support, or participating in the birth of the child.

Breathing techniques

Breathing techniques are an important part of nonpharmacologic pain relief and are taught in most childbirth preparation classes. They distract the woman from the pain of the contractions and also help to relax the abdominal muscles. When a woman is focusing on slow-paced, rhythmic breathing, she's less likely to concentrate on the pain she's experiencing.

Easing pain one breath at a time

The most common breathing technique used is the Lamaze method. Originally developed in Russia and based on Pavlov's conditioning studies, the Lamaze method was popularized by Ferdinand Lamaze, a French physician. The method incorporates the theory that women can learn to use controlled breathing to reduce the pain felt during labor through the use of stimulus-response conditioning.

In Lamaze, the woman is encouraged to direct her attention to a focal point, such as a spot on the wall, at the first sign of a contraction. This focus creates a visual stimulus that goes directly to the woman's brain. The woman then takes a deep cleansing breath, which is followed by rhythmic breathing. During the contraction, the woman's partner provides a series of commands or verbal encouragements to provide an auditory stimulus to her brain.

Relief at your fingertips

The rhythmic breathing is followed by effleurage (a light fingertip massage) that the woman or her partner performs on the abdomen or thighs. The massage introduces a tactile stimulus that goes directly to her brain, calming the nerves and promoting relaxation. The rate of effleurage is slow and remains constant, even though the rate of breathing may change. (See *Effective effleurage patterns*, page 350.)

It isn't too late to educate

If a woman hasn't attended childbirth preparation classes and hasn't received instruction in breathing and relaxation techniques, the techniques can be taught to her while she's in the early stages of labor. Although techniques learned under these circumstances usually aren't as effective, they may at least help to delay the use of analgesics.

Breathing on so many levels

Different levels of breathing are used depending on the intensity of the contractions. The woman's coach assists in determining the level of breathing by resting a hand on her abdomen or watching a contraction monitor. As the strength of the contraction changes, the coach calls out the key words that act as commands to the woman.

At the start and finish of each breathing exercise, the woman takes a cleansing breath—she breathes in slowly and deeply and then exhales in the same manner. This decreases the chance of hyperventilation during rapid breathing and also helps to maintain adequate oxygen supply for the fetus.

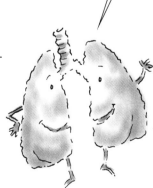

A cleansing breath decreases the chance of hyperventilation and helps maintain the fetus's oxygen supply.

First level

At the first level, the woman uses slow chest breathing. These full respirations should be done at a rate of 6 to 12 breaths/minute. The woman is instructed to use this level of breathing for early contractions.

Effective effleurage patterns

Effleurage is a light fingertip massage that the woman or her partner performs on her abdomen or thighs during contractions. This illustration shows the tracing patterns used for effleurage.

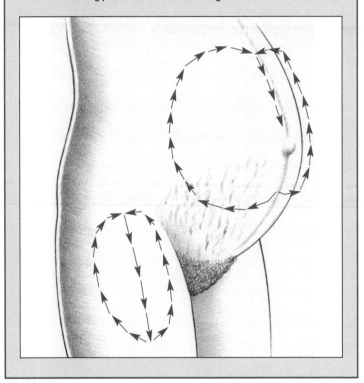

Second level

At the second level, breathing should be heavy enough so that the rib cage expands but light enough so that the diaphragm barely moves. The rate of respirations is up to 40 breaths/minute. The second level of breathing is recommended when cervical dilation is 4 to 6 cm.

Third level

The third level involves shallow, sternal breathing level. The rate is 50 to 70 breaths/minute. As the respirations become faster, the exhalation must be a little stronger than the inhalation to promote good air exchange and prevent hyperventilation. The woman can achieve a stronger exhalation than inhalation if she practices saying "out" with each exhalation. The woman should use this level of breathing for contractions that occur during the transition phase of labor. To help prevent the oral mucosa from drying out during such rapid breathing, instruct the woman to keep the tip of her tongue against the roof of her mouth.

Fourth level

At the fourth level, the woman should use a "pant-blow" pattern of breathing by taking three or four quick breaths in and out and then forcefully exhaling. The breathing pattern is "hee-hee-hee-hoo" (shallow breath, shallow breath, shallow breath, long exhalation). This type of breathing is often referred to as "choo-choo" breathing because it sounds like a train.

Fifth level

At the fifth level, the woman should perform continuous chest panting. Breaths are shallow and occur at about 60 breaths/ minute. This type of breathing can be used during strong contractions or during the second stage of labor to prevent the woman from pushing before full dilation.

Heat and cold application

Heat application to the lower back is considered effective in reducing labor pain. A heating pad, moist compress, warm shower, or tub bath can significantly aid relaxation if the membranes are still intact. Applying a cool washcloth to the woman's forehead and providing ice chips to relieve dry mouth are other measures that can increase the woman's comfort level.

Counterpressure

Counterpressure is the application of firm or forceful pressure, using the heel of the hand or fist, to the woman's lower back or sacrum during a contraction. It relieves back pain during labor by countering the pressure of the fetus against the mother's back.

The amount of force applied varies, depending on the patient. Some women prefer considerable force during a contraction, whereas others prefer firm support on the back. The exact spot for applying pressure also varies from woman to woman and may change throughout the labor. If the partner is using considerable force on the back, suggest that he hold the front of the woman's hipbone to help maintain his balance.

Transcutaneous electrical nerve stimulation

TENS is the stimulation of large-diameter neural fibers via electric currents to alter pain perception. Although not documented as being a significant factor in reducing the pain caused by uterine contractions, TENS may be effective in reducing the extreme back pain that some women have during contractions.

Hypnosis

Hypnosis, though used infrequently, can provide a satisfactory method of pain relief for the woman who follows hypnotic suggestions. The woman must meet with the hypnotherapist several times during her pregnancy for evaluation and conditioning. If it's determined that she's a good candidate for this method of pain relief, she's given a posthypnotic suggestion that she'll experience either reduced pain during labor or no pain at all.

Acupuncture and acupressure

Acupuncture and acupressure are also methods of pain relief that are sometimes used during labor. Acupuncture is the stimulation of key trigger points with needles. It isn't necessary for the trigger points to be near the affected organ because their activation causes the release of endorphins, which reduce the perception of pain. Acupressure is finger pressure or massage at the same trigger points. Holding and squeezing the hand of a woman in labor may trigger the point most commonly used for acupuncture and acupressure during labor.

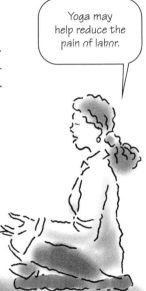

Yoga may help reduce the pain of labor.

Yoga

Yoga uses a series of deep breathing exercises, body stretching postures, and meditation to promote relaxation, slow the respiratory rate, lower blood pressure, improve physical fitness, reduce stress, and ease anxiety. It may be helpful in reducing the pain of labor though the ability to relax the body and possibly through the release of endorphins that may occur.

Pharmacologic pain relief

Pharmacologic pain relief during labor includes analgesia and regional or local anesthesia. These approaches differ in the degree to which pain sensation is decreased. The main goals of using medication during labor are to relax the woman and relieve her discomfort without having a significant effect on her contractions, pushing efforts, or the fetus.

The right amount at the right time

Almost all medications given during labor have an effect on the fetus because they cross the placental barrier, so it's important to give as little medication as possible. It's also important that medications be given at the proper time. When given after 5 cm dilation in a primipara or after 3 cm dilation in a multipara, medications can speed the progress of labor because the woman can focus on working with the contractions rather than against them. If given too early in labor, medications can slow or stop the contractions. If given within 1 hour of birth, the neonate is likely to experience neuromuscular, respiratory, and cardiac depression after delivery.

Know your drugs

The nurse must be familiar enough with anesthetic and analgesic agents to answer a patient's questions, assist the anesthesiologist and obstetrician, and identify adverse maternal, fetal, and neonatal effects quickly.

Opioids

Opioids are commonly used during labor because they significantly reduce pain. Common anesthetic agents used during labor are opioids such as meperidine (Demerol), butorphanol (Stadol), and nalbuphine (Nubain). Some opioids have additional effects that are beneficial during labor, such as relaxing the cervix, which facilitates dilation. However, opioids depress the central nervous system of the fetus, which may lead to respiratory depression. In a preterm neonate or one who is already compromised in some way, this could be fatal. If a neonate is born with respiratory depression, an opioid antagonist such as naloxone (Narcan) can be given to counteract the effects of the opioid. This medication should be readily available whenever an opioid is given to the mother during labor.

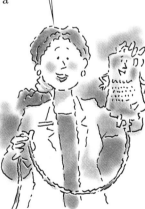

Opioids may cause respiratory depression in the fetus.

Labor's feel-good drug

Meperidine is commonly used to relieve labor pains because of its sedative and antispasmodic actions. It also gives the mother feelings of well-being and euphoria, while helping to relax the cervix. Meperidine is given when the mother is more than 3 hours from birth so that there's less risk of respiratory depression in the fetus.

Given in so many ways

Meperidine can be given I.V., I.M., or intrathecally (injected into the subarachnoid space of the spinal cord), although the intrathecal route isn't successful in all women. This drug may also be self-administered by the woman during labor with the use of a patient-controlled analgesic pump.

In on the action

When given I.M., meperidine usually begins to act within 30 minutes; when administered I.V., it acts within 5 minutes. Its effects last approximately 3 to 4 hours. The possible maternal or fetal adverse effects from meperidine are drowsiness, nausea, vomiting, respiratory depression, and maternal hypotension.

More and more

Other opioids that are given I.V. or I.M. during labor to provide pain relief include Nubain and Stadol. These drugs also pose a possible risk of respiratory depression in the neonate and most slow labor if given too early.

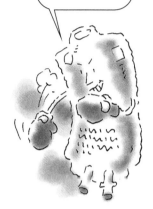

Are you ready for some of this action, labor pains?

Regional anesthesia

Regional anesthesia is used to block specific nerve pathways that pass from the uterus to the spinal cord. It relieves pain by making the nerve unable to conduct pain sensations. This form of anesthesia allows the woman to be completely awake, aware of what's happening, and—depending on the region anesthetized—aware of contractions, which gives her the opportunity to push at the appropriate time.

Regional results

Although regional anesthetics aren't injected into the maternal circulatory system, they still can produce adverse effects in the neonate, such as flaccidity, bradycardia, hypotension, and convulsions; however, these effects aren't as common or severe as with systemic anesthetics.

Lumbar epidural anesthesia is the method of regional anesthesia most frequently used for labor and delivery. A less commonly used method is spinal anesthesia, used primarily for cesarean deliveries and in emergency situations.

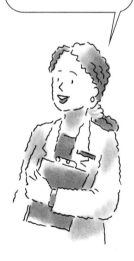

Regional anesthesia makes the nerves unable to conduct pain sensations.

Lumbar epidural anesthesia

Lumbar epidural anesthesia (also known as an *epidural block*) is the injection of a narcotic medication, such as fentanyl (Sublimaze), bupivacaine (Marcaine), or a lidocaine-like drug, through a needle or catheter into the epidural space (the vacant space just outside the membrane in the lumbar region containing the cerebrospinal fluid that bathes the spinal column and brain). When the drug is administered into this space, it anesthetizes the nerves that carry pain signals from the uterus and perineum to the brain,

A closer look at epidural anesthesia

This illustration shows the placement of the epidural catheter used for injecting pain-relieving medication into the epidural space. This process anesthetizes the nerves that carry pain signals from the uterus and perineum to the brain.

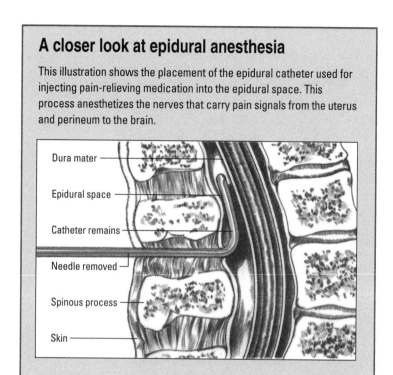

Dura mater

Epidural space

Catheter remains

Needle removed

Spinous process

Skin

thus dulling or eliminating the perception of pain for the woman. Women with preexisting medical conditions, such as heart disease, diabetes, and PIH, tend to choose this method because it makes labor almost pain-free, which can reduce physical and emotional stress. (See *A closer look at epidural anesthesia*.)

The down side, part one

Lumbar epidural anesthesia is relatively safe, but it can lower the woman's blood pressure, which can decrease the flow of blood to the uterus and the placenta. Before receiving lumbar epidural anesthesia, the woman should receive 500 to 1,000 ml of an I.V. solution, such as lactated Ringer's solution, to help prevent hypotension. Avoid administering a glucose solution because of the risk of causing rebound hypoglycemia in the neonate.

Jacking up the pressure

If the woman does become hypotensive, treatment may include placement in the left side-lying position, oxygen administration, increased I.V. fluids, and administration of a medication, such as ephedrine, to elevate blood pressure. Monitor FHR closely during periods of maternal hypotension. Fetal distress can occur as a result of reduced blood flow to the placenta from hypotension.

The down side, part two

Lumbar epidural anesthesia can also slow labor if it's given before the cervix is 5 cm dilated. It may also diminish the woman's ability to push because she's unaware of the contractions, which may result in the need for forceps-assisted delivery, vacuum extraction, or cesarean birth.

How it's done

Lumbar epidural anesthesia is administered by an anesthesiologist or nurse anesthetist. The woman is placed on her side or in a sitting position with her back straight. This position is necessary because a back in flexion increases the possibility that the needle will pass through the epidural space into the subarachnoid space.

After the lumbar region of the woman's back is cleaned with an antiseptic and a local anesthetic is injected, a special needle is passed through the L3-L4 space into the epidural space. A catheter is then passed through the needle into the epidural space and taped in place on the skin. The needle is withdrawn, and a syringe is attached to the end of the catheter to create a closed system.

Test the waters

A small dose of the anesthetic is injected through the catheter, and the woman is observed to make sure that the catheter is in the proper position and the desired effect is obtained. When this is ascertained, the initial dose of the anesthetic is given. The anesthetic takes effect within 10 to 15 minutes and lasts from 40 minutes to 2 hours. An infusion pump is used and the anesthetic is infused at a slow, continuous rate. Close observation of the woman is necessary to avoid a toxic reaction from too much anesthetic.

Step up to the baseline

Here's what you should do during the procedure:
• Perform baseline vital signs and assess FHR before the epidural is initiated.
• If your facility requires that the patient be placed on a continuous ECG monitor, apply the leads and obtain a baseline ECG.
• Monitor the patient for signs of adverse reactions to the narcotic, such as a change in sedation level, respiratory depression, or itching. Also monitor the patient for adverse effects of the local anesthetic, which may include numbness in the arms, hands, or around mouth; ringing in the ears; seizure activity; nausea and vomiting; and metallic taste.
• Once you've determined that the patient isn't experiencing adverse reactions to the test, monitor maternal vital signs every 5 minutes for 20 minutes, then every 15 minutes for 45 min-

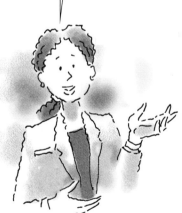

A small dose of anesthetic is injected through the catheter before the initial dose. This verifies catheter placement and patient response.

utes, and then every 30 minutes for the duration of the epidural and labor, or according to your facility's protocol.

Ins and outs

• Monitor the woman's intake and output because the woman can't feel the sensations associated with a full bladder. Encourage the woman to void at least once every 2 hours, and regularly palpate for bladder distention.
• Monitor FHR and observe for fetal distress, which can result from maternal hypotension.

Spinal anesthesia

With spinal anesthesia, a local anesthetic is injected into the cerebrospinal fluid in the subarachnoid space at the third or fourth lumbar interspace. Recently, the use of spinal anesthesia has significantly declined, having been replaced by lumbar epidural anesthesia. Currently, spinal anesthesia is used almost exclusively for cesarean birth.

For spinal anesthesia administration, place the woman in a side-lying or sitting position with her head bent forward and her back flexed as much as possible. If she's lying down, make sure that her head and upper body are higher than her abdomen and legs so that the anesthetic doesn't rise too high in the spinal canal.

The down side

As with epidural anesthesia, hypotension is a possible adverse effect of spinal anesthesia. Preventive measures should be taken before injecting anesthetic, and the woman should be closely monitored afterward.

Other disadvantages of spinal anesthesia include the possibility of a spinal headache, the risk of transient complete motor paralysis, increased incidence and degree of hypotension, and urine retention.

Local anesthesia

Local anesthesia is used only for pain relief during the actual birth of the fetus because it doesn't provide relief from the pain of contractions. It's used for a vaginal delivery when there isn't time for other types of anesthesia, after labor pain was relieved by the use of narcotics (which can't be given within 1 hour of the birth), or when a woman who was using nonpharmacologic pain relief during labor needs more relief during birth.

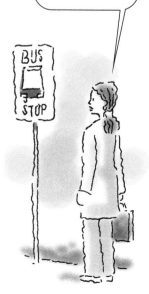

Let's see...which route is best? The local can be used for pain relief during birth but doesn't run during labor.

For when labor keeps going and going and going

In most cases, the pressure of the fetal head on the perineum causes a natural anesthesia, making local anesthesia administration unnecessary. However, after hours of exhaustive labor, many women need this relief, especially if an episiotomy is to be performed.

Local infiltration

Local infiltration is the injection of a local anesthetic (usually lidocaine) into the superficial perineal nerves. It's commonly used in preparation for or before suturing an episiotomy; however, anesthesia with this method isn't as effective as a pudendal block. (See *Local infiltration location*.)

There are no significant risks to local infiltration except rare allergic reactions and inadvertent intravascular injections. However, some practitioners believe that injection may weaken the perineal tissue and increase the likelihood of tearing.

Nursing interventions

Nursing interventions during labor and delivery focus on providing the woman comfort and support. Here's what you should do:
- To promote the woman's comfort and general body cleanliness, advise her to take a warm shower or, if her membranes haven't ruptured, a Jacuzzi or a tub bath. If she can't walk, perform a sponge or bed bath with meticulous perineal care.
- To increase the woman's comfort and reduce the risk of infection, change her gown and sheets whenever they become soiled. Also be sure to change the disposable underpad, especially after a vaginal examination. Wipe the woman's face and neck with a cool, clean washcloth, especially during the transition phase of labor.

Comforts of home

- To increase the woman's feelings of comfort and well-being, advise her to use her own toiletries, if available.
- To maintain throat and mouth moisture, offer the woman frequent sips of water or allow her to suck on some ice, hard candy, or a washcloth saturated with ice water. Provide mouth care during labor, and encourage the woman to brush her teeth or use mouthwash to freshen her breath.
- To moisturize and heal dry, cracked lips, help the woman to apply lip balm or petroleum jelly to her lips.
- To give the woman a sense of control over her pain, teach her about the possible causes of back pain during labor and the coping strategies that she can use.

Local infiltration location

Local infiltration is the injection of a local anesthetic (usually lidocaine [Xylocaine]) into the superficial perineal nerves. This illustration shows the location of the injection.

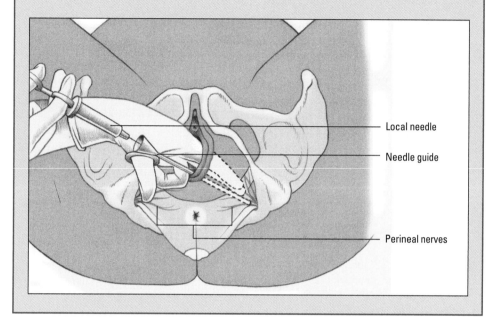

Local needle

Needle guide

Perineal nerves

• To help the woman relax during labor, teach her to use relaxation techniques and slow, paced breathing (not less than one-half the normal respiratory rate) between contractions.
• To help maintain relaxation during the later part of labor and prevent hyperventilation, advise her to increase her respiratory rate (not more than twice the normal rate) and to modify her breathing pattern during contractions.

Under pressure

• To reduce the woman's pain and promote her comfort, show her partner how to apply firm counterpressure with the heel of one hand to the sacral area.
• To prevent feelings of helplessness during a difficult labor, encourage the woman to let her partner know the amount and location of counterpressure that relieves the most pain. Feedback allows the partner to relieve pain most effectively.
• To allow the pressure of the fetus to fall away from the patient's back, help the woman assume a side-lying, upright forward-leaning, or hands-and-knees position.

• To promote the woman's comfort and further anterior rotation of the fetus (if the fetus is in the occiput posterior position), help the patient change positions at least every 30 minutes — from side-lying to hands-and-knees to the opposite side-lying positions.
• To reduce back discomfort, apply a warm, moist towel; an ice bag; or a covered rubber glove filled with ice chips, to the woman's lower back.

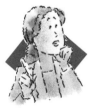

Quick quiz

1. Which option isn't a primary factor in determining the presentation of the fetus during birth?
A.   Fetal attitude
B.   Fetal heart rate
C.   Fetal lie
D.   Fetal position

Answer: B. The primary factors that determine fetal presentation are fetal attitude, lie, and position.

2. In the LOA and ROA fetal positions, the presenting part is the:
A.   olecranon.
B.   chin.
C.   occiput.
D.   buttocks.

Answer: C. The occiput is the presenting part in the LOA and ROA fetal positions.

3. Which of the following drugs is a common ripening agent?
A.   Cervidil
B.   Pitocin
C.   Sublimaze
D.   Stadol

Answer: A. Cervidil is commonly used to ripen the cervix. The drug initiates the breakdown of the collagen that keeps the cervix tightly closed.

4. Transition is part of which stage of labor?
A.   First stage
B.   Second stage
C.   Third stage
D.   Fourth stage

Answer: A. The first stage of labor is divided into three phases: latent, active, and transition.

5.   In which order do the cardinal movements of labor occur?
   A.   Flexion, extension, internal rotation, external rotation, descent, expulsion
   B.   Descent, flexion, internal rotation, extension, external rotation, and expulsion
   C.   Descent, internal rotation, flexion, external rotation, extension, expulsion
   D.   Descent, extension, internal rotation, flexion, external rotation, expulsion

Answer: B. The cardinal movements of labor occur in this order: descent, flexion, internal rotation, extension, external rotation, and expulsion.

6.   Which of the following signs isn't a sign of true labor?
   A.   Bloody show
   B.   Painful uterine contractions
   C.   Lightening
   D.   Rupture of the membranes

Answer: C. Lightening is a preliminary sign of labor—not a sign of true labor.

7.   Before the administration of an epidural anesthetic, the woman should receive 500 to 1,000 ml of which I.V. solution?
   A.   Normal saline solution
   B. D_5W
   C. D_5W in lactated Ringer's solution
   D.   Lactated Ringer's solution

Answer: D. Lactated Ringer's solution should be administered before a woman receives epidural anesthesia.

8.   Which uncommon fetal attitude results in a brow presentation?
   A.   Partial extension
   B.   Complete extension
   C.   Moderate flexion
   D.   Complete flexion

Answer: A. Partial extension is an uncommon fetal attitude that results in a brow presentation through the birth canal.

Scoring

☆☆☆ If you answered all eight questions correctly, super! When it comes to handling the challenges of labor, you deliver.

☆☆ If you answered six or seven questions correctly, great work! You're presenting to the head of the class.

☆ If you answered fewer than six questions correctly, keep a positive attitude! You'll ace the next quick quiz.

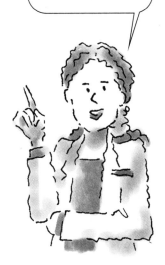

Now that you've labored through the chapter on labor and birth, you're ready to move on to the chapter on labor and birth complications.

8

Complications of labor and birth

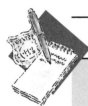

Just the facts

In this chapter, you'll learn:

♦ various complications that can occur with labor and birth

♦ ways to assess and detect problems occurring with labor and birth

♦ treatment and management of various complications.

A look at complications

Although labor usually proceeds without problems, about 8% of births involve complications. A problem can arise at any point in the labor process and can involve uterine contractions, the fetus, or the birth canal.

Stress stinks, honesty works

Emotional support is essential for the mother and her birthing partner during labor and birth. Even when labor and birth progress normally, the process is stressful and usually lengthy. It's important to periodically assure the laboring woman that everything is going well and that she and the neonate are fine, as appropriate. When a complication arises, stress increases and honesty and sincerity remain just as important.

The importance of being careful

Because complications can occur at any point in the process, the mother and fetus need to be carefully monitored. Careful monitoring of the mother and fetus is important for several reasons. A malpositioned fetus is a major factor in birth complications. Nurses can be instrumental in identifying a malpositioned fetus and helping avoid complications. For example, early detection of signs and symptoms of uterine rupture can help decrease maternal mor-

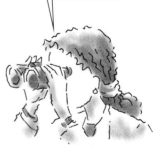

Identifying a malpositioned fetus is one thing a nurse can do to help avoid complications.

bidity during labor. When working with a monitoring device, be sure to explain its importance to the patient and her partner. (See *Tips for electronic monitoring.*)

C is for "complication"

In addition to problems arising from the condition of the mother or fetus, medical interventions to prevent or manage complications can cause other problems. One of the most invasive of these interventions is cesarean birth, in which a surgical incision is made in the abdominal and uterine walls for delivery of the neonate. Because this procedure is commonly performed, many times as a result of other complications, it's listed below with other birth complications.

Amniotic fluid embolism

Amniotic fluid embolism occurs as rarely as 1 in 8,000 births. Occurring during labor or during the postpartum period, amniotic fluid embolism happens when amniotic fluid is forced into an open maternal uterine blood sinus due to some defect in the membranes themselves or after membrane rupture or partial premature separation of the placenta. Solid particles then enter the maternal circulation and travel to the lungs, causing pulmonary embolism. Amniotic fluid embolism isn't preventable and requires prompt intervention and lifesaving treatment.

What causes it

Possible risk factors for amniotic fluid embolism include:
• oxytocin administration
• abruptio placentae
• polyhydramnios.

How it's detected

Signs of amniotic fluid embolism are dramatic. The woman, who's commonly in strong labor when the problem occurs, may sit up suddenly and grasp her chest. She may also complain of a sharp pain in her chest and an inability to breathe. In assessment, her color markedly pales and then turns the typical bluish gray associated with pulmonary embolism and lack of blood flow to the lungs.

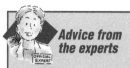

Advice from the experts

Tips for electronic monitoring

When applying an external electronic fetal and uterine monitoring device, remember to explain monitoring and why it must be used to the woman in labor to ensure compliance with the technology. Also, to avoid causing the patient distraction and stress, explain in advance that the alarms may sound even when everything is going smoothly.

Don't forget
When reading the monitor pattern, remember:
• to assess the mother and fetus to verify what the various patterns suggest
• that the woman may move as a result of pain or a desire to adjust her position
• that patient movement may result in artifacts on the tracings that require monitor adjustment.

What to do

Prognosis of the mother and fetus depends on the size of the emboli and the skill and speed of the emergency interventions. Immediate management of this complication includes oxygen administration by face mask or cannula. Because vital organs are deprived of oxygen supply due to the emboli, within minutes the woman develops cardiopulmonary arrest, necessitating cardiopulmonary resuscitation (CPR). Even so, CPR may be ineffective because, despite providing oxygen transport to organs, it does nothing to remove the emboli. If the emboli aren't removed, blood can't circulate to the lungs. Death may occur within minutes.

Here are some other facts you should consider:
- Even if the initial insult (the emboli) is resolved, disseminated intravascular coagulation (DIC) is highly likely from the presence of particles in the bloodstream, further complicating the patient's condition.
- If the patient survives initial emergency procedures, she'll need continued management (such as endotracheal intubation) to maintain pulmonary function and therapy with fibrinogen to counteract DIC.
- Prompt transfer to the intensive care unit (ICU) is necessary.
- The prognosis for the fetus is guarded because reduced placental perfusion results from the severe drop in maternal blood pressure.
- The fetus may be delivered immediately by cesarean birth or vaginally using forceps.

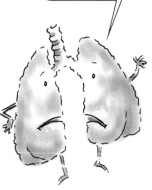

If the emboli aren't removed, I don't get the blood I need, and death can occur.

Cephalopelvic disproportion

A narrowing, or *contraction*, of the birth canal, which can occur at the inlet, midpelvis, or outlet, causes a disproportion between the size of the fetal head and the pelvic diameters, or cephalopelvic disproportion (CPD). CPD results in failure of labor to progress.

Other problems

In addition, malpositioning can occur because the fetus's head isn't engaged in the pelvis. Malpositioning can lead to further complications. For example, if membranes rupture, the risk of cord prolapse increases significantly.

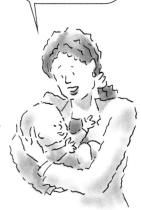

CPD is a disproportion between the size of the fetal head and the pelvic diameters.

What causes it

A small pelvis is a major contributing factor in CPD. The small size of the pelvis may be the result of rickets in the early life of the mother or a genetic predisposition.

A perfect fit

In primigravidas, the fetal head normally engages with the pelvic brim at weeks 36 to 38 of pregnancy. When this event occurs before labor begins, it's assumed that the pelvic inlet is adequate. Engagement of the head proves that the head fits into the pelvic brim and indicates that the head will probably also be able to pass through the midpelvis and through the outlet.

Inlets and outlets

Inlet contraction occurs when the narrowing of the anteroposterior diameter (from the symphysis pubis to the sacral prominence) is less than 11 cm or a maximum transverse diameter (between the ischial spines) is 12 cm or less. In outlet contraction, the transverse diameter narrows at the outlet to less than 11 cm. The outlet measurement is the distance between the ischial tuberosities. Because this measurement is easy to take during the expectant mother's prenatal visits, the health care team can anticipate and prepare for outlet contraction before labor begins.

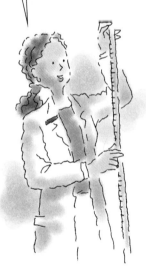

Measuring the distance between the ischial tuberosities is easy during prenatal visits and it helps to anticipate and prepare for outlet contraction before labor begins.

How it's detected

When engagement doesn't occur in a primigravida, a problem exists. This problem may be a fetal abnormality, such as a larger-than-usual head, or a pelvic abnormality, as in a smaller-than-usual pelvis. It's important to note that engagement doesn't usually occur in multigravidas until labor begins. In this situation, a previous delivery of a full-term neonate vaginally without problems is substantial proof that the birth canal is considered adequate.

Rule of mum

Every primigravida should have pelvic measurements taken and recorded before week 24. Based on these measurements and the assumption that the fetus will be of average size, a decision can be made about the possibility of vaginal delivery.

What to do

If the pelvic measurements are borderline or just adequate, especially the inlet measurement, and the fetal lie and position are good, the woman's doctor or nurse-midwife may allow a trial labor to determine whether labor can progress normally. A trial labor may be allowed to continue if descent of the presenting part and dilation of the cervix are occurring. In other words, normal labor and delivery are occurring and no complications have been detected.

Giving it a try

If trial labor is anticipated, the following nursing measures are important:

• Monitor fetal heart sounds and uterine contractions continuously if possible to detect any abnormalities promptly.
• Make sure that the woman's urinary bladder is kept as empty as possible, such as by urging her to void every 2 hours, to allow the fetal head to use all the space available, making delivery possible.
• After rupture of the membranes, assess fetal heart rate (FHR) carefully. If the fetal head is still high, alterations in FHR may indicate an increased danger of prolapsed cord and fetal anoxia.
• Monitor progress of labor. After 6 to 12 hours, if fetal descent and cervical dilation can't be documented or fetal distress occurs at any time, the woman should be scheduled for a cesarean birth.
• Keep in mind that a woman undertaking trial labor may feel she'll be unable to complete the process, which may lead her to feel she's being needlessly subjected to pain. Emphasize that it's best for the baby to be born vaginally, if possible.
• If the trial labor fails and cesarean delivery is scheduled, explain why the procedure is necessary and why it's a better alternative for the baby at that point.
• A woman having a trial labor may feel as if she's on trial herself. She may feel she's being judged and may be self-conscious if labor doesn't go as well as hoped.
• When dilation doesn't occur, the woman may feel discouraged and inadequate, as if she's somehow at fault. A woman may not be aware how much she wanted the trial labor to work until she's told that it isn't working.
• Remember to support the support person. He or she may also be frightened and feel helpless when a problem occurs.
• Assure the parents that a cesarean birth isn't an inferior method of birth. Remind them that it's an alternative method. In this instance, it's the method of choice, allowing them to achieve their goal of a healthy mother and a healthy child.

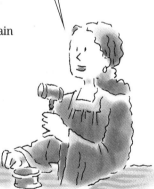

If trial labor fails, the woman may feel that she's being judged a failure, too. Remind her that cesarean birth is the best way to deliver a healthy baby.

Cesarean birth

Also known as *cesarean section* or *cesarean delivery*, cesarean birth is one of the oldest surgical procedures known. It may be performed as a planned surgery or an emergency procedure when vaginal birth isn't possible. (See *Cesarean factors*.)

Follow the plan

A cesarean birth is usually planned when the patient has had a previous cesarean birth and a vaginal birth after cesarean (VBAC) isn't recommended. It's considered elective because the patient and her health care provider choose the date that the cesarean birth will be performed based on her due date and the maturity of the fetus.

Still dangerous

Of course, because it's an invasive surgical procedure, cesarean birth is considered more hazardous than vaginal birth. Thus, it's only performed when the health and safety of the mother or fetus are in jeopardy. In addition, cesarean birth is generally contraindicated when there's a documented dead fetus. In this situation, labor can be induced to avoid an unnecessary surgical procedure.

On the rise

The incidence of cesarean birth is on the rise. In the United States, between 9% and 16% of pregnancies end in cesarean birth. In perinatal centers that care for mothers with high-risk deliveries, the

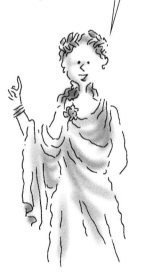

Cesarean birth is necessary when vaginal birth isn't possible.

Cesarean factors

Cesarean birth may be a planned or an emergency procedure. Factors that lead to cesarean birth may be maternal, placental, or fetal in nature.

Maternal
• Cephalopelvic disproportion
• Active genital herpes or papilloma
• Previous cesarean birth by classic incision
• Disabling conditions, such as severe pregnancy-induced hypertension and heart disease, that prevent pushing to accomplish the pelvic division of labor

Placental
• Placenta previa
• Premature separation of the placenta

Fetal
• Transverse fetal lie
• Extremely low fetal size
• Fetal distress
• Compound conditions, such as macrosomic fetus in a breech lie

rate has risen to as high as 25%. Some theories have attributed this rise to recent medical and technologic advances in fetal and placental surveillance and care. However, nurse-midwifery birthing services have a lower incidence of cesarean birth than more mainstream hospital services. Some suggest that the midwifery model of continuous support during labor may be a reason for the difference.

Other possible influences include:
• combination of the increasing safety of cesarean birth and the use of fetal monitors, which provide for early detection of fetal problems that would necessitate cesarean birth
• doctors becoming increasingly skilled in the procedure, while not acquiring comparable experience in alternative methods, such as external cephalic version and exercises to encourage a breech presentation to move into a vertex presentation
• doctors' fears of malpractice suits, which may result when a fetus is allowed to be delivered vaginally and then discovered to have suffered anoxia.

In the United States, about 15% of all pregnancies and about 25% of high-risk pregnancies end in cesarean birth.

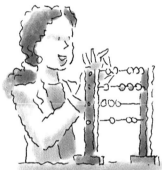

Double trouble

Occasionally, a woman may refuse to submit to a cesarean birth. Because women have a right to decide if they'll undergo surgery, the right to refuse the procedure is respected. In some instances, however, a court order to go ahead with the procedure may be obtained when cesarean birth is seen as necessary for the life of the fetus as well as the mother. Nurses working in labor and delivery units should be aware of the opinion of their agency's ethics committee on this issue and should also be aware of the proper channels to take should this situation arise.

Body system effects

Because cesarean birth requires a surgical procedure, it can result in systemic effects, including thrombophlebitis from interference in the body's natural stress response as well as alterations in body defenses, circulatory function, organ function, self-image, and self-esteem.

Stress response

Whenever the body is subjected to stress, either physical or psychological, it responds by trying to preserve function of all major body systems. This response includes the release of epinephrine and norepinephrine from the adrenal medulla. Norepinephrine release leads to peripheral vasoconstriction, which forces blood to the central circulation and increases blood pressure. Epinephrine causes changes resulting in:

- increased heart rate
- bronchial dilation
- elevation of blood glucose levels.

These responses are considered normal and are elicited when the person is tensed. The body is then ready for action with an increased heart rate and lung function as well as glucose for energy.

Antagonize, not minimize

However, these responses may antagonize anesthetic action aimed at minimizing body activity in the mother undergoing a cesarean birth. In addition, the stress response may result in reduced blood supply to the patient's lower extremities. The pregnant patient is prone to thrombophlebitis due to the stasis of blood flow; the stress response compounds this potential, greatly increasing the risk of thrombophlebitis. Combined with other effects of stress on major body systems, the stress response can significantly increase the risks associated with surgery.

Altered body defenses

The skin is the first line of defense against bacterial invasion. When the skin is incised for a surgical procedure, as in cesarean birth, this important line of defense is automatically lost. In addition, if cesarean birth is performed after membranes have been ruptured for hours, the woman's risk of infection doubles. Of course, precautions should be taken to minimize the risk to the patient through strict adherence to sterile technique during surgery and the days following the procedure.

Altered circulatory function

During cesarean birth, blood vessels are incised, a consequence of even the simplest surgical procedure. A surgical wound results in blood loss that, if extensive, can lead to hypovolemia and decreased blood pressure. When blood pressure decreases, inadequate perfusion of body tissues results, especially if the problem isn't recognized and corrected quickly. The amount of blood lost in cesarean birth is relatively high compared with vaginal birth. Pelvic vessels are usually congested with blood needed to supply the placenta. When pressure is placed on these vessels, blood loss occurs freely. During a vaginal birth, a woman may loose up to 500 ml of blood. This loss increases dramatically to 1,000 ml with a cesarean birth.

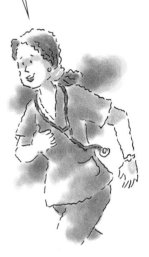

The stress response ensures that the body is ready for action with increased heart rate, lung function, and glucose for energy.

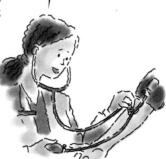

Decreased blood pressure results in inadequate perfusion — especially in cesarean birth, in which blood loss is greater than in other procedures.

Altered organ function

Like any body organ, the uterus may respond to being manipulated, cut, or repaired with a temporary disruption in function. Pressure from edema or inflammation can occur as fluid moves into the injured area. This normal response can further impair function of the uterus. In addition, handling of the uterus may result in a decrease in its ability to contract, which can lead to postpartum hemorrhage. Because complications may not be evident during the procedure, close assessment of the uterus is required in the postoperative period as well as an assessment of total body function to determine the degree of disruption.

What about the others

In addition to effects on the uterus, other organs may be directly affected. For example, to reach the uterus, the bladder must be displaced anteriorly. To perform the cesarean birth, pressure must be exerted on the intestine, possibly leading to paralytic ileus or halting of intestinal function. Because of these manipulating events, uterine, bladder, intestine, and lower circulatory function must be carefully assessed after a cesarean birth to detect complications early and avert potential problems.

Altered self-image or self-esteem

Surgical procedures almost always leave incisional scars that are noticeable to some extent afterward. In some situations, the resulting scar from a cesarean birth may be quite noticeable, such as when a horizontal incision is performed across the lower abdomen. The appearance of this scar may cause the woman to feel self-conscious later. She may also experience decreased self-esteem. This decrease may stem from a belief that she's marked as someone who can't give birth vaginally.

Incision types

Depending on the type of cesarean incision, a patient may be able to deliver vaginally after previously delivering by cesarean birth. Recent studies suggest that VBAC is becoming an increasingly successful alternative to elective cesarean birth. The type of incision chosen depends on the presentation of the fetus and the speed with which the procedure can be performed. In general, there are two types of cesarean incisions: classic and low-segment.

Classic cesarean incision

In a classic cesarean incision, the incision is made vertically through the abdominal skin and the uterus. It's made high on the uterus in the case of a placenta previa to avoid cutting the placenta. The result of this incision type is a wide skin scar that runs through the active contractile portion of the uterus. This scarring pattern carries an additional risk of complication in future pregnancies. Because this type of scar could cause uterine rupture during labor, it's likely that the woman won't be able to have a subsequent vaginal birth.

> Classic doesn't always mean good. A classic cesarean incision may eliminate the option of vaginal birth in subsequent pregnancies.

Low-segment incision

Low-segment incision is the most common type of cesarean incision. Unlike the classic incision, a low-segment incision is made horizontally across the lower abdomen just over the symphysis pubis and occurs horizontally across the uterus just over the cervix. This incision type is also referred to as *Pfannenstiel's incision* or a *bikini incision* because even a low-cut bathing suit should cover it. Because it's made through the nonactive portion of the uterus, or the part of the uterus that contracts minimally, it's less likely to cause rupture in subsequent labors. Thus, the low-segment incision makes it possible for a woman to attempt VBAC. Other advantages of this incision type include:
• decreased blood loss
• ease of suturing
• minimal postpartum uterine infection risk
• decreased risk of postpartum GI complications.

The downside

The major disadvantage of this incision is that it takes longer to perform. So if the cesarean must be done in a hurry, such as in an emergency, low-segment incision becomes impractical because of time constraints.

No assumptions, please

Sometimes a skin incision is made horizontally and the uterine incision is made vertically, or vice versa. Thus, during a future pregnancy, don't assume that a small skin incision indicates a small uterine incision.

What causes it

Cesarean birth is indicated when labor or vaginal birth carries an unacceptable risk for the mother or fetus, such as in CPD and transverse lie or other malpresentations. It may also be necessary if induction is contraindicated or difficult or if advanced labor increases the risk of morbidity and mortality.

The most common reasons for cesarean birth are:
• malpresentation of the fetus (such as shoulder or face presentation)
• evidence of fetal intolerance of labor stress
• CPD in which the pelvis is too small to accommodate the fetal head
• certain cases of toxemia or preeclampsia
• previous cesarean birth, especially with a classic incision
• inadequate progress in labor (failure of induction).

Fetus in distress

Conditions causing fetal distress can also indicate a need for cesarean birth. These conditions include:
• living fetus with prolapsed cord
• fetal hypoxia
• abnormal FHR patterns
• unfavorable intrauterine environment, such as from infection
• moderate to severe rhesus factor (Rh) isoimmunization.

Mom needs help

Less commonly, maternal conditions may necessitate cesarean birth. These conditions include:
• complete placenta previa
• abruptio placentae
• placenta accreta
• malignant tumors
• chronic diseases in the mother in which delivery is indicated before term.

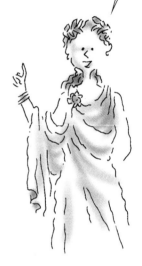

Cesarean birth is indicated when labor or vaginal birth carries an unacceptable risk for the mother or fetus.

How it's detected

Special tests and monitoring procedures provide early indications of the need for cesarean birth:
• Magnetic resonance imaging (MRI) or X-ray pelvimetry reveals CPD and malpositioning.
• Ultrasonography shows pelvic masses that interfere with vaginal birth and fetal position.
• Auscultation of FHR (by fetoscope, Doppler unit, or electronic fetal monitor) determines acute fetal intolerance of labor.

What to do

In preparation for cesarean birth, an anesthetic is administered. Patients may have general or regional anesthetic, depending on the extent of maternal or fetal distress. The woman is then positioned on the operating table. A towel may be placed under her left hip to help relocate abdominal contents so that they're up and away from the surgical field. This can also assist in lifting the uterus off the vena cava, promoting better circulation to the fetus as well as maternal blood return.

Blocking bacteria as well as the view

A metal screen or some other type of shielding may be placed at the patient's shoulder level and covered with a sterile drape. This not only serves as a courtesy to help obstruct the patient's view of the necessary surgical incision but also helps to block the flow of bacteria from the woman's respiratory tract to the incision site. Placement of the drape also blocks the support person's line of vision, preventing additional anxiety and fear that may arise from the sight of blood.

Support for the support

The support person is usually positioned at the mother's head. The incision area on the patient's abdomen is then scrubbed, and drapes are placed around the area of incision so that only a small area of skin is left exposed. In many cases, watching a cesarean birth is the first surgery the father or support person has witnessed. Thus, the person may be too overwhelmed by the whole event or too interested in the procedure to be of optimum support. He or she may become concerned about the amount of manipulation and cutting that occurs before the uterus itself is cut, assuming fetal distress isn't extreme. Remember to prepare the patient and support person for what they might see. This can help avert too much shock or surprise as well as promote open discussion about how much they would like to see or not see.

> Remember to prepare the patient and support person for what they might see in the operating room.

The down side

Possible maternal complications of cesarean birth include:
- respiratory tract infection
- wound dehiscence
- thromboembolism
- paralytic ileus
- hemorrhage
- genitourinary tract infection
- bowel, bladder, or uterine injury.

Before surgery

Preoperative care measures involve both the mother and fetus. Here are some measures you should take:
• Assess maternal and fetal status frequently until delivery, as your facility's policy directs.
• If ordered, make sure that an ultrasound has been obtained. The doctor may have ordered the test to determine fetal position.
• Explain cesarean birth to the patient and her partner, and answer any questions they may have.
• Provide reassurance and emotional support to help improve the self-esteem and self-concept of the mother and her partner. Remember that a cesarean birth is commonly performed after hours of labor, resulting in an exhausted patient and partner. Be brief but clear and stress the essential points about the procedure.
• For a scheduled cesarean birth, discuss the procedure with both parents and provide preoperative teaching.
• Observe the mother for signs of imminent delivery.
• Demonstrate use of the incentive spirometer, and have the patient practice deep breathing. Review splinting measures to decrease incisional pain with deep breathing and coughing.
• Restrict food and fluids after midnight if a general anesthetic is ordered to prevent aspiration vomitus.
• Prepare the patient by shaving her from below the breasts to the pubic region and the upper quarter of the anterior thighs as indicated. Scrub and shave the abdomen and the symphysis pubis as ordered.
• Make sure the patient's bladder is empty, use an indwelling urinary catheter as ordered, and check for flow and patency. Tell the mother that the catheter may remain in place for 24 hours or longer.
• Administer ordered preoperative medication.
• Give the mother an antacid to help neutralize stomach acid if ordered.
• Start an I.V. infusion for fluid replacement therapy using the patient's nondominant hand if required. Use an 18G or larger catheter to allow blood administration through the I.V. if needed.
• Make sure the doctor has ordered typing and crossmatching of the mother's blood and that 2 units of blood are available.

Promote bonding between mom and baby by letting the mother see, touch, and hold her baby as soon as possible after delivery.

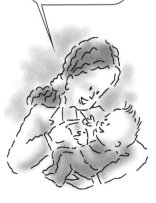

After surgery

Postoperative care measures of the mother and child include:
• As soon as possible, allow the mother to see, touch, and hold her neonate, either in the delivery room or after she recovers from the general anesthetic. Contact with the neonate promotes bonding.

- Check the perineal pad and abdominal dressing on the incision every 15 minutes for 1 hour, then every half-hour for 4 hours, every hour for 4 hours, and finally every 4 hours for 24 hours.
- Perform fundal checks at the same intervals. Gently assess the fundus.
- Check the dressing frequently for bleeding, and report it immediately. Be sure to keep the incision clean and dry.
- Monitor vital signs every 5 minutes until stable. Then check vital signs when you evaluate perineal and abdominal drainage.
- The doctor may order oxytocin mixed in with the first 1,000 to 2,000 ml of I.V. fluids infused to promote uterine contraction and decrease the risk of hemorrhage. Make sure the I.V. is patent and monitor the patient carefully for effects of the medication.
- Monitor intake and output as ordered. Expect the mother to receive I.V. fluids for 24 to 48 hours.
- Make sure the catheter is patent and urine flow is adequate. When the catheter is removed, make sure that the woman can void without difficulty and that urine color and amount are adequate.
- Maintain a patent airway for the mother and the neonate.
- Encourage the mother to cough and deep-breathe and use the incentive spirometer to promote adequate respiratory function.
- If a general anesthetic was used, remain with the patient until she's responsive.
- If regional anesthetic was used, monitor the return of sensation to the legs.
- Help the mother to turn from side to side every 1 to 2 hours.
- If ordered, show the patient how to administer patient-controlled analgesia.
- Administer pain medication as ordered, and provide comfort measures for breast engorgement as appropriate.
- If the mother wants to breast-feed, offer encouragement and help.
- Recognize afterpains in multiparas and monitor the effects of pain medication. Timing of administration of pain medication and breast-feeding may need to be coordinated so that the neonate won't receive as much of the sedating effect.
- Promote early ambulation to prevent cardiovascular and pulmonary complications. Remember to assist the mother initially and make sure she doesn't suffer from orthostatic hypotension. Warn her that lochia may flow freely when she moves from a supine to an upright position.

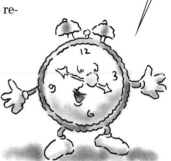

After cesarean delivery, check the perineal pad and abdominal dressing every 15 minutes for 1 hour, every half-hour for 4 hours, every hour for 4 hours, and finally every 4 hours for 24 hours.

Going home

Home care instructions should also be provided to the patient who has had a cesarean birth, including:

• Instruct the patient to immediately report hemorrhage, chest or leg pain (possible thrombosis), dyspnea, or separation of the wound's edges.
• Tell her to also report signs and symptoms of infection, such as fever, difficulty urinating, and flank pain.
• Remind the patient to keep her follow-up appointment. At that time, she can talk to the doctor about using contraception and resuming intercourse.

Fetal presentation or position

Problems can occur with the fetus's presentation or position during labor and delivery. Although most fetuses move into the proper birthing position, alternative positions and presentations can occur, making vaginal delivery difficult and, in some situations, impossible.

Problematic presentations and positions

Some presentations and positions that can be problematic include occipitoposterior position, breech presentation, face presentation, and transverse lie. A fifth type of presentation, called *brow presentation*, is rarely seen. (See *A briefing on brow presentation*.)

Occipitoposterior position

In about one-tenth of labors, the fetal position may be posterior rather than the traditional anterior position. When this occurs, the occiput, assuming the presentation is vertex, is directed diagonally and posteriorly, right occipitoposterior or left occipitoposterior. In these positions, during internal rotation, the fetal head must rotate through not the normal 90-degree arc but an arc of approximately 135 degrees.

This rotation through the 135-degree arc may not be possible if the fetus is above average size or isn't in good flexion or if contractions are ineffective. Ineffective contractions may occur in:
• uterine dysfunction from maternal exhaustion
• fetal head arrested in the transverse position (transverse arrest).

1-2-3 rotate!

If rotation through the 135-degree arc doesn't occur but the fetus has reached the midportion of the pelvis, he may be rotated manually to an anterior position with forceps and then delivered. As an alternative, cesarean delivery may be preferred because the risk of a midforceps maneuver exceeds the risk of cesarean delivery. If

A briefing on brow presentation

A brow presentation (the rarest of the presentations) may occur with a multipara or in an individual with relaxed abdominal muscles. Here are some key points about this type of presentation:
• It almost invariably results in obstructed labor because the head becomes jammed in the brim of the pelvis as the occipitomental diameter presents.
• Unless the presentation spontaneously corrects, cesarean birth is necessary to safely deliver the neonate.
• Because brow presentation leaves extreme ecchymotic bruising on the neonate's face and head, his parents may need additional reassurance that he's healthy.

midforceps are used for birth, the woman is at risk for reproductive tract lacerations, hemorrhage, and infection in the postpartum period.

Breech presentation

Most fetuses are in a breech presentation early in pregnancy. However, in approximately 97% of pregnancies, the fetus turns to a cephalic presentation by week 38. Although the fetal head is the widest single diameter, the fetus's buttocks (breech), plus the lower extremities, takes up more space. The fundus, being the largest part of the uterus, promotes fetal turning so that the buttocks and lower extremities are within it. Additionally, some evidence suggests that a breech presentation is less likely to occur if a woman assumes a knee-chest position for approximately 15 minutes three times per day during pregnancy.

Styles of breech from frank to complete

There are several types of breech presentations:
• frank breech—in which the buttocks are the presenting part and the legs are extended and rest on the fetal chest
• footling breech—which can be either one foot (single-footling) or both feet (double-footling breech) and the thighs or lower legs aren't flexed
• complete breech—in which the fetal thighs are flexed on the abdomen and both the buttocks and the tightly flexed feet are against the cervix.

Danger, danger

Breech presentation is more hazardous than a cephalic presentation because there's a greater risk of:
• anoxia from a prolapsed cord
• traumatic injury to the after-coming head, which can result in intracranial hemorrhage or anoxia
• fracture of the spine or arm
• dysfunctional labor
• early rupture of the membranes because of the poor fit of the presenting part
• meconium aspiration (the inevitable contraction of the fetal buttocks from cervical pressure commonly causes meconium to be extruded into the amniotic fluid before birth).

Same stages

In a breech birth, the same stages of flexion, descent, internal rotation expulsion, and external rotation occur as in a cephalic birth. (See *A look at breech birth*.)

Turn, turn, turn

An alternative to vaginal or cesarean birth of a fetus in breech presentation is a method called *external cephalic version*. In this method, the fetus is manually turned from a breech to a cephalic position before birth. Use of external version can decrease the number of cesarean births due to breech presentations by about 40%. To turn the fetus:

The breech and vertex of the fetus are located and grasped transabdominally by an examiner's hands on the woman's abdomen.

Gentle pressure is then exerted to rotate the fetus. The fetus must be moved in a forward direction to a cephalic lie. (See *A look at external cephalic version,* page 380.)

> In external cephalic version, the fetus is manually turned from a breech presentation to a cephalic position before birth.

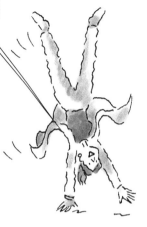

A look at breech birth

A breech presentation follows the same stages of descent, flexion, and rotation as a cephalic presentation.

As the breech fetus enters the birth canal, descent and external rotation occur, as shown below.

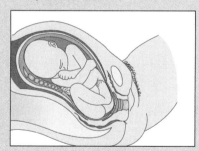

If the presenting part is the buttocks, the health care provider reaches up into the birth canal and pulls the legs down and out, as shown below. The breech delivery continues as the shoulders turn and present in the anteroposterior diameter of the mother's pelvis.

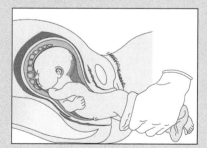

The head is then delivered by laying the neonate across the health care provider's left hand while two fingers are placed in the neonate's mouth and the other hand is placed on the back of the neck to apply gentle pressure to flex the head fully, as shown below. At the same time, gentle upward and outward traction is applied to the shoulders. An assistant may need to gently apply external abdominal wall pressure to ensure that head flexion occurs.

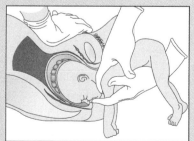

A look at external cephalic version

In external cephalic version, a health care provider manually rotates the fetus. The fetus is rotated by external pressure to a cephalic lie, aiding the possibility of a normal vaginal delivery.

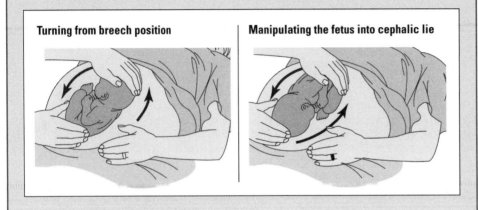

Turning from breech position

Manipulating the fetus into cephalic lie

Face presentation

In a face presentation, the chin, or *mentum*, is the presenting part. Although this presentation is rare, when it does occur, birth usually can't proceed because the diameter of the presenting part is too large for the maternal pelvis.

In your face

Face presentation is considered a warning sign because its cause is always some abnormality in the fetus or mother.

Transverse lie

Transverse lie occurs when the fetus lays horizontal to the uterus. Because there's no firm presenting part, a vaginal delivery isn't possible.

What causes it

Contributing factors depend on the specific fetal presentation or position.

Occipitoposterior position

Posterior positions tend to occur in women with these pelvic structures:

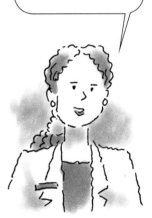

It may be difficult to face, but a face presentation results from some abnormality in the fetus or mother.

- android pelvis
- anthropoid pelvis
- contracted pelvis.

Breech presentation

Breech presentation may occur for various reasons:
- gestational age less than 40 weeks
- fetal abnormality from anencephaly, hydrocephalus, or meningocele
- hydramnios, which allows free fetal movement so the fetus doesn't have to engage for comfort
- congenital anomaly of the uterus, such as a midseptum, that traps the fetus in a breech position
- space-occupying mass in the pelvis that doesn't allow engagement, such as a fibroid tumor of the uterus and placenta previa
- pendulous abdomen in the mother that occurs when the abdominal muscles are lax, which may cause the uterus to fall so far forward that the head comes to lie outside the pelvic brim, causing breech presentation
- multiple gestation in which the presenting fetus can't turn to a vertex position.

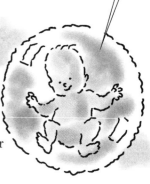

Gestational age less than 40 weeks can contribute to breech presentation.

Face presentation

A fetus in a posterior position, instead of flexing the head as labor proceeds, may extend the head, resulting in a face presentation. The situations in which this occurs include:
- a woman with a contracted pelvis
- placenta previa
- relaxed uterus of a multipara
- prematurity
- hydramnios
- fetal malformation.

Transverse lie

Transverse lie occurs in these conditions:
- a woman with a pendulous abdomen
- a uterine mass, such as fibroid tumor, that obstructs the lower uterine segment
- contraction of the pelvic brim
- congenital uterine abnormalities
- hydramnios
- hydrocephalus or other gross abnormalities that prevent the head from engaging

- prematurity
- room for free fetal movement in the uterus
- multiple gestation (particularly in a second twin)
- short umbilical cord
- placenta previa
- fetal abnormalities.

> Multiple gestation can cause transverse lie, especially in a second twin.

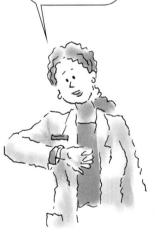

How it's detected

Detection of abnormalities depends on the specific type of fetal position or presentation abnormality.

Occipitoposterior position

On assessment, a posteriorly presenting head will be found to not fit the cervix as snugly as one occurring in an anterior position. Because this increases the risk of prolapse of the umbilical cord, the position of the fetus should be confirmed on vaginal examination or by sonogram.

A posterior position may also be suspected when dysfunctional labor patterns occur, such as:
- prolonged active phase
- arrested descent
- fetal heart sounds heard best at the lateral sides of the abdomen.

Getting into position

Most fetuses presenting in posterior positions rotate during labor, and birth can proceed normally. This scenario is most common when the fetus is of average size and in good flexion. This rotation is also aided by forceful uterine contractions causing the fetus to rotate through the large arc. The fetus arrives at a good birth position for the pelvic outlet in these situations and can be delivered satisfactorily. The fetus may experience slightly increased molding and caput formation.

> Posterior position may be suggested by a prolonged active phase.

Drawing it out

One of the drawbacks to the posterior position is the duration of the labor process. Because the arc of rotation is greater, it's common for the labor to be somewhat prolonged. Labor pain is also different in this type of positioning. Because the fetal head rotates against the sacrum, the woman may experience pressure and pain in her lower back from sacral nerve compression during labor.

Breech presentation

Breech presentation is detected by these findings:
- Fetal heart sounds are commonly heard high in the abdomen.
- Leopold's maneuvers identify the fetal head in the uterine fundus.
- Vaginal examination reveals the presence of the buttocks or the foot (or both) as the presenting part, although, if the breech is complete and firmly engaged, the tightly stretched gluteal muscles may be mistaken on vaginal examination for a head and the cleft between the buttocks may be mistaken for the sagittal suture line.
- Ultrasound reveals the position of the fetus and provides information on pelvic diameter, fetal skull diameter, and the existence of placenta previa.

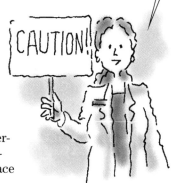

Make sure that you don't mistake tightly stretched gluteal muscles for a head during vaginal examination for breech presentation.

Face presentation

When a face presentation is suspected, a sonogram can be performed to confirm the position of the fetus. If indicated, measurements of the pelvic diameters are made. Other signs of face presentation include:
- fetus's head that feels more prominent than normal with no engagement apparent during Leopold's maneuvers
- fetus's head and back that are both felt on the same side of the uterus with Leopold's maneuvers
- difficulty outlining the fetus's back (because it's concave)
- fetal heart tones heard on the side of the fetus where feet and arms can be palpated (in extremely concave back, which causes transmission of fetal heart tones to the forward-thrust chest)
- vaginal examination that reveals the nose, mouth, or chin as the presenting part.

Transverse lie

A transverse lie is usually obvious on inspection, when the ovoid of the uterus is found to be more horizontal than vertical. Other detection methods include:
- Leopold's maneuvers, which make it easier to palpate the fetus in a transverse lie position
- sonogram, which confirms transverse lie and provides other information (such as pelvic size).

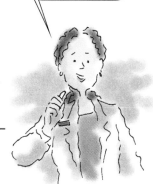

How you should intervene depends on the specific presentation and position.

What to do

Management of fetal position or presentation abnormalities depends on the specific type of abnormality.

Occipitoposterior position

Because labor pain may be intense when a fetus is in the occipito-posterior position, management can be a challenge. Commonly, the laboring woman asks for medication for relief of the intense pressure on and pain in her back. Consider alternative methods to help relieve back pressure, such as those mentioned here:
• Place pressure on the sacrum, such as with a back rub, or suggest a position change to relieve some of the pain.
• Apply heat or cold, depending on which is more successful in obtaining relief.
• Ask the woman to lie on the side opposite the fetal back or maintain a hands-and-knees position to help the fetus rotate.
• Encourage the woman to void approximately every 2 hours to keep the bladder empty to avoid impeding the descent of the fetus and additional discomfort.
• Because of the commonly lengthy labor, be aware of how long it has been since the patient last ate. During a long labor, she may need I.V. glucose solutions to replace glucose stores used for energy.

Something else to consider

Here are some other considerations for the woman delivering a baby in the occipitoposterior position:
• During labor, the woman needs a great deal of support to prevent her from becoming panicked over the length of the labor. In addition, you should provide practical, step-by-step explanations of what's happening.
• Be aware that the woman who's best prepared for labor is commonly the most frightened when deviations occur because she realizes that her labor isn't going "by the book" or as described by her birthing instructor. Provide frequent reassurance to her that, although the labor is long, her pattern of labor is still within safe, controlled limits.

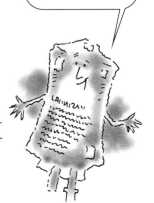

Because labor can be long, be aware of the last time the woman ate. She may need I.V. glucose to replace glucose used for energy.

Breech presentation

If the fetus in a breech presentation can be born vaginally, when full dilation is reached, the woman is allowed to push and the breech, trunk, and shoulders are delivered. Here's what else you can expect:
• As the breech spontaneously emerges from the birth canal, it's steadied and supported by a sterile towel held against the neonate's inferior surface.
• The shoulders present toward the outlet, with their widest diameter anteroposterior. If the shoulders don't deliver readily, the arm of the posterior shoulder may be drawn down by passing two

fingers over the neonate's shoulder and down the arm to the elbow and then sweeping the flexed arm across the neonate's face and chest and out.
• The other arm is then delivered in the same way. External rotation is allowed to occur to bring the head into the best outlet diameter.

Everything comes to a head

Birth of an aftercoming head involves a great deal of judgment and skill. Here's how it's done:
• To aid delivery of the head, the trunk of the neonate is usually straddled over the doctor's right forearm.
• The doctor places two fingers of his right hand in the neonate's mouth.
• The doctor slides his left hand into the mother's vagina, palm down, along the neonate's back.
• Pressure is applied to the occiput to flex the head fully.
• Gentle traction applied to the shoulders (upward and outward) delivers the head.

Pied Piper

An aftercoming head may also be delivered using Piper forceps to control the flexion and rate of descent. (See *Using Piper forceps*, page 386.)

Head hazards

Birth of the head is the most hazardous part of a breech birth. Here are some complications to consider:
• Because the umbilicus comes before the head, a loop of cord passes down alongside the head and automatically becomes compressed. This compression is due to the pressure of the head against the pelvic brim.
• With a cephalic presentation, molding to the confines of the birth canal occurs over hours. With a breech birth, this pressure change occurs instantaneously. Tentorial tears can occur as a result of this pressure change. These tears may cause gross motor malfunction, mental problems, or lethal damage to the fetus.
• The neonate may be delivered suddenly to decrease the duration of cord compression. Doing so, however, may result in an intracranial hemorrhage.
• A neonate delivered gradually in order to reduce the possibility of intracranial injury may suffer hypoxia.

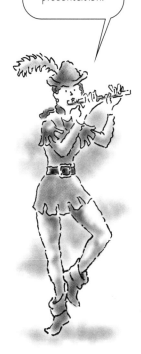

Piper forceps control the flexion and rate of descent of a fetus in breech presentation.

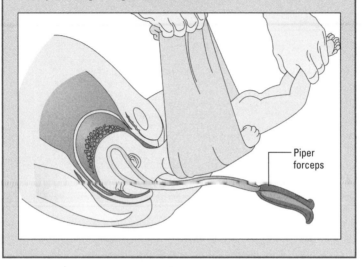

Using Piper forceps

Occasionally, the fetal head can't be easily delivered in a breech presentation. Piper forceps may be used to apply traction directly to the head, preventing damage to the fetal neck.

Piper forceps

What happened?

Parents and health care providers usually inspect a breech baby a little more closely than a baby from a normal delivery for many reasons:

• The cause of the breech birth may be unknown. The parents and the person who makes the initial physical assessment of the neonate may look for the reason that made the presentation breech.

• Remember that a neonate who was delivered in a frank breech position may resume his fetal position. He may keep his legs extended and at the level of the face for the first 2 to 3 days of life.

• The neonate who presented in a footling breech may keep the legs extended in a footling position for the first few days.

• Be sure to point out these possible positions to the parents to avoid undue worry or a misinterpretation of the neonate's unusual posture.

Alternate version

If external cephalic version is performed before the birth to turn the fetus to a cephalic position, remember the following considerations:

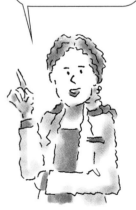

Parents and the health care team usually inspect a breech baby a little more closely than a baby from a normal delivery.

• FHR and, possibly, ultrasound should be recorded continuously.
• A tocolytic agent may be administered to help relax the uterus.
• Provide support to the woman to help her tolerate the discomfort from the pressure experienced during the procedure.
• Women who are Rh-negative should receive Rh immunoglobulin in case minimal bleeding occurs.

Aversion to version

Contraindications to external cephalic version include:
• multiple gestation
• severe oligohydramnios
• contraindications to vaginal birth
• a nuchal cord
• unexplained third-trimester bleeding (possibly suggesting placenta previa).

Face presentation

If the chin is anterior and the pelvic diameters are within normal limits, the fetus in face presentation may be delivered without difficulty. However, certain complications must be considered:
• There may be a long first stage of labor because the face doesn't mold well to make a snugly engaging part.
• If the chin is posterior, cesarean delivery is the optimal method of birth because a vaginal birth would require posterior-to-anterior rotation, which could take a long time. In addition, such rotation can result in uterine dysfunction or a transverse arrest.

Edema dilemma

Babies born after a face presentation have a great deal of facial edema and may be purple from ecchymotic bruising. Additional considerations include:
• Lip edema may be so severe that the neonate can't suck for 1 or 2 days.
• The neonate may need gavage feedings to obtain enough fluid until he can suck effectively.
• The neonate must be observed closely for a patent airway.
• The neonate is usually transferred to a neonatal ICU for the first 24 hours.
• Assure the parents that the edema will disappear in a few days and causes no long-term effects.

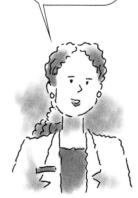

Assure parents that facial edema will disappear in a few days and causes no long-term effects.

Transverse lie

A mature fetus in a transverse lie position can't be delivered vaginally. Although the membranes usually rupture at the beginning of labor, there's no firm presenting part. Thus, the cord or arm may prolapse or the shoulder can come down and obstruct the cervix. Cesarean delivery is mandatory in this instance. Thus, to manage transverse lie presentation, follow the care measures for cesarean delivery.

Fetal size

The size of the fetus may be an indication of a difficult delivery. In general, a fetus who weighs more than 4,500 g (9.9 lb) may lead to a difficult delivery. An abnormally large fetal size may pose a problem at birth because it can cause fetal pelvic disproportion or uterine rupture from obstruction. The risk of perinatal mortality in larger neonates is substantially higher than in normal-sized neonates (15% versus 4%). The large neonate born vaginally also has a higher-than-normal risk of:

- cervical nerve palsy
- diaphragmatic nerve injury
- fractured clavicle because of shoulder dystocia.

Mom, too

During the postpartum period, the mother has an increased risk of hemorrhage because an overdistended uterus may not contract as readily.

Shoulder dystocia

Shoulder dystocia is increasing in incidence along with the increasing average weight of neonates. The problem occurs at the second stage of labor when the fetal head is born but the shoulders are too broad to enter the pelvic outlet. This situation can cause vaginal or cervical tears in the mother or cord compression leading to a fractured clavicle or brachial plexus injury in the fetus.

> Shoulder dystocia is increasing in incidence along with the increasing average weight of neonates.

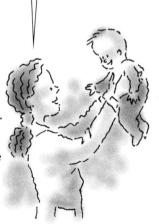

What causes it

Large fetuses are most common in women who are diabetic. Large babies are also associated with multiparity, because each neonate born to a woman tends to be slightly heavier and larger than the one born just before. Shoulder dystocia is most apt to occur in babies of women with diabetes, multiparas, and in postdate pregnancies.

How it's detected

Although fetus size can usually be detected using palpation, the size of the fetus may be missed in an obese woman because the fetal contours are difficult to palpate. Also, just because she's obese doesn't mean the woman has a larger-than-usual pelvis; in fact, her pelvis may be small. Pelvimetry or sonography is the best way to compare fetal size with the woman's pelvic capacity.

Head and...shoulders?

Shoulder dystocia, however, commonly isn't identified until the head has been born. The wide anterior shoulder then seems to lock beneath the symphysis pubis. Shoulder dystocia may be suspected earlier if:
- second stage of labor is prolonged
- arrest of descent occurs
- the head, when it appears on the perineum (crowning), retracts instead of protruding with each contraction (turtle sign).

What to do

If the fetus is so large that the child can't be delivered vaginally, cesarean delivery becomes the method of choice. In shoulder dystocia, measures may include:
- asking the woman to flex her thighs sharply on her abdomen to widen the pelvic outlet and help the anterior shoulder deliver
- applying suprapubic pressure to help the shoulder escape from beneath the symphysis pubis.

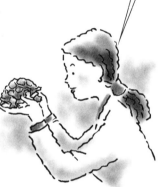

Shoulder dystocia should be suspected if the head of the fetus appears on the perineum and then retracts with each contraction. This is known as the turtle sign.

Ineffective uterine force

Uterine contractions force the moving fetus through the birth canal. Usually, contractions are initiated at one pacemaker point in the uterus. When a contraction occurs, it sweeps down over the uterus, encircling it. Repolarization then occurs, a low resting tone is achieved, and another pacemaker-activated contraction begins. This process is aided by:
- hormones — adenosine triphosphate, estrogen, and progesterone
- electrolytes — calcium, sodium, and potassium
- proteins — actin and myosin
- epinephrine and norepinephrine
- oxytocin
- prostaglandins.

Ineffective = increased mortality

Although about 95% of labors are completed with contractions following a predictable, normal course, ineffective labor can occur. The incidence of maternal puerperal infection and hemorrhage and infant mortality is higher in women who have a prolonged labor than in those who don't. Therefore, it's vital to recognize and prevent ineffective labor.

Although effective labor can become ineffective at any time, there are two general types:

 primary (at beginning of labor)

 secondary (later in labor).

Be productive

Abnormal labor can produce anxiety, fear, or discouragement in the woman as well as her partner. You should provide continuous explanations of what's happening to the woman and her support person. (See *Helping your patient reduce stress*.) In addition, there are some measures you

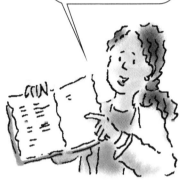

> It's important to recognize and prevent ineffective labor because prolonged labor increases the risk of maternal infection and hemorrhage as well as infant mortality.

Advice from the experts

Helping your patient reduce stress

Stress results from and can lead to or increase dysfunctional labor. If a woman is tense or frightened during labor, her cervix won't dilate as rapidly, making labor prolonged.

Employ these management techniques to help your patient and her partner reduce stress:

• Ask directly if the woman has any concerns.
• Offer explanations of all procedures.
• Make the support person just as welcome and comfortable as the woman herself.
• Ask questions such as, "Is labor what you thought it would be?" to both the woman and her support person to help them express concerns.
• Remember that pain is exhausting and rest promotes adequate cervical dilation. Encour-

age the patient to rest or sleep (if possible) in between the contractions.
• Encourage the use of nonpharmacologic comfort measures.
• Employ comfort measures, such as breathing with the woman, giving back rubs, changing sheets, and using cool washcloths. If breathing exercises are effective, the need for analgesia (which can lead to hypotonic contractions) can be reduced.
• Urge the woman to lie on her side so the uterus is lifted off the vena cava to promote comfort, increase blood supply to the uterus, and prevent hypotension.
• If a woman is more comfortable lying supine, place a hip roll under one buttock to tip her pelvis and move the uterus to the side.

Take charge!

Promoting productive labor

Some measures used to promote productive labor can help avoid serious complications from ineffective labor. Consider the following measures for a patient suffering from abnormal labor.

Glucose stores
Because labor is work, it can cause a woman to deplete her glucose stores. To investigate this possibility:
• On a patient's admission to a birthing room, ask the time of her last meal to help determine if she's at risk for depleting her glucose stores. Alert the doctor or nurse-midwife to this possibility.
• If the patient is still in early labor, she may be allowed to drink some high-carbohydrate fluid such as orange juice. I.V. fluid therapy may also be initiated to provide glucose for energy.
• Most doctors and nurse-midwives also allow women to have lollipops or hard candy to suck on during labor to supply additional glucose.

Fluid replacement
Many women don't want to receive I.V. fluid therapy during labor. Some perceive it as losing control over their bodies or having the naturalness of labor and birth taken away.

Take these measures to allay your patient's concerns:
• Explain the purpose of I.V. fluid therapy before arriving with the bag of fluid and tubing.
• When inserting the I.V. catheter device, try to use an insertion site in the woman's nondominant hand.
• Assure the patient that she can be out of bed and walking as well as turn freely or move about during labor as desired because none of these acts should interfere with the infusion.

can employ to try to promote a more productive labor. (See *Promoting productive labor.*)

When the force isn't with you

Complications due to ineffective uterine force can impede the natural course of labor. These complications include:
• hypertonic contractions
• hypotonic contractions
• uncoordinated contractions. (See *Comparing and contrasting contractions*, page 392.)

Hypertonic contractions

Hypertonic uterine contractions are marked by an increased resting tone to more than 15 mm Hg. Even so, the intensity of contractions may be no stronger than with hypotonic contractions. Hypertonic contractions tend to occur frequently. They're most commonly

Three major complications impede the natural course of labor: hypertonic, hypotonic, and uncoordinated contractions.

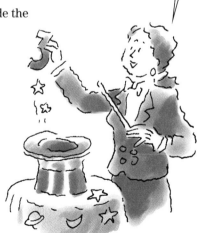

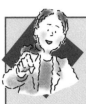

Take charge!

Comparing and contrasting contractions

Below are illustrations of the different uterine activity types. Depending on your assessment, you may need to intervene to promote adequate labor contractions.

Typical contractions
Typical uterine contractions occur every 2 to 5 minutes during active labor and typically last 30 to 90 seconds.

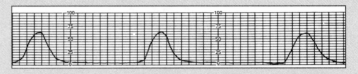

Hypotonic contractions
Hypotonic contractions are evident by a rise in pressure of no more than 10 mm Hg during a contraction.

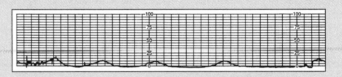

Hypertonic contractions
Hypertonic contractions don't allow the uterus to rest between contractions, as shown by a resting pressure of 40 to 50 mm Hg.

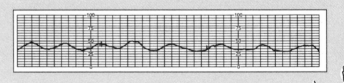

seen in the latent phase of labor, and may result in precipitous labor. (See *Precipitous labor.*)

Hypotonic contractions

Contractions are termed *hypotonic* when the number or frequency of contractions is low. For example, they might not increase beyond two or three in a 10-minute period. The strength of contractions doesn't rise above 25 mm Hg.

Utter exhaustion

Hypotonic contractions tend to increase the length of labor because so many of them are necessary to achieve cervical dilation. This can result in exhaustion of the mother as well as of the organs involved. This exhaustion can lead to:
• ineffective contraction of the uterus, increasing the woman's chance for postpartum hemorrhage

Precipitous labor

Precipitous labor and birth occur when uterine contractions are so strong that the woman delivers with only a few rapidly occurring contractions. It's commonly defined as labor completed within less than 3 hours. Such rapid labor may occur with multiparity. It may also follow induction of labor by oxytocin or when an amniotomy is performed.

Dangerous force

In precipitous labor, contractions may be so forceful that they lead to premature separation of the placenta, placing the mother and fetus at risk for hemorrhage. The woman may also sustain injuries such as lacerations of the birth canal from the forceful delivery. Precipitous labor is also disconcerting and the woman may feel as if she has lost control.

Rapid labor poses an additional risk to the fetus as well. Subdural hemorrhage may result from the sudden release of pressure on the head.

Graphic evidence

A precipitous labor can be detected from a labor graph. This can occur during the active phase of dilation, when the rate is greater than 5 cm/hour (1 cm every 12 minutes) in a nullipara and more than 10 cm/hour (1 cm every 6 minutes) in a multipara. If this situation occurs, a tocolytic may be administered to reduce the force and frequency of contractions.

Even shorter next time

Because labors tend to be quicker with subsequent pregnancies, inform the multiparous woman by week 28 of pregnancy that her labor might be shorter than a previous one. She should plan for appropriately timed transportation to the hospital or alternative birthing center. When labor begins, alert a woman who has had a prior precipitous labor and birth that she may deliver this way again. When preparing for delivery, both grand multiparas and women with histories of precipitous labor should have the birthing room converted to birth readiness before full dilation. Then birth can be accomplished in a controlled surrounding.

• risk of infection in the uterus and the fetus because of the extended period of cervical dilation.

Uncoordinated contractions

Uncoordinated contractions occur erratically, such as one on top of another followed by a long period without any. The lack of a regular pattern to contractions makes it difficult for the woman to rest or to use breathing exercises between contractions. Uncoordinated contractions may occur so closely together that they don't allow good filling time.

What causes it

The causes of ineffective uterine force depend on the type of dysfunction.

Hypertonic contractions

Hypertonic contractions occur because the muscle fibers of the myometrium don't repolarize after a contraction, making it ready to accept a new pacemaker stimulus. They can occur when more than one pacemaker is stimulating the contractions, unlike the normal single stimulus found with normally occurring contractions. Oxytocin administration may also cause hypertonic contractions. (See *Hypertonic contractions and oxytocin.*)

Hypotonic contractions

Hypotonic contractions usually occur during the active phase of labor. They may occur when:
• analgesia has been administered too early (before cervical dilation of 3 to 4 cm)
• bowel or bladder distention is present, preventing descent or firm engagement
• the uterus is overstretched due to multiple gestation, larger-than-normal single fetus, hydramnios, or grand multiparity.

> Hypertonic contractions can occur when more than one pacemaker stimulates contractions. It's like trying to ride two waves at once. Yikes!

Hypertonic contractions and oxytocin

When assessing the patient receiving oxytocin, monitor for hypertonic uterine contractions. These contractions can be as high as 100 mm Hg in intensity. With these contractions, the fetus may experience late decelerations and fetal heart rate increases, as depicted below.

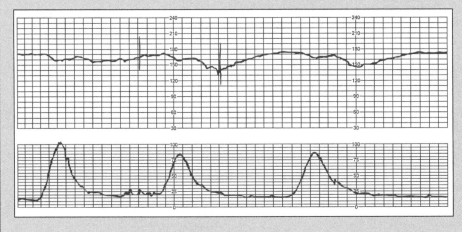

Uncoordinated contractions

With uncoordinated contractions, more than one pacemaker may initiate contractions. In addition, receptor points in the myometrium act independently of the pacemaker.

How it's detected

Ineffective uterine force is determined through physical examination and monitoring. Signs and symptoms depend on the type of dysfunction.

Hypertonic contractions

Hypertonic contractions are determined by the presence of painful uterine contractions that are either palpated or observed on an electronic monitor. On the electronic monitor, these uterine contractions show a high resting tone, and a lack of relaxation between contractions is also present. Fetal monitoring may even reveal bradycardia and fetal distress in the form of late decelerations because the absence of uterine relaxation doesn't allow the best possible uterine filling, which results in diminished oxygenation to the fetus. The woman won't be able to relax between contractions and may find it difficult to breathe with her contractions. These contractions are painful because the myometrium becomes tender as a result of inadequate relaxation.

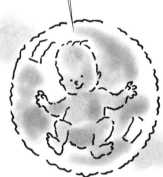

Hypertonic contractions can cause me distress. Impaired uterine filling means that there's less oxygen coming my way.

Hypotonic contractions

Hypotonic contractions usually aren't abnormally painful because they aren't intense. However, pain is subjective; one woman's interpretation of uterine contractions may be different from another. Thus, some women may interpret these contractions as very painful.

Lack of progress

Hypotonic contractions are detected by lack of labor progression and cervical dilation. The contractions are insufficient to dilate the cervix and won't register as intense on an electronic uterine contraction monitoring strip.

Uncoordinated contractions

Uncoordinated contraction patterns may be detected with the application of a fetal and uterine external monitor. Monitoring allows assessment of the rate, pattern, resting tone, and fetal response to contractions, revealing an abnormal pattern. Usually this pattern may be detected within 15 minutes; however, a longer time may be necessary to show the disorganized pattern in early labor.

What to do

Management of ineffective uterine force depends on the type of dysfunction. Emotional support and other comfort measures are essential. Medication such as oxytocin may be required. (See *Oxytocin adverse effects* and *Preventing oxytocin complications*.) Cesarean delivery may be necessary if other measures are unsuccessful.

Hypertonic contractions

Any woman whose pain seems out of proportion to the quality of her contractions should have both a uterine and fetal external monitor applied for at least a 15-minute interval to ensure the resting phase of the contractions is adequate and to determine that the fetal pattern isn't showing late deceleration.

For good measures

Other management measures include:
• promoting rest

Oxytocin adverse effects

When administering oxytocin, be aware of its possible adverse effects and intervene to avoid complications. Adverse effects include:
• dizziness
• headache
• nausea and vomiting
• tachycardia
• hypotension
• fetal bradycardia or tachycardia
• hypertonic contractions
• decreased urine output.

Preventing oxytocin complications

Oxytocin infusion can cause excessive uterine stimulation—leading to hypertonicity, tetany, rupture, cervical or perineal lacerations, premature placental separation, fetal hypoxia, or rapid forceful delivery—and fluid overload—leading to seizures and coma. To help prevent these complications, follow these guidelines.

Excessive uterine stimulation
• Administer oxytocin with a volumetric pump and use piggyback infusion so that the drug may be discontinued, if necessary, without interrupting the main I.V. line.
• Every 15 minutes, monitor uterine contractions, intrauterine pressure, fetal heart rate, and the character of blood loss.
• If contractions occur less than 2 minutes apart, last 90 seconds or longer, or exceed 50 mm Hg, stop the infusion, turn the patient onto her side (preferably the left), and notify the

doctor. Contractions should occur every 2½ to 3 minutes, followed by a period of relaxation.
• Keep magnesium sulfate (20% solution) available to relax the myometrium.

Fluid overload
• To identify fluid overload, monitor the patient's intake and output, especially in prolonged infusion of doses above 20 milliunits/minute.
• The risk of fluid overload also increases when oxytocin is given in hypertonic saline solution after abortion.

- providing analgesia with a drug such as morphine
- possibly inducing sedation so the woman can rest
- possibly administering morphine to relax hypertonicity
- comfort measures, such as changing the linen and the patient's gown, darkening room lights, and decreasing noise and stimulation.

If it isn't working

If decelerating FHR, an abnormally long first stage of labor, or lack of progress with pushing (second stage arrest) occurs, cesarean delivery may be necessary. The woman and her support person need to understand that, although the contractions are strong, they are, in reality, ineffective and aren't achieving cervical dilation.

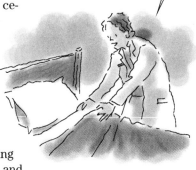

Comfort measures for hypertonic contractions include changing the patient's linens and gown, dimming lights, and decreasing noise and stimulation.

Hypotonic contractions

Management of hypotonic contractions includes these considerations:
- If hypotonicity is the only abnormal factor (including ruling out CPD or poor fetal presentation by sonogram), then rest and fluid intake should be encouraged.
- If the membranes haven't ruptured spontaneously, rupturing them at this point may be helpful.
- Oxytocin may be administered I.V. to augment labor by causing the uterus to contract more effectively.
- If hypertension occurs, discontinue oxytocin and notify the doctor.

Uncoordinated contractions

Management of uncoordinated contractions includes these considerations:
- Oxytocin administration may be helpful in uncoordinated labor to stimulate a more effective and consistent pattern of contractions with a better, lower resting tone.
- If hypertension occurs, discontinue oxytocin and notify the doctor.

If hypertension occurs, discontinue oxytocin and notify the doctor.

Multiple gestation

A woman with multiple gestations usually causes excitement in the labor room. Additional personnel are needed for the birth. Nurses are needed to attend to possibly immature neonates. Additional pediatricians or neonatal nurse practitioners are required.

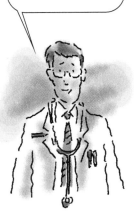

The woman may get lost in all this activity and may be more frightened than excited.

Multiple gestations may be delivered by cesarean birth to decrease the risk of anoxia to a subsequent fetus. This problem is more common in multiple gestations of three or more because of the increased incidence of cord entanglement and premature separation of a placenta.

Twin positions

Most twin pregnancies present with both twins in the vertex position. This is followed in frequency by vertex and breech, breech and vertex, and then breech and breech. (See *Twin presentations*.)

What causes it

Multiple gestation may occur spontaneously, especially with a history of twins or multiple births in the family. It may also occur with fertility medications, which cause multiple ova to be released simultaneously, thus increasing the chances of fertilization of more than one ovum.

How it's detected

Multiple gestation may be suspected when several FHRs are auscultated, the mother is larger than average for ges-

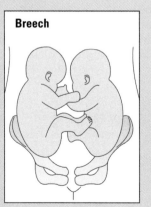

Fertility drugs increase the risk of multiple gestation.

Twin presentations

There are four types of twin presentations. These types are illustrated below.

Vertex	Vertex and breech	Breech	Vertex and transverse lie

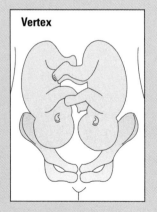

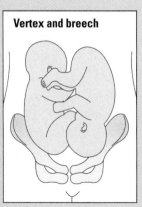

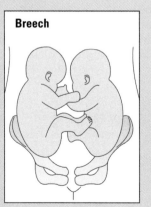

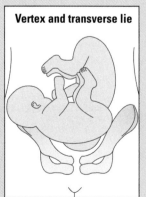

tational age of the fetus, or when palpation reveals multiple fetuses. Multiple gestation is confirmed by ultrasound.

Multiple gestations of three or more have extremely varied presentations after the birth of the first child. The lie of the second fetus is usually determined by external abdominal palpation and sonogram.

What to do

If the presentation isn't vertex, external version is attempted to make it so. If external version isn't successful, a decision for a breech delivery or cesarean delivery must be made. If a woman with multiple gestation is to deliver vaginally, she's usually instructed to come to the hospital early in labor. Here are some other considerations:

• The first stage of labor won't differ greatly from that of a single-gestation labor but coming to a hospital early may make labor seem long.

• Urge the woman to spend the early hours of labor engaged in an activity such as playing cards to make the time pass more quickly.

• Analgesia administration is given conservatively so it won't compound any respiratory difficulties the neonates may have at birth because of their immaturity.

• Oxytocin infusion may be initiated to assist uterine contractions and shorten the time span between the births. It's usually begun after the first fetus is delivered.

• Nitroglycerine may be administered to relax the uterus.

• Support breathing exercises to minimize the need for analgesia or anesthesia. Remember that multiple pregnancies commonly end before they're full-term, so the woman may not yet have practiced breathing exercises. The early hours of labor are an excellent opportunity to practice breathing.

• Try to monitor each FHR by a separate fetal monitor if possible.

Multiple complications

Complications, such as those listed here, are common in multiple gestation:

• Because the babies are usually small, firm head engagement may not occur, which increases the risk of cord prolapse after rupture of the membranes.

• Uterine dysfunction from a long labor may occur.

• An overstretched uterus may result and could cause ineffective labor.

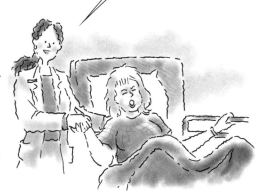

Help the patient practice breathing exercises to minimize the need for pharmacologic pain relief.

• Premature separation of the placenta after the birth of the first child is more common in multiple gestation. When separation occurs, there's sudden, profuse bleeding at the vagina, causing a risk of exsanguination for the woman.
• Because of the multiple fetuses, abnormal fetal presentation may occur.
• Anemia and pregnancy-induced hypertension occur at higher-than-usual incidences in multiple gestation. Hematocrit and blood pressure should be monitored closely during labor.
• After the birth, the uterus can't contract, placing the woman at risk for hemorrhage from uterine atony.
• Separation of the first placenta may cause loosening of the additional placentas. If a common placenta is involved, the fetal heart sounds of the other fetuses immediately register distress. Careful FHR monitoring is essential. If separation occurs, the fetuses must be delivered immediately to avoid fetal death.

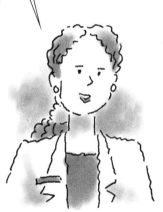

Multiple gestation puts the patient at greater risk for anemia and pregnancy-induced hypertension.

After the event

Keep in mind the following points after the birth of multiple neonates:
• The neonates need careful assessment to determine their true gestational age and if twin-to-twin transfusion has occurred.
• Some parents worry that the hospital will confuse their neonates through improper identification. Review with them the careful measures that are taken to ensure correct identification.
• Despite preparations for a multiple birth, the woman may have difficulty believing she has given birth to multiple neonates. She may find it helpful to discuss her feelings with you as well as view all her neonates together to become accustomed to the idea.
• The parents may be unable to inspect the neonates thoroughly immediately after the birth because of low birth weight and the danger of hypothermia. Bonding time should be promoted as soon as possible to dispel any fears they have that the babies are less than perfect.

Placental abnormalities

The normal placenta weighs in at approximately 500 g (1⅛ lb) and is 15 to 20 cm (5⅞″ to 7⅞″) in diameter and 1.5 to 3 cm (⅝″ to 1⅛″) thick. Its weight is approximately one-sixth that of the fetus. Problems can occur with the size of the placenta or the blood vessels connected to it. Other abnormalities can involve the placement of the umbilical cord or placental attachment. Types of abnormalities include:
• battledore placenta

- placenta accreta
- placenta circumvallata
- placenta succenturiata
- vasa previa
- velamentous cord insertion. (See *Abnormal placental formations*, page 402.)

What causes it

Abnormalities may be present for several reasons. For example, a placenta may be unusually enlarged in a woman with diabetes. In certain diseases, such as syphilis or erythroblastosis, the placenta may be so large that it weighs half as much as the fetus. The placenta may be wider in diameter if the uterus has scars or a septum, possibly because it was forced to spread out to find implantation space.

Well, that depends...

Other causes of placental abnormalities depend on the type of abnormality:

- *Battledore placenta* has no known cause.
- *Placenta accreta* is caused by a defect in decidua formation from implantation over uterine scars or in the lower segment of the uterus.
- *Placenta circumvallata* has no known cause, although formation of insufficient chorion frondosum, subchorial infarcts, and an abnormally implanted blastocyst causes part of the fetal surface to be covered by the decidua.
- *Placenta succenturiata* is caused when a group of villi distant to the placenta fail to degenerate and implantation is superficial or confined to a specific site so that attachment of the trophoblast also occurs on the opposing wall. This condition can occur in the case of a bicornuate uterus.
- *Vasa previa* is caused by rotation of the inner cell mass and body stalk, which aligns in an eccentric insertion.
- In *velamentous cord insertion*, the umbilical cord inserts into the membrane, causing the vessels to run between the amnion and chorion before entering the placenta. This condition most likely occurs during implantation.

> Battledore placenta has no known cause.

How it's detected

Placental abnormalities usually aren't detected until after the birth of the placenta. Both the umbilical cord and placenta are examined. However, if sudden painless bleeding occurs with the beginning of cervical dilation, vasa previa should be suspected. Sonogram confirms this diagnosis.

Abnormal placental formations

Abnormal placental formations occur for various reasons, some of which are unknown. The types of abnormal placental formations and their clinical significance are discussed below.

On the border

In *battledore placenta*, the umbilical cord is attached marginally, rather than centrally. It can lead to preterm labor, fetal distress, and bleeding from cord compression or vessel rupture.

Battledore placenta

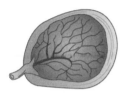

Deeply attached

In *placenta accreta*, an unusually deep attachment of the placenta to the uterine myometrium doesn't allow the placenta to loosen and deliver as it should. Attempts to remove it manually may lead to extreme hemorrhage. This abnormality is associated with placenta previa, which can lead to severe maternal hemorrhage, uterine perforation, and subsequent hysterectomy.

Missing a membrane

In *placenta circumvallata,* the chorion membrane that usually begins at the edge of the placenta and spreads to envelop the fetus is missing on the fetal side of the placenta. In this condition, the umbilical cord may enter the placenta at the usual midpoint with large vessels spreading out from there. However, the vessels end abruptly at the point where the chorion folds back onto the surface. This abnormality can lead to spontaneous abortion, abruptio placentae, preterm labor, placental insufficiency, and intrapartum and postpartum hemorrhage.

Placenta circumvallata

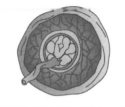

Accessories included

In *placenta succenturiata,* one or more accessory lobes are connected to the main placenta by blood vessels. Identify this abnormality through careful examination of the placenta after birth because the small lobes may be retained in the uterus, leading to severe maternal postpartum hemorrhage.

Placenta succenturiata

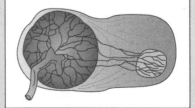

Cord cuts in front

In *vasa previa*, velamentous insertion of the cord is present and the unprotected and fragile umbilical vessels cross the internal os and lie in front of the presenting fetal head. This abnormal insertion may cause the cord to be delivered before the fetus, possibly causing the vessels to tear with cervical dilation, leading to hemorrhage.

Smaller separations

Velamentous cord insertion occurs when the cord separates into small vessels that reach the placenta by spreading across a fold of amnion. This form of cord insertion is found most commonly in multiple gestation and may be associated with fetal abnormalities. This condition can lead to vessel tearing and hemorrhage because the vessels are unprotected as they travel through the amnion and chorion before they form the cord.

Velamentous cord insertion

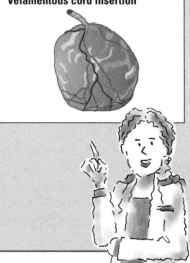

What to do

Some placental abnormalities require immediate attention, whereas others may not be significant. For example, if the patient has a placenta succenturiata, the remaining lobes must be removed from the uterus manually. This is done to prevent maternal hemorrhage from poor uterine contraction.

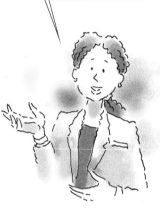

Because some routine care measures can cause problems, be sure to inspect for placental abnormalities first.

Look before you touch

Some abnormalities must be detected before routine care may be performed. For example, before inserting any instrument (such as an internal fetal monitor), fetal and placental structures must be identified to prevent problems. For example, accidental tearing of a vasa previa can result in sudden fetal blood loss. If vasa previa is identified, cesarean delivery of the neonate is necessary.

Abnormalities such as placenta accreta require more intense treatment. Placenta accreta requires a hysterectomy or treatment with methotrexate (Rheumatrex) to destroy the still attached tissue.

Preterm labor and delivery

When labor begins earlier in gestation than normal, it's considered preterm. As with normal labor, in preterm labor, rhythmic uterine contractions produce cervical change. This change may occur after fetal viability but before fetal maturity. It usually occurs between the 20th and 37th week of gestation. Premature labor is a major cause of perinatal morbidity and mortality. Neonatal complications may include respiratory distress syndrome and intracranial bleeding. Only 5% to 10% of pregnancies end prematurely; however, about 75% of these pregnancies result in neonatal death.

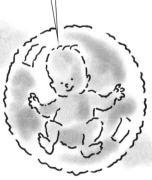

Sometimes I decide to greet the world before I'm mature.

Weight and length = outcome

The outcome of the fetus depends on birth weight and length of gestation:
• Neonates weighing less than 1 lb, 10 oz (737.1 g) and born at fewer than 26 weeks' gestation have a survival rate of about 10%.
• Neonates weighing 1 lb, 10 oz to 2 lb, 3 oz (992.2 g) and born at 27 to 28 weeks' gestation have a survival rate of more than 50%.
• Neonates weighing 2 lb, 3 oz to 2 lb, 11 oz (1,219 g) and born at more than 28 weeks' gestation have a 70% to 90% survival rate.

What causes it

Causes of preterm labor include:
- PROM (30% to 50% of cases)
- hydramnios
- fetal death.

When mom is at risk

Numerous maternal risk factors also increase the incidence of preterm labor, including:
- pregnancy-induced hypertension
- chronic hypertensive vascular disease
- placenta previa
- abruptio placentae
- incompetent cervix
- abdominal surgery
- trauma
- structural anomalies of the uterus
- infections (such as group B streptococci)
- genetic defect in the mother.

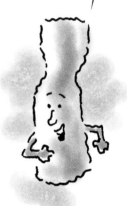

Sometimes it's just written in the genes. Genetically imprinted information may warn the fetus that its environment is unsuitable — leading to preterm labor.

Other contributors

Other factors that may cause preterm labor include:
- stimulation of the fetus via heredity — genetically imprinted information tells the fetus that nutrition is inadequate and that a change in environment is required for well-being, thus provoking the onset of labor
- sensitivity to the hormone oxytocin — labor begins because the myometrium becomes hypersensitive to oxytocin, the hormone that usually induces uterine contractions.

How it's detected

As with labor at term, preterm labor produces:
- rhythmic uterine contractions
- cervical dilation and effacement
- possible rupture of the membranes
- expulsion of the cervical mucus plug
- bloody discharge.

Combination confirmation

Preterm labor is confirmed by the combined results of:
- prenatal history indicating 20th to 37th week of gestation
- ultrasonography (if available) showing the position of the fetus in relation to the mother's pelvis

• vaginal examination confirming progressive cervical effacement and dilation
• electronic fetal monitoring showing rhythmic uterine contractions
• possible ambulatory home monitoring with a tocodynamometer to identify preterm contractions
• differential diagnosis excluding Braxton Hicks contractions and urinary tract infection.

What to do

Treatment of premature labor aims to suppress labor when tests show:
• immature fetal pulmonary development
• cervical dilation of less than 4 cm
• absence of factors that contraindicate continuation of pregnancy.

Let's be conservative

Here are some conservative measures to suppress labor:
• A patient in preterm labor requires bed rest, close observation for signs of fetal or maternal distress, and comprehensive supportive care.
• During attempts to suppress preterm labor, make sure the patient maintains bed rest and administer medications as ordered.
• Because sedatives and analgesics may be harmful to the fetus, administer them sparingly. Minimize the need for these drugs by providing comfort measures, such as frequent repositioning and good perineal and back care.
• Avoid preterm labor by successfully identifying patients at risk. Such patients should comply with the prescribed home treatment.
• Ensure that the woman is taking proper preventive measures, such as good prenatal care, adequate nutrition, and proper rest.
• Insertion of a purse-string suture (cerclage) can reinforce an incompetent cervix at 14 to 18 weeks' gestation to avoid preterm delivery in a patient with a history of this disorder.
• Women at risk can be treated at home and have their contractions monitored via telephone hookup.

Drug details

Pharmacologic measures to suppress labor include:
• *terbutaline (Brethine)* — to stimulate the beta$_2$-adrenergic receptors and inhibit contractility of uterine smooth muscle. When administering this drug, monitor blood pressure, pulse rate, respirations, FHR, and uterine contraction pattern.

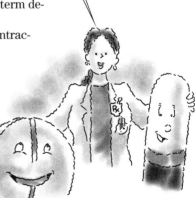

Pharmacologic measures to suppress labor include terbutaline and magnesium sulfate.

• *magnesium sulfate*—to relax the myometrium and stop contractions.

Monitoring measures

Careful monitoring is essential throughout therapy. The usual monitoring of uterine contractions and fetal heart tones should be conducted. Additional measures include:

• If a uterine relaxant is to be given I.V., perform a baseline electrocardiogram (ECG).

• During therapy, monitor laboratory test results to detect hypokalemia, hypoglycemia, or decreased hematocrit. Report abnormal findings to the doctor.

• Monitor the patient's cardiac status continuously and report arrhythmias.

• Check the patient's blood pressure and pulse every 10 to 15 minutes initially, then every 30 minutes or as ordered.

• Notify the doctor if her pulse rate exceeds 140 beats/minute or if her blood pressure falls 15 mm Hg or more.

• If the patient complains of palpitations or chest pain or tightness, decrease the drug dosage and notify the doctor immediately.

• Keep emergency resuscitation equipment nearby.

• Assess pulmonary status every hour during I.V. therapy, and report crackles or increased respirations.

• Monitor intake and output and notify the doctor if urine output drops below 50 ml/hour as pulmonary edema may result.

• If signs of pulmonary edema develop, place the patient in high-Fowler's position, administer oxygen as ordered, and notify the doctor.

• For 1 to 2 hours after I.V. therapy, monitor the patient's vital signs, intake and output, and fetal heart sounds.

• Perform serial ECGs as ordered.

• Immediately report tachycardia, hypotension, decreased urine output, or diminished or absent fetal heart sounds.

• Watch for maternal adverse reactions to magnesium sulfate administration, including drowsiness, slurred speech, flushing, decreased reflexes, decreased GI motility, and decreased respirations.

• Watch for fetal and neonatal adverse effects of magnesium sulfate use, including central nervous system depression, decreased respirations, and decreased sucking reflex.

• Carry out thorough patient teaching to ensure patient understanding and compliance with treatment. (See *Teaching the patient about preterm labor.*)

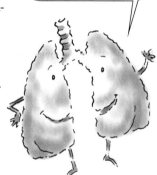

Be sure to assess pulmonary status every hour during I.V. therapy, and report crackles or increased respirations.

Education edge

Teaching the patient about preterm labor

Here are some guidelines for teaching a patient about preterm labor:
• Reassure the patient that drug effects on her neonate should be minimal.
• Tell the patient to notify the doctor immediately if she experiences sweating, chest pain, or increased pulse rate.
• Teach her to check her pulse before oral drug administration. If her pulse exceeds 130 beats/minute, she shouldn't take the drug and should notify the doctor.
• Emphasize the importance of immediately reporting contractions, lower back pain, cramping, or increased vaginal discharge.
• Instruct her to report other adverse reactions requiring a reduction in drug dosage, such as headache, nervousness, tremors, restlessness,
nausea, and vomiting.
• Tell her to notify the doctor if her urine output decreases or if she gains more than 5 lb (2.3 kg) in 1 week.
• Tell her to take her temperature every day and to report fever to the doctor because it may be a sign of infection.
• Advise her to take oral doses of the drug with food (to avoid GI upset) and take the last dose several hours before bedtime (to avoid insomnia).
• Encourage her to remain in bed as much as possible.
• Tell her to avoid preparing her breasts for breast-feeding until about 2 weeks before her due date because this can stimulate the release of oxytocin and initiate contractions.

Preterm delivery

It may be in the best interest of the fetus or the mother and fetus to allow preterm labor to progress and delivery to ensue. Maternal factors that jeopardize the mother and fetus, making preterm delivery the lesser risk, include:
• intrauterine infection
• abruptio placentae
• severe preeclampsia.

Factors that jeopardize the fetus can become more significant as pregnancy nears term, and so preterm delivery may be more favorable. These factors include:
• placental insufficiency
• isoimmunization
• congenital anomalies.

Ideal situation

Ideally, treatment of active preterm labor should take place in a perinatal intensive care center, where the staff is specially trained to handle this situation. The neonate can also remain

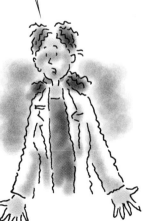

Such factors as intrauterine infection, abruptio placentae, and severe preeclampsia can place the fetus and mother at risk, making preterm delivery the better option.

close to his parents, promoting bonding. Community hospitals commonly lack the facilities for special neonatal care and transfer the neonate alone to a perinatal center.

Part of a team

Treatment and delivery require an intensive team effort focusing on:
• continuous assessment of the fetus's health through fetal monitoring
• unless contraindicated, administration of antenatal steroids to assist fetal lung development
• maintenance of adequate hydration through I.V. fluids.

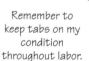

Treatment and delivery of a preterm neonate require a team effort.

Constant concerns

Also keep in mind:
• Morphine (Duramorph) and meperidine (Demerol) may cause fetal respiratory depression. They should be administered only when necessary and in the smallest possible dose.
• Amniotomy should be avoided, if possible, to prevent cord prolapse or damage to the fetus's tender skull.
• The preterm neonate has a lower tolerance for the stress of labor and is much more likely to become hypoxic than the term neonate.
• If necessary, administer oxygen to the patient through a nasal cannula.
• Observe fetal response to labor through continuous monitoring.
• Continually reassure the patient throughout labor to help reduce her anxiety.
• Monitor fetal and maternal response to local and regional anesthetics.
• Pushing between contractions is ineffective and can damage the premature neonate's soft skull.
• Throughout labor, keep the patient informed of her progress and the condition of the fetus.
• Inform the parents of their neonate's condition. Describe his appearance and explain the purpose of supportive equipment.
• As necessary, before the parents leave the facility with the neonate, refer them to a community health nurse who can help them adjust to caring for a preterm neonate.

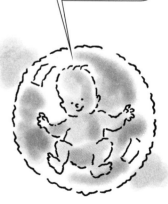

Remember to keep tabs on my condition throughout labor.

Umbilical cord anomalies

Umbilical cord anomalies include absence of an umbilical artery and an unusually long or short umbilical cord.

Absent artery

A normal umbilical cord contains one vein and two arteries. The presence of a single umbilical artery is caused by atrophy of a previously normal artery, presence of the original artery of the body stalk, or agenesis of one of the umbilical arteries. The absence of one of the umbilical arteries has been associated with congenital heart and kidney defects because the insult that caused the loss of the vessel probably led to an insult to other mesoderm germ layer structures as well.

The long...

An unusually long cord can be compromised more easily because of its greater tendency to twist or knot. When this happens, the natural pulsations of the blood through the vessels and the muscular vessel walls usually keep the blood flow adequate. A long cord that wraps around the fetus's neck is called a *nuchal cord*. If the cord is wrapped tightly enough to restrict blood flow to the fetus, it may cause stillbirth.

...and short of it

An unusually short umbilical cord can result in premature separation of the placenta or an abnormal fetal lie. It can also result in fetal asphyxia because of traction on the umbilical cord as the fetus descends.

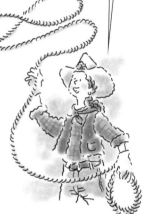

A cord that's either too long or too short can be a problem.

What causes it

The cause of differences in cord length is unknown. Some researchers suggest that reduced fetal activity, such as in the case of twinning (monoamniotic and conjoined), may be a cause as well as a genetic failure of the cord to elongate. However, the cause of unusual inversions of the cord into the placenta may be a result of rotation of the body stalk (which becomes the cord) as it implants into the placenta. The degree of rotation determines how far the umbilical cord will be from the center of the placenta.

How it's detected

Cord length abnormalities and abnormal cord insertion can be detected using ultrasound. However, detection of other umbilical cord abnormalities is only possible upon inspection of a cord at birth. Inspection should take place immediately, before the cord begins to dry because drying distorts the appearance.

What to do

Document the number of vessels present. The neonate with only two vessels needs to be observed carefully for other defects during the neonatal period.

Umbilical cord prolapse

In umbilical cord prolapse, a loop of the umbilical cord slips down in front of the presenting fetal part. This prolapse may occur at any time after the membranes rupture, especially if the presenting part isn't fitted firmly into the cervix. It happens in 1 out of 200 pregnancies. (See *Prolapse patterns.*)

What causes it

Prolapse tends to occur more commonly with the following conditions:
- PROM
- fetal presentation other than cephalic
- placenta previa
- intrauterine tumors that prevent the presenting part from engaging
- small fetus
- CPD that prevents firm engagement
- hydramnios
- multiple gestation.

Perhaps prolapse has occurred if the membranes have ruptured but the presenting part doesn't firmly engage.

How it's detected

Signs of prolapse include a sudden variable deceleration FHR pattern with the cord then visible at the vulva. To rule out cord prolapse, auscultate heart sounds immediately after rupture of the membranes (occurring spontaneously or by amniotomy).

Prolapse patterns

Prolapse of the umbilical cord may occur in two ways: outwardly prolapsed or hidden. Regardless of the type of prolapse, it means that the fetal nutrient supply is compromised. Both types of prolapse can be detected by fetal monitoring.

Hidden prolapse
The cord still remains within the uterus but is prolapsed.

Outward prolapse
The cord can be seen at the vulva.

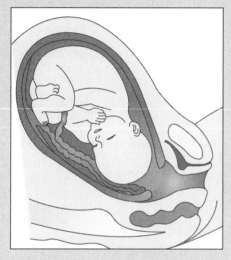

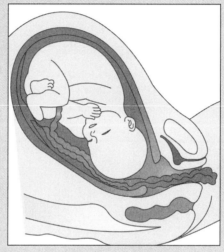

Perhaps it's prolapse

Signs of hypoxia and fetal distress suggest prolapse. In rare instances, the cord may be felt as the presenting part on vaginal examination. It can also be identified in this position on sonogram.

What to do

Cord prolapse leads to immediate cord compression because the fetal presenting part presses against the cord at the pelvic brim. Management is aimed toward relieving pressure on the cord, thereby relieving the compression and avoiding fetal anoxia.

Here are some points that you should consider if this occurs:
• If vaginal examination reveals the cord as the presenting part, cesarean delivery is necessary before rupture of the membranes occurs. Otherwise, with rupture, the cord prolapses down into the vagina.

- A gloved hand may be placed in the vagina. This is done to manually elevate the fetal head off the cord.
- The woman may be placed in a knee-chest or Trendelenburg's position, which causes the fetal head to fall back from the cord.
- Administering oxygen at 10 L/minute by face mask to the mother is also helpful.
- A tocolytic agent may be used to reduce uterine activity and pressure on the fetus.
- If the cord has prolapsed so far that it's exposed to room air, drying begins, leading to atrophy of the umbilical vessels. If this happens, don't attempt to push any exposed cord back into the vagina. This may add to the compression and further cause knotting or kinking. Cover any exposed portion with a sterile saline compress to prevent drying.
- If the cervix is fully dilated at the time of the prolapse, the doctor may choose to deliver the neonate quickly, possibly with forceps, to prevent a period of anoxia.
- If dilation is incomplete, the birth method of choice is upward pressure on the presenting part by a practitioner's hand in the woman's vagina to keep pressure off the cord until a cesarean delivery can be performed.

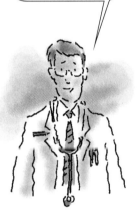

If the cervix is fully dilated at the time of prolapse, I may choose to deliver the neonate quickly to prevent a period of anoxia.

Uterine rupture

Rupture of the uterus during labor is a rare occurrence. It happens in about 1 in 1,500 births. A uterus ruptures when it undergoes more strain than it can sustain. If the situation isn't relieved, uterine rupture and death of the fetus may occur. In the placental stage, massive maternal hemorrhage may result because the placenta is loosened but then can't deliver, preventing the uterus from contracting. Uterine rupture accounts for as many as 5% of all maternal deaths. When it occurs, fetal death results 50% of the time.

The viability of the fetus depends on the extent of the rupture and the time that elapses between the rupture and abdominal extraction. The woman's prognosis depends on the extent of the rupture and blood loss. It's inadvisable for a woman to conceive again after a rupture of the uterus unless it occurred in the inactive lower segment.

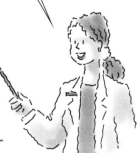

Fetal death results in about 50% of all cases of uterine rupture.

What causes it

The most common cause of uterine rupture is previous cesarean birth, such as when a vertical scar from a previous incision is present. It can also be from hysterotomy repair. Contributing factors include:

- prolonged labor
- faulty presentation
- multiple gestation
- use of oxytocin
- obstructed labor
- traumatic maneuvers using forceps or traction.

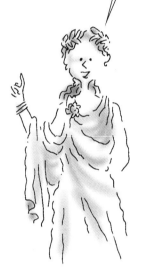

Previous cesarean birth is the most common cause of uterine rupture.

How it's detected

Strong uterine contractions that occur without any cervical dilation are a sign of impending rupture. A more specific sign, called a *pathologic retraction ring*, is an indentation that appears across the abdomen over the uterus just before rupture.

The things about rings

Two types of retraction rings can occur in abnormal labor:

Bandl's ring—This sign is evident at the junction of the upper and lower uterine segments. It usually appears during the second stage of labor as a horizontal indentation across the abdomen. It's formed by excessive retraction of the upper uterine segment. The uterine myometrium is much thicker above the ring than below it.

constricting ring—This sign can occur at any point in the myometrium and at any time during labor. When it occurs in early labor, it's usually the result of uncoordinated contractions. Causes may include obstetric manipulation or administration of oxytocin. In a constricting ring, the fetus is gripped by the constricting ring and can't advance beyond that point. The undelivered placenta is also held at that point.

Retraction rings are confirmed by sonogram. Such a finding is extremely serious and should be reported promptly.
- Administration of I.V. morphine or the inhalation of amyl nitrite may relieve the retraction ring.
- A tocolytic may be administered to halt contractions.

Complete rupture

If the rupture is complete, here are some changes you can expect:
- The woman experiences a sudden, severe pain during a strong labor contraction and then contractions stop.
- The patient may report a tearing sensation and hemorrhaging may occur from the torn uterus into the abdominal cavity and pos-

sibly into the vagina. Rupture goes through endometrium, myometrium, and peritoneum.
- Signs of shock begin immediately, including rapid, weak pulse; falling blood pressure; cold and clammy skin; and respiratory distress.
- The woman's abdomen changes in contour. Two distinct swellings are visible: the retracted uterus and the extrauterine fetus.
- Fetal heart sounds become absent.

Incomplete rupture

If the rupture is incomplete, the signs are less dramatic:
- The woman may experience only a localized tenderness.
- She may complain of a persistent aching pain over the area of the lower segment.
- Fetal heart sounds, lack of contractions, and the woman's vital signs gradually reveal fetal and maternal distress. (See *Signs of uterine rupture*.)

What to do

The uterus at the end of pregnancy is a highly vascular organ. This makes uterine rupture an immediate emergency situation. It's comparable to a splenic or hepatic rupture. Most likely, a cesarean delivery is performed to ensure safe birth of the fetus. Manual removal of the placenta under general anesthesia may be necessary in the event of placental-stage pathologic retraction rings. The following measures are also indicated:
- Administer emergency fluid replacement therapy as ordered.
- Anticipate use of I.V. oxytocin to attempt to contract the uterus and minimize bleeding.
- Prepare the woman for a possible laparotomy as an emergency measure to control bleeding and effect a repair.
- The doctor, with consent, may perform a hysterectomy (removal of the damaged uterus) or tubal ligation at the time of the laparotomy. Explain to the patient that these procedures result in loss of childbearing ability.
- The woman may have difficulty giving her consent at this time because it isn't known whether the fetus will live.
- If blood loss is acute, the woman may be unconscious from hypotension. If this is the case, her support person must give consent, relying on the information provided by the operating surgeon to decide whether a functioning uterus can be saved.
- Be prepared to offer information and support and to inform the support person about the fetal outcome, the extent of the surgery, and the woman's safety as soon as possible.

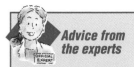

Advice from the experts

Signs of uterine rupture

Signs and symptoms of uterine rupture require prompt recognition and intervention. Intervene immediately to save the life of the mother and fetus. Signs and symptoms include:
- severe abdominal pain
- halt in contractions
- absent fetal heart rate
- possible vaginal bleeding
- falling blood pressure
- rapid weak pulse.

Give time for grief

- Expect the parents to go through a grieving process for not only the loss of this child (as applicable) but also the loss of having future children through pregnancies.
- Allow them time to express these justifiable emotions without feeling threatened.

Uterine inversion

Uterine inversion is a rare phenomenon in which the uterus turns inside out. It occurs in about 1 in 15,000 births. It may occur after the birth of the neonate, especially if traction is applied to the uterine fundus when the uterus isn't contracted. It may also occur when there's insertion of the placenta at the fundus, so that during birth, the passage of the fetus pulls the fundus down.

A matter of degrees

Uterine inversion can range from first-degree (incomplete) inversion, in which the corpus extends to the cervix but not beyond the cervical ring, to third-degree (complete) inversion. In complete inversion, the inverted uterus extends into the perineum. An additional condition, called *total uterine inversion*, involves total inversion of the uterus and the vagina.

What causes it

Causes of uterine inversion occur during the third stage of labor and include:
- excessive cord traction
- excessive fundal pressure.

How it's detected

Signs of inversion include:
- a large, sudden gush of blood from the vagina
- inability to palpate the fundus in the abdomen
- signs of blood loss (hypotension, dizziness, paleness, diaphoresis)
- signs of shock (such as increased heart rate and decreased blood pressure) if the loss of blood continues unchecked for more than a few minutes

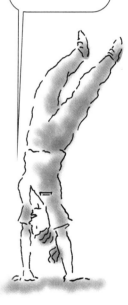

Uterine inversion is a rare phenomenon in which the uterus turns inside out.

• inability of the uterus to contract, resulting in continued bleeding (a woman could exsanguinate within a period as short as 10 minutes).

What to do

When exsanguination is imminent, follow these measures:
• Never attempt to replace the inversion because without good pelvic relaxation this may only increase bleeding.
• Never attempt to remove the placenta if it's still attached because this only creates a larger bleeding area.
• Administering an oxytocic drug only compounds the inversion.
• Start an I.V. fluid line if one isn't present. Use a large-gauge needle because blood must be replaced. Open an existing fluid line to achieve optimal fluid flow for fluid volume replacement.
• Administer oxygen by mask, and assess vital signs.
• Be prepared to perform CPR if the woman's heart fails from the sudden blood loss.
• The woman should immediately receive general anesthesia or, possibly, nitroglycerine or a tocolytic drug I.V. to relax the uterus.
• The delivering doctor or nurse-midwife replaces the fundus manually.
• Oxytocin is administered after manual replacement helps the uterus to contract into place.
• Because the uterine endometrium was exposed, the woman requires antibiotic therapy postpartum to prevent infection.

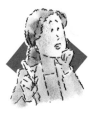

Quick quiz

1. Maternal factors indicating the need for cesarean delivery include:
    A.   transverse fetal lie.
    B.   previous cesarean delivery with bikini incision.
    C.   active genital herpes.
    D.   hypotension.

Answer: C. Maternal factors for cesarean delivery include CPD, active genital herpes or papilloma, previous cesarean delivery by classic incision, and disabling conditions, such as severe hypertension of pregnancy or heart disease, that prevent pushing to accomplish the pelvic division of labor.

2.   Contraindications for cesarean delivery include:
   A.   papilloma.
   B.   fetal distress.
   C.   transverse fetal lie.
   D.   dead fetus.

Answer: D. Cesarean delivery is generally contraindicated when there's a documented dead fetus. In this situation, labor can be induced to avoid a surgical procedure.

3.   The presence of meconium in the amniotic fluid before birth may indicate:
   A.   breech presentation.
   B.   transverse lie.
   C.   abruptio placentae.
   D.   placenta previa.

Answer: A. In breech presentation, the inevitable contraction of the fetal buttocks from cervical pressure typically causes meconium to be extruded into the amniotic fluid before birth. This, unlike meconium staining that occurs from fetal anoxia, isn't a sign of fetal distress but is expected from the buttock pressure.

4.   The child born in breech presentation is at risk for:
   A.   hypotension.
   B.   hypoxia.
   C.   intracranial hemorrhage.
   D.   infection.

Answer: C. A danger of breech birth is intracranial hemorrhage. With a cephalic presentation, molding to the confines of the birth canal occurs over hours. With a breech birth, pressure changes occur instantaneously. The neonate who's delivered suddenly to reduce the amount of time of cord compression may, therefore, suffer an intracranial hemorrhage.

5.   Administration of oxytocin should be discontinued when:
   A.   contractions are less than 2 minutes apart.
   B.   contractions are stronger than 50 mm Hg.
   C.   contractions are less than 50 seconds long.
   D.   contractions are irregular.

Answer: B. General guidelines for oxytocin use include that contractions should occur no more than every 2 minutes, shouldn't be stronger than 50 mm Hg, and shouldn't last longer than 70 seconds.

6. With the administration of magnesium sulfate, the woman should be observed for:
- A. hyperactivity.
- B. flushing.
- C. increased reflexes.
- D. increased respirations.

Answer: B. Magnesium sulfate relaxes the myometrium. It also produces maternal adverse effects, such as drowsiness, slurred speech, flushing, decreased reflexes, decreased GI motility, and decreased respirations.

Scoring

☆☆☆ If you answered all six items correctly, bravo! You've got a handle on a complicated subject.

☆☆ If you answered five items correctly, excellent! You're on your way to an uncomplicated understanding of labor complications.

☆ If you answered fewer than five items correctly, no sweat. Reviewing the chapter again should induce a perfect understanding!

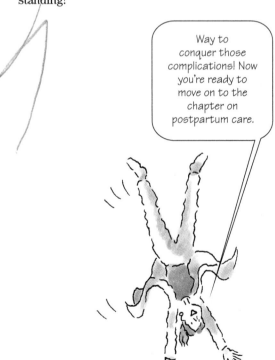

Way to conquer those complications! Now you're ready to move on to the chapter on postpartum care.

9

Postpartum care

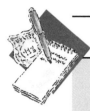

Just the facts

In this chapter, you'll learn:

♦ physiologic and psychological changes that occur during the postpartum period

♦ key components of a postpartum assessment

♦ nursing care measures required during the postpartum period

♦ physiologic events that occur during lactation

♦ two feeding methods, including their advantages and disadvantages.

A look at postpartum care

The postpartum period, or *puerperium,* refers to the 6- to 8-week period after delivery during which the mother's body returns to its prepregnant state. Some people refer to this period as the *fourth trimester of pregnancy.* Many physiologic and psychological changes occur in the mother during this time. Nursing care should focus on helping the mother and her family adjust to these changes and on easing the transition to the parenting role.

Physiologic changes

Two types of physiologic changes occur during the postpartum period: retrogressive changes and progressive changes.

Getting back to normal

Retrogressive changes involve returning the body to its prepregnancy state. Retrogressive reproductive system changes include:

- shrinkage and descent of the uterus into its prepregnancy position in the pelvis
- sloughing of the uterine lining and development of lochia
- contraction of the cervix and vagina
- recovery of vaginal and pelvic floor muscle tone.

Theory of involution

After delivery, the uterus gradually decreases in size and descends into its prepregnancy position in the pelvis — a process known as *involution*. Involution normally begins immediately after delivery, when the firmly contracted uterus lies midway between the umbilicus and symphysis pubis. Soon after, the uterus rises to the umbilicus or slightly above it. After the first postpartum day, the uterus begins its descent into the pelvis at the rate of 1 cm/day (or 1 fingerbreadth/day), or slightly less for the patient who has had a cesarean delivery. By the 10th postpartum day, the uterus lies deep in the pelvis — either at or below the symphysis pubis — and it can't be palpated.

Contraction is key

If the uterus fails to contract or remain firm during involution, uterine bleeding or hemorrhage can result. At delivery, placental separation exposes large uterine blood vessels. Uterine contraction acts as a tourniquet to close these blood vessels at the placental site. Fundal massage, the administration of synthetic oxytocics, and the release of natural oxytocics during breast-feeding help to maintain or stimulate contraction.

All systems under-go

Other body systems undergo retrogressive changes as well. These alterations include:
- reduction in pregnancy hormones, such as human chorionic gonadotropin, human placental lactogen, progestin, estrone, and estradiol
- extensive diuresis, which rids the body of excess fluid and reduces the added blood volume of pregnancy
- gradual rise in hematocrit, which occurs as excess fluid is excreted
- reactivation of digestion and absorption
- eventual fading of striae gravidarum (stretch marks), chloasma (pigmentation on face and neck), and linea nigra (pigmentation on abdomen)
- gradual return of tone to the abdominal muscles, wall, and ligaments
- return of vital signs to normal parameters
- weight loss due to rapid diuresis and lochial flow

Don't worry about me. In the postpartum period, I slowly but surely regain my muscle tone.

• recession of varicosities (although they may never return completely to prepregnancy appearance).

In addition, estrogen and progesterone production drops abruptly after delivery and follicle-stimulating hormone (FSH) production rises, resulting in the gradual return of ovulation and the menstrual cycle.

Making progress

Progressive changes involve the building of new tissues, primarily those that occur with lactation and the return of menstrual flow. In the postpartum period, fluid accumulates in the breast tissue in preparation for breast-feeding and breast tissue increases in size as breast milk forms. The changes associated with lactation are discussed in more detail later in this chapter.

Psychological changes

The postpartum period is a time of transition for the new mother and her family. Even if the couple has other children, each family member must adjust to having a neonate in the family. The mother, in particular, undergoes many psychological changes during this time in addition to the changes that are occurring in her body.

Don't let the phases faze you

The mother goes through three distinct phases of adjustment in the postpartum period:

 taking in

 taking hold

 letting go.

In the past, each phase of the postpartum period encompassed a specific time span, with women progressing through the phases sequentially. However, with today's shorter hospitalizations for childbirth, women move through the phases more quickly and sometimes even experience more than one phase at a time. (See *Phases of the postpartum period*, page 422.)

Building relationships

The mother and her family undergo other changes as well. Ideally, these changes lead to the development of parental love for the neonate and positive relationships among all family members.

Not all change is good

In some cases, negative psychological reactions may also occur. For example, a mother may feel let down because the neonate is

Phases of the postpartum period

The chart below summarizes the three phases of the postpartum period.

Phase	Maternal behavior and tasks
Taking in (1 to 2 days after delivery)	• Contemplation of her recent birth experience • Assumption of passive role and dependence on others for care • Verbalization about labor and birth • Sense of wonderment when looking at the neonate
Taking hold (2 to 7 days after delivery)	• Increased independence in self-care • Strong interest in caring for the neonate that's often accompanied by a lack of confidence about her ability to provide care
Letting go (about 7 days after delivery)	• Adaption to parenthood and definition of new role as parent and caregiver • Abandonment of fantasized image of neonate and acceptance of real image • Recognition of neonate as a separate entity • Assumption of responsibility and care for the neonate

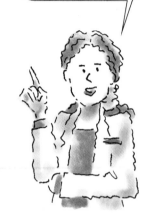

Taking in, taking hold, and letting go. Some women move through the phases more quickly than others.

now the center of attention or she may feel disappointed because the neonate doesn't meet her preconceived expectations.

A mother may also feel overwhelming sadness for no discernible reason; these feelings are commonly termed *postpartum blues* or *baby blues*. A mother with postpartum blues may experience emotional lability, a let-down feeling, crying for no apparent reason, headache, insomnia, fatigue, restlessness, depression, and anger. These feelings most commonly peak around the 5th postpartum day and subside by the 10th postpartum day. (See *Battling the baby blues.*)

First contact

Early contact and interaction between the parents, the neonate, and other siblings — including rooming in and sibling visitation — encourages bonding and helps integrate the neonate into the family.

Education edge

Battling the baby blues

For most women, having a baby is a joyous experience. However, childbirth leaves some women feeling sad, depressed, angry, anxious, and afraid. Commonly called postpartum blues or baby blues, these feelings affect about 70% to 80% of women after childbirth. In most cases, they occur within the first few days postpartum and then disappear on their own within a few days.

More than the blues
Unfortunately, about 10% of women experience a more profound problem called *postpartum depression.* In these cases, maternal feelings of depression and despair last longer than a few weeks and are so intense that they interfere with the woman's daily activities. Postpartum depression can occur after any pregnancy; it isn't specifically associated with first pregnancies. It commonly requires counseling to resolve.

Possible causes of postpartum depression include:
• doubt about the pregnancy
• recent stress, such as loss of a loved one, a family illness, or a recent move
• lack of a support system
• unplanned cesarean birth (may leave the woman feeling like a failure)
• breast-feeding problems, especially if a new mother can't breast-feed or decides to stop
• sharp drop in estrogen and progesterone levels after childbirth, possibly triggering depression in the same way that much smaller changes in hormone levels can trigger mood swings and tension before menstrual periods
• early birth of neonate (may cause woman to feel unprepared)
• unresolved issues of not being able to be the "perfect" mother
• feeling of failure if the mother believes that she should instinctively know how to care for her neonate
• disappointment over sex of neonate or other characteristics (neonate isn't as mother imagined).

Help is on the way
To help your patient with postpartum blues, tell her to:
• get plenty of rest
• ask for help from her family and friends
• take special care of herself
• spend time with her partner
• call her doctor if her mood doesn't improve after a few weeks and she has trouble coping (this may be a sign of a more severe depression).

Be sure to explain to the patient that many new mothers feel sadness, fear, anger, and anxiety after having a baby. These feelings don't mean that she's a failure as a woman or as a mother. They indicate that she's adjusting to the changes that follow birth. Reassure her that this experience is common and doesn't indicate that she's mentally ill.

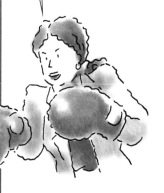

You can help your patient battle the baby blues by providing care and reassurance.

Postpartum assessment

As with any assessment, a postpartum assessment consists of a patient history and a physical examination.

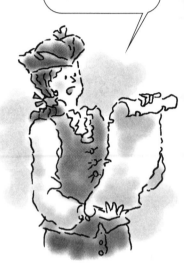

Hear ye! Hear ye! Your postpartum patient history should focus on the patient's pregnancy, labor, and birth events.

Patient history

Your postpartum patient history should focus on the patient's pregnancy, labor, and birth events. You should be able to find much of this information on the medical record. For example, the medical record should contain information about:
• problems experienced, such as pregnancy-induced hypertension or gestational diabetes
• time of labor onset and admission to the labor and delivery area
• types of analgesia and anesthesia used
• length of labor
• time of delivery
• time of placenta expulsion and appearance of the placenta
• sex, weight, and status of the neonate.
    You'll need this information to plan the mother's care and promote maternal-neonate bonding

Another reliable source

Don't rely on the medical record as your sole source of information. Always ask the mother to describe the events and fill in the details in her own words. This is also a good way to find out her emotions and feelings about pregnancy and childbirth.

    Also ask the mother about her family and lifestyle, including support systems, other children, other people living in the home, her occupation, her community environment, and her socioeconomic level. This information can help you determine whether additional support, follow-up, or education about self-care and neonatal care are needed.

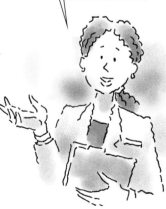

Medical records don't tell the whole story. Ask the mom to fill in the blanks.

Physical examination

In most cases, you don't need to do a complete physical examination in the postpartum period because the mother already had an assessment early in the labor process. However, you should complete a review of systems, covering the following areas:
• general appearance
• skin

- eyes, including color of conjunctivae (an indicator of possible anemia or excessive blood loss at birth)
- energy level, including level of activity and fatigue
- pain, including location, severity, and aggravating factors, such as sitting and walking
- GI elimination, including bowel sounds, passage of flatus, and hemorrhoids
- fluid intake
- urinary elimination, including the time and amount of first voiding
- peripheral circulation.
    In addition, you'll need to assess these four critical areas:
- breasts
- uterus
- lochia
- perineum.

Breasts

Inspect and then palpate the breasts, noting size, shape, and color. At first, the breasts should feel soft and secrete a thin, yellow fluid called *colostrum*. However, as they fill with milk — usually around the third postpartum day — they should begin to feel firm and warm, eventually becoming large and reddened with taut, shiny skin. Between feedings, the entire breast may be tender, hard, and tense on palpation. A low-grade temperature (under 101° F [38.3° C]) isn't uncommon between days 2 to 5, but it shouldn't last for more than 24 hours. (See *Engorgement or something else?* page 426.)

Land of nodule

A small, firm nodule in the breast may be caused by a temporarily blocked milk duct or milk that hasn't flowed forward into the nipple. This problem generally corrects itself when the neonate breast-feeds. Be sure to reassess the breast after the neonate feeds to determine if the problem has resolved, and report your findings — including the location of the nodule — to the doctor.

Also, inspect the nipples for cracks, fissures, or caked breast milk. Don't squeeze the nipples or manipulate them too much. Squeezing can be painful, and manipulation can cause cracks or breaks in the skin, providing an entry for organisms and leading to infection.

Uterus

During your examination, palpate the uterine fundus to determine uterine size, degree of firmness, and rate of descent, which is measured in fingerbreadths above or below the umbilicus. Un-

Memory jogger

To help you remember what to evaluate during a postpartum assessment, think of the words **BUBBLE HE.**

Breasts

Uterus

Bowel

Bladder

Lochia

Episiotomy

Homan's sign

Emotions

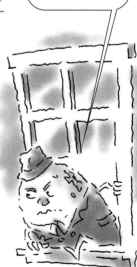

I'm just looking for a way in! That's my opportunity to cause infection.

Education edge

Engorgement or something else?

Engorgement, which may result from venous and lymphatic stasis and alveolar milk accumulation, causes the entire breast to appear reddened and to feel warm, firm, and tender. Encourage the woman to perform frequent and regular breast-feedings to help prevent this problem.

Something else

If the warmth, tenderness, and redness are localized to only one portion of the breast and the patient has a fever, suspect *mastitis*—inflammation of the glands or milk ducts.

Mastitis occurs postpartum in about 1% of mothers. It usually results from a pathogen that passes from the infant's nose or pharynx into breast tissue through a cracked nipple. Teach the mother about mastitis, and warn her to call the doctor immediately if she has any signs or symptoms.

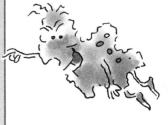

Mastitis man strikes again!

less the doctor orders otherwise, perform fundal assessments every 15 minutes for the first hour after delivery, every 30 minutes for the next 2 to 3 hours, every hour for the next 4 hours, every 4 hours for the rest of the first postpartum day, and then every 8 hours until the patient is discharged.

Pain at the incision site makes fundal assessment especially uncomfortable for the patient who has had a cesarean birth. In such cases, provide pain medication beforehand as ordered. Be aware that the doctor may order fundal assessment less frequently than usual, especially if oxytocin is being administered I.V.

Ready, set, palpate!

Before palpating the uterus, explain the procedure to the patient and provide privacy. Wash your hands and then put on gloves. Also, ask the patient to void. A full bladder makes the uterus boggier and deviates the fundus to the right of the umbilicus or +1 or +2 above the umbilicus. When the bladder is empty, the uterus should be at or close to the level of the umbilicus.

Next, lower the head of the bed until the patient is lying supine or with her head slightly elevated. Expose the abdomen for palpation and the perineum for inspection. Watch for bleeding, clots, and tissue expulsion while massaging the uterus.

Performing palpation

To palpate the uterine fundus, follow these steps:
• Gently compress the uterus between both hands to evaluate its firmness. (See *Feeling the fundus.*)

Advice from the experts

Feeling the fundus

A full-term pregnancy stretches the ligaments supporting the uterus, placing it at risk for inversion during palpation and massage. To guard against this, place one hand against the patient's abdomen at the symphysis pubis level, as shown below. This steadies the fundus and prevents downward displacement. Then place the other hand at the top of the fundus, cupping it, as shown below.

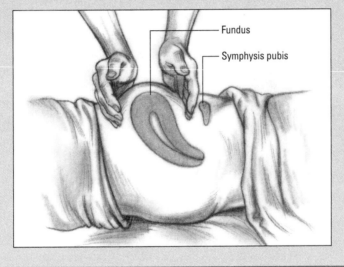

Fundus

Symphysis pubis

• Note the level of the fundus above or below the umbilicus in centimeters or fingerbreadths.
• If the uterus seems soft and boggy, gently massage the fundus with a circular motion until it becomes firm. Without digging into the abdomen, gently compress and release your fingers, always supporting the lower uterine segment with your other hand. Observe the vaginal drainage during massage.
• Massage long enough to produce firmness but not discomfort. You may also encourage the patient to massage her fundus for 10 to 15 seconds every 15 minutes. This is usually necessary only for a few hours.
• Notify the doctor immediately if the uterus fails to contract and heavy bleeding occurs. If the fundus becomes firm after massage, keep one hand on the lower uterus and press gently toward the pubis to expel clots. (See *Complications of fundal palpation*, page 428.)

Remember the bladder

When assessing the uterine fundus, also assess for bladder distention. A distended bladder can impede the downward descent of the uterus by pushing it upward and, possibly, to the right side. If the bladder is distended and the patient is unable to urinate, you may need to catheterize her.

Lochia

After birth, the outermost layer of the uterus becomes necrotic and is expelled. This vaginal discharge — called *lochia* — is similar to menstrual flow and consists of blood, fragments of the decidua, white blood cells (WBCs), mucus, and some bacteria.

Assessing lochia flow

Lochia is commonly assessed in conjunction with fundal assessment. (See *Three types of lochia.*)

Help the patient into the lateral Sims' position. Be sure to check under the patient's buttocks to make sure that blood isn't pooling there. Then remove the patient's perineal pad and evaluate the character, amount, color, odor, and consistency (presence of clots) of the discharge. Before removing the perineal pad, make sure that it isn't sticking to any perineal stitches. Otherwise, tearing may occur, possibly increasing the risk of bleeding.

On the lookout

Here's what to look for when assessing lochia:
• *Amount* — Although it varies, the amount of lochia is typically comparable to the amount during menstrual flow. A woman who's breast-feeding may have less lochia. Also, a woman who has had a cesarean birth may have a scant amount of lochia; however, lochia shouldn't be absent. Lochia should be present for at least 3 weeks postpartum. Lochia flow increases with activity; for example, when the patient gets out of bed the first several times (due to pooled lochia being released) or when she lifts a heavy object or walks up stairs (due to an actual increase in the amount of lochia). If your patient saturates a perineal pad in less than an hour, this is considered excessive flow, and you should notify the doctor.
• *Color* — Lochia typically is described as lochia rubra, serosa, or alba, depending on the color of the discharge. Lochia color depends on the postpartum day. A sudden change in color — for example, from pink back to red — suggests new bleeding or retained placental fragments.
• *Odor* — Lochia should smell similar to menstrual flow. A foul or offensive odor suggests infection.

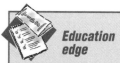

Education edge

Complications of fundal palpation

Because the uterus and its supporting ligaments are tender after birth, pain is the most common complication of fundal palpation and massage. Excessive massage can stimulate premature uterine contractions, causing undue muscle fatigue and leading to uterine atony or inversion. Lack of lochia may signal a clot blocking the cervical os. Heavy bleeding may result if a position change dislodges the clot. Take the patient's vital signs frequently to assess for hypovolemic shock.

• *Consistency*—Lochia should be clot free. Evidence of large clots indicates poor uterine contraction and requires further assessment.

Perineum and rectum

The pressure exerted on the perineum and rectum during birth results in edema and generalized tenderness. Some areas of the perineum may be ecchymotic, caused by the rupture of surface capillaries. Sutures for an episiotomy or laceration may also be present. Hemorrhoids are also commonly seen.

What's your position?

Assessment of the perineum and rectum mainly involves inspection and is performed at the same time that you assess the lochia. Help the patient into the lateral Sims' position. This position provides better visibility and causes less discomfort for the patient with a mediolateral episiotomy. A back-lying position can also be used for patients with midline episiotomies. Make sure you have adequate light for inspection.

Checking down under

Lift the patient's buttocks and observe for intactness of skin, positioning of the episiotomy (if one was performed), and appearance of sutures (from episiotomy or laceration repair) and the surrounding rectal area. Keep in mind that the edges of an episiotomy are usually sealed 24 hours after delivery. Note ecchymosis, hematoma, erythema, edema, drainage or bleeding from sutures, a foul odor, or signs of infection. Also, observe for the presence of hemorrhoids.

Perineal care

Perineal assessment also includes perineal care. The goals of postpartum perineal care are to relieve discomfort, promote healing, and prevent infection by cleaning the perineal area. Perform perineal care in conjunction with a perineal assessment and after the patient voids or has a bowel movement.

Two methods of providing perineal care are generally used: a water-jet irrigation system or a peri bottle. In either case, help the patient walk to the bathroom or place her on a bedpan; then wash your hands and put on gloves.

Water-jet system

If you're using a water-jet irrigation system, follow these steps:

Three types of lochia

Lochia color, which typically changes throughout the postpartum period, may be categorized as:
• *lochia rubra*—red vaginal discharge that occurs from approximately day 1 to day 3 postpartum
• *lochia serosa*—pinkish or brownish discharge that occurs from approximately day 4 to day 10 postpartum
• *lochia alba*—creamy white or colorless vaginal discharge that occurs from approximately day 10 to day 14 postpartum (although it may continue for up to 6 weeks).

- Insert the prefilled cartridge containing the antiseptic or medicated solution into the handle, and push the disposable nozzle into the handle until you hear it click into place.
- Help the patient sit on the toilet or bedpan.
- Place the nozzle parallel to the perineum and turn on the unit.
- Rinse the perineum for at least 2 minutes from front to back.
- Turn off the unit, remove the nozzle, and discard the cartridge.
- Dry the nozzle and store as appropriate for later use.

Peri bottle

If you're using a peri bottle for perineal care, follow these steps:
- Fill the bottle with cleaning solution (usually warm water).
- Help the patient sit on the toilet or bedpan.
- Tell her to pour the solution over her perineal area.
- After completion, help the patient off the toilet or remove the bedpan.
- Pat the perineal area dry, and help the patient apply a new perineal pad.

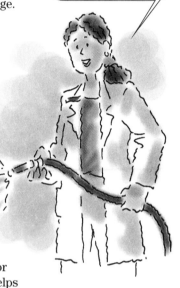

Water-jet irrigation and other irrigation methods help to relieve discomfort, promote healing, and prevent infection.

Hot and cold comfort

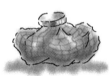

During perineal care, note if the patient complains of pain or tenderness. If she does, you may need to apply ice or cold packs to the area for the first 24 hours after birth. This helps reduce perineal edema and prevent hematoma formation, thereby reducing pain and promoting healing.

Cold therapy isn't effective after the first 24 hours. Instead, heat is recommended because it increases circulation to the area. Forms of heat include a perineal hot pack (dry heat) or a sitz bath (moist heat).

Sitz right down

For extensive lacerations, such as third or fourth degree lacerations, the doctor may order a sitz bath to aid perineal healing, provide comfort, and reduce edema. Because of shortened hospitalization time, you may need to teach the patient how to use a sitz bath at home. (See *Using a sitz bath*.)

Postpartum care measures

Ongoing assessment is crucial during the postpartum period. Continue to assess the patient's vital signs, uterine fundus, lochia, breasts, and perineum as ordered. Administer medications as ordered to relieve discomfort from the episiotomy or from uterine

Education edge

Using a sitz bath

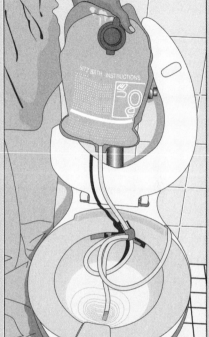

A sitz bath allows the postpartum patient to immerse her perineal area in warm or hot water without the bother of taking a complete bath. It relieves discomfort and promotes wound healing by cleaning the perineum and anus, increasing circulation, and reducing inflammation. It also helps relax local muscles.

How it's done

Tell the patient to follow these steps to use a sitz bath correctly:

• Assemble the equipment and wash your hands.

• Empty your bladder.

• Fill the basin to the specified line with water at the prescribed temperature (usually 100° to 105° F [37.8° to 40.6° C]). Be sure to check the water temperature frequently to ensure therapeutic effects.

• Place the basin under the commode seat, clamp the irrigation tubing to block water flow, and fill the irrigation bag with water of the same temperature as that in the basin.

• To create flow pressure, hang the bag above your head on a hook, towel rack, or edge of a door.

• Remove and dispose of your perineal pad and then sit on the basin.

• If your feet don't reach the floor and the weight of your legs presses against the edge of the equipment, place a small stool under your feet. Also place a folded towel or small pillow against your lower back.

• Cover your shoulders and knees with blankets or a robe to prevent chilling.

• Open the clamp on the irrigation tubing to allow a stream of water to flow continuously. Refill the bag with water of the correct temperature, as needed, and continue to regulate the flow.

• After approximately 15 to 20 minutes, clamp the tubing and rest for a few minutes before arising to prevent dizziness and lightheadedness.

• Pat the perineal area dry from front to back, and apply a new perineal pad (by holding the bottom sides or ends).

• Dispose of soiled materials properly. Empty and clean the sitz bath according to the manufacturer's directions.

• Report any changes in drainage amount or characteristics, lightheadedness, perspiration, weakness, nausea, or irregular heart rate.

contractions, incisional pain, or breast engorgement and assess for therapeutic effectiveness. Encourage the patient to rest after delivery and throughout the postpartum period to prevent exhaustion.

A-voiding catheterization

Assess the patient's urinary elimination. The patient should void within 6 to 8 hours after delivery. If she doesn't, help her urge to void by administering analgesics as ordered, pouring warm water over the perineum, placing the patient's hands in warm water, or running water for the patient to hear (the sound may encourage the urge to void). If all attempts fail, the patient may need to be catheterized.

Flatus foreshadows function

Finally, assess bowel function. Elimination is typically a good indicator of bowel function. The patient should have a bowel movement 1 to 2 days after delivery to avoid constipation. However, a patient who has eaten nothing by mouth for 12 to 24 hours and then has a cesarean birth may not have a bowel movement for several days. In these cases, flatus may be a better indicator of bowel function.

Encourage the patient to drink plenty of fluids and eat high-fiber foods to prevent constipation. If necessary, the doctor may order stool softeners or laxatives. If the patient has hemorrhoids, cool witch hazel compresses may be helpful. Don't use suppositories if the patient has a 3rd or 4th degree laceration.

You should drink plenty of fluids and eat high-fiber foods to prevent constipation.

Patient teaching

Because of the short length of stay for most postpartum women, patient teaching is essential. Teaching should focus on maternal self-care activities and neonatal care. (See *Postpartum maternal self-care.*)

Lactation

Lactation refers to the production of breast milk, the preferred source of nutrition for a neonate. All patients experience the physiologic changes that occur with lactation and breast milk production regardless of whether they plan to breast-feed.

Physiology of lactation

During pregnancy, a hormone called *prolactin* prepares the woman's breasts to secrete milk. Other hormones, progesterone and estrogen, interact to suppress milk secretion while developing

Education edge

Postpartum maternal self-care

When teaching your patient about self-care for the postpartum period, be sure to include these topic areas and instructions.

Personal hygiene
• Change perineal pads frequently, removing them from the front to the back and disposing of them in a plastic bag.
• Perform perineal care each time that you urinate or move your bowels.
• Monitor your vaginal discharge; it should change from red to pinkish brown to clear or creamy white before stopping altogether. Notify your doctor if the discharge returns to a previous color, becomes bright red or yellowish green, suddenly increases in amount, or develops an offensive odor.
• Follow your doctor's instructions about using sitz baths or applying heat to your perineum.
• Shower daily.

Breasts
• Wear a firm, supportive bra.
• If nipple leakage occurs, use clean gauze pads or nursing pads inside your bra to absorb the moisture.
• Inspect your nipples for cracking, fissures, or soreness, and report any areas of redness, tenderness, or swelling.
• Wash breasts daily with clear water when showering and dry with a soft towel or allow to air dry. Don't use soap on your breasts because soap is drying.
• If you're breast-feeding and your breasts become engorged, allow your baby to suck at the breast or use warm compresses or stand under a warm shower for relief. If you aren't breast-feeding, apply cool compresses several times per day.

Activity and exercise
• Balance rest periods with activity, get as much sleep as possible at night, and take frequent rest periods or naps during the day.
• Check with your doctor about when to begin exercising.
• If your vaginal discharge increases with activity, elevate your legs for about 30 minutes. If the discharge doesn't decrease with rest, call your doctor.

Nutrition
• Increase your intake of protein and calories.
• Drink plenty of fluids throughout the day, including before and after breast-feeding.

Elimination
• If you have the urge to urinate or move your bowels, don't delay doing so. Urinate at least every 2 to 3 hours. This helps keep the uterus contracted and decreases the risk of excessive bleeding.
• Report any difficulty urinating, burning, or pain to your doctor.
• Drink plenty of liquids and eat high-fiber foods to prevent constipation.
• Follow your doctor's instructions about the use of stool softeners or laxatives.

Sexual activity and contraception
• Remember that breast-feeding isn't a reliable method of contraception. Discuss birth control options with your doctor.
• Ask your doctor when you can resume sexual activity and contraceptive measures. Most couples can resume having sex within 3 to 4 weeks after delivery, or possibly as soon as lochia ceases.
• Use a water-based lubricant if necessary
• Expect a decrease in intensity and rapidity of sexual response for about 3 months after delivery.
• Perform Kegel exercises to help strengthen your pelvic floor muscles. To do this, squeeze your pelvic muscles as if tying to stop urine flow, and then release them.

Sleeping positions
• To aid uterine involution, lie on your abdomen. This position tips the uterus into its natural forward position and also provides support to the abdominal muscles.
• Avoid lying on your side in the knee-chest position until at least the third postpartal week or, better yet, until after the 6-week postpartal examination. (*Note:* The knee-chest position may cause the vagina to open, possibly allowing air to enter through the still slightly open cervical os. The air can pass through the still open blood sinuses in the uterus and enter the circulatory system, placing the woman at risk for an air embolism.

the breasts for lactation. Estrogen causes the breasts to grow by increasing their fat content. Progesterone causes lobule growth and develops the alveolar (acinar) cells' secretory capacity.

After birth, the mother's estrogen and progesterone levels drop abruptly. This drop in hormones triggers the release of prolactin from the anterior pituitary, which starts the cycle of synthesis and secretion of milk (See *A closer look at lactation.*)

Breast milk composition

From about the fourth month of pregnancy until the first 3 to 4 days after delivery, the acinar cells produce and secrete colostrum. Colostrum is a thick, sticky, golden-yellow fluid that contains protein, sugar, fat, water, minerals, vitamins, and maternal antibodies. It's easy for the neonate to digest because it's high in protein and low in sugar and fat. It also provides completely adequate nutrition for the neonate. The high protein level of colostrum aids in the binding of bilirubin and also has a laxative effect, which promotes early passage of the neonate's first stool called *meconium.*

Got milk?

On about the second to fourth postpartum day, colostrum is replaced by mature breast milk. During this time, the woman experiences copious amounts of breast milk. The composition of this breast milk changes with each feeding. As the neonate nurses, the bluish-white foremilk that contains part skim and part whole milk provides primarily protein, lactose, and water-soluble vitamins to the neonate. Hind-milk, or cream, is produced within the first 10 to 20 minutes of nursing. It contains denser calories from fat. This transitional breast milk is replaced by true or mature breast milk by around the 10th day after delivery.

Lactation and the menstrual cycle

After delivery of the placenta, estrogen and progesterone production ceases. As a result, the pituitary gland increases the production of FSH, which eventually leads to ovulation and resumption of the menstrual cycle.

Here we go again

Most lactating women begin menstruating again in about 3 months. Ovulation may occur by the end of the first month postpartum, or it may not occur for one or more menstrual cycles. Woman who aren't lactating usually resume menstruating in 6 to 10 weeks. Approximately one-half of these women ovulate with the first menstrual cycle.

A closer look at lactation

After delivery of the placenta, the drop in progesterone and estrogen levels stimulates the production of prolactin. This hormone stimulates milk production by the acinar cells in the mammary glands.

Nerve impulses, caused by the neonate sucking at the breast, travel from the nipple to the hypothalamus, resulting in the production of prolactin-releasing factor. This factor leads to additional production of prolactin and, subsequently, more milk production.

Go with the flow

Milk flows from the acinar cells through small tubules to the lactiferous sinuses (small reservoirs located behind the nipple). This milk, called *foremilk*, is thin, bluish, and sugary and is constantly forming. It quenches the neonate's thirst but contains little fat and protein.

When the neonate sucks at the breast, oxytocin is released, causing the sinuses to contract. Contraction pushes the milk forward through the nipple to the neonate. In addition, release of oxytocin causes the smooth muscles of the uterus to contract.

That let-down feeling

Movement of the milk forward through the nipple is termed the let-down reflex and may be triggered by things other than the infant sucking at the breast. For example, women have reported that hearing their baby cry or thinking about him causes this reflex.

Once the let-down reflex occurs and the neonate has fed for 10 to 15 minutes, new milk — called *hind milk* — is formed. This milk is thicker, whiter, and contains higher concentrations of fat and protein. Hind milk contains the calories and fat necessary for the neonate to gain weight, build brain tissue, and be more content and satisfied between feedings.

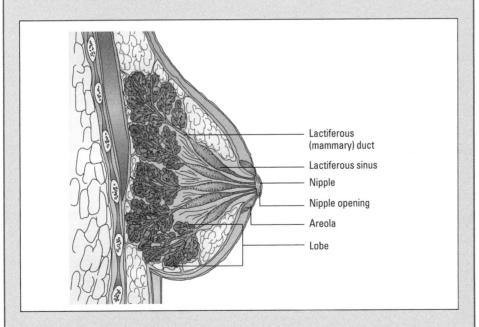

Lactiferous (mammary) duct

Lactiferous sinus

Nipple

Nipple opening

Areola

Lobe

Neonatal nutrition

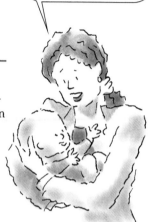

Although breast-feeding is the safest, simplest, and least expensive way to provide complete neonate nourishment, it's contraindicated in some cases.

Human milk consumed through breast-feeding is considered optimal for neonates. Despite this, not all mothers can or choose to breast-feed. Medical conditions, cultural background, anxiety, drug abuse, and various other factors can prevent a woman from breast-feeding. Furthermore, some neonates can't take in enough breast milk through breast-feeding to meet nutritional needs. Some breast milk may be insufficient in calcium, protein, and essential vitamins, especially for premature neonates. In these cases, bottle-feeding with formula is an acceptable alternative.

Breast-feeding

Breast-feeding is considered the safest, simplest, and least expensive way to provide complete neonate nourishment. The American Academy of Pediatrics and the American Dietetic Association recommend breast-feeding exclusively for the first 4 to 6 months and then in combination with infant foods until age 1.

Contrary to popular belief

Breast-feeding is contraindicated if the mother:
- has herpes lesions on her nipples
- is receiving such medications as methotrexate (Folex PFS) or lithium (Eskalith) that pass into the breast milk and may harm the neonate
- is on a restricted diet that interferes with adequate nutrient intake and subsequently affects the quality of milk produced
- has breast cancer
- has a severe chronic condition, such as active tuberculosis, human immunodeficiency virus infection, or hepatitis.

Breast-feeding is also contraindicated if the neonate has galactosemia (inability to digest lactose in milk).

Advantages

Breast-feeding is advantageous for the mother and the neonate. (See *Benefits of breast-feeding*.)

Maternal benefits include:
- protection against breast cancer
- assistance in uterine involution due to the release of oxytocin
- empowerment (as the woman learns to master the skill)
- less preparation time and less cost.

More good news about breast-feeding

Breast milk is also highly beneficial for the neonate. For example, it reduces the risk of infection because it contains:
- immunoglobulin A — an antibody that prevents foreign proteins from being absorbed by the neonate's GI tract
- lactoferrin — an iron-binding protein that interferes with bacterial growth
- lysozyme — an enzyme that actively destroys bacteria
- leukocytes — WBCs that protect against common respiratory infections
- macrophages — cells that produce interferon, which offers protection from viral invasion.

In addition, breast-feeding is advantageous to the neonate for these reasons:
- Breast milk promotes rapid brain growth because it contains large amounts of lactose, which is easily digested and can be rapidly converted to glucose.
- Breast milk's protein and nitrogen contents provide foundations for neurologic cell building.
- Breast milk contains adequate electrolyte and mineral composition for the neonate's needs without overloading the neonate's renal system.

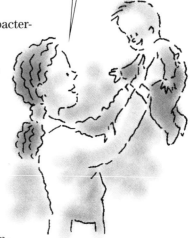

Breast-feeding is awesome! It reduces your risk of infection.

Benefits of breast-feeding

It's a well-known fact that breast-feeding is best for babies. Here are some of the reasons.

Passive immunity
Human milk provides passive immunity. Colostrum is the first fluid secreted from the breast (occurs within the first few days of life) and provides immune factor and protein to the new baby. Many components of breast milk protect against infection — it contains antibodies (especially immunoglobulin A) and white blood cells that protect the baby from some forms of infection. Breast-fed babies also experience fewer allergies and intolerances.

Easily digestible
Breast milk provides essential nutrients in an easily digestible form. It contains lipase, which breaks down dietary fat, making it easily available to the baby's system.

Brain booster
The lipids in breast milk are high in linoleic acid and cholesterol, which are needed for brain development.

Low protein content
Cow's milk contains proportionally higher concentrations of electrolytes and protein than are needed by human babies. It must be cleared by the immature kidneys and thus isn't recommended until after a baby is at least 12 months old.

Convenient and cheap
Breast-feeding saves time and money in buying and preparing formula.

- Breast-feeding improves the neonate's ability to regulate calcium and phosphorus levels.
- The sucking mechanism associated with breast-feeding reduces dental arch malformations.
- A breast-fed neonate's GI tract contains large amounts of *Lactobacillus bifidus*, a beneficial bacterium that prevents the growth of harmful organisms.

On the contrary

Contrary to some people's beliefs, breast-feeding isn't a reliable form of contraception. In addition, evidence doesn't suggest that breast-feeding aids in weight loss after pregnancy.

Maternal nutrition and breast-feeding

Nutritional needs for a woman who's breast-feeding are only slightly different from those during her pregnancy. Folate and iron needs decrease after giving birth, and energy requirements increase.

Fueling milk production

While breast-feeding, a healthy woman should consume 2,300 to 2,700 calories/day, approximately 500 calories/day more than prepregnancy recommendations. If maternal intake is poor, which can occur when a lactating woman is dieting, the nutrient intake in her breast milk may become inadequate.

Water hydrant

Adequate hydration encourages ample milk production, so it's important for new mothers to drink plenty of fluids — 2 to 3 qt (2 to 3 L)/day. The mother should also drink one 8-oz glass of fluid each time she breast-feeds to ensure she stays hydrated. Water and such beverages as fruit juices and milk are good choices to maintain adequate hydration.

Keep contaminants out!

Most substances that the mother ingests are secreted into her milk. Therefore, beverages containing alcohol and caffeine should be limited or avoided because they may be harmful to the neonate. In addition, it's important to check with a pediatrician before taking any medication. Some researchers believe that components of the maternal food may contribute to colic or the neonate's fussiness.

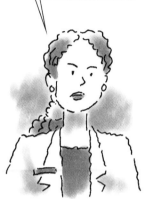

No matter what your grandmother says, breast-feeding will NOT prevent pregnancy!

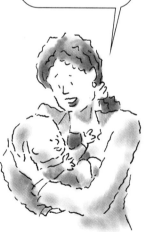

Lactation requires more energy! Now isn't the time for mom to cut calories.

Breast-feeding assistance

Even women who have previously breast-fed can benefit from assistance and instruction. The key is helping the patient to relax, which encourages the let-down reflex.

Breast-feeding should occur as soon as possible after birth. However, this may not be possible, especially if the woman is overly fatigued or if a complication has developed.

Don't get comfy yet

When assisting with breast-feeding, explain the procedure and provide privacy. Encourage the mother to drink a beverage before and during or after breast-feeding to ensure adequate fluid intake, which maintains milk production. Also encourage her to use the bathroom and change the neonate's diaper before breast-feeding begins so that feeding is uninterrupted. Then wash your hands and instruct the mother to do the same.

Now, take a load off

Now, help her find a comfortable position. (See *Breast-feeding positions*, page 440.) Then follow these instructions:
• Have the mother expose one breast and rest the nape of the neonate's neck in the crook of her arm, supporting his back with her forearm.
• Urge the mother to relax to encourage the let-down reflex. Tell her that she may feel a tingling sensation when the reflex occurs and that milk may drip or spray from her breasts. Explain that the reflex may also be initiated by hearing the neonate's cry.
• Inform her that uterine cramping may occur during breast-feeding until her uterus returns to its original size.
• Guiding the mother's free hand, have her place her thumb on top of the exposed breast's areola and her first two fingers beneath it, forming a C. Have her turn the neonate so that his entire body faces the breast.
• Tell the mother to stroke the neonate's cheek with her finger or the neonate's mouth with her nipple. This stimulates the rooting reflex. Emphasize that she should touch the cheek closest to the exposed breast. Touching the other cheek may cause the neonate to turn his head toward the touch and away from the breast.
• When the neonate opens his mouth and roots for the nipple, instruct the mother to move him onto the breast so that he gets as much of the areola as possible into his mouth. This helps him to exert sufficient pressure with his lips, gums, and cheek muscles on the milk sinuses below the areola.
• Show the mother how to check for occlusion of the neonate's nostrils by the breast. If this happens, she should reposition the

Encourage a breast-feeding mother to drink a beverage before breast-feeding as well as during or after to ensure adequate fluid intake, which maintains milk production.

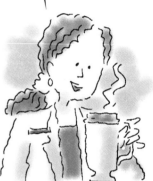

Education edge

Breast-feeding positions

The position a mother uses when breast-feeding should be comfortable and efficient. Explain to the mother that changing positions periodically alters the neonate's grasp on the nipple and helps to prevent contact friction on the same area. As appropriate, suggest these three popular feeding positions.

Cradle position	**Side-lying position**	**Football position**
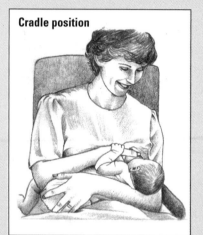	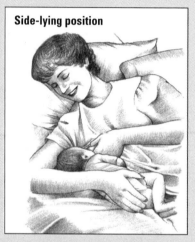	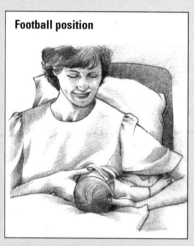
The mother cradles the neonate's head in the crook of her arm. Tell her to place a pillow on her lap for the neonate to lie on. Also tell her to place a pillow behind her back; this provides comfort and also puts her breasts in the correct position for feeding.	Tell the mother to lie on her side with her stomach facing the neonate's. As the neonate's mouth opens, she should pull him toward the nipple. Tell her to place a pillow or rolled blanket behind the neonate's back to prevent him from moving or rolling away from the breast.	Sitting with a pillow in front of her, the mother places her hand under the neonate's head. As the neonate's mouth opens, she pulls the neonate's head near her breast. This position may be more comfortable for the woman who has had a cesarean birth.

neonate to give him room to breathe. The tip of his nose should touch the breast but not be mashed into it. The baby will breathe out of the sides of his nose.

• Suggest that the mother breast-feed for 15 minutes on each breast for the first 24 hours after birth. After that, the best advice is to never break a good latch. Remember: The neonate doesn't start receiving fat-and-protein-rich hind milk until after 15 minutes of feeding.

• To switch to the other breast, instruct the mother to slip a finger into the side of the neonate's mouth to break the seal, and then move him to the other breast.

Burping basics

Because some neonates swallow large amounts of air when feeding, encourage the mother to burp the neonate after emptying the first breast and again at the end of the feeding. Before burping, remind the mother to place a protective cover, such as a cloth diaper or washcloth, under the neonate's chin. The most common way to burp an neonate is to place him over one shoulder and gently pat or rub his back to help expel ingested air.

A burp is a burp is a burp

Some mothers have trouble supporting the neonate's head while patting or rubbing his back. This position may be especially awkward with small neonates because they lack the ability to control their heads. In these cases, suggest the sitting position for burping. (See *Sitting up for burping*, page 442.) A third acceptable position is placing the neonate prone across the mother's lap.

Taking a breather

When the mother finishes breast-feeding, instruct her to place the neonate in bed, either lying on his back or on his side with a towel roll for support. She should let her nipples air dry for about 15 minutes after breast-feeding.

To make sure that both breasts are completely emptied, advise the mother to begin the next feeding using the breast on which the neonate finished this feeding. To help her remember, she can put a safety pin on her bra strap on the side last used.

Quelling concerns

Mothers commonly have questions about breast-feeding, including how often the neonate should feed, how much the neonate is getting, and what to do if the neonate is too sleepy to breast-feed. Reassure the mother that breast-feeding schedules aren't carved in stone and that developing a schedule that both she and her baby feel comfortable with takes time.

Feed me, feed me!

During the first few days of life, a neonate is usually fed as often as he's hungry, possibly every 2 hours. This helps to ensure that the neonate is satisfying his sucking needs and is receiving the necessary fluid and nutrients. Frequent feeding also helps to maintain the mother's milk supply because frequent emptying stimulates more milk production.

A neonate's behavior helps to determine if he's getting enough breast milk. If he's content between feedings, wets approximately

> The most common way to burp a baby is to place him over one shoulder and gently pat or rub his back. This helps to expel ingested air.

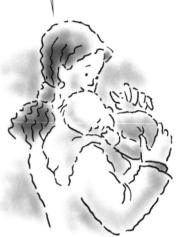

Advice from the experts

Sitting up for burping

If the mother indicates that placing the neonate over her shoulder for burping is awkward, suggest this alternative:

• Hold the neonate in a sitting position on your lap.

• Lean the neonate forward against one hand and support his head and neck with the index finger and thumb of that same hand, as shown at right.

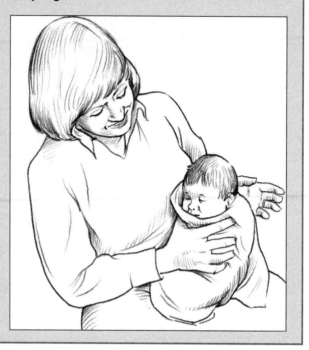

> It's been 2 hours. Looks as if it might be time for another feeding.

6 to 8 diapers per day, and gains weight, then he's probably receiving adequate nutrition.

Whetting his appetite

Sometimes neonates seem to be uninterested or fall asleep when breast-feeding. If the neonate shows little interest in breast-feeding, assure the mother that the baby may need several days to learn and adjust. If the neonate is sleepy, suggest that the mother try rubbing the baby's feet, unwrapping his blanket, changing the diaper, or changing her position or the neonate's. She may also manually express a little milk and allow the neonate to taste it. (See *Manual breast milk expression.*)

Keep up the good work!

Always encourage the mother's breast-feeding efforts. To boost these efforts, urge her to eat balanced meals, to drink at least eight 8-oz glasses of fluid daily, and to nap daily for at least the

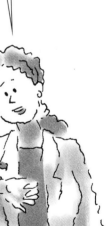

first 2 weeks after giving birth. Answer her questions about breast-feeding and provide instructional materials if available. Always provide a patient who's breast-feeding information and instructions related to possible complications. (See chapter 10, Complications of the postpartum period, for more in-depth information on complications.) Contact a lactation consultant as appropriate.

Before discharge, tell the mother about local breast-feeding and parenting support groups such as La Leche League International.

Daddy dearest

To involve the father, have him change the neonate's diaper before feeding or burp the neonate afterwards. Even young children can get involved by helping with burping.

Bottle-feeding with breast milk

In some cases, a mother may need to be away from her neonate but still desires to provide breast milk. The mother may also need to express breast milk when her breasts are engorged. Although

---

Manual breast milk expression

Manually expressing breast milk can enhance milk production and ensure an adequate supply. It's especially helpful for mothers who have problems with engorgement or those who must be away from their infants for several hours. (A mother who works outside the home or is away on a regular basis may find an electric pump quicker and more efficient.)

Express yourself

To help the mother manually express breast milk, follow these steps:

• Make sure that a clean collection container is available and that you and the patient have washed your hands.

• Explain the procedure to the patient, have her sit in a comfortable position, and provide privacy.

• Tell her to place her dominant hand on one breast with the thumb positioned on the top

and the fingers below and at the outer limit of the areola.

• Instruct her to press her thumb and fingers inward toward her chest while holding the collection container with her opposite hand directly under the nipple.

• Tell the patient to move her thumb and fingers forward, using gentle pressure in a milking type motion. Caution her not to use too much pressure because this can injure breast tissue. Milk should flow out of the nipple and into the collection container.

• Encourage the patient to move her thumb and fingers around the breast, using the same motion, to ensure complete emptying.

• Advise the patient to cover the container and place the milk in the refrigerator if it will be used within 24 hours; if not, she should freeze it.

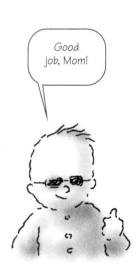

Good job, Mom!

the breasts can be expressed by hand, pumping is the most efficient method.

Breast pumping

Breast pumping involves the use of suction created with a manual cylinder pump or a battery-powered or electric pump to stimulate lactation. It's used when the mother and neonate are separated or while illness temporarily incapacitates one or the other.

A breast pump can also relieve engorgement, collect milk for a premature neonate with a weak sucking reflex, reduce pressure on sore or cracked nipples, or reestablish the milk supply. The mother can also use a pump to collect milk when she's unable to manually express it.

Preparing to pump

Before teaching the mother to use a breast pump:
• Assemble the equipment according to the manufacturer's instructions.
• Explain the procedure to the patient.
• Provide privacy.
• Wash your hands and instruct the patient to wash hers.
• Help the patient into a comfortable position and urge her to relax.

Tell the patient to drink a beverage before and after pumping. If the patient's breasts are engorged, instruct her to apply warm compresses for 5 minutes or take a warm shower.

There's more than one way to get pumped.

Manual cylinder pump

To use a manual cylinder pump, instruct the patient to place the flange or shield against her breast with the nipple in the center of the device. Then have her pump each breast by moving the outer cylinder back and forth in a pistonlike motion. She should continue until the breast is empty and then repeat the procedure on the other breast.

Battery-powered or electric pump

To use a battery-powered or electric pump, instruct the patient to set the suction regulator on low. Tell her to hold the collection unit upright to prevent milk from being sucked into the machine. Have her place the shield against her breast with the nipple in the center. She should turn on the machine and adjust the suction regulator to a comfortable pressure.

Warn her to start with the least amount of suction to prevent nipple damage and then gradually increase the suction. Instruct her to check the operator's manual to see the pressure setting at which the pump functions most efficiently.

Keep on pumping

Tell the patient to pump each breast for 5 to 8 minutes or until the spray grows scant. Then she should massage her breasts for 1 to 2 minutes or apply warm compresses. Next, pump each breast again for 3 to 5 minutes, massage or reapply the compresses, and then pump again for 2 to 3 minutes. Usually, 8 oz can be pumped within 15 to 30 minutes.

When she's finished, show the patient how to remove the shield from the breast by inserting a finger between the breast and the shield to break the vacuum seal. Then return the suction regulator to the low setting and turn off the machine.

Freeze, store, or enjoy right now?

After using either type of pump, the patient should let her nipples air dry for about 15 minutes. She should also disassemble the removable parts of the pump and clean them according to the manufacturer's directions.

If she plans to store or freeze the milk, have her fill a sterile plastic bottle with milk from the cylinder or collection unit. Place the milk in the refrigerator or freezer immediately. Always label the collected milk with the date, the time of collection, and the amount. Write the neonate's name on the label, if necessary. If the neonate is going to drink the milk right away, show the patient how to attach a rubber nipple to the cylinder or collection unit.

> Store fresh pumped breast milk in the fridge for 5 days or freeze it for up to 6 months. But once you defrost it (in the fridge, of course), use it within 24 hours.

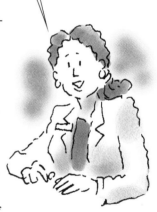

Bottle-feeding with formula

Formula-feeding is a reliable and nutritionally adequate method of feeding for neonates whose mothers are unable to breast-feed or who choose not to. Commercial formulas very closely resemble human milk.

Types of formulas

Commercial formulas typically provide 20 calories per ounce when diluted properly and are classified as milk-based, soy-based, and elemental. Milk-based formulas, such as Enfamil and Similac, are usually prescribed. Some of these formulas are lactose free, so they can be used for neonates with galactosemia or lactose intolerance.

Health food for babies

Soy-based formulas, such as Isomil and Nursoy, are used for babies who are allergic to cow's milk protein. Elemental formulas are commonly prescribed for babies who have protein allergies or fat malnutrition. With these formulas, the amount of fat, protein, and carbohydrates is modified. However, all commercial formulas simulate the nutritional content of human milk along with providing additional vitamins.

Formula x four

Commercial formulas may be supplied in one of four forms:
• powdered — to be combined with water
• condensed liquid — must be diluted
• ready to feed
• disposable, individually prepared bottles.

The powdered form is the least expensive; whereas, individually prepared bottles are most expensive but easiest to use. Most health care facilities use individually prepared bottles. Tell parents about the forms of formula available so they can choose what's most convenient for them.

Formula-feeding assistance

Each day, an infant requires 2.5 to 3 ounces of fluid per pound of body weight (150 to 200 ml/kg) and 50 to 55 calories per pound of body weight (100 to 120 kcal/kg). Because commercial formulas consistently provide 20 calories per ounce, only the infant's fluid needs are used to determine the amount of each feeding. Unlike breast-feeding, you can measure the amount of formula consumed.

Until about age 4 months, most infants need 6 feedings per day. After this, the number of feedings drops, but the amount at each feeding increases because the baby starts to eat cereal, fruits, and vegetables.

Prefeeding prep

When bottle-feeding a neonate, or helping the mother with bottle-feeding, know the type of formula that's ordered and how it's supplied. If you're using a commercially prepared formula, uncap the formula bottle and make sure that the seal isn't broken to ensure sterility and freshness. If the seal is broken, discard the formula. If the seal isn't broken, remove it.

Next, screw on the nipple and cap. Keep the protective sterile cap over the nipple until the neonate is ready to feed. If you're preparing formula, follow the manufacturer's directions or the

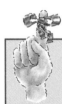

Memory jogger

To easily determine the amount of milk an infant should take in at each feeding, add 2 to 3 oz to the infant's age (in months). So, for example:
• A 1-month-old should take 3 to 4 oz at each feeding.
• A 4-month-old should take 6 to 7 oz.
• A 5-month-old should take 7 to 8 oz.

doctor's prescription. Administer the formula at room temperature or slightly warmer.

Bottle-feeding blow by blow

Teach the mother and other family members to follow these steps when bottle-feeding the neonate:

• After washing your hands and preparing the formula, invert the bottle and shake some formula on your wrist to test the formula's temperature and the patency of the nipple hole. The formula should drip freely but not stream out. If the hole is too large, the neonate may aspirate formula; if it's too small, the extra sucking effort may tire him before he can empty the bottle.

• Sit comfortably in a semireclining position and cradle the neonate in one arm to support his head and back. This position allows swallowed air to rise to the top of the stomach where it's more easily expelled. If the neonate can't be held, sit by him and elevate his head and shoulders slightly.

• Place the nipple in the neonate's mouth on top of his tongue, but not so far back that it stimulates the gag reflex. He should begin to suck, pulling in as much nipple as is comfortable. If he doesn't start to suck, stroke him under the chin or on his cheek, or touch his lips with the nipple to stimulate the sucking reflex.

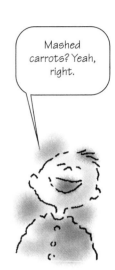

Mashed carrots? Yeah, right.

Tilting does the trick

• As the neonate feeds, tilt the bottle upward to keep the nipple filled with formula and to prevent him from swallowing air. Watch for a steady stream of bubbles in the bottle. This indicates proper venting and flow of formula.

• If the neonate pushes out the nipple with his tongue, reinsert the nipple. Expelling the nipple is a normal reflex. It doesn't necessarily mean that the neonate is full.

• Always hold the bottle for a neonate. If left to feed himself, he may aspirate formula or swallow air if the bottle tilts or empties. In older infants, experts also link bottle propping with an increased incidence of otitis media and dental caries.

• Be sure to interact with the neonate during feeding.

• Burp the neonate after each ½ oz of formula because he'll usually swallow some air even when fed correctly. Use the same positions previously described for breast-feeding.

• After feeding and burping the neonate, place him on his back as recommended by the American Association of Pediatricians. This position reduces the incidence of sudden infant death syndrome.

• Don't worry if the baby regurgitates some of the feeding. Neonates are prone to regurgitation because of an immature cardiac sphincter. Regurgitation is merely an overflow and shouldn't

be confused with vomiting—a more complete emptying of the stomach accompanied by symptoms not associated with feeding.
• Discard any remaining formula and properly dispose of all equipment.

Too much or not enough

A neonate tires if he feeds too long, and his sucking needs aren't met if he doesn't feed long enough. In some cases, you or the mother may need to change the size of the nipple or nipple hole and thus change the duration of the feeding. Additionally, be sure to note how much formula is in the bottle before and after the feeding. Use the calibrations along the side of the container to calculate the amount of formula consumed.

At home, go with the flow

Teach parents and other family members how to prepare and (if required) sterilize formula, bottles, and nipples. Although most health care facilities have a feeding schedule, advise the mother to switch to a more flexible demand-feeding schedule when at home. Warn her that the neonate may not feed well on his first day home because of the new activity and environment.

I've got those burping-up-my-feeding blues.

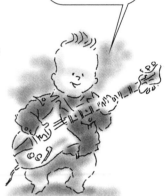

Breast care

A mother who plans to breast-feed should prepare her breasts as directed by the doctor. After the neonate's birth, she'll need to maintain breast tissue integrity. Although postpartum care varies for breast-feeding and non-breast-feeding women, some guidelines are similar.

For breast-feeding women

Provide these instructions to a woman who's breast-feeding her neonate:
• Using your fingers—not a washcloth—wash your areolae and nipples. Use only water to avoid washing away the natural oils and keratin.
• If your nipples are sore or irritated, apply ice compresses to them just before breast-feeding. This numbs them, making them less sensitive and easier for the neonate to grasp
• To help prevent tenderness, lubricate the nipple with a few drops of expressed breast milk before feeding.
• Place breast pads over your nipples to collect milk, and replace the pads often to reduce the risk of infection. Breasts often leak during the first few weeks you're breast-feeding.

• Be alert for a slight temperature elevation and an increase in breast size, warmth, and firmness 2 to 5 days after birth. This signals that breast milk is coming in.
• Wear a well-fitting support bra to help control engorgement.
• Apply warm compresses, massage the breasts, take a warm shower, or express some milk before feeding if your breasts are engorged and the neonate can't latch on to the nipple.

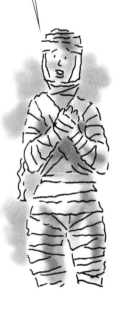

This oughta' prevent engorgement.

For non-breast-feeding women

Provide these instructions to a woman who isn't breast-feeding her neonate:
• Clean your breasts with water only or with soap if necessary.
• Wear a supportive bra to help minimize engorgement and decrease nipple stimulation.
• To minimize further milk production, avoid stimulating the nipples or manually expressing milk.
• Use analgesics (if ordered), ice packs, or a breast binder to minimize engorgement.

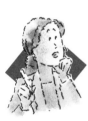

Quick quiz

1. Which of the following changes would you identify as a progressive physiologic change in the postpartum period?
    A.   Lactation
    B.   Lochia
    C.   Uterine involution
    D.   Diuresis

Answer: A. Lactation is an example of a progressive physiologic change that occurs during the postpartum period.

2. Which behavior would you expect to assess during the taking-in phase?
    A.   Strong interest in caring for the neonate
    B.   Redefinition of new role
    C.   Insecurity about ability to provide neonatal care
    D.   Passivity with dependence on others

Answer: D. During the taking-in phase, the patient assumes a passive role, relying on others for care.

3. Where would you expect to assess the uterine fundus in a patient who's 2 days postpartum?

A. 2 cm above the level of the umbilicus
B. At the level of the symphysis pubis
C. Approximately 2 cm below the umbilicus
D. 2 cm above the symphysis pubis

Answer: C. The uterus descends at a rate of about 1 cm/day. The fundus of a woman who's 2 days postpartum should be 2 cm below the umbilicus.

4. At the patient's 6-week follow-up appointment, you should assess:
A. lochia rubra.
B. lochia serosa.
C. lochia alba.
D. absence of lochia.

Answer: D. By 6 weeks, lochia usually has ceased. Lochia rubra typically lasts from days 1 to 3 postpartum; lochia serosa, from days 3 to 10; and lochia alba, from days 10 to 14.

5. Lactation is stimulated by:
A. estrogen.
B. prolactin.
C. progesterone.
D. FSH.

Answer: B. Prolactin is the hormone responsible for stimulating lactation.

6. Which measure would the woman who isn't breast-feeding use to minimize engorgement?
A. Cold compresses
B. Manual expression
C. Warm showers
D. Nipple stimulation

Answer: A. For the woman who isn't breast-feeding, cold compresses help to minimize engorgement.

Scoring

☆☆☆ If you answered all six questions correctly, hooray! You've taken in quite a bit of information on postpartum care.

☆☆ If you answered four or five questions correctly, way to go! You have more than a fundal-mental knowledge of the subject.

☆ If you answered fewer than four questions correctly, no problem. Sit down, feed yourself the information in this chapter again, and milk it for all it's worth. You'll be up to speed in no time.

Complications of the postpartum period

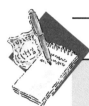

Just the facts

In this chapter, you'll learn:

♦ major complications that can occur during the postpartum period, including risk factors for each

♦ ways to identify complications based on key assessment findings

♦ treatments that are appropriate for each complication

♦ appropriate nursing interventions for each complication.

A look at postpartum complications

Although the postpartum period is a time of many physiologic and psychological changes and stressors, these changes are usually considered good changes—not unhealthy. During this time, the mother, the neonate, and other family members interact and grow as a family.

A cluster of complications

However, complications can develop due to a wide range of factors, such as blood loss, trauma, infection, or fatigue. Some common postpartum complications include postpartum hemorrhage, puerperal infection, mastitis, and deep vein thrombosis (DVT). Your keen nursing skills can help to prevent problems or detect them early before they cause more stress or seriously interfere with the parent-child relationship.

> It isn't that complicated. Postpartum complications can occur for a number of reasons.

Postpartum hemorrhage

Postpartum hemorrhage — any blood loss from the uterus that exceeds 500 ml during a 24-hour period — is the major cause of maternal mortality. The danger of postpartum hemorrhage is greatest during the first hour after birth. During this time, the placenta has detached, leaving the highly vascular yet denuded uterus widely exposed. The risk continues to be high for 24 hours after birth.

After vaginal birth, blood loss of up to 500 ml is considered acceptable, although this amount may vary among health care facilities. The acceptable range for blood loss after cesarean birth is usually between 1,000 and 1,200 ml.

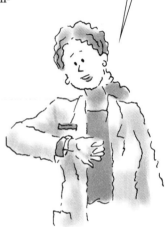

The patient is in greatest danger of postpartum hemorrhage during the first hour after birth.

Complicating the matter

A patient who has a birth complicated by any of these factors should be observed for the possibility of developing a postpartum hemorrhage:
- abruptio placentae
- missed abortion
- placenta previa
- uterine infection
- placenta accreta
- uterine inversion
- severe preeclampsia
- amniotic fluid embolism
- intrauterine fetal death.

What a difference a day makes

Postpartum hemorrhage is classified as early or late, depending on when it occurs. *Early postpartum hemorrhage* is blood loss in excess of 500 ml that occurs during the first 24 hours postpartum. *Late postpartum hemorrhage* is uterine blood loss in excess of 500 ml that occurs during the remaining 6-week postpartum period but after the first 24 hours.

What causes it

Uterine atony, lacerations, retained placenta or placental fragments, and disseminated intravascular coagulation (DIC) are the most common causes of postpartum hemorrhage.

Relax — don't do it!

The primary cause of postpartum hemorrhage, especially early postpartum hemorrhage, is uterine atony (uterine relaxation).

Relaxation is risky

Risk factors for uterine atony include:
- multiple pregnancy
- polyhydramnios
- delivery of a macrosomic neonate, usually more than 9 lb (4.1 kg)
- use of magnesium sulfate during labor
- multifetal pregnancy
- delivery that was rapid or required operative techniques, such as forceps or vacuum suction
- injury to the cervix or birth canal, such as from trauma, lacerations, or hematoma development
- use of oxytocin to initiate or augment labor or prolonged use of tocolytic agents
- dystocia (dysfunctional labor)
- previous history of postpartum hemorrhage
- use of deep analgesia or anesthesia
- infection, such as chorioamnionitis or endometritis.

> When the uterus relaxes, meaning it fails to contract properly, blood loss can occur. It's the primary cause of postpartum hemorrhage.

When the uterus doesn't contract properly, vessels at the placental site remain open, allowing blood loss. Any condition that interferes with the ability of the uterus to contract can lead to uterine atony and, subsequently, postpartum hemorrhage. (See *Relaxation is risky.*)

Blame it on lacerations

Lacerations of the cervix, birth canal, or perineum can also lead to postpartum hemorrhage. Cervical lacerations may result in profuse bleeding if the uterine artery is torn. This type of hemorrhage usually occurs immediately after delivery of the placenta, while the patient is still in the delivery area. Suspect lacerations when bleeding persists but the uterus is firm.

Stuck on you

Entrapment of a partially or completely separated placenta by an hourglass-shaped uterine constriction ring (a condition that prevents the entire placenta from expelling) can cause placental fragments to be retained in the uterus. Poor separation of the placenta is common in preterm births of usually 20 to 24 weeks' gestation.

The reason for abnormal adherence is unknown but it may result from the implantation of the zygote in an area of defective en-

etrium. This abnormal implantation leaves a zone of separa-
between the placenta and the decidua. If the fragment is
, bleeding may be apparent in the early postpartum period. If
ragment is small, however, bleeding may go unnoticed for
several days, after which time the woman suddenly has a large
amount of bloody vaginal discharge.

To clot or not to clot

DIC is a fourth cause of postpartum hemorrhage. Any woman is at
risk for DIC after childbirth. However, it's more common in
women with abruptio placentae, missed abortion, placenta previa,
uterine infection, placenta accreta, uterine inversion, severe
preeclampsia, amniotic fluid embolism, or intrauterine fetal death.

What to look for

Bleeding is the key assessment finding for postpartum hemorrhage. It can occur suddenly in large amounts or over time, as
seeping or oozing of blood. Expect a patient with postpartum hemorrhage to saturate perineal pads more quickly than usual.

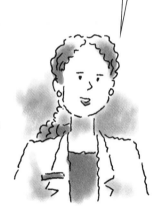

Bleeding is the key assessment finding for postpartum hemorrhage.

Soft and boggy

When uterine atony is the cause, the uterus feels soft and relaxed. The bladder may be distended, displacing the uterus to the
right or left side of midline and preventing it from contracting
properly. The fundus may also be pushed upward.

A cut above

When a laceration is the cause of postpartum hemorrhage, you
may notice bright-red blood with clots oozing continuously from
the site and a uterus that remains firm.

Left behind

Bleeding caused by a retained placenta or placental fragments
usually starts as a slow trickle, oozing, or frank hemorrhage. In
the case of retained placental fragments, also expect to find the
uterus soft and noncontracting.

The fourth culprit: DIC

When the patient's bleeding is continuous and uterine atony, lacerations, and retained placenta or fragments have been ruled out,
coagulation problems may be the cause of the bleeding.

The shocking truth

If blood loss is sufficient, the patient exhibits signs and symptoms
of hypovolemic shock, such as increasing restlessness, light-

headedness, and dizziness as cerebral tissue perfusion decreases. Inspection may also reveal pale skin, decreased sensorium, and rapid, shallow respirations. Urine output usually falls below 25 ml/hour. Palpation may disclose rapid, thready peripheral pulses and cool skin that becomes cold and clammy.

Auscultation of blood pressure usually detects a mean arterial pressure below 60 mm Hg and a narrowing pulse pressure. Capillary refill at the nail beds is delayed 3 to 5 seconds.

What tests tell you

Diagnostic testing reveals a decrease in hemoglobin level and hematocrit. The patient's hemoglobin level typically decreases 1 to 1.5 g/dl and hematocrit drops 2% to 4% from baseline. If the patient has retained placental fragments, you may also find that serum human chorionic gonadotropin levels are elevated.

Coagulating the matter

When DIC is the cause of postpartum hemorrhage, platelet and fibrinogen levels are decreased and clotting times (prothrombin time [PT] and partial thromboplastin time [PTT]) are prolonged. Blood tests also reveal decreased fibrinogen levels and fragmented red blood cells (RBCs). Fibrinolysis increases and then decreases. Coagulation factors are decreased, with decreased antithrombin III, an increased D-dimer test, and a normal or prolonged euglobulin lysis time.

How it's treated

Treatment of postpartum hemorrhage focuses on correcting the underlying cause and instituting measures to control blood loss and to minimize the extent of hypovolemic shock.

Pump up the tone

For the patient with uterine atony, initiate uterine massage. The goal is to increase uterine tone and contractility to minimize blood loss. If clots are present, they should be expressed. If the patient's bladder is distended, she should try to empty her bladder because a distended bladder prevents the uterus from fully contracting. If these efforts are ineffective or fail to maintain the uterus in a contracted state, oxytocin (Pitocin) or methylergonovine (Methergine) may be given I.M. or I.V. to produce sustained uterine contractions. Prostaglandins (Carboprost Tromethamine) can also be given I.M. to promote strong, sustained uterine contractions.

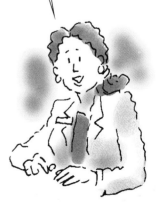

Treatment of postpartum hemorrhage focuses on correction of the underlying cause.

Source search

If the uterus is firm and contracted and the bladder isn't distended, the source of the bleeding must still be identified. Perform visual or manual inspection of the perineum, vagina, uterus, cervix, and rectum. A laceration requires sutures. If a hematoma is found, treatment may involve observation, cold therapy, ligation of the bleeding vessel, or evacuation of the hematoma. Depending on the extent of fluid loss, replacement therapy may be indicated.

Remove the stragglers

Retained placental fragments typically are removed manually or, if manual extraction is unsuccessful, via dilation and curettage (D&C). If the placenta is adhered to the uterine wall or has implanted into the myometrium, a hysterectomy may need to be performed to stop uterine bleeding.

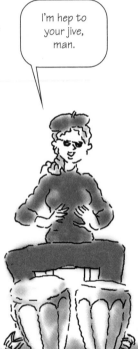

I'm hep to your jive, man.

Supportive to specific

Successful management of DIC requires prompt recognition and adequate treatment of the underlying disorder. Treatment may be supportive (for example, when the underlying disorder is self-limiting) or highly specific. If the patient isn't actively bleeding, supportive care alone may reverse DIC. Active bleeding may require administration of blood, fresh-frozen plasma, platelets, or packed RBCs to support hemostasis.

Heparin (Hep-loc) therapy for DIC is controversial. It may be used early in the disease to prevent microclotting but may be considered a last resort in the patient who's actively bleeding. If thrombosis occurs, heparin therapy is usually mandatory. In most cases, it's administered in combination with transfusion therapy.

Making up for lost fluids

Emergency treatment relies on prompt and adequate blood and fluid replacement to restore intravascular volume and to raise blood pressure and maintain it above 60 mm Hg. Rapid infusion of normal saline or lactated Ringer's solution and, possibly, albumin or other plasma expanders may be needed to expand volume adequately until whole blood can be matched.

What to do

Close, frequent assessment is crucial to prevent complications or allow early identification and prompt intervention should hemorrhage occur.

Here are other steps you should take in case of postpartum hemorrhage:

• Assess the patient's fundus and lochia frequently to detect changes. Notify the doctor if the fundus doesn't remain contracted or if lochia increases.

• Perform fundal massage, as indicated, to assist with uterine involution. Stay with the patient, frequently reassessing the fundus to ensure that it remains firm and contracted. Keep in mind that the uterus may relax quickly when massage is completed, placing the patient at risk for continued hemorrhage.

• If you suspect postpartum hemorrhage, weigh perineal pads to estimate blood loss. (See *One to one.*)

• Turn the patient onto her side and inspect under the buttocks for pooling of blood. If necessary, weigh disposable bed linen pads and add this to the weight of the perineal pads to more accurately assess blood loss.

• Inspect the perineal area closely for oozing from possible lacerations.

• Monitor vital signs frequently for changes, noting trends such as a continuously rising pulse rate and a drop in blood pressure. Report changes immediately. (See *Managing low blood pressure*, page 458.)

• Assess intake and output, and report urine output less than 30 ml/hour. Encourage the patient to void frequently to prevent bladder distention from interfering with uterine involution. If she can't void, you may need to insert an indwelling urinary catheter.

A shocking development

Here are the steps you should take if the patient develops signs and symptoms of hypovolemic shock:

Advice from the experts

One to one

When weighing perineal pads to assess for postpartum hemorrhage, use this rule of thumb:

1 g of weight is approximately equal to 1 ml of fluid.

To ensure accuracy, always weigh the dry perineal pad first and then subtract this amount from the weight of the soiled perineal pad to determine the correct weight. For example, suppose a dry perineal pad weighs 10 g and a soiled perineal pad weighs 300 g. The actual weight of the soiled pad would be 290 g, which equals 290 ml of blood loss.

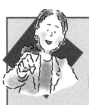

Take charge!

Managing low blood pressure

If the patient's systolic blood pressure drops below 80 mm Hg, increase the oxygen flow rate and notify the doctor immediately. Systolic blood pressure below 80 mm Hg usually results in inadequate coronary artery blood flow, cardiac ischemia, arrhythmias, and further complications of low cardiac output.

Another ominous sign
Notify the doctor and increase the infusion rate if the patient has a progressive drop in blood pressure (30 mm Hg or less from baseline) accompanied by a thready pulse. This usually signals inadequate cardiac output from reduced intravascular volume. Assess the patient's level of consciousness. As cerebral hypoxia increases, the patient becomes more restless and confused.

• Begin an I.V. infusion with normal saline solution or lactated Ringer's solution delivered through a large-bore (14G to 18G) catheter. Assist with insertion of a central venous line and a pulmonary artery catheter for hemodynamic monitoring.
• Administer colloids (albumin) and blood products, as ordered.
• Monitor the patient for fluid overload.
• Monitor for signs and symptoms of infection, such as increased temperature, foul smelling lochia, or redness and swelling of the incision.
• Record blood pressure, pulse and respiratory rates, and peripheral pulse rates every 15 minutes until stable.
• Monitor cardiac rhythm continuously.
• Monitor the patient's central venous pressure, right atrial pressure, pulmonary artery pressure, pulmonary artery wedge pressure, and cardiac output at least hourly or as ordered.
• During therapy, assess skin color and temperature and note any changes. Cold, clammy skin may signal continuing peripheral vascular constriction and progressive shock.
• Monitor capillary refill and skin turgor.
• Watch for signs of impending coagulopathy, such as petechiae, bruising, and bleeding or oozing from gums or venipuncture sites.
• Anticipate the need for fluid replacement and blood component therapy, as ordered.
• Obtain arterial blood samples to measure arterial blood gas (ABG) levels. Administer oxygen by nasal cannula, face mask, or airway to ensure adequate tissue oxygenation. Adjust the oxygen flow rate as ABG measurements indicate.

If the patient develops hypovolemic shock, begin an I.V. infusion of normal saline or lactated Ringer's solution.

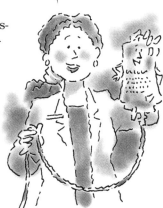

- Obtain venous blood specimens as ordered for a complete blood count, electrolyte measurements, typing and crossmatching, and coagulation studies.
- If the patient has received I.V. oxytocin for treatment of uterine atony, continue to assess the fundus closely. The action of oxytocin, although immediate, is short in duration, so atony may recur. Monitor for nausea and vomiting.
- Monitor the patient for hypertension if methylergonovine is administered.
- If the doctor orders I.M. administration of prostaglandin, be alert for possible adverse effects, such as nausea, diarrhea, tachycardia, headache, fever, and hypertension.
- Provide emotional support to the patient, and explain all procedures to help alleviate fear and anxiety.
- Monitor the patient's level of consciousness (LOC) for signs of hypoxia (decreased LOC).
- Prepare the patient for possible treatments, such as bimanual massage, surgical repair of lacerations, or D&C.

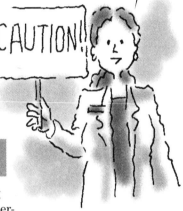

If prostaglandin is administered, watch for such adverse effects as diarrhea, tachycardia, fever, and hypertension.

Puerperal infection

Infection during the puerperal period (immediately following childbirth) is a common cause of childbirth-related death. Puerperal infection affects the uterus and structures above it with a characteristic fever pattern. It can result in endometritis, parametritis, pelvic and femoral thrombophlebitis, and peritonitis.

In the United States, puerperal infection develops in about 6% of maternity patients. The prognosis is good in these cases with treatment. There are also certain precautions you can take to prevent puerperal infection. (See *Preventing puerperal infection,* page 460.)

What causes it

Microorganisms that commonly cause puerperal infection include group A, B, or G hemolytic streptococcus, *Gardnerella vaginalis, Chlamydia trachomatis,* and coagulase-negative staphylococci. Less common causative agents are *Clostridium perfringens, Bacteroides fragilis,* Klebsiella, *Proteus mirabilis,* Pseudomonas, *Staphylococcus aureus,* and *Escherichia coli.*

> ## Preventing puerperal infection
>
> Here are some steps that you can take to help prevent puerperal infection in your postpartum patient:
> - Adhere to standard precautions at all times.
> - Maintain aseptic technique when assisting with or performing a vaginal examination. Limit the number of vaginal examinations performed during labor. Wash your hands thoroughly after each patient contact.
> - Instruct all pregnant patients to call their doctors immediately when their membranes rupture. Warn them to avoid intercourse after rupture of or leakage from the amniotic sac.
> - Keep the episiotomy site clean, and teach the patient how to maintain good perineal hygiene.
> - Screen personnel and visitors to keep people with active infections away from maternity patients.

Normal unless predisposed

Most of these organisms are considered normal vaginal flora. However, they can cause puerperal infection in the presence of the following predisposing factors:
- prolonged (more than 24 hours) or premature rupture of the membranes
- prolonged (more than 24 hours) or difficult labor, allowing bacteria to enter while the fetus is still in utero
- frequent or unsterile vaginal examinations or unsterile delivery
- delivery requiring the use of instruments, which may traumatize the tissue, providing an entry portal for microorganisms
- internal fetal monitoring, which may introduce organisms when electrodes are placed
- retained products of conception (such as placental fragments), which cause tissue necrosis and provide an excellent medium for bacterial growth
- hemorrhage, which weakens the patient's overall defenses
- maternal conditions, such as anemia, diabetes mellitus, immunosuppression, or debilitation from malnutrition, that lower the woman's ability to defend against microorganism invasion
- cesarean birth (places patient at 20-fold increase risk for puerperal infection)
- existence of localized vaginal infection or other type of infection at delivery, which allows direct transmission of infection
- bladder catheterization
- episiotomy or lacerations

I was considered normal before I got in with the wrong crowd.

- epidural anesthesia
- history of urinary tract infection
- pneumonia
- venous thrombosis.

What to look for

A characteristic sign of puerperal infection is fever (at least 100.4° F [38° C]) that occurs during the first 10 days postpartum (except during the first 24 hours) and lasts for 2 consecutive days. The fever can spike as high as 105° F (40.6° C) and is commonly accompanied by chills, headache, malaise, restlessness, and anxiety.

Care to accompany me?

Accompanying signs and symptoms depend on the extent and site of infection and may include:
- *localized perineal infection* — pain, elevated temperature, edema, redness, firmness, and tenderness at the wound site; sensation of heat; burning on urination; discharge from the wound; or separation of the wound
- *endometritis* — heavy, sometimes foul-smelling lochia; tender, enlarged uterus; backache; severe uterine contractions persisting after childbirth; fever greater than 100.4° F; chills; and increased pulse rate
- *parametritis (pelvic cellulitis)* — vaginal tenderness and abdominal pain and tenderness (pain may become more intense as infection spreads).

Spreading far and wide

The inflammation may remain localized, may lead to abscess formation, or may spread through the blood or lymphatic system. Widespread inflammation may cause these conditions, signs, and symptoms:
- *septic pelvic thrombophlebitis* — severe, repeated chills and dramatic swings in body temperature; lower abdominal or flank pain; and, possibly, a palpable tender mass over the affected area, which usually develops near the second postpartum week
- *peritonitis* — rigid, boardlike abdomen with guarding (usually the first sign); elevated body temperature; tachycardia (greater than 140 beats/minute); weak pulse; hiccups; nausea; vomiting; diarrhea; and constant, possibly excruciating, abdominal pain.

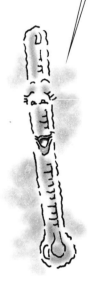

A fever of at least 100.4° F that lasts for 48 hours is a characteristic sign of puerperal infection.

What tests tell you

Development of the typical clinical features — especially fever for 48 hours or more after the first postpartum day — suggests a diagnosis of puerperal infection. Uterine tenderness is also highly suggestive. Typical clinical features usually suffice for a diagnosis of endometritis and peritonitis. In parametritis, pelvic examination shows induration without purulent discharge.

You're so cultured

A culture of lochia, incisional exudate (from cesarean incision or episiotomy), uterine tissue, or material collected from the vaginal cuff that reveals the causative organism may help confirm the diagnosis. However, such cultures are generally contaminated with vaginal flora and aren't considered helpful. A sensitivity test is also done to determine if the proper antibiotic has been administered.

White cell uprising

Normal white blood cell (WBC) count during pregnancy is 5,000 to 15,000 µl. WBCs can increase to 30,000 µl during labor due to the stress response and decreases after recovery. A sudden increase of 30% above the baseline WBC count over a 6-hour period or the presence of bands in the differential WBC count is a sign of infection after birth. Erythrocyte sedimentation rate may also be elevated.

How it's treated

Treatment of puerperal infection usually begins with I.V. infusion of a broad-spectrum antibiotic. This controls the infection and prevents its spread while you await culture results. After identifying the infecting organism, the doctor may prescribe a more specific antibiotic. (An oral antibiotic may be prescribed after discharge.)

Ancillary measures include analgesics for pain, antiseptics for local lesions, and antiemetics for nausea and vomiting from peritonitis.

Stick to the standards

A mother with a contagious disease is usually placed in a private room and should be isolated, even from her neonate. Some hospitals allow the neonate to stay in the room with the mother, while others place the neonate in an isolette before it returns to the nursery to keep it isolated from the other neonates.

If the mother isn't contagious, she doesn't need to be in isolation but you should follow standard precautions. Follow the

Memory jogger

To help you remember what to look for when assessing an episiotomy site or a laceration, think REEDA:

Redness

Erythema and Ecchymosis

Edema

Drainage or Discharge

Approximation (of wound edges).

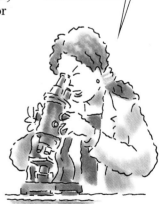

A culture may help confirm puerperal infection if it isn't contaminated with vaginal flora.

guidelines of the Centers for Disease Control and Prevention and your facility to determine whether isolation precautions are necessary.

A break from breast-feeding?

Whether the mother can continue breast-feeding, if applicable, depends on the type of antibiotic she's receiving and her physical ability to breast-feed. A mother can't breast-feed if she's receiving metronidazole (Flagyl) or acyclovir (Zovirax). If she plans to breast-feed after her course of antibiotics, help her to pump her breasts and discard the breast milk produced while she's on the medication.

Support, surgery, and drugs

Supportive care includes bed rest, adequate fluid intake, I.V. fluids when necessary, and measures to reduce fever. Surgery may also be necessary to remove remaining products of conception or retained placental fragments or to drain local lesions such as an abscess in parametritis.

If the patient develops septic pelvic thrombophlebitis, treatment consists of heparin anticoagulation for about 10 days in conjunction with broad-spectrum antibiotic therapy.

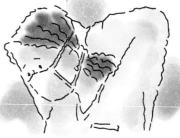

Be sure to follow standard precautions even if your patient isn't contagious.

What to do

If your postpartum patient develops an infection, perform these interventions:
- Monitor vital signs every 4 hours (or more frequently depending on the patient's condition).
- If the patient has a wound, place her in a high Fowler's to semi-Fowler's position to promote drainage.
- Assess capillary refill and skin turgor as well as mucous membranes.
- Assess intake and output closely.
- Enforce strict bed rest.
- Provide a high-calorie, high-protein diet to promote wound healing.
- Provide fluids (3,000 to 4,000 ml), unless otherwise contraindicated.
- Encourage the patient to void frequently, which empties the bladder and helps to prevent infection.
- Inspect the perineum often. Assess the fundus and palpate for tenderness (subinvolution may indicate endometritis). Note the amount, color, and odor of vaginal drainage and document your observations.

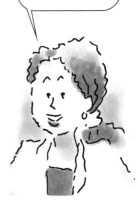

Prevention is best, but prompt treatment runs a close second.

- Encourage the patient to change perineal pads frequently, removing them from front to back. Help her change pads, if necessary. Be sure to wear gloves when helping the patient change a perineal pad.
- Administer antibiotics and analgesics, as ordered. Assess and document the type, degree, and location of pain as well as the patient's response to analgesics. Give the patient an antiemetic to relieve nausea and vomiting, as needed.
- Provide sitz baths or warm or cool compresses for local lesions, as ordered.
- Change bed linens, perineal pads, and underpads frequently.
- Provide warm blankets and keep the patient warm.
- Thoroughly explain all procedures to the patient and her family. Offer reassurance and emotional support.
- If the mother is separated from her neonate, reassure her often about his progress. Encourage the father to reassure the mother about the neonate's condition as well.

Mastitis

Mastitis is a parenchymatous inflammation of the mammary glands that disrupts normal lactation. It occurs postpartum in about 1% of women, mainly in primiparas who are breast-feeding. It occurs only occasionally in nonlactating females. The prognosis for a woman with mastitis is good.

What causes it

Mastitis develops when a pathogen — usually from the nursing neonate's nose or pharynx — invades breast tissue through a fissured or cracked nipple. The pathogen that most commonly causes mastitis is *Staphylococcus aureus;* less frequently, *Staphylococcus epidermidis* and beta-hemolytic streptococci are the culprits. Rarely, mastitis may result from disseminated tuberculosis or the mumps virus.

Predisposing factors include a fissure or abrasion on the nipple, blocked milk ducts, and an incomplete let-down reflex, usually due to emotional trauma. Blocked milk ducts can result from wearing a tight-fitting bra or waiting prolonged intervals between breast-feedings.

What to look for

Mastitis may develop anytime during lactation, but it usually begins 1 to 4 weeks postpartum with fever (101° F [38.3° C], or higher in acute mastitis), chills, malaise, and flulike symptoms. Mastitis is generally unilateral and localized but, in some cases, both breasts or the entire breast is affected.

Inspection and palpation may uncover redness, swelling, warmth, hardness, tenderness, nipple cracks or fissures, and enlarged axillary lymph nodes. Unless mastitis is treated adequately, it may progress to breast abscess.

Which kind is it?

Mastitis must be differentiated from normal breast engorgement, which generally starts with the onset of lactation (day 2 to day 5 postpartum). During this time, the breasts undergo changes similar to those in mastitis and body temperature may also be elevated.

Engorgement may be mild, causing only slight discomfort, or severe, causing considerable pain. A severely engorged breast can prevent a neonate from feeding properly because he can't latch on to the nipple of the swollen, rigid breast.

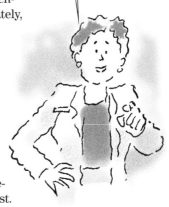

If mastitis isn't treated adequately and promptly, it can progress to breast abscess.

What tests tell you

Cultures of expressed breast milk are used to confirm generalized mastitis; cultures of breast skin are used to confirm localized mastitis. These cultures are also used to determine antibiotic therapy. Differential diagnosis should exclude breast engorgement, breast abscess, viral syndrome, and a clogged duct.

How it's treated

Antibiotic therapy, the primary treatment for mastitis, generally consists of oral cephalosporins or either cloxacillin (Cloxapen) or dicloxacillin (Dynapen) to combat staphylococcus. Azithromycin (Zithromax) or vancomycin (Vancocin) may be used for patients who are allergic to penicillin. Although symptoms usually subside 2 to 3 days after treatment begins, antibiotic therapy should continue for 10 days.

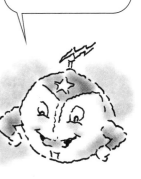

Antibiotics to the rescue! Antibiotic therapy is the primary treatment for mastitis.

Other appropriate measures include analgesics for pain and, on the rare occasions when antibiotics fail to control the infection and mastitis progresses to breast abscess, incision and drainage of the abscess.

What to do

Here's what you should do to treat a patient with mastitis:
• Explain mastitis to the patient and why infection control measures are necessary.
• Establish infection control measures for the mother and neonate to prevent the spread of infection to other nursing mothers.
• Obtain a complete patient history, including a drug history, especially allergy to penicillin.
• Administer antibiotic therapy, as ordered.
• Assess and record the cause and amount of discomfort. Give analgesics, as needed.
• Reassure the mother that breast-feeding during mastitis won't harm her neonate because he's the source of the infection.
• Tell the mother to offer the neonate the affected breast first to promote complete emptying and prevent clogged ducts. However, if an open abscess develops, she must stop breast-feeding with this breast and use a breast pump until the abscess heals. She should continue to breast-feed on the unaffected side.
• Suggest applying a warm, wet towel to the affected breast or taking a warm shower to relax and improve her ability to breast-feed. Cold compresses may also be used to relieve discomfort.
• Advise the patient to wear a supportive bra.
• Provide good skin care.
• Show the patient how to position the neonate properly to prevent cracked or sore nipples.
• Tell the patient to empty her breasts as completely as possible with each feeding.
• Tell the patient to get plenty of rest and drink sufficient fluids to help combat fever.

An ounce of prevention

Before your breast-feeding patient leaves the hospital, teach her about breast care and how to prevent mastitis. (See *Preventing mastitis.*)

Education edge

Preventing mastitis

With today's shortened hospital stays for childbirth, postpartum teaching is more important than ever. If your patient is breast-feeding, be sure to include these instructions about breast care and preventing mastitis in your teaching plan:
• Wash your hands after using the bathroom, before touching your breasts, and before and after every breast-feeding.
• If necessary, apply a warm compress or take a warm shower to help facilitate milk flow.
• Position the neonate properly at the breast, and make sure that he grasps the nipple and entire areola area when feeding.
• Empty your breasts as completely as possible at each feeding.
• Alternate feeding positions and rotate pressure areas.
• Release the neonate's grasp on the nipple before removing him from the breast.
• Expose your nipples to the air for part of each day.
• Drink plenty of fluids, eat a balanced diet, and get sufficient rest to enhance the breast-feeding experience.
• Don't wait too long between feedings or wean the infant abruptly.

Deep vein thrombosis

DVT, also called *deep vein thrombophlebitis*, is an inflammation of the lining of a blood vessel that occurs in conjunction with clot formation. It typically occurs at the valve cusps because venous stasis encourages the accumulation and adherence of platelets and fibrin.

Thrombophlebitis usually begins with localized inflammation (phlebitis), but this rapidly provokes thrombus formation. Rarely, venous thrombosis develops without associated inflammation of the vein (phlebothrombosis).

Any vein will do

DVT can affect small veins, such as the lesser saphenous vein, or large veins, such as the iliac, femoral, pelvic, and popliteal veins and the vena cava. It's more serious than superficial vein thrombophlebitis because it affects the veins deep in the leg musculature that carry 90% of the venous outflow from the leg.

What causes it

DVT may be idiopathic, but it's more likely to occur along with certain diseases, treatments, injuries, or other factors. In the postpartum woman, DVT most commonly results from an extension of endometritis.

Risky business

Risk factors for developing DVT in the postpartum period include:
- history of varicose veins
- obesity
- previous DVT
- multiple gestations
- increased age (older than age 30)
- family history of DVT
- smoking
- cesarean birth
- multiparity.

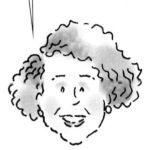

Being older than age 30 increases my risk of developing DVT during the postpartum period.

Compounding the risk

These risk factors are compounded by specific occurrences during labor and delivery. For example, blood clotting increases postpartally as a result of elevated fibrinogen levels. Also, pressure from the fetal head during pregnancy and delivery causes veins in the lower extremities to dilate, leading to venous stasis. Finally, lying in the lithotomy position for a long time with the lower extremities in stirrups promotes venous pooling and stasis.

Bad news x 2

During the postpartum period, two major types of DVT may occur: femoral or pelvic. Pelvic DVT runs a long course, usually 6 to 8 weeks. (See *Comparing femoral and pelvic DVT.*)

What to look for

The signs and symptoms for femoral and pelvic DVT differ, but both types require careful assessment.

Femoral DVT

With femoral thrombophlebitis, the patient's temperature increases around the 10th day postpartum. Other signs and symptoms include malaise; chills; and pain, stiffness, or swelling in a leg or in the groin.

With leg swelling, the affected extremity appears reddened or inflamed, edematous below the level of the obstruction, and possi-

Comparing femoral and pelvic DVT

The table below outlines the major differences between femoral and pelvic deep vein thrombosis (DVT), including the vessels affected, time of onset, assessment findings, and treatment.

Characteristic	Femoral DVT	Pelvic DVT
Vessels affected	• Femoral • Saphenous • Popliteal	• Ovarian • Uterine • Hypogastric
Onset	Approximately 10th day postpartum	Approximately 14th to 15th day postpartum
Assessment findings	• Associated arterial spasm, making leg appear milky-white or drained • Edema • Fever • Malaise • Diminished peripheral pulses • Positive Homans' sign • Chills • Pain • Redness and stiffness of affected leg • Shiny white skin on extremity	• Extremely high fever • Chills • General malaise • Possible pelvic abscess
Treatment	• Bed rest • Elevation of affected extremity • Never massaging affected area • Anticoagulants • Moist heat applications • Analgesics	• Complete bed rest • Anticoagulants • Antibiotics • Incision and drainage if abscess develops

bly shiny and white. This white appearance may be related to an accompanying arterial spasm, which results in a decrease in arterial circulation to the area. When measured, the thigh and calf of the affected leg are typically larger than the unaffected extremity.

Man, Homan oh man!

Pain may occur in the calf of the affected leg when the foot is dorsiflexed. This finding — called a positive Homans' sign — suggests DVT but isn't a reliable indicator. Even if the patient is negative for Homans' sign, the possibility of an obstruction can't be ruled out. Always elicit Homans' sign passively; active dorsiflexion could lead to embolization of a clot.

What's your sign?

A positive Rielander's sign (palpable veins inside the thigh and calf) or Payr's sign (calf pain when pressure is applied on the inside of the foot) also suggests femoral DVT.

Pelvic DVT

The patient with pelvic DVT appears acutely ill with a sudden onset of a high fever, severe repeated chills, and general malaise. In most cases, body temperature fluctuates widely. The patient may complain of lower abdominal or flank pain, and you may be able to palpate a tender mass over the affected area

What tests tell you

Diagnosis of DVT is based on these characteristic test findings:
* *Doppler ultrasonography* identifies reduced blood flow to a specific area and obstruction to venous flow, particularly in iliofemoral DVT
* More sensitive than ultrasonography in detecting DVT, *plethysmography* shows decreased circulation distal to the affected area.
* *Venography* usually confirms the diagnosis and shows filling defects and diverted blood flow.

How it's treated

Treatment for DVT includes bed rest, with elevation of the affected arm or leg; application of warm, moist compresses; and administration of analgesics, antibiotics, and anticoagulants. After the acute episode subsides, the patient may begin to ambulate while wearing antiembolism stockings (applied before she gets out of bed).

Bring on the meds

Drug therapy typically includes anticoagulants to prolong clotting time, starting with heparin for 5 to 7 days and then changing to another anticoagulant, such as warfarin (Coumadin), for 3 months.

For lysis of acute, extensive DVT, treatment should include streptokinase if the risk of bleeding doesn't outweigh the potential benefits of thrombolytic treatment.

Kicking the treatment up a notch

Rarely, DVT may cause complete venous occlusion, which requires venous interruption through simple ligation, vein plication, or clipping. Embolectomy may be done if clots are being shed to

Education edge

Preventing DVT

Incorporate the instructions below in your teaching plan to reduce a woman's risk of developing deep vein thrombosis (DVT):

• Check with your doctor about using a side-lying or back-lying (supine recumbent) position for birth instead of the lithotomy position (on your back with your legs in stirrups). These alternative positions reduce the risk of blood pooling in the lower extremities.

• If you must use the lithotomy position for birth, ask a health care provider to pad the stirrups well so that you put less pressure on your calves.

• Change positions frequently if on bed rest.

• Avoid deeply flexing your legs at the groin or sharply flexing your knees.

• Don't stand in one place for too long or sit with your knees bent or legs crossed. Elevate your legs slightly to improve venous return.

• Don't wear garters or constrictive clothing.

• Wiggle your toes and perform leg lifts while in bed to minimize venous pooling and help increase venous return.

• Walk as soon as possible after birth.

• Wear antiembolism or support stockings as ordered. Put them on before getting out of bed in the morning.

the pulmonary and systemic vasculature and other treatments are unsuccessful.

Caval interruption with transvenous placement of an umbrella filter can trap emboli, preventing them from traveling to the pulmonary vasculature. If the patient develops a pulmonary embolism, heparin may be initiated until the embolism resolves; then subcutaneous heparin or an oral anticoagulant may be continued for 6 months.

Pelvic DVT in particular

In addition, treatment for pelvic DVT focuses on complete bed rest and administration of antibiotics along with anticoagulants. If the patient develops a pelvic abscess, a laparotomy for incision and drainage may be done. Because this procedure may cause tubal scarring and may interfere with fertility, the patient may need additional surgery later to remove the vessel before becoming pregnant again.

What to do

Prevention of DVT is key. Assess the patient for risk factors, and teach her ways to reduce her risk. (See *Preventing DVT.*)

In addition, because postpartal DVT commonly results from an endometrial infection:
- be alert to signs and symptoms of endometritis
- notify the doctor if signs and symptoms of endometritis occur
- institute treatment promptly, as ordered.

Fighting back

To combat DVT, take the following measures:
- Enforce bed rest as ordered, and elevate the patient's affected arm or leg. If you use pillows for elevation of a leg, place the pillows so that they support its entire length to avoid compressing the popliteal space.
- Apply warm compresses or a covered aquathermia pad to increase circulation to the affected area and to relieve pain and inflammation.
- Give analgesics to relieve pain as ordered.
- Assess uterine involution and note any changes in fundal consistency such as the inability to remain firm or contracted
- Monitor vital signs closely, at least every 4 hours or more frequently if indicated. Report changes in pulse rate or blood pressure as well as temperature elevations.
- Administer I.V. anticoagulants as ordered, using an infusion monitor or pump to control the flow rate, if necessary. Have an anticoagulant antidote, such as protamine sulfate (for heparin therapy), readily available.
- Because neither heparin nor warfarin is excreted in significant amounts in breast milk, breast-feeding is allowed.
- If the mother is hospitalized, have her pump her breast milk for the neonate.
- Administer antibiotic and antipyretic therapy for the patient with pelvic DVT.
- Mark, measure, and record the circumference of the affected extremity at least once daily, and compare it to the other extremity. To ensure accuracy and consistency of serial measurements, mark the skin over the area and measure at the same spot daily.
- Obtain coagulation studies, such as International Normalized Ratio (INR), PTT, and PT, as ordered. Keep in mind that therapeutic anticoagulation values usually are considered to be 1½ to 2 times the control value; INR should be between 2 and 3.5.

I'm knocking out DVT!

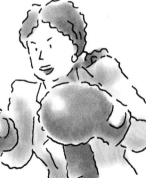

On the lookout for lochia

- Monitor the patient for increased amounts of lochia. Encourage her to change perineal pads frequently, and weigh the pads to estimate the amount of blood loss.

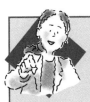

Take charge!

Dealing with pulmonary embolism

A woman with deep vein thrombosis is at high risk for developing a pulmonary embolism. Be alert for the classic signs and symptoms of pulmonary embolism, such as:
• chest pain
• dyspnea
• tachypnea
• tachycardia
• hemoptysis
• sudden changes in mental status
• hypotension.

Also, be vigilant in monitoring for the following problems, which may occur along with the classic signs and symptoms:
• chills
• fever
• abdominal pain
• signs and symptoms of respiratory distress, including tachypnea, tachycardia, restlessness, cold and clammy skin, cyanosis, and retractions.

Nip it in the bud

A pulmonary embolism is a life-threatening event that can lead to cardiovascular collapse and death. You should intervene at once if pulmonary embolism is suspected. Follow these steps:
• Elevate the head of the bed to improve the work of breathing.
• Administer oxygen via face mask at 8 to 10 L per minute, as ordered.
• Begin I.V. fluid administration, as ordered.
• Monitor oxygen saturation rates continuously via pulse oximetry.
• Obtain arterial blood gas samples for analysis as ordered to evaluate gas exchange

• Assess vital signs frequently, as often as every 15 minutes.
• Anticipate the need for continuous cardiac monitoring to evaluate for arrhythmias secondary to hypoxemia and for insertion of a pulmonary artery catheter to evaluate hemodynamic status and gas exchange
• Administer emergency drugs, such as dopamine (Intropin) for pressure support and morphine (Duramorph) for analgesia, as ordered
• Expect the patient to be transferred to the critical care unit
• Administer analgesics without aspirin for pain relief
• Administer anticoagulants or thrombolytics, as ordered.

• Watch for signs and symptoms of bleeding, such as tarry stools, coffee-ground vomitus, and ecchymoses. Note oozing of blood at I.V. sites, and assess gums for excessive bleeding. Report positive findings to the doctor immediately.
• Assess the patient for signs and symptoms of pulmonary emboli, such as crackles, dyspnea, hemoptysis, sudden changes in mental status, restlessness, and hypotension. (See *Dealing with pulmonary embolism*.)
• Provide emotional support to the woman and her family, and explain all procedures and treatments.
• Prepare the patient for surgery, if indicated.
• Emphasize the importance of follow-up blood studies to monitor anticoagulant therapy.
• If the patient is discharged on heparin therapy, teach her or a family member how to give subcutaneous injections. If additional

assistance is required, arrange for a home health care referral and follow-up.

• Teach the patient how to properly apply and use antiembolism stockings. Tell her to report any complications, such as toes that are cold or blue.

• To prevent bleeding, encourage the patient to avoid medications that contain aspirin and to check with the doctor before using any over-the-counter medications. Teach the patient the signs and symptoms of bleeding, such as easy bruising or blood in the urine or stool.

• Tell her to use a soft toothbrush and an electric razor to prevent tissue damage and bleeding.

• Advise her to use contraception because oral anticoagulants are teratogenic.

• Tell the patient not to increase her vitamin K intake while taking oral anticoagulants because vitamin K counteracts the anticoagulant effects.

• Stress that the patient should report her history of DVT to the doctor if she becomes pregnant again so that preventative measures can be started early.

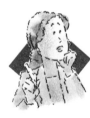

Quick quiz

1. What is considered the major cause of early postpartum hemorrhage?

    A.   Uterine atony
    B.   Perineal laceration
    C.   Retained placental fragments
    D.   DIC

Answer: A. Although all of the above complications are possible causes of postpartum hemorrhage, uterine atony (relaxation of the uterus) is considered the primary and most common cause of early postpartum hemorrhage.

2. If a patient's perineal pad weighs 100 g, you would estimate the blood loss as:

    A.   50 ml.
    B.   100 ml.
    C.   150 ml.
    D.   200 ml.

Answer: B. One gram of weight is approximately equivalent to 1 ml of fluid. Therefore, the blood loss estimate for a perineal pad weighing 100 g would be approximately 100 ml.

3. Which finding would lead you to suspect that a woman has developed hypovolemic shock secondary to postpartum hemorrhage?
    A.   Respiratory rate of 22 breaths/minute
    B.   Pale-pink, moist skin
    C.   Urine output below 25 ml/hour
    D.   Bounding peripheral pulses

Answer: C. A urine output below 25 ml/hour suggests hypovolemic shock secondary to decreased renal perfusion. Other findings include rapid and shallow respirations; pale, cold, clammy skin; rapid, thready peripheral pulses; mean arterial pressure below 60 mm Hg; and narrowed pulse pressure.

4. Which factor predisposes a patient to a puerperal infection?
    A.   External fetal monitoring during labor
    B.   Rupture of membranes 15 hours ago
    C.   Labor lasting 20 hours
    D.   Cesarean birth

Answer: D. A cesarean birth increases a woman's risk for puerperal infection by as much as 20 times. The use of internal fetal monitoring, prolonged (more than 24 hours) or premature rupture of membranes, and prolonged (more than 24 hours) or difficult labor also increase the risk for puerperal infection.

5. A patient reports foul-smelling lochia with strong uterine contractions persisting after birth. Her temperature has been elevated, ranging from 102.2° (39° C) to 104° F (40° C), for the past 2 days. Her uterus is firm but tender, and her abdomen is soft with no guarding noted. You would suspect:
    A.   localized perineal infection.
    B.   peritonitis.
    C.   endometritis.
    D.   parametritis.

Answer: C. Endometritis may cause heavy, foul-smelling lochia; a tender, enlarged uterus; backache; severe uterine contractions that persist after childbirth; and elevated temperature for 2 or more days after the first 24 hours.

6. Which microorganism most commonly causes mastitis?
    A.   *Staphylococcus aureus*
    B.   *Staphylococcus epidermis*
    C.   Beta hemolytic streptococcus
    D.   Mumps virus

Answer: A. Although all are possible causative organisms, Staphylococcus aureus is the most common. Mastitis caused by the mumps virus is rare.

7. If your patient has DVT, for which complication should you watch?

    A.   Endometritis
    B.   Pulmonary embolism
    C.   Hematoma
    D.   Mastitis

Answer: B. A possible life threatening complication of DVT, pulmonary embolism occurs when the clot breaks off and travels to the pulmonary vascular bed, interfering with gas exchange.

Scoring

☆☆☆ If you answered all seven questions correctly, awesome, dude! You're a favorite for next year's Complications Cup.

☆☆ If you answered five or six questions correctly, right on! You've retained a significant number of fragments from the chapter and are ready to move on to chapter 11.

☆ If you answered fewer than five questions correctly, no worries. A little more studying and you'll be competing with the big boys.

Assessment and care of the neonate

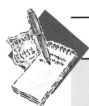

Just the facts

In this chapter, you'll learn:

♦ changes that occur in the neonate after birth

♦ the proper way to perform a neonatal assessment

♦ nursing interventions critical to neonatal care.

Adapting to extrauterine life

After birth, a neonate must quickly adapt to extrauterine life, even though many of the neonate's body systems are still developing. During this time of adaptation, the nurse must be aware of normal neonatal physiologic characteristics and assessment findings in order to detect possible problems and initiate appropriate interventions. (See *Physiology of the neonate*, page 478.)

Respiratory system

The major adaptation for the neonate is that he must breathe on his own rather than depend on fetal circulation. At birth, air is substituted for the fluid that filled the neonate's respiratory tract in the alveoli during gestation. In a normal vaginal delivery, some of this fluid is squeezed out during birth. After delivery, the fluid is absorbed across the alveolar membrane into the capillaries.

At first breath

The onset of the neonate's breathing is stimulated by several factors:
• low blood oxygen levels
• increased blood carbon dioxide levels
• low blood pH
• temperature change from the warm uterine environment to the cooler extrauterine environment.

Physiology of the neonate

This chart provides a summary of the physiologic characteristics of a neonate after birth, including adaptations the neonate must make to cope with extrauterine life.

Body system	Physiology after birth
Cardiovascular	• Functional closure of fetal shunts occurs. • Transition from fetal to postnatal circulation occurs.
Respiratory	• Onset of breathing occurs as air replaces the fluid that filled the lungs before birth.
Renal	• System doesn't mature fully until after the first year of life; fluid imbalances may occur.
Gastrointestinal	• System continues to develop. • Uncoordinated peristalsis of the esophagus occurs. • The neonate has a limited ability to digest fats.
Thermogenic	• The neonate is more susceptible to rapid heat loss due to acute change in environment and thin layer of subcutaneous fat. • Nonshivering thermogenesis occurs. • The presence of brown fat (more in mature neonate; less in premature neonate) warms the neonate by increasing heat production.
Immune	• The inflammatory response of the tissues to localize infection is immature.
Hematopoietic	• Coagulation time is prolonged.
Neurologic	• Presence of primitive reflexes and time in which they appear and disappear indicate the maturity of the developing nervous system.
Hepatic	• The neonate may demonstrate jaundice.
Integumentary	• The epidermis and dermis are thin and bound loosely to each other. • Sebaceous glands are active.
Musculoskeletal	• More cartilage is present than ossified bone.
Reproductive	• Females may have a mucoid vaginal discharge and pseudomenstruation due to maternal estrogen levels. • In males, testes descend into the scrotum. • Small, white, firm cysts called *epithelial pearls* may be visible at the tip of the prepuce. • Genitals may be edematous if the neonate presented in breech position.

Noise, light, and other sensations related to the birth process may also influence the neonate's initial breathing.

Delicate and developing

Although the neonate can breathe on his own, his respiratory system isn't as developed as an adult's system. The neonate is an obligatory nose breather. In addition, the neonate has a relatively large tongue whereas the trachea and glottis are small.

Other significant differences between a neonate's respiratory system and an adult's system include:
- airway lumens that are narrower and collapse more easily
- respiratory tract secretions that are more abundant
- mucous membranes that are more delicate and susceptible to trauma
- alveoli that are more sensitive to pressure changes
- capillary network that's less developed
- rib cage and respiratory musculature that are less developed.

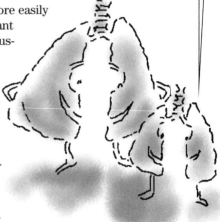

My mucous membranes are more susceptible to trauma than yours.

Cardiovascular system

The neonate's first breath triggers the start of several cardiopulmonary changes that help him transition from fetal circulation to postnatal circulation. During this transition, the foramen ovale, ductus arteriosis, and ductus venosus close. These closures allow blood to start flowing to the lungs.

Ovale to no avail

When the neonate takes his first breath, the lungs inflate. When the lungs are inflated, pulmonary vascular resistance to blood flow is reduced and pulmonary artery pressure drops. Pressure in the right atrium decreases, and the increased blood flow to the left side of the heart increases the pressure in the left atrium. This change in pressure causes the foramen ovale (the fetal shunt between the left and right atria) to close. Increased blood oxygen levels then influence other fetal shunts to close.

From ducts to ligaments

The ductus arteriosus, located between the aorta and pulmonary artery, eventually closes and becomes a ligament. The ductus venosus, between the left umbilical vein and the inferior vena cava, closes because of vasoconstriction and lack of blood flow; then it also becomes a ligament. The umbilical arteries and vein and the hepatic arteries also constrict and become ligaments.

Renal system

After birth, the renal system is called into action because the neonate can no longer depend on the placenta to excrete waste products. However, the renal system function doesn't fully mature until after the first year, which means that the neonate is at risk for chemical imbalances. The neonate's limited ability to excrete drugs because of renal immaturity, coupled with excessive neonatal fluid loss, can rapidly lead to acidosis and fluid imbalances.

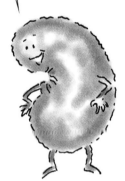

> Because the neonate's renal system hasn't fully matured yet, the neonate can easily develop acidosis and fluid imbalances.

Gastrointestinal system

At birth, the neonate's GI system isn't fully developed because normal bacteria aren't present in the digestive tract. The lower intestine contains meconium, which usually starts to pass within 24 hours. It appears greenish black and viscous.

Ongoing developments

As the GI system starts to develop, these characteristics appear:
• audible bowel sounds 1 hour after birth
• uncoordinated peristaltic activity in the esophagus for the first few days of life
• limited ability to digest fats because amylase and lipase are absent at birth
• frequent regurgitation because of an immature cardiac sphincter.

Thermogenic system

Among the many adaptations that occur after birth, the neonate must regulate his body temperature by producing and conserving heat. This can be difficult for the neonate because he has a thin layer of subcutaneous fat and his blood vessels are closer to the surface of the skin. In addition, the neonate's vasomotor control is less developed, his body surface area to weight ratio is high, and his sweat glands have minimal thermogenic function until he's age 4 weeks or older.

Where's the heat?

The neonate's body also has to work against four routes of heat loss:

 convection—the flow of heat from the body to cooler air

radiation—the loss of body heat to cooler, solid surfaces in close proximity of (but not in direct contact with) the neonate

evaporation—heat loss that occurs when liquid is converted to a vapor

conduction—the loss of body heat to cooler substances in direct contact with the neonate.

Warming things up

To maintain body temperature, the neonate must produce heat through a process called *nonshivering thermogenesis*. This involves an increase in the neonate's metabolism and oxygen consumption. Thermogenesis mainly occurs in the heart, liver, and brain. Brown fat (brown adipose tissue) is another source of thermogenesis that's unique to the neonate.

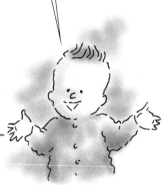

Thermogenesis is the production of heat. It helps me maintain my body temperature.

Immune system

The neonatal immune system depends largely on three immunoglobulins: immunoglobulin (Ig) A, IgG, and IgM.

Fighting infection with shear numbers

IgG (which can be detected in the fetus at 3 months' gestation) is an immunoglobulin consisting of bacterial and viral antibodies. It's the most abundant immunoglobulin and is found in all body fluids. In utero, IgG crosses from the placenta to the fetus. After birth, the neonate produces his own IgG during the first 3 months while the leftover maternal antibodies in the neonate break down.

The enforcer of bacterial growth

IgA, an immunoglobulin that limits bacterial growth in the GI tract, is produced gradually. Maximum levels of IgA are reached during childhood. The neonate obtains IgA from maternal colostrum and breast milk.

First responder

IgM, found in blood and lymph fluid, is the first immunoglobulin to respond to infection. It's produced at birth, and by age 9 months the IgM level in the neonate reaches the level found in adults.

Still in training

Even though these immunoglobulins are present in the neonate, the inflammatory response of the tissues to localized infection is still immature. All neonates, especially those born prematurely, are at high risk for infection during the first several months of life.

Hematopoietic system

In the neonatal hematopoietic system, blood volume accounts for 80 to 85 ml/kg of body weight. Immediately after birth, the neonatal blood volume averages 300 ml; however, it can drop as low as 100 ml depending on how long the neonate remains attached to the placenta via the umbilical cord. In addition, neonatal blood has a prolonged coagulation time because of decreased levels of vitamin K.

Neurologic system

The neurologic system at birth isn't completely integrated, but it's developed enough to sustain extrauterine life. Most functions of this system are primitive reflexes. The full-term neonate's neurologic system should produce equal strength and symmetry in responses and reflexes. Diminished or absent reflexes may indicate a serious neurologic problem, and asymmetrical responses may indicate that trauma, such as nerve damage, paralysis, or fracture, occurred during birth.

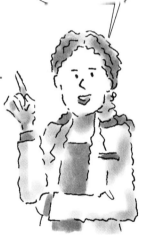

Most functions of the neonate's neurologic system are primitive reflexes.

Hepatic system

Jaundice (yellowing of the skin) is a major concern in the neonatal hepatic system. It's caused by hyperbilirubinemia, a condition that occurs when serum levels of unconjugated bilirubin increase because of increased red blood cell lysis, altered bilirubin conjugation, or increased bilirubin reabsorption from the GI tract.

A mellow yellow

Jaundice resulting from physiologic hyperbilirubinemia occurs in 50% of full-term neonates and 80% of preterm neonates. It's a mild form of jaundice that appears after the first 24 hours of extrauterine life and usually disappears in 7 days (9 or 10 days in preterm neonates). However, if bilirubin levels rise, pathologic conditions such as kernicterus may develop.

Shades of an underlying condition

Jaundice resulting from pathologic hyperbilirubinemia is evident at birth or within the first 24 hours of extrauterine life. It may be caused by hemolytic disease, liver disease, or severe infection. Prognosis varies depending on the cause.

Education edge

Protecting neonates from the sun

Neonates are more susceptible to the harmful effects of the sun because the amount of melanin (pigment) in the skin is low at birth. Teach parents the importance of avoiding sun exposure by giving them these tips:

• Keep a hat with a visor on the neonate when outside.

• Make sure that the hood of the stroller covers the neonate.

• Use a blanket to shade the neonate from the sun when necessary.

• Be especially careful in the car. Sun roofs and windows may expose the neonate to too much sun. Use commercially available window shades and visors.

Integumentary system

At birth, all of the structures of the integumentary system are present, but many of their functions are immature. The epidermis and dermis are bound loosely to each other and are very thin. In addition, the sebaceous glands are very active in early infancy because of maternal hormones. (See *Protecting neonates from the sun.*)

Musculoskeletal system

At birth, the skeletal system contains more cartilage than ossified bone. The process of ossification occurs very rapidly during the first year of life. The muscular system is almost completely formed at birth.

Reproductive system

The ovaries of the female neonate contain thousands of primitive germ cells. These germ cells represent the full potential for ova. The number of ova decreases from birth to maturity by about 90%. After birth, the uterus undergoes involution and decreases in size and weight because, in utero, the fetal uterus enlarges from the effects of maternal hormones.

For 90% of male neonates, the testes descend into the scrotum after birth. However, spermatogenesis doesn't occur until puberty.

At birth, the skeletal system contains more cartilage than ossified bone.

Neonatal assessment

Neonatal assessment includes initial and ongoing assessments, a head-to-toe physical examination, and neurologic and behavioral assessments.

Initial assessment

The initial neonatal assessment involves draining secretions, assessing abnormalities, and keeping accurate records. To complete an initial assessment, follow these steps:
• For infection control purposes, all caregivers should wear gloves when assessing or caring for a neonate until after his initial bath.
• Ensure a proper airway by suctioning, and administer oxygen as needed.
• Dry the neonate under the warmer while keeping his head lower than his trunk (to promote the drainage of secretions)
• Apply a cord clamp, and monitor the neonate for abnormal bleeding from the cord; check the number of cord vessels.
• Observe the neonate for voiding and meconium; document the first void and stools.
• Assess the neonate for gross abnormalities and clinical manifestations of suspected abnormalities.
• Continue to assess the neonate by using the Apgar score criteria even after the 5-minute score is received.
• Obtain clear footprints and fingerprints. (In some facilities, the neonate's footprints are kept on a record that also includes the mother's fingerprints.)
• Apply identification bands with matching numbers to the mother (one band) and the neonate (two bands) before they leave the delivery room. Some facilities also give the father or significant other an identification band.
• Promote bonding between the mother and the neonate by putting the neonate to the mother's breast or having the mother and neonate engage in skin to skin contact.

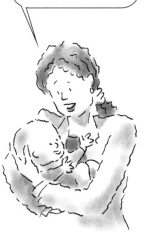

Skin to skin contact helps promote bonding between the mother and neonate.

Apgar scoring

During the initial examination of a neonate, expect to calculate an Apgar score and make general observations about the neonate's appearance and behavior. Developed by anesthesiologist Dr. Virginia Apgar in 1952, Apgar scoring evaluates neonatal heart rate, respiratory effort, muscle tone, reflex irritability, and color. Evaluation of each category is performed 1 minute after birth and again

Recording the Apgar score

Use this chart to determine the neonatal Apgar score at 1 minute and 5 minute intervals after birth. For each category listed, assign a score of 0 to 2, as shown. A total score of 7 to 10 indicates that the neonate is in good condition; 4 to 6, fair condition (the neonate may have moderate central nervous system depression, muscle flaccidity, cyanosis, and poor respirations); 0 to 3, danger (the neonate needs immediate resuscitation, as ordered).

Sign	Apgar score		
	0	1	2
Heart rate	Absent	Less than 100 beats/minute	More than 100 beats/minute
Respiratory effort	Absent	Slow, irregular	Good crying
Muscle tone	Flaccid	Some flexion and resistance to extension of extremities	Active motion
Reflex irritability	No response	Grimace or weak cry	Vigorous cry
Color	Pallor, cyanosis	Pink body, blue extremities	Completely pink

at 5 minutes after birth. Each item has a maximum score of 2 and a minimum score of 0. The final Apgar score is the sum total of the five items; a maximum score is 10.

Evaluation at 1 minute quickly indicates the neonate's initial adaptation to extrauterine life and whether resuscitation is necessary. The 5-minute score gives a more accurate picture of his overall status. (See *Recording the Apgar score*.)

First and foremost

Assess heart rate first. If the umbilical cord still pulsates, you can palpate the neonate's heart rate by placing your fingertips at the junction of the umbilical cord and the skin. The neonate's cord stump continues to pulsate for several hours and is a good, easy place (next to the abdomen) to check heart rate. You can also place two fingers or a stethoscope over the neonate's chest at the fifth intercostal space to obtain an apical pulse. For accuracy, the heart rate should be counted for 1 full minute.

Second to one

Next, check the neonate's respiratory effort, the second most important Apgar sign. Assess the neonate's cry, noting its volume

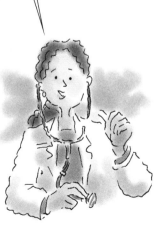

The neonate's cord stump is a good, easy place to check heart rate.

and vigor. Then auscultate his lungs, using a stethoscope. Assess his respirations for depth and regularity. If the neonate exhibits abnormal respiratory responses, begin neonatal resuscitation according to the guidelines of the American Heart Association and the American Academy of Pediatrics. Then use the Apgar score to judge the progress and success of resuscitation efforts. (See *Monitoring for effects of sedation.*)

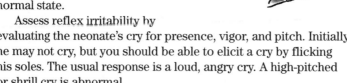

Nice volume. Love the vigor. I give you 2 points toward your total Apgar score.

Move along to the muscles

Determine muscle tone by evaluating the degree of flexion in the neonate's arms and legs and their resistance to straightening. This can be done by extending the limbs and observing their rapid return to flexion—the neonate's normal state.

Assess reflex irritability by evaluating the neonate's cry for presence, vigor, and pitch. Initially he may not cry, but you should be able to elicit a cry by flicking his soles. The usual response is a loud, angry cry. A high-pitched or shrill cry is abnormal.

Now give the Apgar some skin!

Finally, observe skin color for cyanosis. A neonate usually has a pink body with blue extremities. This condition, called *acrocyanosis*, appears in about 85% of normal neonates 1 minute after birth. Acrocyanosis results from decreased peripheral oxygenation caused by the transition from fetal to independent circulation. When assessing a nonwhite neonate, observe for color changes in the mucous membranes of the mouth, conjunctivae, lips, palms, and soles.

Gestational age and birth weight

Perinatal mortality and morbidity are related to gestational age and birth weight. Classifying a neonate by both weight and gestational age provides a more accurate method for assessing mortality risk and offers guidelines for treatment. The neonate's age and weight classifications should also be considered during future assessments.

How old are you now?

The clinical assessment of gestational age classifies a neonate as *preterm* (less than 37 weeks' gestation), *term* (37 to 42 weeks' gestation), or *postterm* (42 weeks' gestation or longer). The Ballard scoring system uses physical and neurologic findings to estimate a

Take charge!

Monitoring for effects of sedation

Closely observe a neonate whose mother has received heavy sedation just before delivery. Even if he has a high Apgar score at birth, he may exhibit secondary effects of sedation later. Be alert for respiratory depression or unresponsiveness.

neonate's gestational age within 1 week, even in extremely premature neonates. This evaluation can be done at any time between birth and 42 hours after birth, but the greatest reliability is between 30 and 42 hours after birth. (See *Ballard gestational-age assessment tool.*)

(Text continues on page 490.)

Ballard gestational-age assessment tool

To use this tool, evaluate and score the neuromuscular and physical maturity criteria, total the score, and then plot the sum in the maturity rating box to determine the neonate's corresponding gestational age.

Posture

With the neonate supine and quiet, score as follows:
- Arms and legs extended = 0
- Slight or moderate flexion of hips and knees = 1
- Moderate to strong flexion of hips and knees = 2
- Legs flexed and abducted, arms slightly flexed = 3
- Full flexion of arms and legs = 4

Square window

Flex the hand at the wrist. Measure the angle between the base of the thumb and the forearm. Score as follows:
- > 90 degrees = −1
- 90 degrees = 0
- 60 degrees = 1
- 45 degrees = 2
- 30 degrees = 3
- 0 degrees = 4

Arm recoil

With the neonate supine, fully flex the forearm for 5 seconds, then fully extend by pulling the hands and releasing. Observe and score the reaction according to this criteria:
- Remains extended 180 degrees or random movements = 0
- Minimal flexion (140 to 180 degrees) = 1
- Small amount of flexion (110 to 140 degrees) = 2
- Moderate flexion (90 to 110 degrees) = 3
- Brisk return to full flexion (< 90 degrees) = 4

Popliteal angle

With the neonate supine and the pelvis flat on the examining surface, use one hand to flex the leg and then the thigh. Then use the other hand to extend the leg. Score the angle attained:
- 180 degrees = −1
- 160 degrees = 0
- 140 degrees = 1
- 120 degrees = 2
- 100 degrees = 3
- 90 degrees = 4
- < 90 degrees = 5

Scarf sign

With the neonate supine, take his hand and draw it across the neck and as far across the opposite shoulder as possible. You may assist the elbow by lifting it across the body. Score according to the location of the elbow:
- Elbow reaches or nears level of opposite shoulder = −1
- Elbow crosses opposite anterior axillary line = 0
- Elbow reaches opposite anterior axillary line = 1
- Elbow at midline = 2
- Elbow does not reach midline = 3
- Elbow does not cross proximate axillary line = 4

Heel to ear

With the neonate supine, hold his foot with one hand and move it as near to the head as possible without forcing it. Keep the pelvis flat on the examining surface. Score as shown in the chart.

(continued)

Ballard gestational-age assessment tool *(continued)*

NEUROMUSCULAR MATURITY

Neuromuscular maturity sign	Score							Record score here
	−1	**0**	**1**	**2**	**3**	**4**	**5**	
Posture	—						—	
Square window (wrist)	>90°	90°	60°	45°	30°	0°	—	
Arm recoil	—	180°	140° to 180°	110° to 140°	90° to 100°	<90°	—	
Popliteal angle	180°	160°	140°	120°	100°	90°	<90°	
Scarf sign							—	
Heel to ear							—	

Total neuromuscular maturity score [ ]

Ballard gestational-age assessment tool (continued)

PHYSICAL MATURITY

Physical maturity sign	Score							Record score here
	−1	**0**	**1**	**2**	**3**	**4**	**5**	
Skin	Sticky, friable, transparent	Gelatinous, red, translucent	Smooth, pink; visible vessels	Superficial peeling or rash; few visible vessels	Cracking; pale areas; rare visible vessels	Parchment-like; deep cracking; no visible vessels	Leathery, cracked, wrinkled	
Lanugo	None	Sparse	Abundant	Thinning	Bald areas	Mostly bald	—	
Plantar surface	Heel-to-toe 40 to 50 mm: −1; < 40 mm: −2	> 50 mm; no crease	Faint red marks	Anterior transverse crease only	Creases over anterior two-thirds	Creases over entire sole	—	
Breast	Imperceptible	Barely perceptible	Flat areola; no bud	Stippled areola; 1- to 2-mm bud	Raised areola; 3- to 4-mm bud	Full areola; 5- to 10-mm bud	—	
Eye and ear	Lids fused, loosely: −1; tightly: −2	Lids open; pinna flat, stays folded	Slightly curved pinna; soft, slow, recoil	Well-curved pinna; soft but ready recoil	Formed and firm; instant recoil	Thick cartilage; ear stiff	—	
Genitalia (male)	Scrotum flat, smooth	Scrotum empty; faint rugae	Testes in upper canal; rare rugae	Testes descending; few rugae	Testes down; good rugae	Testes pendulous; deep rugae	—	
Genitalia (female)	Clitoris prominent; labia flat	Prominent clitoris; small labia minora	Prominent clitoris; enlarging minora	Majora and minora equally prominent	Majora large; minora small	Majora cover clitoris and minora	—	

Total physical maturity score

(continued)

Ballard gestational-age assessment tool *(continued)*

SCORE *Neuromuscular:* _____ *Physical:* _____ Total maturity score: _____	Total maturity score	−10	−5	0	5	10	15	20	25	30	35	40	45	50
	Gestational age (weeks)	20	22	24	26	28	30	32	34	36	38	40	42	44

GESTATIONAL AGE (Weeks)
By dates: _____
By ultrasound: _____
By score: _____

Adapted with permission from Ballard, J.L., et al. "New Ballad Score, expanded to include extremely premature infants," *Journal of Pediatrics* 119(3):417-23, 1991. Used with permission from Mosby–Year Book, Inc.

Too small, too big, just right

Normal birth weight is 2,500 g (5 lb, 8 oz) or greater. A neonate is considered to have a low birth weight if he weighs between 1,500 g (3 lb, 5 oz) and 2,499 g. A neonate of very low birth weight ranges between 1,000 g (2 lb, 3 oz) and 1,499 g. A neonate weighing less than 1,000 g has an extremely low birth weight.

Postnatal growth charts are used to assess the neonate based on head circumference, weight, length, and gestational age. Neonates who are small for gestational age have a birth weight less than the 10th percentile on postnatal growth charts; weight appropriate for gestational age signifies a birth weight within the 10th and 90th percentiles; and weight large for gestational age means a birth weight greater than the 90th percentile. (See *Caring for a preterm neonate*.)

Ongoing assessment

Ongoing neonatal physical assessment includes observing and recording vital signs and administering prescribed medications. To perform ongoing assessment, follow these steps:
- Assess the neonate's vital signs.
- Measure and record the neonate's vital statistics.
- Administer prescribed medications such as vitamin K (AquaME-PHYTON), which is a prophylactic to the transient deficiency of coagulation factors II, VII, IX, and X.
- Administer erythromycin ointment (Ilotycin), the drug of choice for neonatal eye prophylaxis, to prevent damage and blindness

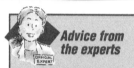
Advice from the experts

Caring for a preterm neonate

When caring for a preterm neonate, be alert for problems — even if the neonate is of average size. A preterm neonate who's an appropriate weight for his gestational age is more prone to respiratory distress syndrome, apnea, patent ductus arteriosus with left-to-right shunt, and infection. A preterm neonate who's small for his gestational age is more likely to experience asphyxia, hypoglycemia, and hypocalcemia.

Reviewing normal neonatal vital signs

The list below includes the normal ranges for neonatal vital signs.

Respiration
- 30 to 50 breaths/minute

Heart rate (apical)
- 110 to 160 beats/minute

Temperature
- Rectal: 96° to 99.5° F (35.6° to 37.5° C)
- Axillary: 97.5° to 99° F (36.4° to 37.2° C)

Blood pressure
- Systolic: 60 to 80 mm Hg
- Diastolic: 40 to 50 mm Hg

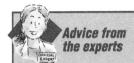

Advice from the experts

Counting neonatal respirations

When counting a neonate's respiratory rate, observe abdominal excursions rather than chest excursions. Auscultation of the chest or placing the stethoscope in front of the mouth and nares are other ways to count respirations.

from conjunctivitis caused by *Neisseria gonorrhoeae* and *Chlamydia*; treatment is required by law.
- Perform laboratory tests.
- Monitor glucose levels and hematocrit (test results aid in assessing for hypoglycemia and anemia).

Vital signs

Measuring vital signs establishes the baseline of any neonatal assessment. Vital signs include the respiratory rate, heart rate (taken apically), and the first neonatal temperature (this is taken rectally to verify rectal patency). Subsequent temperature readings are axillary to avoid injuring the rectal mucosa. Blood pressure readings may be assessed by sphygmomanometer or by palpation or auscultation. An electronic vital signs monitor may be used. (See *Reviewing normal neonatal vital signs*.)

Determining respiratory rate

Observe respirations first, before the neonate becomes active or agitated. Watch and count respiratory movements for 1 minute and record the result. A normal respiratory rate is usually between 30 and 50 breaths/minute. Also, note any signs of respiratory distress, such as cyanosis, tachypnea, sternal retractions, grunting, nasal flaring, or periods of apnea. Short periods of apnea (less than 15 seconds) are characteristic of the neonate. (See *Counting neonatal respirations*.)

Assessing heart rate

Use a pediatric stethoscope to determine the neonate's apical heart rate. Place the stethoscope over the apical impulse on the fourth or fifth intercostal space at the left midclavicular line over the cardiac apex. To ensure an accurate measurement, count the beats for 1 minute. A normal heart rate ranges from 110 to 160 beats/minute. Variations during sleeping and waking states are normal.

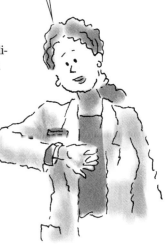

To ensure an accurate measurement when assessing the neonate's heart rate, count beats for 1 minute.

Taking a rectal temperature

The technique for taking a rectal temperature in a neonate is relatively simple. With the neonate lying in a supine position, place a diaper over the penis (if applicable) and firmly grasp his ankles with your index finger between them. Then insert a lubricated thermometer into the rectum, no more than ½″ (1.3 cm). Place your palm on his buttocks, and hold the thermometer between your index and middle fingers. If resistance is met while inserting the thermometer, withdraw the thermometer and notify the doctor.

Hold it

Hold a mercury thermometer in place for 3 minutes and an electronic thermometer in place until the temperature registers. Remove the thermometer and record the result.

Body temperature in neonates is less constant than in adults and can fluctuate during the course of a day, without reason. The normal range for a rectal temperature is 96° to 99.5° F (35.6° to 37.5° C).

Taking an axillary temperature

To take an axillary temperature, make sure that the axillary skin is dry. Place the thermometer in the axilla and hold it along the outer aspect of the neonate's chest between the axillary line and the arm. Hold the thermometer in place until the temperature registers. Normal axillary temperature is 97.5° to 99° F (36.4° to 37.2° C).

Reassess axillary temperature in 15 to 30 minutes if the first measurement registers outside the normal range. If the temperature remains abnormal, notify the doctor.

The low-down on low temperatures

Decreased temperatures by either the rectal or axillary route could suggest:
• prematurity
• infection
• low environmental temperature
• inadequate clothing
• dehydration.

Why it may be high

Possible reasons for increased temperatures include:
- infection
- high environmental temperature
- excessive clothing
- proximity to heating unit or direct sunlight
- drug addiction
- diarrhea and dehydration.

Determining blood pressure

If possible, measure a neonate's blood pressure when he's in a quiet or relaxed state. Make sure that the blood pressure cuff is small enough for the neonate (cuff width should be about one-half the circumference of the neonate's arm). Then wrap the cuff one or two fingerbreadths above the antecubital or popliteal area. With the stethoscope held directly over the chosen artery, hold the cuffed extremity firmly to keep it extended and inflate the cuff no faster than 5 mm Hg/second.

Normal systolic readings are 60 to 80 mm Hg and normal diastolic readings are 40 to 50 mm Hg. A drop in systolic blood pressure (about 15 mm Hg) during the first hour after birth is common. Crying and movement result in blood pressure changes.

From top to bottom

Compare blood pressures in the upper and lower extremities at least once to detect abnormalities. Remember that blood pressure readings from the thigh will be approximately 10 mm Hg higher than the arm. If the blood pressure reading in the thigh is the same or lower than the arm, notify the doctor. This could indicate coarctation of the aorta, a congenital heart defect, and should be investigated further.

Size and weight

Size and weight measurements establish the baseline for monitoring growth. Size and weight measurements can also be used to detect such disorders as failure to thrive and hydrocephalus. (See *Average neonatal size and weight,* page 494.)

Measuring head circumference

Head circumference reflects the rate of growth of the head and its contents. To measure head circumference, slide the tape measure under the neonate's head at the occiput and draw the tape around snugly, just above the eyebrows. Normal neonatal head circumference is 13″ to 14″ (33 to 35.5 cm). Cranial molding or caput succedaneum from a vaginal delivery may affect this measurement.

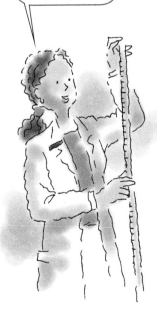

Head circumference should be about 1″ (2.5 cm) larger than chest circumference.

Average neonatal size and weight

In addition to weight, anthropometric measurements include head and chest circumferences and head-to-heel length. These measurements serve as a baseline and show whether neonatal size is within normal ranges or whether there may be a significant problem or anomaly—especially if values stray far from the mean.

Average initial anthropometric ranges are:

- head circumference—13″ to 14″ (33 to 35.5 cm)
- chest circumference—12″ to 13″ (30.5 to 33 cm)
- head to heel—18″ to 21″ (46 to 53 cm)
- weight—2,500 to 4,000 g (5 lb, 8 oz to 8 lb, 13 oz).

Head circumference

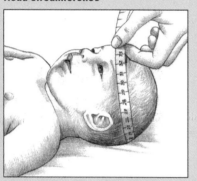

Chest circumference

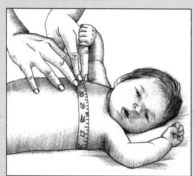

Head-to-heel length

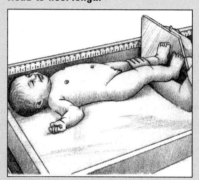

Measuring chest circumference

Measure chest circumference by placing the tape under the back, wrapping it snugly around the chest at the nipple line, and keeping the back and front of the tape level. Take the measurement after the neonate inspires and before he begins to exhale. Normal neonatal chest circumference is 12″ to 13″ (30.5 to 33 cm).

Measuring head-to-heel length

Fully extend the neonate's legs with the toes pointing up. Measure the distance from the heel to the top of the head. A length board may be used, if available. Normal length is 18″ to 21″ (46 to 53 cm).

Weighing the neonate

A neonate should be weighed before a feeding and the scale should be balanced. Remove the diaper and place the neonate in the middle of the scale tray. Keep one hand poised over the neonate at all times. Average weight is 2,500 to 4,000 g (5 lb, 8 oz to 8 lb, 13 oz).

Return the neonate to the crib or examination table. Be sure to document if the neonate had any clothing or equipment on him (such as an I.V.). Take the neonate's weight at the same time each day, if possible. Be careful to prevent heat loss.

Head-to-toe assessment

The neonate should receive a thorough physical examination of each body part. However, before each body part is examined, assess the general appearance and posture of the neonate. Neonates usually lie in a symmetrical, flexed position — the characteristic "fetal position" — as a result of their position while in utero.

Skin

The term neonate has beefy red skin for a few hours after birth. Then the skin turns to its normal color. It commonly appears mottled or blotchy, especially on the extremities.

Findings can be skin deep

Common findings in a neonatal assessment may include:
• acrocyanosis (caused by vasomotor instability, capillary stasis, and high hemoglobin level) for the first 24 hours after birth
• milia (clogged sebaceous glands) on the nose or chin
• lanugo (fine, downy hair) appearing after 20 weeks of gestation on the entire body, except the palms and soles
• vernix caseosa (a white, cheesy protective coating composed of desquamated epithelial cells and sebum)
• erythema toxicum neonatorum (a transient, maculopapular rash)
• telangiectasia (flat, reddened vascular areas) appearing on the neck, upper eyelid, or upper lip
• port-wine stain (nevus flammeus), a capillary angioma located below the dermis and commonly found on the face
• strawberry hemangioma (nevus vasculosus), a capillary angioma located in the dermal and subdermal skin layers indicated by a rough, raised, sharply demarcated birthmark
• sudamina or miliaria (distended sweat glands), which cause minute vesicles on the skin surface, especially on the face
• Mongolian spots, bluish black areas of pigmentation more commonly noted on the back and buttocks of dark-skinned neonates (regardless of race).

Make general observations about the appearance of the neonate's skin in relationship to his activity, position, and temperature. Usually, the neonate is redder when crying or hot. He may also have transient episodes of cyanosis with crying. Cutis marmorata is transient mottling when the neonate is exposed to cooler temperatures.

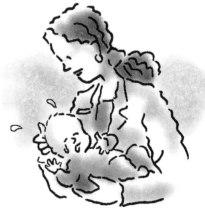

A crying neonate's skin may be redder than normal or temporarily appear cyanotic.

Roll with it, baby

Palpate the skin to assess skin turgor. To do this, roll a fold of skin on the neonate's abdomen between your thumb and forefinger. Assess consistency, amount of subcutaneous tissue, and degree of hydration. A well-hydrated infant's skin returns to normal immediately upon release.

Head

The neonate's head is about one-fourth of its body size. Six bones make up the cranium:
- the frontal bone
- the occipital bone
- two parietal bones
- two temporal bones.

Bands of connective tissue, called *sutures*, lie between the junctures of these bones. At the junction of the sutures are wider spaces of membranous tissue, called *fontanels*.

Fontanel facts

The neonatal skull has two fontanels. The *anterior fontanel* is diamond-shaped and located at the juncture of the frontal and parietal bones. It measures 1⅛″ to 1⅝″ (3 to 4 cm) long and ¾″ (2 cm) to 1⅛″ wide. The anterior fontanel closes in about 18 months. The *posterior fontanel* is triangle-shaped. It's located at the juncture of the occipital and parietal bones and measures about ¾″ across. The posterior fontanel closes in 8 to 12 weeks.

The fontanels should feel soft to touch but shouldn't be depressed. A depressed fontanel indicates dehydration. In addition, fontanels shouldn't bulge. Bulging fontanels require immediate attention because they may indicate increased intracranial pressure. Pulsations in the fontanels reflect the peripheral pulse.

Molding under the pressure

Molding refers to asymmetry of the cranial sutures due to difficulties during vaginal delivery; it isn't seen in neonates born by cesarean delivery. There are two types of cranial abnormalities:
- *Cephalhematoma* occurs when blood collects between a skull bone and the periosteum. It's caused by pressure during delivery and tends to spontaneously resolve in 3 to 6 weeks. A cephalhematoma doesn't cross cranial suture lines.
- *Caput succedaneum* is a localized edematous area of the presenting part of the scalp. It's also caused by pressure during delivery, but disappears spontaneously in 3 to 4 days and can cross cranial suture lines.

Heads up!

The degree of head control the neonate has should also be evaluated during this part of the examination. If neonates are placed down on a firm surface, they'll turn their heads to the side to maintain an open airway. They also attempt to keep their heads in line with their body when raised by their arms. Although head lag is normal in the neonate, marked head lag is seen in neonates with Down syndrome or brain damage and hypoxic infants.

Eyes

Neonates tend to keep their eyes tightly shut. Observe the lids for edema, which is normally present for the first few days of life. The eyes should also be assessed for symmetry in size and shape. Here are some common findings of neonatal eye examination:
• The neonate's eyes are usually blue or gray because of scleral thinness. Permanent eye color is established within 3 to 12 months.
• Lacrimal glands are immature at birth, resulting in tearless crying for up to 2 months.
• The neonate may demonstrate transient strabismus.
• The Doll's eye reflex (when the head is rotated laterally, the eyes deviate in the opposite direction) may persist for up to 10 days.
• Subconjunctival hemorrhages may appear from vascular tension changes during birth.
• The corneal reflex is present but generally isn't elicited unless a problem is suspected.
• The pupillary reflex and the red reflex are present.

Nose

Observe the neonate's nose for:
• shape
• placement
• patency
• bridge configuration.

Because neonates are obligatory nose breathers for the first few months of life, nasal passages must be kept clear to ensure adequate respiration. Neonates instinctively sneeze to remove obstruction. Test the patency of the nasal passages by occluding each naris alternately while holding the neonate's mouth closed. (See *Monitoring for respiratory distress*.)

Take charge!

Monitoring for respiratory distress

Nasal flaring is a serious sign of air hunger from respiratory distress. If you assess nasal flaring or seesaw respirations; pale, gray skin; periods of apnea; or bradycardia, alert the primary health care provider. These may be signs of respiratory distress syndrome.

Mouth and pharynx

The neonate's mouth usually has scant saliva and pink lips. Inspect the mouth for its existing structures. The palate is usually narrow and highly arched. Inspect the hard and soft palates for clefts.

Pearls of wisdom on pearls

Epstein's pearls (pinhead-sized, white or yellow, rounded elevations) may be found on the gums or hard palate. These are caused by retained secretions and disappear within a few weeks or months. The frenulum of the upper lip may be quite thick. Precocious teeth may also be apparent. The pharynx can be best assessed when the neonate is crying. Tonsillar tissue generally isn't visible.

Ears

Assess the neonate's ears for:
- placement on head
- amount of cartilage
- open auditory canal
- hearing.

The neonate's ears are characterized by incurving of the pinna and cartilage deposition. The pinna is usually flattened against the side of the head from pressure in utero. The top of the ear should be above or parallel to an imaginary line from the inner to the outer canthus of the eye. Low-set ears are associated with several syndromes, including chromosomal abnormalities.

Before you go

Procedures to screen for hearing in neonates have become common practice before a neonate leaves the hospital or birthing facility. Testing can detect permanent bilateral or unilateral sensory or conductive hearing loss.

Now hear this!

Auditory assessment is performed by noninvasive, objective, physiologic measures that include otoacoustic emissions or auditory brainstem response. Both testing methods are painless and can be performed while the neonate rests. If the neonate doesn't pass the screening test, the test is usually repeated at age 3 months.

Can you hear me now?

Neck

The neonate's neck is typically short and weak with deep folds of skin. Observe for:

- range of motion
- shape
- abnormal masses.

Also, palpate each clavicle and sternocleidomastoid muscle. Note the position of the trachea. The thyroid gland generally isn't palpable.

Chest

Inspect and palpate the chest, noting:
- shape
- clavicles
- ribs
- nipples
- breast tissue
- respiratory movements
- amount of cartilage in rib cage.

The neonatal chest is characterized by a cylindrical thorax (because the anteroposterior and lateral diameters are equal) and flexible ribs. Slight intercostal retractions are usually seen on inspiration. The sternum is raised and slightly rounded, and the xiphoid process is usually visible as a small protrusion at the end of the sternum.

Breast engorgement from maternal hormones may be apparent, and the secretion of "witch's milk" may occur. Supernumerary nipples may be located below and medial to the true nipples.

Lungs

Normal respirations of the neonate are abdominal with a rate between 30 and 50 breaths/minute. After the first breaths to initiate respiration, subsequent breaths should be easy and fairly regular. Occasional irregularities may occur with crying, sleeping, and feeding.

Hush little baby, don't say a word

It's easiest to auscultate the lung fields when the neonate is quiet. Bilateral bronchial breath sounds should be heard. Crackles soon after birth represent the transition of the lungs to extrauterine life.

Heart

The neonate's heart rate is normally between 110 and 160 beats/minute. Because neonates have a fast heart rate, it's difficult to auscultate the specific components of the cardiac cycle. Heart sounds during the neonatal period are generally of higher pitch, shorter duration, and greater intensity than in later life. The first

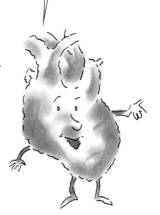

Neonates have a fast heart rate. This may make it difficult to auscultate specific components of the cardiac cycle.

sound is usually louder and duller than the second, which is sharp in quality. Murmurs are commonly heard, especially over the base of the heart or at the third or fourth intercostal space at the left sternal border, due to incomplete functional closure of the fetal shunts.

The apical impulse (point of maximal impulse) is at the fourth intercostal space and to the left of the midclavicular line.

Abdomen

Neonatal abdominal assessment should include:
- inspection and palpation of the umbilical cord
- evaluation of the size and contour of the abdomen
- auscultation of bowel sounds
- assessment of skin color
- observation of movement with respirations
- palpation of internal organs.

Stop, look, listen...

The neonatal abdomen is usually cylindrical with some protrusion. Bowel sounds are heard a few hours after birth. A scaphoid appearance indicates a diaphragmatic hernia. The umbilical cord is white and gelatinous with two arteries and one vein and begins to dry within 1 to 2 hours after delivery.

...and feel

The liver is normally palpable 1″ (2.5 cm) below the right costal margin. Sometimes the tip of the spleen can be felt, but a spleen that's palpable more than ⅓″ (1 cm) below the left costal margin warrants further investigation. Both kidneys should be palpable; this is easiest done soon after delivery, when muscle tone is lowest. The suprapubic area should be palpated for a distended bladder. The neonate should void within the first 24 hours of birth.

Femoral pulses should also be palpated at this point in the examination. Inability to palpate femoral pulses could signify coarctation of the aorta.

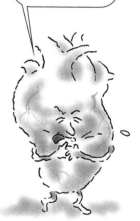

Inability to palpate femoral pulses could signify coarctation of the aorta, a congenital heart defect.

Genitalia

Characteristics of a male neonate's genitalia include rugae on the scrotum and testes descended into the scrotum. Scrotal edema may be present for several days after birth due to the effects of maternal hormones. The urinary meatus is located in one of three places:
- at the penile tip (normal)
- on the dorsal surface (epispadias)
- on the ventral surface (hypospadias).

In the female neonate, the labia majora cover the labia minora and clitoris. These structures may be prominent due to maternal hormones. Vaginal discharge may also occur and the hymenal tag is present.

Extremities

The extremities should be assessed for range of motion, symmetry, and signs of trauma. All neonates are bowlegged and have flat feet. The hips should be assessed for dislocation. Hyperflexibility of joints is characteristic of Down syndrome. Some neonates may have abnormal extremities. They may be polydactyl (more than five digits on an extremity) or syndactyl (two or more digits fused together).

Note the nails

The nailbeds should be pink, although they may appear slightly blue due to acrocyanosis. Persistent cyanosis indicates hypoxia or vasoconstriction.

Reading palms

The palms should have the usual creases. A transverse palmar crease, called a *Simian crease*, suggests Down syndrome.

Expect resistance

Assess muscle tone. Extension of any extremity is usually met with resistance and, upon release, returns to its previously flexed position.

Spine

The neonatal spine should be straight and flat, and the anus should be patent without any fissure. Dimpling at the base of the spine is commonly associated with spina bifida. The shoulders, scapulae, and iliac crests should line up in the same plane.

Neurologic assessment

An examination of the reflexes provides useful information about the neonate's nervous system and his state of neurologic maturation. Some reflexive behaviors in the neonate are necessary for survival whereas other reflexive behaviors act as safety mechanisms.

Reflex revelations

Normal neonates display several types of reflexes. Abnormalities are indicated by absence, asymmetry, persistence, or weakness in these reflexes:

- *sucking* — begins when a nipple is placed in the neonate's mouth
- *Moro's reflex* — when the neonate is lifted above the crib and suddenly lowered; the arms and legs symmetrically extend and then abduct while the fingers spread to form a "C"
- *rooting* — when the neonate's cheek is stroked, the neonate turns his head in the direction of the stroke
- *tonic neck (fencing position)* — when the neonate's head is turned while he's lying in a supine position, the extremities on the same side straighten and those on the opposite side flex
- *Babinski's reflex* — when the sole on the side of the neonate's small toe is stroked and the toes fan upward
- *grasping* — when a finger is placed in each of the neonate's hands, the neonate's fingers grasp tightly enough to be pulled to a sitting position
- *stepping* — when the neonate is held upright with the feet touching a flat surface, he responds with dancing or stepping movements
- *startle* — a loud noise such as a hand clap elicits neonatal arm abduction and elbow flexion and the neonate's hands stay clenched
- *trunk incurvature* — when a finger is run laterally down the neonate's spine, the trunk flexes and the pelvis swings toward the stimulated side
- *blinking* — the neonate's eyelids close in response to bright light
- *acoustic blinking* — both eyes of the neonate blink in response to a loud noise
- *Perez reflex* — when the neonate is suspended prone in one of the health care provider's hands and the thumb of the other hand is moved firmly up the neonate's spine from the sacrum, the neonate's head and spine extend, the knees flex, the neonate cries, and he may empty his bladder.

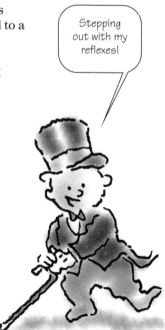

Stepping out with my reflexes!

Behavioral assessment

Behavioral characteristics are an important part of neonatal development. To assess whether a neonate is exhibiting normal behavior, be aware of the neonate's principle behaviors of sleep, wakefulness, and activity (such as crying) as well as his social capabilities and ability to adapt to certain stimuli.

Factors that affect behavioral responses include:
- gestational age
- time of day
- stimuli
- medication.

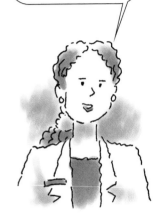

Absent, weak, or constant crying suggests neonatal brain damage.

Why cry?

The neonate should begin life with a strong cry. Variations in this initial cry can indicate abnormalities. For example, a weak, groaning cry or grunt during expiration usually signifies respiratory disturbances. Absent, weak, or constant crying suggests brain damage. A high-pitched shrill cry may be a sign of increased intracranial pressure.

Are you sleeping, are you sleeping?

Another aspect of behavioral assessment is observing the neonate's sleep-wake cycles (the variations in the neonate's consciousness). The nurse should assess how the neonate handles transitions from one state in the cycle to the next.

Six spokes in the sleep-wake cycle

Six specific sleep-activity states have been defined:
- deep sleep — regular breathing, eyes closed, no spontaneous activity
- light sleep — eyes closed, rapid eye movements (REM), random movements and startles, irregular breathing, sucking movements
- drowsy — eyes open, dull, heavy eyelids, variable activity, delayed response to stimuli
- alert — bright, seems focused, minimal motor activity
- active — eyes open, considerable motor activity, thrusting movements, briefly fussy
- crying — high motor activity.

Sleep-wake cycles are highly influenced by the environment.

Social senses

Neonates possess sensory capabilities that indicate their readiness for social interaction. An absence of these behavioral responses is cause for concern:
- sensitivity to light — a neonate opens his eyes when the lights are dim and his responses to movement are noticeable
- selective listening — a neonate tends to exhibit selective listening to his mother's voice

- response to touch—a neonate responds to touch, such as calming when touched softly, suggesting that he's ready to receive tactile messages
- taste preferences—a series of studies have demonstrated that neonates prefer sweet fluids to those that are sour or bitter
- sense of smell—studies have shown that neonates prefer pleasant smells and that they have the ability to learn and remember odors.

Filtering stimuli

Each neonate has a unique temperament and varies in his ability to handle stimuli from the external world. Through habituation, the neonate can control the type and amount of stimuli processed, which decreases his response to constant or repeated stimuli. A neonate presented with new stimuli becomes wide-eyed and alert but eventually shows decreased interest. Habituation enables the neonate to respond to select stimuli, such as human voices, that encourage continued learning about the social world.

The ability to habituate depends on the neonate's:
- state of consciousness
- hunger
- fatigue
- temperament.

Factor this in

These factors also affect behaviors:
- consolability—the ability of the neonate to console himself or be consoled
- cuddliness—the neonate's response to being held
- irritability—how easily a neonate is upset
- crying—the ability of the neonate to communicate different needs with his cry.

Neonatal care

Physical care for the neonate includes:
- protecting from infection and injury
- maintaining a patent airway
- maintaining a stable body temperature
- providing optimum nutrition.

Credé's treatment

Credé's treatment involves instilling 0.5% erythromycin ointment into the neonate's eyes. Its purpose is to prevent gonorrheal conjunctivitis caused by *Neisseria gonorrhoeae*, which the neonate may have acquired from the mother as he passed through the birth canal. Erythromycin provides the antimicrobial effects of a broad-spectrum antibiotic and is also effective against chlamydial infection.

It's the law

Credé's treatment is required by law in all 50 states. Before this treatment, gonorrheal conjunctivitis was a common cause of permanent eye damage and blindness.

Break for bonding

To perform Credé's treatment, you'll need ophthalmic antibiotic ointment as ordered and gloves. Although the drug may be administered in the birthing room, treatment can be delayed for up to 1 hour to allow initial parent-child bonding. Antibiotic prophylaxis may not be effective if the infection was acquired in utero from premature rupture of the membranes.

Credé's treatment can be delayed for up to 1 hour to allow initial parent-child bonding.

Step by step

To perform Credé's treatment, follow these steps:
- Wash your hands, and put on gloves.
- To ensure comfort and effectiveness, shield the neonate's eye's from direct light and tilt his head slightly to the side that will receive the treatment.
- Using your nondominant hand, gently raise the neonate's upper eyelid with your index finger and pull the lower eyelid down with your thumb.
- Using your dominant hand, instill the ointment into the lower conjunctival sac.
- Close and manipulate the eyelids to spread the medication over the eye.
- Repeat the procedure for the other eye.
- A single-dose ointment tube should be used to prevent contamination and the spread of infection.
- If the neonate's parents are present, explain that the procedure is required by state law. Tell them that it may temporarily irritate the neonate's eyes and make him cry but that the effects are transient. (See *Complications of Credé's treatment*.)

Complications of Credé's treatment

Complications of Credé's treatment include chemical conjunctivitis (which may cause redness, swelling, and drainage) or discoloration of the skin around the neonate's eyes. If such complications occur, reassure the parents that these temporary effects will subside within a few days.

Write it down!

Be sure to document Credé's treatment appropriately. If it's done in the delivery room, record the treatment on the delivery room form. If you perform it in the nursery, document it in your notes.

Thermoregulation

Because the neonate has a relatively large surface-to-weight ratio, reduced metabolism per unit area, and small amounts of insulating fat, he's susceptible to hypothermia. The neonate keeps warm by metabolizing brown fat, which has a greater concentration of energy-producing mitochondria in its cells, enhancing its capacity for heat production. This kind of fat is unique to neonates. Brown fat metabolism is effective, but only within a very narrow temperature range.

Without careful external thermoregulation, the neonate may become chilled, which can result in:
• hypoxia
• acidosis
• hypoglycemia
• pulmonary vasoconstriction
• death.

Keep it neutral

The object of thermoregulation is to provide a neutral thermal environment that helps the neonate maintain a normal core temperature with minimal oxygen consumption and caloric expenditure. The core temperature varies with the neonate but is about 97.7° F (36.5° C). Cold stress and its complications can be prevented with proper interventions. (See *Understanding thermoregulators*, page 507.)

To perform thermoregulation, you'll need:
• radiant warmer or incubator (if necessary)
• blankets
• washcloths or towels
• skin probe
• adhesive pad
• water-soluble lubricant
• thermometer
• clothing, including cap.

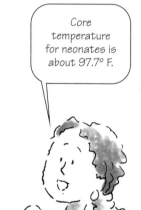

Core temperature for neonates is about 97.7° F.

While you wait

While preparing for the neonate's birth, turn on the radiant warmer in the delivery room and set it to the desired temperature. Warm the blankets, washcloths, or towels under a heat source.

(Text continues on page 507.)

The pregnant woman

As a result of hormonal activity, the breasts may double in size during pregnancy. During this time, fatty tissue is largely replaced by glandular tissue and the mammary glands become capable of secreting milk.

During the third trimester, the fundus reaches the xiphoid process. In addition, the uterus remains oval in shape. It's muscular walls become progressively thinner as it enlarges. In some women, the uterus becomes large enough that the maternal umbilicus everts and protrudes.

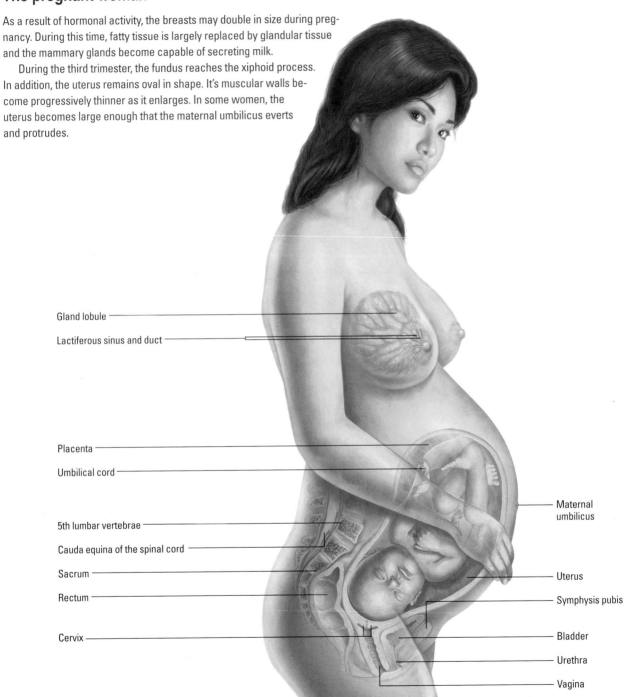

Gland lobule

Lactiferous sinus and duct

Placenta

Umbilical cord

5th lumbar vertebrae

Cauda equina of the spinal cord

Sacrum

Rectum

Cervix

Maternal umbilicus

Uterus

Symphysis pubis

Bladder

Urethra

Vagina

Conditions for cesarean birth

A cesarean birth is removal of the fetus through an abdominal incision. It's a surgical procedure that's performed in certain instances when a vaginal birth would pose a problem to either the mother or the fetus. Conditions that may necessitate cesarean birth include fetal malpresentation, cephalopelvic disproportion (CPD), placenta previa, selected cases of abruptio placentae, and umbilical cord prolapse. A cesarean birth may also be performed in cases of fetal distress.

Fetal malpresentation

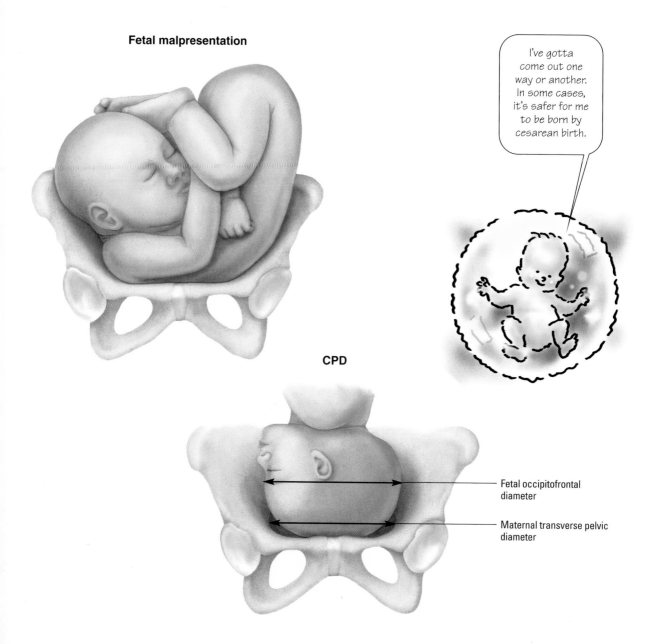

CPD

Fetal occipitofrontal diameter

Maternal transverse pelvic diameter

Placenta previa

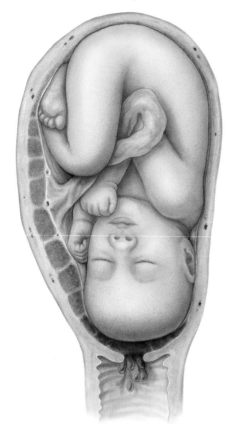

Abruptio placentae

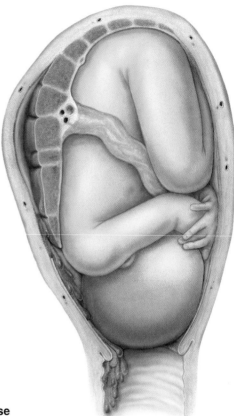

Umbilical cord prolapse

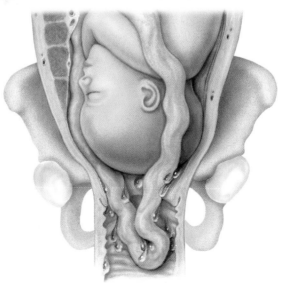

Fetal circulation

Because fetal lungs don't function until after birth, fetal blood is oxygenated by the placenta. Fetal circulation differs from neonatal circulation in that three shunts bypass the liver and the lungs and separate the systemic and pulmonary circulation.
These shunts include:

• ductus venosus — circulatory pathway that allows blood to bypass the liver

• foramen ovale — opening in the interstitial septum that directs blood from the right atrium to the left atrium

• ductus arteriosis — tubular connection that shunts blood away from the pulmonary circulation.

  Because of these shunts, the umbilical vein carries oxygenated blood and the umbilical arteries carries unoxygenated blood.

To head

To arm

Superior vena cava

Foramen ovale

Right atrium

Right lung

Inferior vena cava

Portal vein

Umbilical vein

From placenta

To placenta

Umbilical arteries

Aorta

Ductus arteriosus

Left atrium

Left lung

Aorta

Liver

Ductus venosus

To leg

Understanding thermoregulators

Thermoregulators preserve neonatal body warmth in various ways. A radiant warmer maintains the neonate's temperature by radiation. An incubator maintains the neonate's temperature by conduction and convection.

Temperature settings

Radiant warmers and incubators have two operating modes: *nonservo* and *servo*. The nurse manually sets temperature on nonservo equipment; a probe on the neonate's skin controls temperature settings on servo models.

Other features

Most thermoregulators come with alarms. Incubators have the added advantage of providing a stable, enclosed environment, which protects the neonate from evaporative heat loss.

Radiant warmer

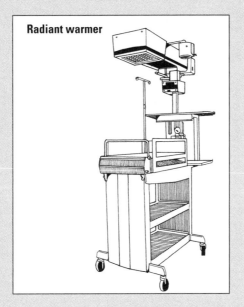

Incubator

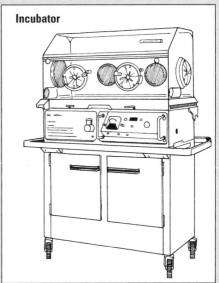

After the arrival

In the birthing room:
• Place the neonate under the radiant warmer, dry him with warm washcloths or towels, then cover his head with a cap to prevent heat loss.
• Perform required procedures quickly and wrap him in the warmed blankets. If his condition permits, give him to his parents to promote bonding.
• Transport the neonate to the nursery in the warmed blankets; use a transport incubator as necessary.

In the nursery:
• Remove the blankets and cap and place the neonate under the radiant warmer.
• Use the adhesive pad to attach the temperature control probe to his skin in the upper-right abdominal quadrant. If the neonate will lie prone, put the skin probe on his back. Don't cover the device with anything because this could interfere with the servo control.
• Take the neonate's rectal temperature on admission, then take axillary temperatures thereafter every 15 to 30 minutes until the

temperature stabilizes, then every 4 hours to ensure stability. (See *Preventing heat loss.*)

Sponge bathe the neonate under the warmer only after his temperature stabilizes and his glucose level is normal. Leave him under the warmer until his temperature remains stable. If the temperature doesn't stabilize, place the neonate under a plastic heat shield or in a warmed incubator, as per facility policy. Check for signs of infection, which can cause hypothermia.

Incubator involvement

Apply a skin probe to a neonate in an incubator as you would for a neonate in a radiant warmer. Move the incubator away from cold walls or objects. Perform all required procedures quickly and close portholes in the hood after completion. If procedures must be performed outside the incubator, do them under a radiant warmer.

To leave the facility or to move to a bassinet, a neonate must be weaned from the incubator by slowly reducing the temperature to that of the nursery. Check periodically for hypothermia. When the neonate's temperature stabilizes, dress him, put him in a bassinet, and cover him with a blanket. Also, be sure to instruct the parents on the importance of maintaining body temperature. (See *Maintaining the neonate's body temperature.*)

Noteworthy items

In your nursing notes, be sure to document:
• the name and temperature of the heat source used
• the neonate's temperature
• complications resulting from use of thermoregulatory equipment.

Oxygen administration

Oxygen relieves neonatal respiratory distress, which can be caused by cyanosis, pallor, tachypnea, nasal flaring, bradycardia, hypothermia, retractions (intercostal, subcostal marginal, suprasternal), hypotonia, hyporeflexia, or expiratory grunting.

Too much of a good thing

No matter how it's administered, oxygen therapy can be hazardous to the neonate. When given in high concentrations and for prolonged periods, it can cause retrolental fibroplasia, which may result in blindness in preterm neonates, and can contribute to bronchopulmonary dysplasia. Because of the neonate's size and special respiratory requirements, oxygen administration commonly requires special techniques and equipment.

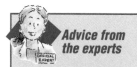
Advice from the experts

Preventing heat loss

Follow these steps to prevent heat loss in the neonate.

Conduction
• Preheat the radiant warmer bed and linen.
• Warm stethoscopes and other instruments before use.
• Before weighing the neonate, pad the scale with a paper towel or a preweighed, warmed sheet.

Convection
• Place the neonate's bed out of a direct line with an open window, fan, or air-conditioning vent.

Evaporation
• Dry the neonate immediately after delivery.
• When bathing the neonate, expose only one body part at a time; wash each part thoroughly, and then dry it immediately.

Radiation
• Keep the neonate and examining tables away from outside windows and air conditioners.

Education edge

Maintaining the neonate's body temperature

To help parents understand the importance of maintaining the neonate's temperature, instruct them to:
• keep the neonate wrapped in a blanket and out of drafts when he isn't in the bassinet
• avoid placing the bassinet next to a window, a fan, an air conditioner, or an air conditioner vent
• keep the stockinette cap on his head because a neonate loses considerable heat through his head
• remove any wet linens from on or around the neonate as soon as possible
• avoid placing the neonate on a cold surface such as a counter without placing a towel or blanket down first.

Hands-on in an emergency

In emergency situations, give oxygen through a manual resuscitation bag and mask of appropriate size until more permanent measures can be initiated.

A method for every occasion

When the neonate merely requires additional oxygen above the ambient concentration, it can be delivered using an oxygen hood. When the neonate requires continuous positive airway pressure (CPAP) to prevent alveolar collapse at the end of an expiration, as in respiratory distress syndrome (hyaline membrane disease), administer oxygen through nasal prongs or an endotracheal (ET) tube connected to a manometer. If the neonate can't breathe on his own, deliver oxygen through a ventilator. Oxygen must be warmed and humidified to prevent hypothermia and dehydration, to which the neonate is especially susceptible.

The right tools for the job

To begin oxygen therapy, you'll need:
• oxygen source (wall, cylinder, or liquid unit)
• compressed air source
• flowmeters
• large and small bore sterile oxygen tubing
• blood gas analyzer
• stethoscope
• nasogastric (NG) tube.
    For handheld resuscitation bag and mask delivery, you'll also need:

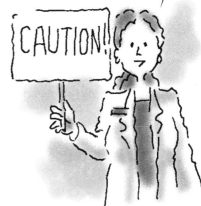

Oxygen must be warmed and humidified to prevent hypothermia and dehydration.

- specially sized mask with handheld resuscitation bag and pressure release valve
- manometer with connectors.
    For delivery via an oxygen hood, also have:
- appropriate sized oxygen hood
- oxygen analyzer.
    For delivery through nasal prongs, other equipment includes:
- nasal prongs
- water-soluble lubricant.
    For CPAP delivery, you'll also need:
- manometer with connectors
- nasopharyngeal or ET tube, or nasal CPAP prongs
- water-soluble lubricant
- hypoallergenic tape.
    For delivery with a ventilator, you'll need:
- ventilator unit with manometer and in-line thermometer
- specimen tubes for arterial blood gas (ABG) analysis
- ET tube
- pulse oximeter or transcutaneous oxygen monitor.

Be prepared

To prepare for oxygen administration, wash your hands and gather and assemble the necessary equipment. To calibrate the oxygen analyzer, turn the analyzer on and read the results. Room air should be about 21% oxygen. Expose the analyzer probe to 100% oxygen, adjust the sensitivity, and recheck the amount of oxygen in room air.

By hand

To use a handheld resuscitation bag and mask:
- Place the assembled resuscitation bag and mask in the crib.
- Turn on the oxygen and compressed air flowmeters and place the mask on the neonate's nose and mouth.
- Check pressure settings and mask size.
- Have another staff member notify the doctor immediately.
- Provide 40 to 60 breaths/minute, using enough pressure to cause a visible rise and fall of the chest. Provide enough oxygen to maintain pink nail beds and mucous membranes.
- Continuously watch the neonate's chest movements and listen to breath sounds, avoiding overventilation. If the neonate's heart rate falls below 100 beats/minute, continue to use the handheld resuscitation bag until the heart rate rises to 100 beats/minute or greater.
- Insert an NG tube to vent air from the neonate's stomach.

By hood

To use an oxygen hood:
• Attach the oxygen hood to the connecting tubing and place an in-line thermometer close to the neonate.
• Activate oxygen and compressed air source, if needed, at ordered flow rates.
• Place the oxygen hood over the neonate's head.
• Measure the amount of oxygen the neonate is receiving with the oxygen analyzer. Be sure to place the analyzer probe close to the neonate's nose.
• Adjust the oxygen to the prescribed amount.

By prongs

When using nasal prongs:
• Match the prong size to the neonate's nose.
• Apply a small amount of water-soluble lubricant to the outside of the prongs.
• Turn on the oxygen and compressed air, if necessary.
• Connect the prongs to the oxygen source.
• Insert the prongs into the nose and secure them.
• Be sure to keep the prongs clean to ensure patency.

By CPAP

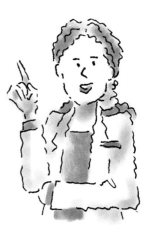

If the neonate needs CPAP to prevent alveolar collapse at the end of each breath (as in respiratory distress syndrome), he may receive this through an ET or nasopharyngeal tube or nasal CPAP prongs. To use CPAP:
• Position the neonate on his back with a rolled towel under his neck to keep the airway open; avoid hyperextending the neck.
• Assist with intubation, if necessary.
• Turn on the oxygen and compressed air source and attach the delivery system to the ET tube or nasal CPAP prongs.
• If an ET tube is in place, confirm placement and tape the tube in place.
• Insert an NG or orogastric tube to keep the stomach decompressed, if ordered. Leave the tube open to air unless the neonate is receiving gavage feedings.
   To use a ventilator:
• Turn on the ventilator and set the controls as ordered.
• Help with ET tube insertion and attach it to the ventilator.
• Confirm placement of the ET tube and tape it securely.
• Watch the manometer to maintain pressure at the prescribed level and monitor the in-line thermometer for correct temperature.

Knowing the know-how

Know how to perform neonatal chest auscultation correctly to pick up subtle respiratory changes. Also, be able to identify signs of respiratory distress and perform emergency procedures. If required, perform chest physiotherapy and percussion, as ordered, and follow with suctioning to remove secretions.

Monitor ABG levels every 15 to 20 minutes (or other reasonable interval) after any changes in oxygen concentration or pressure. If ordered, monitor oxygen perfusion with pulse oximetry, or mixed venous oxygen saturation monitoring. Keep the doctor aware of ABG levels so he can order appropriate changes in oxygen concentration.

As ordered, discontinue oxygen administration when the neonate's fraction of inspired oxygen (FIO_2) is at room air level (20% to 21%) and his arterial oxygen is stable at 60 to 90 mm Hg. Repeat ABG measurements 20 to 30 minutes after discontinuing oxygen and thereafter as ordered by the doctor or by hospital policy.

On the watch

Monitor the neonate for complications of oxygen administration, including:
- signs and symptoms of infection
- hypothermia
- metabolic and respiratory acidosis
- pressure ulcers on the neonate's head, face, and nose
- signs of a pulmonary air leak, including pneumothorax, pneumomediastinum, pneumopericardium, and interstitial emphysema.

Safety first

When administering oxygen, always take safety precautions to avoid fire or explosion. Take measures to keep the neonate warm because hypothermia impedes respiration. (See *Hazards of oxygen therapy.*)

For the record

When documenting oxygen administration, be sure to include:
- respiratory distress requiring oxygen administration
- oxygen concentration given
- oxygen delivery method used
- each change in oxygen concentration
- routine checks of oxygen concentration
- neonate's FIO_2 (as measured by the oxygen analyzer)
- ABG values, noting the time each sample was obtained
- each time suctioning is performed
- amount and consistency of mucus
- type of continuous oxygen monitoring, if any

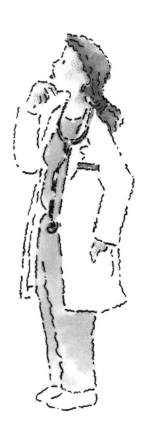

Hazards of oxygen therapy

No matter which system delivers the oxygen, oxygen therapy is potentially hazardous to a neonate. The gas must be warmed and humidified to prevent hypothermia and dehydration. Given in high concentrations over prolonged periods, oxygen can cause retrolental fibroplasia, leading to blindness. With low oxygen concentration, hypoxia and central nervous system damage may occur. Also, depending on how it's delivered, oxygen can contribute to bronchopulmonary dysplasia.

Other worries

Here are some other possible complications of oxygen therapy in neonates:
- Infection or "drowning" can result from over-humidification. Overhumidification, in turn, allows water to collect in tubing, providing a growth medium for bacteria or suffocating the neonate.
- Hypothermia can increase oxygen consumption and can result from administering cool oxygen.
- Metabolic and respiratory acidosis may follow inadequate ventilation.
- Pressure ulcers may develop on the neonate's head, face, and around the nose during prolonged oxygen therapy.
- A pulmonary air leak (pneumothorax, pneumomediastinum, pneumopericardium, interstitial emphysema) may arise spontaneously with respiratory distress or result from forced ventilation.
- Decreased cardiac output may result from excessive continuous positive airway pressure.

- complications
- neonate's condition during oxygen therapy, including respiratory rate, breath sounds, and signs of additional respiratory distress.

Circumcision

Circumcision is the removal of the penile foreskin. It's thought to promote a clean glans, minimize the risk of phimosis (foreskin tightening) later in life, and reduce the risk of penile cancer and cervical cancer in sexual partners. However, after 40 years of research on the risks and benefits of circumcision, the American Academy of Pediatrics has concluded that it can't recommend a policy of routine neonate circumcision. (See *Circumcision and religion*.)

Bells and clamps (but no whistles)

One method of circumcision involves removing the foreskin by using a Yellen clamp to stabilize the penis. With this device, a cone fits over the glans, providing a cutting surface and protecting the glans penis. Another technique uses a plastic circumcision bell (Plastibell) over the glans and a suture that's tied tightly around the base of the foreskin. This method prevents bleeding, and the

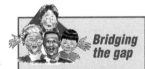

Bridging the gap

Circumcision and religion

For those of Jewish faith, circumcision takes place in a religious ritual called a *Bris Milah*. It's performed by a *mohel* on the 8th day after birth, when the neonate is officially given his name. Because most neonates are sent home before this time, the Bris is rarely done in the hospital.

resultant ischemia causes the foreskin to slough off in 5 to 8 days. It's thought to be painless because it stretches the foreskin, which inhibits sensory conduction.

When it's a no-go

Contraindications to circumcision include:
• illness
• bleeding disorders
• ambiguous genitalia
• congenital penile anomalies, such as hypospadias or epispadias (because the foreskin may be needed for later reconstructive surgery).

Prep the parents

The neonate experiences pain during the circumcision. Explain the procedure to the parents or caregivers, and tell them that a local anesthetic will be administered. The neonate needs to be restricted from feeding for 1 hour before the procedure to reduce the possibility of emesis, aspiration, or both. Tell the parents that it's necessary to restrain the neonate for the procedure. Make sure that the patient has signed a consent form for the procedure (many facilities require this before the circumcision is performed).

Gather what's needed

The following equipment is necessary:
• circumcision tray (contents vary, but usually include circumcision clamps, various sized cones, scalpel, probe, scissors, forceps, sterile basin, sterile towel, and sterile drapes)
• povidone-iodine solution
• restraining board with arm and leg restraints
• sterile gloves
• petroleum gauze
• sterile 4″ × 4″ gauze pads
• anesthetic agent
• optional: sutures, plastic circumcision bell, antimicrobial ointment, topical anesthetic, and overhead warmer.

Be prepared

To prepare for the procedure:
• Assemble the sterile tray and other equipment in the procedure area.
• Open the sterile tray and pour povidone-iodine solution into the sterile basin.
• Using aseptic technique, place sterile 4″ × 4″ gauze pads and petroleum gauze on the sterile tray.

• Arrange the restraining board and direct adequate light on the area.

If a plastic circumcision bell is being used, you won't need a circumcision tray; however, assemble sterile gloves, sutures, restraining board, petroleum gauze and, if ordered, antibiotic ointment.

Set up for the assist

• Place the neonate on the restraining board, and restrain his arms and legs. Don't leave him unattended.
• Assist the doctor as necessary throughout the procedure, and comfort the neonate as needed.
• After putting on sterile gloves, the doctor will clean the penis and scrotum with povidone-iodine, drape the neonate, and administer a local anesthetic.

Clamp champ

When using a Yellen clamp, the doctor:
• applies the Yellen clamp to the penis, loosens the foreskin, and inserts the cone under it to provide a cutting surface for the removal of the foreskin and to protect the penis.
• covers the wound with sterile petroleum gauze to prevent infection and control bleeding.

Over and done

When the procedure is complete, remove the neonate from the restraining board and check for bleeding. His diaper should be changed as soon as he voids. At each diaper change, apply antimicrobial ointment, petroleum jelly, or petroleum gauze until the wound appears healed. (See *Caring for the circumcised neonate.*)

A bell below the belt

When using a plastic circumcision bell, the doctor:
• slides the plastic bell device between the foreskin and the glans penis.
• ties a suture tightly around the foreskin at the coronal edge of the glans.

The foreskin distal to the suture becomes ischemic and then atrophic. After 5 to 8 days, the foreskin drops off with the plastic bell attached, leaving a clean, well-healed excision. No special care is required but the parents should watch for swelling, which may indicate infection or interfere with urination (See *Teaching proper care of a circumcision,* page 516.)

Take charge!

Caring for the circumcised neonate

Here are some points to consider when caring for a neonate who has been circumcised:
• Avoid leaving a circumcised neonate under the radiant warmer after placing petroleum gauze on the penis because the area may burn.
• Apply diapers loosely to prevent irritation.
• If the dressing falls off, clean the wound with warm water to minimize pain on the circumcised area from the urine.
• Don't remove the original dressing until it falls off.
• Check for bleeding every 15 minutes for the first hour and then every hour for the next 24 hours. If bleeding occurs, apply pressure with sterile gauze pads. Notify the doctor if bleeding continues.

Education edge

Teaching proper care of a circumcision

Always be sure to show parents the circumcision before discharge so that they can ask questions. Teach them these tips for proper care of a circumcision:
• Reapply fresh petrolatum gauze after each diaper change, if applicable.
• Don't use premoistened towelettes to clean the penis because they contain alcohol, which can delay healing and cause discomfort.
• Don't attempt to remove exudate that forms around the penis. Removing exudate can cause bleeding.
• Change the neonate's diaper at least every 4 hours to prevent it from sticking to the penis.
• Check to make sure that the neonate urinates after being circumcised. He should have 6 to 10 wet diapers in a 24 hour period. If he doesn't, notify the doctor.
• Wash the penis with warm water to remove urine or feces until the circumcision is healed. Soap can be used after the circumcision has healed.
• Notify the doctor if redness, swelling, or discharge is present on the penis. These signs may indicate infection. Note that the penis is dark red after circumcision and then becomes covered with a yellow exudate in 24 hours.

After the fact

Stay alert for these complications of circumcision:
• urethral fistulae and edema
• infection or bleeding (if a Yellen clamp was used)
• delayed healing or infection, indicated by pus or bloody discharge
• scarring or fibrous bands, from adherence of penile shaft skin to the glans
• incomplete foreskin amputation from use of a plastic circumcision bell.
    In your notes, be sure to document:
• circumcision date and time
• parent teaching provided
• excessive bleeding
• time that the neonate urinates before discharge.

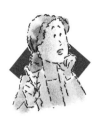

Quick quiz

1. Which factor doesn't stimulate the onset of breathing?
   A.   Decreased carbon dioxide levels
   B.   Increased carbon dioxide levels
   C.   Decreased blood pH
   D.   Decreased blood oxygen levels

Answer: A. Decreased carbon dioxide levels don't stimulate breathing.

2. Which option correctly describes the normal anatomy of the umbilical cord?
   A.   One artery and one vein
   B.   One artery and one ligament
   C.   Two arteries and one vein
   D.   One artery and two veins

Answer: C. The umbilical cord should consist of two arteries and one vein.

3. Apgar scoring evaluates:
   A.   heart rate, respiratory rate, color, blood pressure, and temperature.
   B.   heart rate, respiratory effort, muscle tone, reflex irritability, and color.
   C.   respiratory rate, blood pressure, reflex irritability, muscle tone, and temperature.
   D.   temperature, heart rate, color, muscle tone, and blood pressure.

Answer: B. Apgar scoring involves evaluating the neonate's heart rate, respiratory effort, muscle tone, reflex irritability, and color.

4. A sign of respiratory distress in a neonate is:
   A.   acrocyanosis.
   B.   nasal flaring.
   C.   abdominal movements.
   D.   short periods of apnea (less than 15 seconds).

Answer: B. Nasal flaring is a sign of respiratory distress in the neonate. Acrocyanosis, abdominal movements, and short periods of apnea are all normal findings.

5. Which finding is normal for a neonate's fontanels?
   A.   They're soft to touch.
   B.   They're depressed.
   C.   They're bulging.
   D.   They're closed.

Answer: A. The fontanels should feel soft to the touch.

6.   Where's the apical impulse best assessed on the neonate?
   A.   Second intercostal space, right sternal border
   B.   Fifth intercostal space, left midclavicular line
   C.   Fifth intercostal space, left sternal border
   D.   Apex of the heart

Answer: B. The apical impulse is best assessed at the 4th intercostal space, left midclavicular line.

7.   During which sleep-wake cycle does the neonate experience REM?
   A.   Deep sleep
   B.   Light sleep
   C.   Drowsy
   D.   Crying

Answer: B. During light sleep the eyes are closed and the neonate experiences REM, random movements and startles, irregular breathing, and sucking movements.

Scoring

☆☆☆   If you answered all seven questions correctly, magnificent! You're top-rate with the neonates!

☆☆   If you answered five or six questions correctly, goo goo for you! Now that you've tamed neonates, you're almost ready to tackle toddlers!

☆   If you answered fewer than five questions correctly, don't lose your focus. De-stress, then assess, and you're sure to have success.

High-risk neonatal conditions

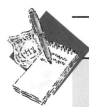
A look at the high-risk neonate

A neonate is considered to be high-risk if he has an increased chance of dying during or shortly after birth or has a congenital or perinatal problem that requires prompt intervention. As medicine continues to develop more treatments for perinatal problems, high-risk neonates are more likely to survive. Many of these neonates have few or no residual effects from the crisis that marked their first hours after birth.

A shaky start

Parents of high-risk neonates may experience grief and difficulty coping as they adjust to their neonate's condition. They may also feel a sense of loss and have difficulty bonding because their neonate isn't the perfect, healthy baby they anticipated. The family of a neonate with a chronic illness or congenital anomaly must find ways to cope with long-term grief and develop strategies to provide the special care the condition will require (and perhaps to balance these care needs with those of other children). If the neonate is stillborn or dies within a few hours or days after birth, family members must complete their bonding with the neonate,

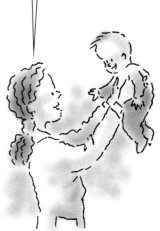

Parents may have difficulty bonding with a high-risk neonate because they feel a sense of loss.

then detach themselves gradually so they can focus again on the family's life and needs.

Although the neonate's condition dictates the specifics of nursing care, the main nursing goals for all high-risk neonates are to:
• ensure oxygenation, ventilation, thermoregulation, nutrition, and fluid and electrolyte balance
• prevent and control infection
• encourage parent-neonate bonding
• provide developmental care.

Drug addiction

Neonatal drug addiction and its associated signs and symptoms of withdrawal result from illicit drug use by the neonate's mother during pregnancy. As in all aspects of health care, care for the drug-addicted neonate should be provided in a nonjudgmental manner, especially because the neonate is an innocent victim of substance abuse by another person.

Lowdown on drug effects

Pregnant women who use illicit drugs are at higher risk for:
• abruptio placentae
• spontaneous abortion
• preterm labor
• precipitous labor
• psychotic responses.

Complications seen in the neonate may include:
• urogenital malformations
• cerebrovascular complications
• low birth weight
• decreased head circumference
• respiratory problems
• death.

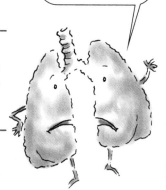

Drug-addicted neonates may have respiratory problems and other serious complications.

What causes it

Neonatal drug addiction can occur if the mother uses illicit drugs while pregnant. These drugs have teratogenic effects, causing abnormalities in embryonic or fetal development.

What to look for

Intrauterine drug exposure may cause obvious physical anomalies, neurobehavioral changes, or withdrawal. Signs and symp-

Opiate withdrawal syndrome

Be alert for these signs and symptoms of opiate withdrawal in the neonate.

Central nervous system
- Seizures
- Tremors
- Irritability
- Increased wakefulness
- High-pitched cry
- Increased muscle tone
- Increased deep tendon reflexes
- Increased Moro reflex
- Increased yawning
- Increased sneezing
- Rapid changes in mood
- Hypersensitivity to noise and external stimuli

GI system
- Poor feeding
- Uncoordinated and constant sucking
- Vomiting
- Diarrhea
- Dehydration
- Poor weight gain

Autonomic nervous system
- Increased sweating
- Nasal stuffiness
- Fever
- Mottling
- Temperature instability
- Increased respiratory rate
- Increased heart rate

toms of a neonate's drug dependence vary and may include physical and behavioral changes. These changes depend on:
- specific drug or combination of drugs used
- dosage
- route of administration
- metabolism and excretion by the mother and fetus
- timing of drug exposure
- length of drug exposure.

Opiates

Clinical presentation of opiate withdrawal in the neonate can last 2 to 3 weeks. Withdrawal signs and symptoms generally include dysfunction of the central nervous system (CNS) and GI system. (See *Opiate withdrawal syndrome*.)

Heroin

Neonates who have been exposed to heroin generally have low birth weights and are small for gestational age. They may also exhibit these signs and symptoms:
- jitters and hyperactivity
- shrill and persistent cry
- frequent yawning or sneezing

- increased deep tendon reflexes
- decreased Moro reflex
- poor feeding and sucking
- increased respiratory rate
- vomiting
- diarrhea
- hypothermia or hyperthermia
- increased sweating
- abnormal sleep cycle.

Methadone

Withdrawal from methadone resembles that from heroin but tends to be more severe and prolonged. It includes:
- increased incidence of seizures
- disturbed sleep patterns
- higher birth weight in neonates who are appropriate size for gestational age
- higher risk of sudden infant death syndrome.

Marijuana

Neonates born to mothers who used marijuana while pregnant tend to be born at earlier gestations. An increased incidence of precipitous labor and meconium staining also occurs in this population of neonates. When the mother abuses marijuana and alcohol during pregnancy, there's a fivefold increase in the risk of fetal alcohol syndrome (FAS).

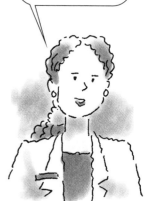

Abusing marijuana and alcohol during pregnancy increases the risk of FAS fivefold.

Amphetamines

Women who use amphetamines while pregnant may have premature neonates or neonates of low birth weight. Other characteristics these neonates may have include:
- drowsiness
- jitters
- respiratory distress soon after birth
- frequent infections
- poor weight gain
- emotional disturbances
- delays in gross motor and fine motor development in early childhood.

What tests tell you

The signs and symptoms of addiction and withdrawal may be mistaken for other common neonatal problems, especially if the mother's drug use is unknown. You'll need to differentiate between neonatal drug withdrawal and CNS irritability caused by infectious or metabolic disorders, such as hypoglycemia or hypocalcemia. You'll also need to rule out hypomagnesemia, hyperthyroidism, CNS hemorrhage, and anoxia.

When it's withdrawal

If the clinical signs and symptoms are consistent with drug withdrawal, obtain specimens of urine and meconium for drug testing. Be aware that urine screening may have a high false negative rate because only neonates with recent exposure test positive. Also keep in mind that although meconium drug testing isn't conclusive if results are negative, this method is more reliable than urine testing.

> **Drugs for withdrawal**
>
> Drugs used to treat withdrawal include:
> - chlorpromazine
> - clonidine
> - diazepam
> - methadone
> - morphine
> - paregoric
> - phenobarbital
> - tincture of opium.

How it's treated

Initial treatment of the neonate who's experiencing withdrawal should be supportive. This includes:
- swaddling
- frequent, small feedings of hypercaloric formula
- observing sleep habits
- observing for temperature instability, weight gain or loss, or changes in clinical status that might suggest another disease process
- fluid and electrolyte replacement
- infection control
- respiratory care
- reducing stimuli.

Treating drugs with drugs

Indications for pharmacologic therapy include:
- seizures
- poor feeding
- diarrhea
- vomiting leading to weight loss and dehydration
- inability to sleep
- fever unrelated to infection.

If pharmacologic therapy is needed, specific therapy from the same drug class is preferred. (See *Drugs for withdrawal.*)

> If pharmacologic therapy is used to treat a neonatal drug addiction, therapy from the same drug class is preferred.

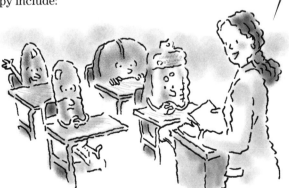

What to do

Nursing interventions for neonatal drug addiction include:
- initiating preventative measures
- identifying neonates at risk
- assessing the neonate
- providing supportive care.

Stop addiction before it starts

Preventing maternal drug use is the ideal approach to eradicating the problem of neonatal drug addiction. Patient teaching and support are essential. To identify a woman and neonate at risk for drug addiction:
- Obtain a detailed maternal prescription and nonprescription drug history.
- Assess the social habits of the parents.

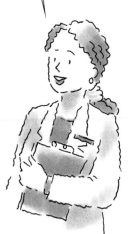

One of the first steps in identifying those at risk for drug addiction is obtaining a detailed drug history.

Screen those on the scene

To screen for drug exposure, perform maternal and neonatal assessments. Maternal findings that may indicate a need for neonatal drug testing include:
- lack of prenatal care
- previous unexplained fetal demise
- precipitous labor
- altered nutrition
- abruptio placentae
- hypertensive episodes
- severe mood swings
- stroke
- myocardial infarction (MI)
- recurrent spontaneous abortions.

Neonatal characteristics that may be associated with maternal drug use include:
- prematurity
- unexplained intrauterine growth retardation
- neurobehavioral abnormalities
- urogenital anomalies
- atypical vascular incidents (stroke, MI, or necrotizing enterocolitis in an otherwise healthy term neonate).

Ongoing neonatal assessment should include monitoring for changes in:
- respiratory system
- reflexes (including suck, swallow, and gag)
- CNS
- feeding and growth
- vital signs.

Aiding the addicted

Supportive care of the neonate with a drug addiction includes:
- maintaining the neonate's airway
- assessing breath sounds frequently
- supporting and monitoring ventilation
- providing supplemental oxygen
- managing mechanical ventilation
- making sure that resuscitative equipment is available
- monitoring pulse oximetry (and arterial blood gas [ABG] studies if pulse oximetry is abnormally low)
- decreasing CNS excitability by keeping the neonate tightly wrapped (swaddling)
- decreasing stimuli by reducing light in the room
- monitoring the neonate with seizures
- preventing trauma
- administering medications as ordered
- promoting rest
- promoting nutritional intake
- feeding in small, frequent amounts with the head elevated and the nipple positioned correctly so that sucking is effective
- maintaining fluid and electrolyte balance
- monitoring intake and output
- giving supplemental fluids as ordered
- evaluating serum electrolytes as ordered
- maintaining skin integrity and providing skin care
- changing the neonate's position
- reporting signs of distress.

Fetal alcohol syndrome

A cluster of birth defects that are caused by in utero exposure to alcohol is referred to as *FAS*. It can result in abnormalities in the CNS, growth retardation, and facial malformations.

What causes it

FAS is caused by the exposure of a fetus to alcohol in utero. Although prenatal alcohol exposure doesn't always result in FAS, the safe level of alcohol consumption during pregnancy isn't known. Alcohol crosses through the placenta and enters the fetal blood supply, and it can interfere with the healthy development of the fetus. In fact, birth defects associated with prenatal alcohol exposure can occur in the first 3 to 8 weeks of pregnancy, before a woman even knows she's pregnant. Variables that affect the extent of damage caused to the fetus by alcohol include the amount of alcohol consumed, the timing of consumption, and the pattern of alcohol use.

What to look for

Affected neonates may display these signs within the first 24 hours of life:
- difficulty establishing respirations
- irritability
- lethargy
- seizure activity
- tremulousness
- opisthotonos
- poor sucking reflex
- abdominal distention.

Overalls

Overall signs of FAS include CNS dysfunction, growth deficiency, and a characteristic set of minor facial abnormalities that tend to normalize as the child grows. (See *Common facial characteristics of FAS*.)

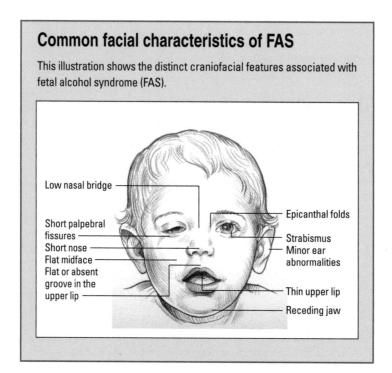

Common facial characteristics of FAS

This illustration shows the distinct craniofacial features associated with fetal alcohol syndrome (FAS).

Low nasal bridge

Short palpebral fissures
Short nose
Flat midface
Flat or absent groove in the upper lip

Epicanthal folds

Strabismus
Minor ear abnormalities

Thin upper lip

Receding jaw

Typical CNS problems for neonates with FAS may include:

- mental retardation
- microcephaly
- poor coordination
- decreased muscle tone
- small brain
- behavioral abnormalities
- irritability.

Growth deficiencies may manifest in a failure to thrive or a disproportionate decrease in adipose tissue. Length and weight in neonates with FAS typically measures 3% less than the average neonate.

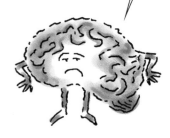

FAS can cause mental retardation and behavioral abnormalities.

Hits to the other systems

Abnormalities may also be seen in the cardiac system, skeletal system, urogenital system, and skin. Potential complications include:

- cardiac murmurs
- limited joint movements
- finger and toe deformities
- aberrant palmar creases
- kidney defects
- labial hypoplasia
- hemangiomas.

As children and adults, individuals with FAS also commonly display:

- defects in intellectual functioning
- difficulties with learning, memory, attention, and problem solving
- problems with mental health
- difficulties with social interaction.

What tests tell you

Identifying clinical problems and assessment findings characteristic of FAS leads to diagnosis. Respiratory distress and neurologic dysfunction may be present. Feeding difficulties may also be noted. Radiographic studies may be used to reveal renal or cardiac defects.

How it's treated

Treatment of FAS is supportive and depends on the individual neonate. The initial difficulties may be managed by preventing stimulation that may precipitate seizures, administering sedative or anticonvulsant medications, and providing supportive measures. Because the effects of alcohol in utero vary, care must be individualized to focus on the neonate's specific abnormalities and deficits.

What to do

A fundamental nursing intervention for FAS is helping to prevent it. This can be achieved by:
- increasing public awareness
- increasing women's access to prenatal care
- providing educational programs
- screening women of reproductive age for alcohol problems
- using appropriate resources and strategies for decreasing alcohol use.

FASe out respiratory problems

Caring for neonates with FAS involves preventing or treating respiratory distress.
- Place the neonate on a cardiac monitor and set the alarms.
- Assess breath sounds frequently and be alert for signs of distress.
- Suction as needed.
- Place the neonate in a position in which he displays the least distress.

EmFASize nutrition

Special emphasis should be placed on following weight gain, assessing feeding behaviors, and devising strategies to increase nutritional intake.
- Encourage feeding to promote bonding with the parents.
- Elevate the neonate's head during and after feeding.
- Evaluate different nipples.
- Burp the neonate well during and after feedings.
- Monitor the neonate's weight.
- Measure intake and output.

FAScillitate bonding

To promote mother-neonate attachment:
- Encourage visits.
- Encourage physical contact.
- Educate parents about the neonate's complications.
- Provide emotional support.

Gestational size variations

Whether they're preterm, term, or postterm, neonates are classified by weight in three ways:

👆 Large for gestational age (LGA) neonates are above the 90th percentile for weight.

✌️ Appropriate for gestational age (AGA) neonates are between the 10th and 90th percentile for weight.

🤟 Small for gestational age (SGA) neonates are below the 10th percentile for weight.

What causes it

Variations in gestational size are caused by different factors.

SGA neonates

Factors that can contribute to a neonate being SGA include:
- congenital malformations
- chromosomal anomalies
- maternal infections
- pregnancy-induced hypertension (PIH)
- advanced maternal diabetes due to decreased blood flow to the placenta
- intrauterine malnutrition due to poor placental function or maternal malnutrition
- maternal smoking
- maternal drug or alcohol use
- multiple gestation.

LGA neonates

Neonates may become LGA because of genetic factors. For example, neonates tend to be larger if they're male, if their parents are larger, or if the mother is a multipara. Neonates of mothers with diabetes also tend to be LGA because high maternal glucose levels stimulate continued insulin production by the fetus. This constant state of hyperglycemia leads to excessive growth and fat deposition.

High glucose levels in mothers with diabetes can result in LGA neonates.

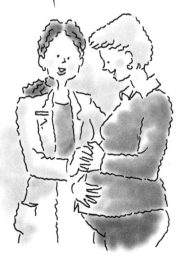

What to look for

Assessment findings depend on whether the neonate is SGA or LGA.

SGA neonates

SGA neonates fall below the 10th percentile for weight and are more likely to experience respiratory distress and hypoxia. They may also appear wide-eyed and alert at birth because of prolonged prenatal hypoxia. In addition, SGA neonates are prone to meconium aspiration because fetal hypoxia allows meconium to pass through a relaxed anal sphincter, thus causing the neonate to experience reflexive gasping. Hypoglycemia can occur in SGA neonates and can be noted from birth to day 4 of life. Decreased subcutaneous fat and a large ratio of body surface area to weight put the SGA neonate at risk for problems with thermoregulation.

LGA neonates

Neonates are considered LGA if they are above the 90th percentile for weight. They generally weigh more than 4,000 g (8 lb, 13 oz) and appear plump and full-faced. The LGA neonate may experience hypoxia during labor and be exposed to excessive trauma, such as fractures and intracranial hemorrhage, during vaginal delivery. Hypoglycemia may be noted at birth and during the transition period.

What tests tell you

Neonates of mothers with diabetes should have laboratory work to determine their hematocrit and glucose, calcium, and bilirubin levels. They should also be monitored for hypoglycemia, hyperbilirubinemia, and respiratory distress syndrome.

How it's treated

Treatment of gestational age size abnormalities varies depending on whether the neonate is SGA or LGA.

SGA neonates

Treatment of the SGA neonate should be supportive and individualized with nutrition being the primary focus. SGA neonates have higher caloric needs and benefit from frequent

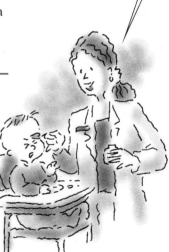

SGA neonates have higher caloric needs and benefit from frequent feedings.

feedings. Care of the SGA neonate also includes glucose monitoring and careful respiratory assessments.

LGA neonates

During delivery of an LGA neonate, the mother may need additional help, such as an episiotomy, change in position, or the use of forceps or a vacuum. After birth, glucose monitoring and evaluation of jaundice is essential in LGA neonates. Any birth traumas also need to be managed.

What to do

Nursing interventions for SGA and LGA neonates include:
- supporting respiratory efforts
- providing a neutral thermal environment
- protecting the neonate from infection
- providing appropriate nutrition
- maintaining adequate hydration
- conserving the neonate's energy
- assessing glucose level
- preventing skin breakdown
- facilitating growth and development
- keeping parents informed
- providing support to the entire family.

Human immunodeficiency virus infection

Today, pregnant women have the opportunity to be tested for human immunodeficiency virus (HIV). Such testing has led to an increase in the number of neonates known to be exposed to HIV, which in turn has allowed for early diagnosis and treatment.

What causes it

HIV can be transmitted to the neonate in one of three ways:

 transplacentally during pregnancy

during labor and delivery

through breast-milk.

> ### Risk factors for perinatal transmission of HIV
>
> Neonatal and maternal factors can contribute to perinatal transmission of the human immunodeficiency virus (HIV).
>
> **Neonatal factors**
> - Bacterial infection
> - Being the first-born twin
> - Breast-feeding
> - Prematurity
>
> **Maternal factors**
> - Chorioamnionitis
> - Low CD4+ count
> - High CD8+ count
> - High viral load
> - New onset of disease
> - Ongoing drug abuse
> - Prolonged or complicated labor

Risk factors for perinatal transmission can be either maternal or neonatal. (See *Risk factors for perinatal transmission of HIV.*)

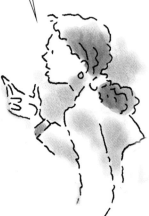

Physical findings of HIV infection aren't usually present at birth, but they may develop later.

What to look for

Most neonates exposed to HIV are born at term and are of AGA. Normal physical findings are usually present. Physical findings, such as adenopathy or hepatosplenomegaly, are absent at birth because HIV infection is believed to occur at delivery. These findings may develop later and suggest HIV infection.

What tests tell you

The Centers for Disease Control and Prevention recommend testing for HIV within 48 hours of birth, at age 1 to 2 months, and again at age 3 to 6 months. Two positive tests at different ages are required to make a positive diagnosis. Diagnostic tests used to detect HIV include HIV deoxyribonucleic acid (DNA) polymerase chain reactions (PCR), HIV P24 antigen assay, HIV antibody, HIV culture, and immunologic testing.

PCR preferred

The HIV DNA PCR test is the preferred method for diagnosing HIV in neonates. It's highly sensitive and specific. Positive results can be detected in 93% of infected neonates by day 14 of life. This test should be performed at birth and between ages 1 and 2 months. The test should be repeated at age 4 months if the infant remains asymptomatic and the previous test results were negative.

Assay you, assay me

HIV P24 antigen assay may be used to assess HIV infection in infants older than one month, but the sensitivity is less than PCR testing. The absence of the P24 antigen, however, doesn't rule out HIV infection.

Antibody home?

The HIV antibody test uses enzyme-linked immunoabsorbent assay and Western blot analysis to determine whether HIV antibodies are present as a result of exposure to the virus. However, this test doesn't differentiate between maternal and neonatal infection. In addition, diagnosis can be complicated by the presence of the maternal, anti-HIV immunoglobulin (Ig) G antibody in the neonate. Because of this complication, cord blood should never be used for HIV testing.

A positive HIV antibody test obtained at age 18 months (after the maternal IgG in the neonate has broken down) indicates infection. For infants exposed to HIV whose previous testing was negative, a final HIV antibody test at age 24 months is recommended.

An uncommon culture

An HIV culture is a test that isn't readily available. It's also expensive to perform, requires a large blood sample, and the results may not be available for 2 to 4 weeks. If performed, an HIV culture should be taken at birth and again between ages 1 and 2 months. If the initial result is positive, the test should be repeated immediately to confirm. If an infant remains asymptomatic after testing negative, repeat the HIV culture at age 4 months.

More monitoring

Immunologic testing, including lymphocyte subsets (CD4+, CD8+, CD4+–CD8+ ratio) and quantitative immunoglobulins (IgG, IgM, IgA) should be performed on all neonates born to HIV-positive mothers. Children born to HIV-infected mothers should also undergo hematologic monitoring. This includes assessing complete blood count (CBC), differential leukocyte count, and platelet count during the first 6 months of life. Monitoring should continue in infected children and in those whose infection status is undetermined at age 6 months.

To be free of HIV

A neonate is considered uninfected with HIV when:
- no physical findings consistent with HIV are present
- immunologic test results are negative
- virologic tests are negative
- after 12 months, two or more HIV antibody tests are negative.

How it's treated

To help prevent perinatal transmission of HIV, zidovudine (Retrovir) is given to HIV-positive women during the second and third trimesters of pregnancy as well as during labor and delivery. The drug is also given to neonates born to HIV-positive mothers during the first 6 weeks of life. Such treatment has been shown to dramatically decrease perinatal transmission of HIV. Zidovudine therapy is discontinued at age 6 weeks. (See *Complications of zidovudine therapy in the neonate*.)

But wait, there's more

After zidovudine therapy is completed, prophylaxis for *Pneumocystis carinii* pneumonia (PCP) should start. PCP prophylaxis is recommended for all neonates born to HIV-infected women—regardless of the infant's initial test results—because PCP infection commonly occurs between ages 3 and 6 months, when many HIV-exposed infants haven't yet been identified as being infected. PCP prophylaxis should continue until at least age 12 months—even if the infant's infection status hasn't been determined.

Co-trimoxazole (Bactrim) is the recommended chemoprophylaxis regimen for PCP in infants. When initiating therapy, first obtain a baseline CBC, differential leukocyte count, and platelet count. These measurements should be checked monthly while the infant receives prophylaxis treatment. If this regimen isn't tolerated, dapsone may be used.

What to do

Whether the HIV-infected woman is delivering vaginally or by cesarean birth, follow standard precautions. Be sure to wear gloves, a gown, and protective eyewear. Prompt and careful removal of blood and amniotic fluid from the neonate's skin is important. Isolation, however, isn't required. Inform the mother that breast-feeding isn't recommended, and instruct her and her family on caring for the neonate exposed to HIV. (See *Caring for a neonate exposed to HIV*.)

Hydrocephalus

Hydrocephalus is an excessive accumulation of cerebrospinal fluid (CSF) within the ventricular spaces of the brain. This accumulation of fluid forces the ventricles to dilate, which can put harmful pressure on brain tissue. Such pressure on brain tissue and cere-

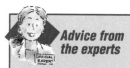

Advice from the experts

Complications of zidovudine therapy in the neonate

Zidovudine may cause transient anemia. To monitor for this adverse effect, a complete blood count and differential leukocyte count should be performed at birth as a baseline and again at ages 4 and 6 weeks.

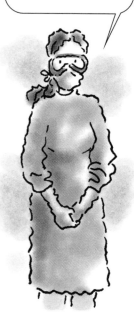

If a pregnant woman is infected with HIV, follow standard precautions during delivery.

bral blood vessels may lead to ischemia and, eventually, cell death.

Are we communicating?

Hydrocephalus may be communicating or noncommunicating. *Communicating* hydrocephalus occurs because CSF isn't absorbed properly. *Noncommunicating* hydrocephalus occurs because normal CSF flow is obstructed. Congenital hydrocephalus is present at birth. Acquired hydrocephalus develops at the time of birth or later in life.

What causes it

The cause of hydrocephalus isn't exactly known. Possible causes include:
- genetic inheritance
- neural tube defects, such as spina bifida and encephalocele
- complications of premature birth such as intraventricular hemorrhage
- meningitis
- tumors
- traumatic head injury
- subarachnoid hemorrhage
- prenatal maternal infections.

What to look for

Assessment findings vary. Be aware that a neonate's ability to tolerate the accumulation of CSF differs from an adult's — the neonate's skull can expand because the sutures haven't yet closed.

On the lookout

Findings in neonates that may suggest hydrocephalus include:
- rapid increase in head circumference or an unusually large head size disproportionate to neonate's growth
- distended scalp veins
- bulging fontanels
- thin, shiny, fragile-looking scalp skin
- downward deviation of the eyes ("sunsetting" eyes)
- sluggish pupils with unequal response to light
- seizures
- high-pitched, shrill cry
- irritability
- projectile vomiting

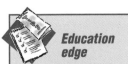

Education edge

Caring for a neonate exposed to HIV

When teaching a woman and her family about caring for a neonate exposed to human immunodeficiency virus (HIV), emphasize the need for:
- frequent follow-up
- testing to determine infection status
- zidovudine administration to decrease the risk of infection
- prophylaxis for *Pneumocystis carinii* pneumonia
- taking precautions to prevent the spread of HIV infection.

Patient teaching should also include signs of possible HIV infection in the neonate, including:
- recurrent infections
- unusual infections
- failure to thrive
- hematologic manifestations
- renal disease
- neurologic manifestations.

• feeding problems (because the head is 1⅛″ [3 cm] larger than the chest).

In addition, the neonate may cry when picked up or rocked and be quiet when still.

What tests tell you

Hydrocephalus is diagnosed by clinical assessment and imaging techniques, such as:
• ultrasound
• computed tomography
• magnetic resonance imaging
• pressure monitoring techniques.

The appropriate diagnostic tool should be chosen based on age, clinical presentation, and presence of known or suspected abnormalities of the brain or spinal cord.

How it's treated

Hydrocephalus is commonly treated with the surgical insertion of a shunt. The shunt, consisting of a catheter and a valve, leads from a ventricle in the brain to the peritoneum or an atrial chamber of the heart, thus allowing CSF to drain to an area where it can be absorbed into the circulation. The valve maintains one-way flow and regulates the rate at which CSF is drained.

Aw shunts

Potential complications of shunt systems include:
• mechanical failure
• infection
• obstruction
• need to lengthen or replace catheter.

Patients with surgically implanted shunt systems require regular medical follow-up.

What to do

The neonate with diagnosed or suspected hydrocephalus must be observed carefully for signs of increasing intracranial pressure (ICP). The nurse must be alert for:
• irritability
• lethargy
• seizure activity
• altered vital signs
• altered feeding behavior.

If hydrocephalus is suspected, be on the lookout for signs of increasing ICP.

Flexible and frequent feedings

Another aspect of nursing care for the neonate with hydrocephalus is maintaining adequate nutrition. Keep feeding schedules flexible to help accommodate for various procedures. Offer small, frequent feedings, and allow extra time for feeding in case the neonate has difficulty.

Support after surgery

Postoperative care involves:
- positioning the neonate on the side opposite the shunt
- observing for signs of increased ICP
- monitoring intake and output carefully
- preventing infection
- providing skin care.

On the home front

Hydrocephalus poses risks to the neonate's cognitive and physical development. The prospect of dealing with chronic disabilities or delayed development can be overwhelming to parents. Providing support to the family is crucial to helping them cope. Allow them to express their concerns, and refer them to appropriate resources and rehabilitation services, as needed.

Hyperbilirubinemia

Hyperbilirubinemia is an excess of bilirubin in the blood that results in elevated serum bilirubin levels and mild jaundice. Hyperbilirubinemia can be physiologic (with jaundice being the only symptom) or pathologic (resulting from an underlying disease). (See *Ethnic groups susceptible to physiologic jaundice*.)

Physiologic hyperbilirubinemia is self-limiting. It usually resolves in 7 to 10 days. Prognosis for pathologic hyperbilirubinemia varies, depending on the cause. If left untreated, hyperbilirubinemia may result in kernicterus, a neurologic syndrome caused by unconjugated bilirubin depositing in the brain cells. Survivors may develop cerebral palsy, epilepsy, or mental retardation, or they may have only minor after effects, such as perceptual-motor disabilities and learning disorders.

What causes it

As erythrocytes break down at the end of their neonatal life cycle, hemoglobin separates into globin (protein) and heme (iron) fragments. Heme fragments form unconjugated bilirubin. Unconjugat-

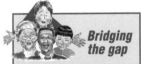

Bridging the gap

Ethnic groups susceptible to physiologic jaundice

Physiologic jaundice tends to be more common and more severe in individuals of Chinese, Japanese, Korean, or Native American descent. Individuals from these ethnic groups have a mean peak of unconjugated bilirubin that's about twice the average level.

ed bilirubin then binds with albumin and is transported to liver cells to conjugate with glucuronide and form direct bilirubin. During this process, unconjugated bilirubin may escape to extravascular tissue, causing hyperbilirubinemia.

Developing news

Several factors may affect whether a neonate develops hyperbilirubinemia:

• Certain drugs (such as aspirin, tranquilizers, and sulfonamides) or conditions (such as hypothermia, anoxia, hypoglycemia, and hypoalbuminemia) can disrupt conjugation and usurp albumin-binding sites.

• Decreased hepatic function can result in reduced bilirubin conjugation.

• Increased erythrocyte production or breakdown or Rh or ABO incompatibility can accompany hemolytic disorders.

• Maternal enzymes present in breast milk can inhibit the neonate's glucuronosyltransferase conjugating activity.

What to look for

The predominant sign of hyperbilirubinemia is jaundice, which doesn't become clinically apparent until serum bilirubin levels reach about 7 mg/100 ml.

Physiologic hyperbilirubinemia

Physiologic hyperbilirubinemia typically develops within 2 to 3 days after birth in 50% of term neonates and within 3 to 5 days after birth in 80% of preterm neonates. It generally disappears by day 7 in term neonates and by day 9 or 10 in preterm neonates. Throughout physiologic jaundice, the serum unconjugated bilirubin level doesn't exceed 12 mg/100 ml.

Pathologic hyperbilirubinemia

Pathologic hyperbilirubinemia may appear anytime after the first day of life and persists beyond 7 days with serum bilirubin levels greater than 12 mg/100 ml in a term neonate, 15 mg/100 ml in a preterm neonate, or increasing more than 5 mg/100 ml in 24 hours.

What tests tell you

Jaundice and elevated levels of serum bilirubin confirm hyperbilirubinemia. Inspection of the neonate in a well-lit room (without yellow or gold lighting) reveals yellowish skin coloration, particularly in the sclerae. To verify jaundice, press the skin on the cheek or abdomen lightly with one finger, then release pressure and observe skin color immediately. Signs of jaundice necessitate measuring and charting serum bilirubin levels every 4 hours. Testing may include direct and indirect bilirubin levels, particularly for pathologic hyperbilirubinemia. Bilirubin levels that are excessively elevated or vary daily suggest a pathologic process.

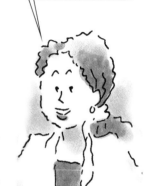

If bilirubin levels are excessively high or vary daily, suspect pathologic hyperbilirubinemia.

Connecting the cause

Identifying the underlying cause of hyperbilirubinemia requires:
- a detailed patient history (including prenatal history)
- a detailed family history (paternal Rh factor, inherited red blood cell defects)
- present status of the neonate (immaturity, infection)
- blood testing of the neonate and mother (blood group incompatibilities, hemoglobin level, direct Coombs' test, hematocrit).

How it's treated

Depending on the underlying cause, treatment may include:
- exchange transfusions
- phototherapy
- albumin infusion.

Uneven exchange

An exchange transfusion replaces the neonate's blood with fresh blood (blood that's less than 48 hours old), thus removing some of the unconjugated bilirubin in serum.

Photo albumin

Phototherapy uses fluorescent light to decompose bilirubin in the skin by oxidation. Implemented after the initial exchange transfusion, phototherapy is usually discontinued after bilirubin levels fall below 10 mg/100 ml and continue to decrease for 24 hours. (See *Performing phototherapy*, page 540.)

Other therapy for excessive bilirubin levels may include albumin administration (1 g/kg of 25% salt-poor albumin), which provides additional albumin for binding unconjugated bilirubin. This may be done 1 to 2 hours before an exchange transfusion or as a substitute for a portion of the plasma in the transfused blood.

What to do

Nursing interventions for the neonate with hyperbilirubinemia include:

Performing phototherapy

To perform phototherapy, follow these steps:
- Set up the phototherapy unit about 18″ (46 cm) above the neonate's crib and verify placement of the light-bulb shield. If the neonate is in an incubator, place the phototherapy unit at least 3″ (7.6 cm) above the incubator and turn on the lights. Place a photometer probe in the middle of the crib to measure the energy emitted by the lights.
- Explain the procedure to the parents.
- Record the neonate's initial bilirubin level and his axillary temperature.
- Place the opaque eye mask over the neonate's closed eyes and fasten securely.
- Undress the neonate and place a diaper under him. Cover male genitalia with a surgical mask or small diaper to catch urine and prevent possible testicular damage from the heat and light waves.
- Take the neonate's axillary temperature every 2 hours and provide additional warmth by adjusting the warming unit's thermostat.

- Monitor elimination and weigh the neonate twice daily. Watch for signs of dehydration (dry skin, poor turgor, depressed fontanels) and check urine specific gravity with a urinometer to gauge hydration status.
- Take the neonate out of the crib, turn off the phototherapy lights, and unmask his eyes at least every 3 to 4 hours with feedings. Assess his eyes for inflammation or injury.
- Reposition the neonate every 2 hours to expose all body surfaces to the light and to prevent head molding and skin breakdown from pressure.
- Check the bilirubin level at least once every 24 hours—more often if levels rise significantly. Turn off the phototherapy unit before drawing venous blood for testing because the lights may degrade bilirubin in the blood. Notify the doctor if the bilirubin level nears 20 mg/dl in full-term neonates or 15 mg/dl in premature neonates.

- Administer $Rh_0(D)$ immune globulin (human), as ordered, to an Rh-negative mother after amniocentesis or to an Rh-negative mother during the third trimester to prevent hemolytic disease after the neonate is born.
- Assess and record the neonate's jaundice and note the time it began. Report the jaundice and serum bilirubin levels immediately.
- Maintain oral intake. Don't skip feedings because fasting stimulates the conversion of heme to bilirubin.
- Offer extra water to promote bilirubin excretion.
- Reassure parents that most neonates experience some degree of jaundice.
- Explain hyperbilirubinemia, its causes, diagnostic tests, and treatment.
- Explain to the parents that the neonate's stool contains some bile and may be greenish.

Meconium aspiration syndrome

Meconium is a thick, sticky, greenish black substance that constitutes the neonate's first feces. It's present in the bowel of the fetus as early as 10 weeks' gestation. Meconium aspiration syndrome results when the neonate inhales meconium that's mixed with amniotic fluid. It typically occurs while the neonate is in utero or with the neonate's first breath. The meconium partially or completely blocks the neonate's airways so that air becomes trapped during exhalation. Also, the meconium irritates the neonate's airways, making breathing difficult.

In the thick of it

The severity of meconium aspiration syndrome depends on the amount of meconium aspirated and the consistency of the meconium. Thicker meconium generally causes more damage.

Increased effort

Neonates with meconium aspiration syndrome increase their respiratory efforts to create greater negative intrathoracic pressures and improve air flow to the lungs. Hyperinflation, hypoxemia, and acidemia cause increased peripheral vascular resistance. Right-to-left shunting often follows.

What causes it

Meconium aspiration syndrome is commonly related to fetal distress during labor. When a neonate becomes hypoxic, peristalsis increases and the anal sphincter relaxes. Occasionally, healthy neonates pass meconium before birth. In either case, if the neonate gasps or inhales the meconium, meconium aspiration syndrome can develop. The resulting lack of oxygen may lead to brain damage.

Risk factors for meconium aspiration syndrome include:
- maternal diabetes
- maternal hypertension
- difficult delivery
- fetal distress
- intrauterine hypoxia
- advanced gestational age (greater than 40 weeks)
- poor intrauterine growth.

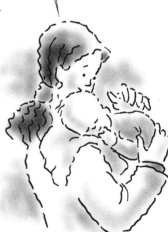

Meconium aspiration syndrome is usually related to fetal distress during labor.

What to look for

Signs and symptoms of meconium aspiration syndrome include:
- dark greenish staining or streaking of the amniotic fluid
- obvious presence of meconium in the amniotic fluid
- skin with a greenish stain (if the meconium was passed long before delivery)
- limp appearance at birth
- cyanosis
- rapid breathing
- labored breathing
- apnea
- signs of postmaturity such as peeling skin and long nails
- low heart rate before birth
- low Apgar score
- hypothermia
- hypoglycemia
- hypocalcemia.

What tests tell you

The most accurate way to diagnose meconium aspiration syndrome is to observe the vocal cords for meconium staining. Assess breath sounds for coarse, crackly sounds, which are common in neonates with meconium aspiration syndrome. ABG analysis helps assess for acidosis (low blood pH and hypoxemia).

Radio for help

A chest radiograph can show patches or streaks of meconium in the lungs and reveal if air is trapped or if hyperinflation has occurred.

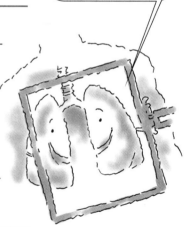

A chest radiograph may reveal patches or streaks of meconium in the lungs.

How it's treated

If meconium aspiration is present or suspected, the neonate's nose and mouth should be suctioned as soon as the head is delivered. Tracheal suctioning may be necessary to remove all of the meconium before the first breath is taken; saline solution may be instilled to remove particularly thick meconium. Close monitoring of the infant is necessary after delivery.

Additional treatments may include:
- chest physiotherapy
- antibiotics
- use of a radiant warmer

Complications of meconium aspiration syndrome

This chart shows potential complications of meconium aspiration syndrome and how they're treated.

Complication	Treatment
Bronchopulmonary dysplasia	• Medication • Oxygen
Pneumothorax	• Chest tube insertion • Oxygen
Aspiration pneumonia	• Surfactant therapy • High-frequency oscillation • Rescue therapy with nitric oxide • Extracorporeal membrane oxygenation

• supplemental oxygen
• mechanical ventilation.

If complications arise, further treatments may be necessary. (See *Complications of meconium aspiration syndrome.*)

What to do

Assess risk factors before delivery, if possible. Other nursing responsibilities include:
• amniotic fluid assessment
• fetal monitoring
• immediate intervention in delivery room
• performing chest physiotherapy
• maintaining thermoregulation
• pulmonary assessment
• administering respiratory support, such as oxygen and mechanical ventilation
• being alert for potential complications
• supporting family members by providing education and reassurance and promoting parent-neonate attachment.

Phenylketonuria

Phenylketonuria (PKU) is a rare hereditary condition. It's characterized by the inability of the body to metabolize phenylalanine, an essential amino acid that's found in protein-containing foods. Excess phenylalanine can affect normal development of the brain and CNS as well as levels of tyrosine, an amino acid that plays a role in the production of melanin, epinephrine, and thyroxine.

What causes it

PKU is inherited as an autosomal recessive trait. Both parents must pass the gene on for the child to be affected. In PKU, there's almost no activity of phenylalanine hydroxylase, an enzyme that helps convert phenylalanine to tyrosine. Phenylalanine accumulates in the blood and urine, resulting in low tyrosine levels. (See *Incidence of PKU.*)

What to look for

Clinical manifestations of PKU in a neonate include:
- seizures
- microcephaly
- hyperactivity
- irritability
- purposeless, repetitive motions
- musty odor from skin and urine excretion of phenylacetic acid
- tremors
- jerking movements of arms and legs
- unusual hand posturing.

PKU phenotypes

Because PKU tends to decrease melanin production, children affected with it have similar phenotypes, including blond hair, blue eyes, and fair skin.

What tests tell you

Diagnostic tests for PKU include:
- enzyme assay to detect whether the parents are carriers of the trait
- chorionic villus sampling during pregnancy to diagnose the fetus prenatally

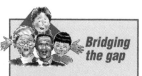

Bridging the gap

Incidence of PKU

Phenylketonuria (PKU) has a high incidence among people of Irish and Scottish descent. Incidence is lower among Blacks and Ashkenazic Jews.

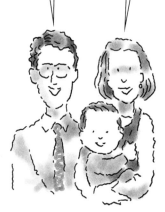

PKU is an autosomal recessive trait that's inherited from both parents.

- PKU screening (mandatory in most states).

The test, not the folk singer

The Guthrie blood test uses a heelstick blood sample from the neonate to screen for PKU. The test detects serum phenylalanine levels of greater than 4 mg/dl (normal level is 2 mg/dl).

How it's treated

Treatment involves maintaining a diet that's extremely low in phenylalanine. Adult women with PKU should strictly adhere to a low phenylalanine diet before and during pregnancy because a strong correlation between maternal phenylalanine levels and improved fetal outcome exists. Increased phenylalanine levels in mothers with PKU can affect embryologic development, causing low birth weight, congenital malformations, microcephaly, and mental retardation.

Eating towards healthy levels

Advise the parents of neonates with PKU to consult with a registered dietitian. A proper diet should meet the neonate's nutritional needs for optimum growth while maintaining a safe phenylalanine level (2 to 8 mg/dl). Phenylalanine levels greater than 10 to 15 mg/dl can lead to brain damage; levels less than 2 mg/dl can lead to protein catabolism and growth retardation.

Foods that can't miss

Special formulas such as Lofenalac are made for infants with PKU. They can be used throughout life as a protein source for individuals with PKU. Foods with low levels of phenylalanine include:
- vegetables
- fruits
- juices
- some cereals, breads, and starches.

Foods to take off the list

To avoid toxicity to the brain and CNS, foods high in phenylalanine should be avoided, including:
- dairy products
- eggs
- meat
- foods or drinks containing aspartame (NutraSweet).

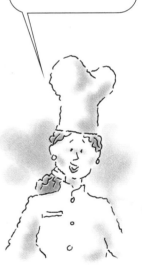

PKU can be controlled with a diet that includes foods low in phenylalanine, such as fruits and vegetables.

What to do

The principle nursing intervention for PKU is teaching the family about dietary restrictions. (See *Teaching parents about PKU*.) Parents also have the burden of knowing that they passed this disorder on to their children. They must make serious decisions regarding future children. Refer these families to genetic counseling.

Prematurity

A neonate is considered premature if he's born before 37 weeks' gestation. The preterm neonate is at risk for complications because the organ systems are immature. The degree of complications depends on gestational age. The closer the neonate is to 40 weeks' gestation, the easier the transition to extrauterine life will be.

What causes it

It may be necessary to deliver a neonate prematurely if evidence of a maternal complication exists. For example, preeclampsia is a condition that can develop in the second or third trimester of pregnancy. Signs of preeclampsia include elevated blood pressure, fluid retention, and protein in the urine. The only treatment for preeclampsia is to deliver the neonate. If left untreated, the mother can suffer severe organ damage and seizures. Kidney disease, heart disease, diabetes, or infection in the mother may also require premature delivery of the neonate.

Additional risk factors for a premature neonate include:
- multiple pregnancy
- adolescent pregnancy
- lack of prenatal care
- substance abuse
- smoking
- previous preterm delivery
- high, unexplained alpha fetoprotein level in second trimester
- abnormalities of the uterus
- cervical incompetence
- premature rupture of membranes
- placenta previa
- PIH.

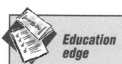

Education edge

Teaching parents about PKU

Parents of neonates with phenylketonuria (PKU) need to have a basic understanding of the disorder. They also need practical suggestions for meal planning because preparing meals can be stressful for parents who have to worry about calculating phenylalanine levels. Be sure to instruct the family on how to:
- eliminate or restrict foods high in phenylalanine
- measure to see if foods are low in phenylalanine
- avoid using artificial sweeteners with aspartame (such as Nutra-Sweet).

What to look for

Premature babies have characteristics that are distinctive at various stages of development. These characteristics can give clues to the neonate's gestational age and physiologic capabilities.

First findings

Initial assessment findings typical of premature neonates include:
- low birth weight
- minimal subcutaneous fat deposits
- proportionally large head in relation to body
- prominent sucking pads in the cheeks
- wrinkled features
- thin, smooth, shiny skin that's almost translucent
- veins that are clearly visible under the thin, transparent epidermis
- lanugo (soft, downy hair) over the body
- sparse, fine, fuzzy hair on the head
- soft, pliable ear cartilage
- minimal creases in the soles and palms
- skull and rib bones that feel soft
- closed eyes
- few scrotal rugae (males)
- undescended testes (males)
- prominent labia and clitoris (females).

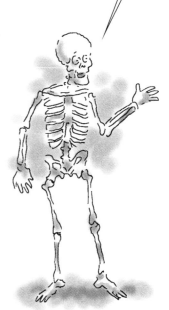

In premature neonates, the skull and rib bones feel soft.

Physical findings

Physical examination findings include:
- inability to maintain body temperature
- limited ability to excrete solutes in the urine
- increased susceptibility to infection
- periodic breathing, hypoventilation, and periods of apnea
- increased susceptibility to hyperbilirubinemia
- increased susceptibility to hypoglycemia
- ability to bring the neonate's elbow across the chest when eliciting the scarf sign
- ability to easily bring the neonate's heel to his ear.

System signs

The neonate's neurologic status is assessed by observing:
- active movements
- response to stimulation
- response to passive movements.
    CNS evaluation may reveal:
- inactivity (although may be unusually active immediately after birth)

- extension of extremities
- absence of suck reflex
- weak swallow, gag, and cough reflexes
- weak grasp reflex.

What tests tell you

These tests may indicate the extent of physiologic maturity and may assist caregivers in the management of the neonate:
- chest X-ray
- ABG analysis
- head ultrasounds
- echocardiography
- eye examination by a retinal specialist
- serum glucose
- serum calcium
- serum bilirubin
- euglobulin lysis time
- CBC.

How it's treated

Premature neonates are cared for by a specially trained staff in the neonatal intensive care unit (NICU). The top priority in treating a premature neonate is supporting the cardiac and respiratory systems as needed. If the neonate isn't breathing or respiratory efforts are poor, an endotracheal tube may be inserted and mechanical ventilation started. Supplemental oxygen may also be given. Medications to increase the heart rate or maintain blood pressure may be administered as part of the resuscitative effort. Other essential interventions include providing thermoregulation and starting I.V. or gavage nutrition.

Three goals

Meticulous care and observation in the NICU is necessary until the neonate:
- receives oral feedings
- maintains body temperature
- weighs about five pounds.

Preemie problems

Certain complications may occur:
- *Respiratory distress syndrome (RDS)* is a leading cause of morbidity and mortality among premature neonates. The lungs lack surfactant, which prevents alveolar collapse at the end of res-

piration. Treatment involves administration of surfactant, oxygen administration, and mechanical ventilation.

• *Intraventricular hemorrhage (IVH)* is bleeding in or around the ventricles of the brain. It's most common in neonates born before 32 weeks' gestation. Damage to brain function and long-term effects vary.

• *Retinopathy of prematurity (ROP)* is a disease caused by abnormal growth of retinal blood vessels. Prematurity may cause abnormal vessels to grow. Supplemental oxygen is also thought to contribute to this growth. ROP can cause mild to severe eye and vision problems. Treatment may involve laser surgery or cryotherapy.

• *Patent ductus arteriosus* occurs when the ductus arteriosus reopens after birth due to lowered oxygen tension associated with respiratory impairment. Treatment involves fluid regulation, respiratory support, administration of indomethacin (Indocin), and surgical ligation (if the neonate doesn't respond to other therapies).

• *Necrotizing enterocolitis (NEC)* is an inflammatory disease of the GI mucosa. (See *A close look at necrotizing enterocolitis.*)

• *Bronchopulmonary dysplasia (BPD)* is also called *chronic lung disease*. The lungs may be less compliant because of the

---

A close look at necrotizing enterocolitis

Necrotizing enterocolitis is an inflammatory disease of the GI mucosa. Here are its causes, pathophysiolgy, and signs as well as tests used to diagnose it and ways in which it's treated.

Causes
• Uncertain; appears to occur in neonates whose GI tract has suffered vascular compromise

Pathophysiology
• Blood flow to gastric mucosa is decreased due to shunting of blood to vital organs.
• Mucosal cells lining the bowel wall die.
• Protective, lubricating mucus isn't secreted.
• Bowel wall is attacked by proteolytic enzymes.
• Bowel wall swells and breaks down.

Signs
• Distended abdomen
• Gastric retention
• Blood in stool or gastric contents
• Lethargy

• Poor feeding
• Hypotension
• Apnea
• Vomiting

Diagnostic tests
• Radiographic studies show intestinal dilation and free air in the abdomen (indicating perforation).
• Laboratory studies show anemia, leukopenia, leukocytosis, electrolyte imbalance.

Treatment
• Prevention
• Discontinuation of enteral feedings
• Nasogastric suction
• Administration of I.V. antibiotics
• Administration of parenteral fluids
• Surgery

damage caused by prematurity, infection, or mechanical ventilation. Treatment involves supplying oxygen, maintaining good nutrition, and preventing respiratory illness.

• *Apnea of prematurity* is a common phenomenon in the premature neonate. It occurs because neurologic and chemical respiratory control mechanisms are immature. The number of apneic spells tends to increase the younger the gestational age of the neonate. The condition can be treated with such medications as theophylline and caffeine.

Additional complications that may occur include:
• infection
• jaundice
• anemia
• hypoglycemia
• delayed growth and development.

What to do

Nursing interventions for the premature neonate should focus on maintaining an environment that's similar to the intrauterine environment. Care should be based on knowledge of the premature neonate's physiologic problems and the need to conserve energy for growth and repair.

Specific nursing responsibilities include:
• rapid initial evaluation
• resuscitative measures, if needed
• thermoregulation
• administration of respiratory support measures
• electronic monitoring
• parenteral fluids, as ordered
• medications, as ordered
• blood specimen analysis, as ordered.

The right touch

Stimulation needs to be individualized to the development and tolerance of each neonate. Touch should be smooth and sure. Stroking and rubbing are discouraged. The head should be supported and the extremities held close to the body during position changes. This type of touch decreases motor disorganization and stress.

Hard to swallow

Premature neonates born before 34 weeks' gestation aren't coordinated enough to maintain the suck, swallow, and breathe regimen necessary for oral feeding. These neonates need to be fed I.V. or by gavage. Be alert for potential complications, such as NEC. Non-

Education edge

Teaching parents of premature neonates

To help the parents of a premature neonate cope with this difficult situation, follow these guidelines:
• Orient them to the neonatal intensive care unit environment and introduce them to all caregivers.
• Orient them to the machinery and monitors that may be attached to their neonate. Reassure them that the staff is alert to alarms as well as the cues of their child.
• Tell them what to expect.
• Teach them the characteristics of a premature neonate.
• Teach them how to handle their neonate.
• Instruct them on feeding, whether it's through gavage, breast, or bottle.
• Inform them of potential complications.
• Offer discharge planning.
• Make appropriate referrals.

nutritive sucking, such as using a pacifier while being fed by gavage, may help to ease the transition to oral feeding that occurs later.

Keep up the communication

Nursing care also involves keeping the parents informed and educated about what's involved in the care of their premature neonate. (See *Teaching parents of premature neonates.*)

Respiratory distress syndrome

RDS occurs when the lungs are immature. It's seen almost exclusively in premature neonates and carries a high risk of long-term respiratory and neurologic complications.

What causes it

RDS is characterized by poor gas exchange and ventilatory failure. It's caused by a lack of pulmonary surfactant, a phospholipid secreted by the alveolar epithelium that normally appears in mature lungs. Surfactant coats the alveoli, keeping them open so that gas exchange can occur. In premature neonates, the lungs may not be fully developed and, therefore, may not have a sufficient amount of surfactant. This leads to:

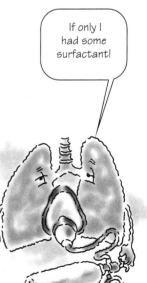

If only I had some surfactant!

- atelectasis
- increased work of breathing
- respiratory acidosis
- hypoxemia.

Changing the flow of the things

As atelectasis worsens, pulmonary vascular resistance increases, which decreases blood flow to the lungs. Blood then shunts from right to left, perpetuating fetal circulation by keeping the foramen ovale and ductus arteriosus patent.

One membrane too many

The alveoli may become necrotic, and the capillaries may become damaged. Ischemia allows fluid to leak into the interstitial and alveolar spaces, causing a hyaline membrane to form. This membrane hinders respiratory function by decreasing the compliance of the lungs.

Risk factors for RDS include:
- prematurity
- maternal diabetes
- stress during delivery that produces acidosis in the neonate.

What to look for

RDS can produce respiratory distress acutely after birth or over a period of a few hours. Initial assessment may reveal:
- increased respiratory rate
- retractions
- satisfactory color
- good air movement on auscultation.

Obvious observations

As respiratory distress becomes more obvious, the nurse may note:
- further increase in respiratory rate
- labored breathing
- more pronounced substernal retractions
- fine rales on auscultation
- expiratory grunting
- nasal flaring
- cyanosis.

It gets worse

If treatment isn't started or if the neonate isn't responding to treatment, the nurse may observe:
- worsening cyanosis

- flaccidity
- unresponsiveness
- apneic episodes
- decreased breath sounds.

What tests tell you

Results of laboratory data, such as hypoxemia, hypercapnia, and acidosis, are nonspecific to RDS. Specific tests must be carried out to evaluate the neonate for complicating factors. These include:
- blood, urine, and CSF cultures
- blood glucose analysis
- serum calcium
- ABG measurements.
    Radiographic evaluation reveals:
- alveolar atelectasis (a diffuse, granular pattern that resembles ground glass) over lung fields
- dilated bronchioles (appear as dark streaks within the granular pattern).

Phospholipid lingo

Prenatal tests can evaluate lung maturity while the fetus is in utero. This is done by evaluating the lecithin and sphingomyelin ratio of the amniotic fluid. Lecithin and sphingomyelin are two surfactant phospholipids. Evaluation of fetal lung maturity gives insight into how the fetus will fare after birth and may precipitate treatment of the mother to delay labor or to mature the neonate's lungs before delivery.

How it's treated

Because RDS is a disease related to gestational age and lung maturity, one management technique is to prevent preterm delivery. If that isn't possible, surfactant production can be stimulated before the neonate is born by administering corticosteroids to the mother before birth.

Supportive steps

RDS treatment after birth is mainly supportive and includes general measures used to treat premature neonates, including:
- thermoregulation
- oxygen administration
- mechanical ventilation, if needed
- prevention of hypotension

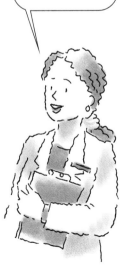

Prevention of preterm delivery decreases the chance that a neonate will suffer from RDS.

- prevention of hypovolemia
- correcting respiratory acidosis by ventilatory support
- correcting metabolic acidosis with the administration of sodium bicarbonate
- parenteral feedings.

Gavage feedings and oral feedings aren't recommended during the acute stage of RDS because such situations that increase respiratory rate or oxygen consumption should be avoided.

Respiratory remedies

Respiratory support can be given by:
- oxygen administration via nasal cannula
- continuous positive airway pressure (CPAP)
- mechanical ventilation.

Sometimes the use of a high-frequency oscillator is needed. Positive end-expiratory pressure (PEEP) may be used via mechanical ventilation. PEEP prevents alveolar collapse during expiration, thereby allowing more time for gas exchange to occur.

The goals of oxygen therapy are to:
- maintain adequate oxygenation to the tissues
- prevent lactic acidosis
- avoid toxic effects of oxygen.

Complications of oxygen therapy and mechanical ventilation may occur despite efforts to prevent them. They include:
- pneumothorax
- pneumomediastinum
- ROP
- BPD
- infection
- IVH.

Myriad of meds

Management of RDS also includes the administration of surfactant. Surfactant can prevent atelectasis and contribute to fluid clearance from the alveoli. Other medications that are commonly used to treat neonates with RDS include antibiotics, sedatives, paralytics, and diuretics.

What to do

Continuous monitoring of the neonate with RDS is essential because of the constant threat of hypoxemia. Nursing responsibilities include:
- collecting blood samples
- monitoring pulse oximetry
- suctioning

- implementing thermoregulation
- monitoring nutrition
- administering medication
- providing mouth and skin care.

Do not disturb

To help decrease oxygen consumption, make efforts to limit how often the neonate with RDS is disturbed. Feeding is generally given parenterally during the acute phase of the disease. Keep the neonate in a dark, quiet, thermal neutral environment as much as possible.

In addition to the general patient teaching for parents of premature neonates, parents of neonates with RDS need to be educated about the syndrome, especially during the acute stage. Refer the parents to social services, a chaplain, and other sources of support as needed.

Transient tachypnea of the neonate

Transient tachypnea of the neonate (TTN) is a mild respiratory problem in neonates. It begins after birth and generally lasts about 3 days. TTN is also known as *wet lungs* or *type II RDS*.

What causes it

TTN results from the delayed absorption of fetal lung fluid after birth. Before birth, the fetus doesn't use his lungs to breathe. Instead, the fetal lungs are filled with fluid. All of the fetus' nutrients and oxygen come from the mother through the placenta. During the birth process, some of the neonate's lung fluid is squeezed out as he passes through the birth canal. After birth, the remaining fluid is pushed out of the lungs as the lungs fill with air. Fluid that remains is later coughed out or absorbed into the blood stream. TTN results when fluid remains in the lungs, forcing the neonate to breathe harder and faster to get adequate oxygen.

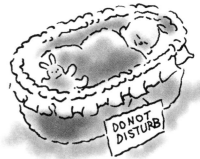

Fluid is usually squeezed out of the neonate's lungs during birth. TTN results if fluid remains in the lungs after birth.

Risk factory

TTN is commonly observed in neonates delivered by cesarean birth. These neonates don't receive the thoracic compression that helps to expel fluid during vaginal delivery. Other risk factors for TTN include:

- premature delivery of the neonate
- smoking during pregnancy
- being born to a mother with diabetes
- size that's SGA.

Neonates who are small or premature, or who were born rapidly by vaginal delivery, may not have received effective squeezing of the thorax to remove fetal lung fluid.

What to look for

Common signs of TTN include:
- increased respiratory rate (greater than 60 breaths/minute)
- labored breathing
- expiratory grunting
- nasal flaring
- retractions
- cyanosis.

These signs typically occur immediately after birth. However, these could also be indicative of a more serious condition; observe the neonate closely.

What tests tell you

Laboratory tests and imaging studies are used to diagnose TTN. For example:
- ABG results may indicate hypoxemia and decreased carbon dioxide levels.
- Increased carbon dioxide levels may be a sign of fatigue and impending respiratory failure.
- Pulse oximetry is used to noninvasively monitor tissue oxygenation and allow titration of supplemental oxygen.
- A CBC may be done to evaluate for signs of infection.
- Chest X-ray, the diagnostic standard for TTN, will reveal streaking which correlates with lymphatic engorgement of retained fetal lung fluid.

Abnormal findings

Abnormalities in diagnostic test results resolve with resolution of the condition, usually within 72 hours.

How it's treated

Specific treatment for TTN depends on:
- the neonate's gestational age, overall health, and medical history
- the extent of respiratory distress

- tolerance of medical therapies
- expectations for the course of the disease.

Be supportive

Care is mainly supportive as the retained lung fluid is reabsorbed. Treatment may involve:

- monitoring heart rate, respiratory rate, and oxygen levels
- providing supplemental oxygen
- maintaining CPAP
- using mechanical ventilation
- providing proper nutrition.

Generally, a neonate with TTN is supported with I.V. fluids or gavage feedings. The increased respiratory rate and increased work of breathing makes oral feeding difficult because the neonate must coordinate the mechanisms of sucking, swallowing, and breathing. The rapid respiratory rate puts the neonate at high risk for aspiration.

Minimal meds

Medication use in TTN is minimal. Antibiotic therapy may be administered until sepsis is ruled out. The regimen usually consists of penicillin (usually ampicillin [Omnipen]) and an aminoglycoside (usually gentamicin [Garamycin]) or a cephalosporin (usually cefotaxime [Claforan]).

What to do

A neonate with TTN may be cared for in an NICU. Nursing interventions include:

- monitoring heart and respiratory rates and oxygenation
- providing respiratory support
- maintaining a neutral thermal environment
- minimizing stimulation by decreasing lights and noise levels
- administering medication, as ordered
- providing proper nutrition
- parental education and emotional support.

Symptoms typically resolve within 72 hours. The neonate usually recovers completely and has no increased risk for further respiratory problems.

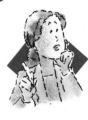

Quick quiz

1.   Testing a neonate for drug exposure while in utero involves collecting and analyzing:

A.   urine and meconium.
B.   blood and urine.
C.   CSF and meconium.
D.   CSF and blood.

Answer: A. Urine and meconium samples are collected when testing a neonate for drug exposure.

2.   Neonates classified as SGA have a birth weight that's:

A.   below the 5th percentile.
B.   below the 10th percentile.
C.   below the 15th percentile.
D.   below the 20th percentile.

Answer: B. Neonates classified as SGA have a birth weight below the 10th percentile.

3.   Which option is a neonatal risk factor for HIV transmission?

A.   Being premature
B.   Being a second-born twin
C.   Being bottle-fed
D.   Being born postterm

Answer: A. Prematurity is neonatal risk factor for HIV infection.

4.   Downward deviation of the eyes ("sunsetting eyes") is a classic assessment finding of:

A.   FAS.
B.   hydrocephalus.
C.   prematurity.
D.   HIV infection.

Answer: B. Downward deviation of the eyes is a characteristic finding in neonates with hydrocephalus.

5.   Which is the most accurate diagnostic tool for meconium aspiration syndrome?

A.   Chest X-ray
B.   ABG analysis
C.   Evaluation of the vocal cords using a laryngoscope
D.   Amniotic fluid testing for meconium

Answer: C. The most accurate way to diagnose meconium aspiration syndrome is to evaluate the vocal cords for meconium staining using a laryngoscope.

6. What's the role of surfactant in the lungs?
   A. It coats the alveoli to help keep them open so that gas exchange can occur.
   B. It increases pulmonary capillary blood flow.
   C. It increases respiratory rate to correct acidemia.
   D. It prevents bronchospasm.

Answer: A. Surfactant is a phospholipid secreted by the alveolar epithelium that coats the alveoli, keeping them open so that gas exchange can occur.

7. Which option isn't a risk factor for TTN?
   A. Prematurity
   B. Delivery by cesarean birth
   C. Being LGA
   D. Smoking during pregnancy

Answer: C. Risk factors for TTN are cesarean delivery, prematurity, smoking during pregnancy, being born to a diabetic mother, and being SGA.

Scoring

☆☆☆ If you answered all seven questions correctly, superb! You bring high-risk neonatal nursing care to new heights.

☆☆ If you answered five or six questions correctly, yeah baby! See you in the NICU!

☆ If you answered fewer than five questions correctly, relax. You may have been a little premature in taking this quick quiz, but you can always review the chapter.

Appendices and index

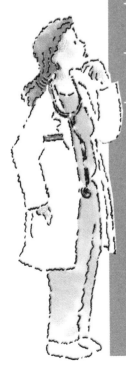

Laboratory values for pregnant and nonpregnant patients

	Pregnant	Nonpregnant
Hemoglobin	11.5 to 14 g/dl	12 to 16 g/dl
Hematocrit	32% to 42%	36% to 48%
White blood cells	5,000 to 15,000/µl	4,500 to 10,000/µl
Neutrophils	60% ±10%	60%
Lymphocytes	34% ±10%	30%
Platelets	150,000 to 350,000/µl	150,000 to 350,000/µl
Serum calcium	7.8 to 9.3 mg/dl	8.4 to 10.2 mg/dl
Serum sodium	Increased retention	136 to 146 mmol/L
Serum chloride	Slight elevation	98 to 106 mmol/L
Serum iron	65 to 120 mcg/dl	75 to 150 mcg/dl
Fibrinogen	450 mg/dl	200 to 400 mg/dl
Red blood cells	1,500 to 1,900/µl	1,600/µl
Fasting blood glucose	Decreased	70 to 105 mg/dl
2-hour postprandial blood glucose	< 140 mg/dl (after a 100 g carbohydrate meal)	< 140 mg/dl
Blood urea nitrogen	Decreased	10 to 20 mg/dl
Serum creatinine	Decreased	0.5 mg/dl to 1.1 mg/dl
Renal plasma flow	Increased by 25%	490 to 700 ml/minute
Glomerular filtration rate	Increased by 50%	88 to 128 ml/minute
Serum uric acid	Decreased	2.0 to 6.6 mg/dl
Erythrocyte sedimentation rate	Elevated during second and third trimesters	20 mm/hour
Prothrombin time	Decreased slightly	11 to 12.5 seconds
Partial thromboplastin time	Decreased slightly during pregnancy and again during second and third stages of labor (indicating clotting at placental site)	60 to 70 seconds

Selected maternal daily dietary allowances

This chart shows selected daily dietary allowances for pregnant and breast-feeding women.

Nutrient	Pregnant women	Breast-feeding women	
		Months 1 through 6	Months 7 through 12
Calcium	1,200 mg	1,200 mg	1,200 mg
Folate	600 mcg	280 mcg	260 mcg
Iodine	175 mcg	200 mcg	200 mcg
Iron	30 mg	18 mg	18 mg
Magnesium	320 mg	310 mg	340 mg
Niacin	17 mg	17 mg	17 mg
Phosphorus	1,200 mg	700 mg	700 mg
Protein	60 g	65 g	62 g
Riboflavin	1.6 mg	1.8 mg	1.7 mg
Selenium	65 mcg	70 mcg	70 mcg
Thiamine (B_1)	1.5 mg	1.6 mg	1.6 mg
Vitamin A	800 mcg	1,300 mcg	1,200 mcg
Vitamin B_6	2.2 mg	2.5 mg	2.5 mg
Vitamin B_{12}	2.2 mcg	2.8 mcg	2.8 mcg
Vitamin C	70 mg	100 mg	100 mg
Vitamin D	10 mcg	10 mcg	10 mcg
Vitamin E	10 mg	11 mg	11 mg
Zinc	15 mg	25 mg	25 mg

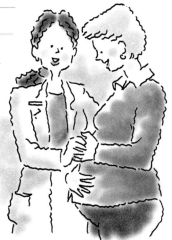

Good nutrition is a vital part of a healthy pregnancy.

Normal neonatal laboratory values

This chart shows laboratory tests that may be ordered for neonates, including the normal ranges for full-term infants. Note that ranges may vary among institutions. Because test results for preterm neonates usually reflect weight and gestational age, ranges for preterm neonates vary.

Test	Normal range
Blood	
Acid phosphatase	7.4 to 19.4 units/L
Albumin	3.6 to 5.4 g/dl
Alkaline phosphatase	40 to 300 units/L (1 week)
Alpha-fetoprotein	up to 10 mg/L, with none detected after 21 days
Ammonia	90 to 150 mcg/dl
Amylase	0 to 1,000 IU/hour
Bicarbonate	20 to 26 mmol/L
Bilirubin, direct	less than 0.5 mg/dl
Bilirubin, total	less than 2.8 mg/dl (cord blood)
0 to 1 day	2.6 mg/dl (peripheral blood)
1 to 2 days	6 to 7 mg/dl (peripheral blood)
3 to 5 days	4 to 6 mg/dl (peripheral blood)
Bleeding time	2 minutes
Arterial blood gases	
ph	7.35 to 7.45
$Paco_2$	35 to 45 mm Hg
Pao_2	50 to 90 mm Hg

Test	Normal range
Blood *(continued)*	
Venous blood gases	
pH	7.35 to 7.45
Pco_2	41 to 51 mm Hg
Po_2	20 to 49 mm Hg
Calcium, ionized	2.5 to 5 mg/dl
Calcium, total	7 to 12 mg/dl
Chloride	95 to 110 mEq/L
Clotting time (2 tube)	5 to 8 minutes
Creatine kinase	10 to 300 IU/L
Creatinine	0.3 to 1 mg/dl
Digoxin level	greater than 2 ng/ml possible; greater than 30 ng/ml probable
Fibrinogen	0.18 to 0.38 g/dl
Glucose	30 to 125 mg/dl
Glutamyltransferase	14 to 331 units/L
Hematocrit	52% to 58%
	53% (cord blood)
Hemoglobin	17 to 18.4 g/dl
	16.8 g/dl (cord blood)
Immunoglobulins, total	660 to 1,439 mg/dl
IgG	398 to 1,244 mg/dl
IgM	5 to 30 mg/dl
IgA	0 to 2.2 mg/dl
Iron	100 to 250 mcg/dl
Iron-binding capacity	100 to 400 mcg/dl

Test	Normal range
Blood (continued)	
Lactate dehydrogenase	357 to 953 IU/L
Magnesium	1.5 to 2.5 mEq/L
Osmolality	270 to 294 mOsm/kg H_2O
Partial thromboplastin time	40 to 80 seconds
Phenobarbital level	15 to 40 mcg/dl
Phosphorus	5 to 7.8 mg/dl (birth)
	4.9 to 8.9 mg/dl (7 days)
Platelets	100,000 to 300,000/µl
Potassium	4.5 to 6.8 mEq/L
Protein, total	4.6 to 7.4 g/dl
Prothrombin time	12 to 21 seconds
Red blood cell count	5.1 to 5.8 (1,000,000/µl)
Reticulocytes	3% to 7% (cord blood)
Sodium	136 to 143 mEq/L
Theophylline level	5 to 10 µg/ml
Thyroid-stimulating hormone	less than 7 microunits/ml
Thyroxine (T_4)	10.2 to 19 mcg/dl
Transaminase	
glutamic-oxaloacetic (aspartate)	24 to 81 units/L
glutamic-pyruvic (alanine)	10 to 33 units/L
Triglycerides	36 to 233 mg/dl
Urea nitrogen	5 to 25 mg/dl
White blood cell (WBC) count	18,000/µl
eosinophils-basophils	3%
immature WBCs	10%
lymphocytes	30%
monocytes	5%
neutrophils	45%

Test	Normal range
Urine	
Casts, WBC	present first 2 to 4 days
Osmolality	50 to 600 mOsm/kg
pH	5 to 7
Phenylketonuria	no color change
Protein	present first 2 to 4 days
Specific gravity	1.006 to 1.008
Cerebrospinal fluid	
Calcium	4.2 to 5.4 mg/dl
Cell count	0 to 15 WBCs/µl 0 to 500 RBCs/µl
Chloride	110 to 120 mg/L
Glucose	32 to 62 mg/dl
pH	7.33 to 7.42
Pressure	50 to 80 mm Hg
Protein	32 to 148 mg/dl
Sodium	130 to 165 mg/L
Specific gravity	1.007 to 1.009

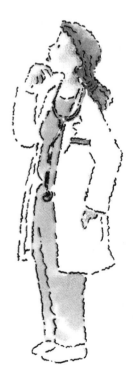

NANDA Taxonomy II codes

The North American Nursing Diagnosis Association (NANDA) endorsed its first nursing diagnosis taxonomic structure, NANDA Taxonomy I, in 1986. This taxonomy has been revised several times, most recently in 2002. The new Taxonomy II has a code structure that's compliant with recommendations from the National Library of Medicine concerning health care terminology codes. The taxonomy that appears here represents the currently accepted classification system for nursing diagnosis.

Nursing diagnosis	Taxonomy II code	Nursing diagnosis	Taxonomy II code
Imbalanced nutrition: More than body requirements	00001	Urge urinary incontinence	00019
Imbalanced nutrition: Less than body requirements	00002	Functional urinary incontinence	00020
Risk for imbalanced nutrition: More than body requirements	00003	Total urinary incontinence	00021
Risk for infection	00004	Risk for urge urinary incontinence	00022
Risk for imbalanced body temperature	00005	Urinary retention	00023
Hypothermia	00006	Ineffective tissue perfusion (specify type: renal, cerebral, cardiopulmonary, gastrointestinal, peripheral)	00024
Hyperthermia	00007		
Ineffective thermo-regulation	00008		
Autonomic dysreflexia	00009	Risk for imbalanced fluid volume	00025
Risk for autonomic dysreflexia	00010	Excess fluid volume	00026
Constipation	00011	Deficient fluid volume	00027
Perceived constipation	00012	Risk for deficient fluid volume	00028
Diarrhea	00013	Decreased cardiac output	00029
Bowel incontinence	00014	Impaired gas exchange	00030
Risk for constipation	00015	Ineffective airway clearance	00031
Impaired urinary elimination	00016	Ineffective breathing pattern	00032
Stress urinary incontinence	00017	Impaired spontaneous ventilation	00033
Reflex urinary incontinence	00018		

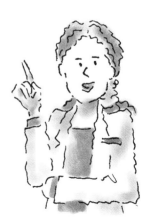

Nursing diagnosis	Taxonomy II code	Nursing diagnosis	Taxonomy II code
Dysfunctional ventilatory weaning response	00034	Caregiver role strain	00061
Risk for injury	00035	Risk for caregiver role strain	00062
Risk for suffocation	00036	Dysfunctional family processes: Alcoholism	00063
Risk for poisoning	00037	Parental role conflict	00064
Risk for trauma	00038	Ineffective sexuality patterns	00065
Risk for aspiration	00039	Spiritual distress	00066
Risk for disuse syndrome	00040	Risk for spiritual distress	00067
Latex allergy response	00041	Readiness for enhanced spiritual well-being	00068
Risk for latex allergy response	00042	Ineffective coping	00069
Ineffective protection	00043	Impaired adjustment	00070
Impaired tissue integrity	00044	Defensive coping	00071
Impaired oral mucous membrane	00045	Ineffective denial	00072
Impaired skin integrity	00046	Disabled family coping	00073
Risk for impaired skin integrity	00047	Compromised family coping	00074
Impaired dentition	00048	Readiness for enhanced family coping	00075
Decreased intracranial adaptive capacity	00049	Readiness for enhanced community coping	00076
Disturbed energy field	00050	Ineffective community coping	00077
Impaired verbal communication	00051	Ineffective therapeutic regimen management	00078
Impaired social interaction	00052	Noncompliance (specify)	00079
Social isolation	00053	Ineffective family therapeutic regimen management	00080
Risk for loneliness	00054		
Ineffective role performance	00055	Ineffective community therapeutic regimen management	00081
Impaired parenting	00056		
Risk for impaired parenting	00057	Effective therapeutic regimen management	00082
Risk for impaired parent/infant/child attachment	00058	Decisional conflict (specify)	00083
Sexual dysfunction	00059		
Interrupted family processes	00060		

Nursing diagnosis	Taxonomy II code	Nursing diagnosis	Taxonomy II code
Health-seeking behaviors (specify)	00084	Dressing or grooming self-care deficit	00109
Impaired physical mobility	00085	Toileting self-care deficit	00110
Risk for peripheral neuro-vascular dysfunction	00086	Delayed growth and development	00111
Risk for perioperative-positioning injury	00087	Risk for delayed development	00112
Impaired walking	00088	Risk for disproportionate growth	00113
Impaired wheelchair mobility	00089	Relocation stress syndrome	00114
Impaired transfer ability	00090	Risk for disorganized infant behavior	00115
Impaired bed mobility	00091	Disorganized infant behavior	00116
Activity intolerance	00092		
Fatigue	00093	Readiness for enhanced organized infant behavior	00117
Risk for activity intolerance	00094	Disturbed body image	00118
Disturbed sleep pattern	00095	Chronic low self-esteem	00119
Sleep deprivation	00096	Situational low self-esteem	00120
Deficient diversional activity	00097	Disturbed personal identity	00121
Impaired home maintenance	00098	Disturbed sensory perception (specify: visual, auditory, kinesthetic, gustatory, tactile, olfactory)	00122
Ineffective health maintenance	00099		
Delayed surgical recovery	00100		
Adult failure to thrive	00101	Unilateral neglect	00123
Feeding self-care deficit	00102	Hopelessness	00124
Impaired swallowing	00103	Powerlessness	00125
Ineffective breast-feeding	00104	Deficient knowledge (specify)	00126
Interrupted breast-feeding	00105	Impaired environmental interpretation syndrome	00127
Effective breast-feeding	00106		
Ineffective infant feeding pattern	00107	Acute confusion	00128
Bathing or hygiene self-care deficit	00108	Chronic confusion	00129

Nursing diagnosis	Taxonomy II code	Nursing diagnosis	Taxonomy II code
Disturbed thought processes	00130	Risk for situational low self-esteem	00153
Impaired memory	00131	Wandering	00154
Acute pain	00132	Risk for falls	00155
Chronic pain	00133	Risk for sudden infant death syndrome	00156
Nausea	00134	Readiness for enhanced communication	00157
Dysfunctional grieving	00135		
Anticipatory grieving	00136	Readiness for enhanced coping	00158
Chronic sorrow	00137		
Risk for other-directed violence	00138	Readiness for enhanced family processes	00159
Risk for self-mutilation	00139	Readiness for enhanced fluid balance	00160
Risk for self-directed violence	00140		
Posttrauma syndrome	00141	Readiness for enhanced knowledge (specify)	00161
Rape-trauma syndrome	00142		
Rape-trauma syndrome: Compound reaction	00143	Readiness for enhanced management of thera- peutic regimen	00162
Rape-trauma syndrome: Silent reaction	00144	Readiness for enhanced nutrition	00163
Risk for posttrauma syndrome	00145	Readiness for enhanced parenting	00164
Anxiety	00146		
Death anxiety	00147	Readiness for enhanced sleep	00165
Fear	00148		
Risk for relocation stress syndrome	00149	Readiness for enhanced urinary elimination	00166
Risk for suicide	00150	Readiness for enhanced self-concept	00167
Self-mutilation	00151		
Risk for powerlessness	00152		

Glossary

aberration:
a deviation from what's typical or normal

acme:
the peak of a contraction

adnexal area:
accessory parts of the uterus, ovaries, and fallopian tubes

agenesis:
failure of an organ to develop

amnion:
the inner of the two fetal membranes that forms the amniotic sac and houses the fetus and the fluid that surrounds it in utero

amniotic:
relating to or pertaining to the amnion

amniotic fluid:
fluid surrounding the fetus, derived primarily from maternal serum and fetal urine

amniotic sac:
membrane that contains the fetus and fluid during gestation

analgesic:
pharmacologic agent that relieves pain without causing unconsciousness

anesthesia:
use of pharmacologic agents to produce partial or total loss of sensation, with or without loss of consciousness

anomaly:
an organ or a structure that's malformed or in some way abnormal due to structure, form, or position

artificial insemination:
mechanical deposition of a partner's or donor's spermatozoa at the cervical os

autosomes:
any of the paired chromosomes other than the X and Y (sex) chromosomes

basal body temperature:
temperature when body metabolism is at its lowest, usually below 98° F (36.7° C) before ovulation and above 98° F after ovulation

Bishop score:
method of assessing cervical dilation, effacement, station, consistency, and position to determine readiness for induction of labor

c-peptide:
an enzyme predictor of early hyperinsulinemia

cephalocaudal development:
principle of maturation that development proceeds from the head to the tail (rump)

chorion:
the fetal membrane closest to the uterine wall; gives rise to the placenta and is the outer membrane surrounding the amnion

conduction:
loss of body heat to a solid, cooler object through direct contact

congenital disorder:
disorder present at birth that may be caused by genetic or environmental factors

convection:
loss of body heat to cooler ambient air

corpus luteum:
yellow structure formed from a ruptured graafian follicle that secretes progesterone during the second half of the menstrual cycle; if pregnancy occurs, the corpus luteum continues to produce progesterone until the placenta assumes that function

cotyledon:
one of the rounded segments on the maternal side of the placenta, consisting of villi, fetal vessels, and an intervillous space

cryptorchidism:
undescended testes

cul-de-sac:
pouch formed by a fold of the peritoneum between the anterior wall of the rectum and the posterior wall of the uterus; also known as *Douglas' cul-de-sac*

decidua:
mucous membrane lining of the uterus during pregnancy that's shed after birth

dilation:
widening of the external cervical os

dizygotic:
pertaining to or derived from two fertilized ova, or zygotes (as in dizygotic twins)

doll's eye sign:
movement of a neonate's eyes in a direction opposite to which the head is turned; this reflex typically disappears after 10 days of extrauterine life

Down syndrome:
abnormality involving the occurrence of a third chromosome, instead of the normal pair (trisomy 21), that characteristically results in mental retardation and altered physical appearance

dystocia:
difficult labor

effleurage:
gentle massage to the abdomen during labor for the purpose of relaxation and distraction

effacement:
thinning and shortening of the cervix

embryo:
conceptus from the time of implantation to 8 weeks

endometrium:
inner mucosal lining of the uterus

engagement:
descent of the fetal presenting part to at least the level of the ischial spines

Epstein's pearls:
small, white, firm epithelial cysts on the neonate's hard palate

evaporation:
loss of body heat that occurs as fluid on the body surface changes to a vapor

fetus:
conceptus from 8 weeks until term

follicle-stimulating hormone:
hormone produced by the anterior pituitary gland that stimulates the development of the graafian follicle

fontanelle:
space at the junction of the sutures connecting fetal skull bones

gamete intrafallopian tube transfer:
placement of an ovum and spermatozoa into the end of the fallopian tube via laparoscope; also called *in vivo fertilization*

gene:
factor on a chromosome responsible for the hereditary characteristics of the offspring

general anesthesia:
use of pharmacologic agents to produce loss of consciousness, progressive central nervous system depression, and complete loss of sensation

hematoma:
collection of blood in the soft tissue

hereditary disorder:
disorder passed from one generation to another

heterozygous:
presence of two dissimilar genes at the same site on paired chromosomes

Homans' sign:
calf pain on leg extension and foot dorsiflexion that's an early sign of thrombophlebitis

homozygous:
presence of two similar genes at the same site on paired chromosomes

human chorionic gonadotropin:
hormone produced by the chorionic villi that serves as the biologic marker in pregnancy tests

hyperinsulinemia:
prediabetic state marked by insulin resistance and commonly seen in polycystic ovarian syndrome

hypoxia:
reduced oxygen availability to tissues or fetus

increment:
period of increasing strength of a uterine contraction

induction of labor:
artificial initiation of labor

informed consent:
written consent obtained by the doctor after the patient has been fully informed of the planned treatment, potential adverse effects, and alternative management choices

intensity:
the strength of a uterine contraction (if measured with an intrauterine pressure device, measured and recorded in millimeters of mercury [mm Hg]; if measured externally, a relative measurement may be used)

interval:
period between the end of one uterine contraction and the beginning of the next uterine contraction

intervillous space:
irregularly-shaped areas in the maternal portion of the placenta that are filled with blood and serve as the site for maternal-fetal gas, nutrient, and waste exchange

in vitro fertilization:
fertilization of an ovum outside the body, followed by reimplantation of the blastocyte into the woman

involution:
reduction of uterine size after delivery; may take up to 6 weeks

karyotype:
schematic display of the chromosomes within a cell arranged to demonstrate their numbers and morphology

lanugo:
downy, fine hair that covers the fetus between 20 weeks of gestation and birth

lecithin:
a phospholipid surfactant that reduces surface tension and increases pulmonary tissue elasticity; presence in amniotic fluid is used to determine fetal lung maturity

lecithin-sphingomyelin ratio:
measurement of the relation of lecithin (which rises sharply around 35 weeks' gestation) and sphingomyelin (which remains stable) that's used as an indicator of fetal lung maturity; also known as *L/S ratio*

leukorrhea:
white or yellow vaginal discharge

lie:
relationship of the long axis of the fetus to the long axis of the pregnant patient

linear terminalis:
imaginary line that separates the true pelvis from the false pelvis

local anesthesia:
blockage of sensory nerve pathways at the organ level, producing loss of sensation only in that organ

lochia:
discharge after delivery from sloughing of the uterine decidua

luteinizing hormone:
hormone produced by the anterior pituitary gland that stimulates ovulation and the development of the corpus luteum

meiosis:
process by which germ cells divide and decrease their chromosomal number by one-half

mifepristone:
a progesterone antagonist that prevents implantation of fertilized egg; also called *RU-486*

mitosis:
process of somatic cell division in which a single cell divides but both of the new cells have the same number of chromosomes as the first

molding:
shaping of the fetal head caused by shifting of sutures in response to pressure exerted by the maternal pelvis and birth canal during labor and delivery

myometrium:
middle muscular layer of the uterus that's made up of three layers of smooth, involuntary muscles

neonate:
an infant between birth and the 28th day

nidation:
implantation of the fertilized ovum in the uterine endometrium

Nitrazine paper:
a treated paper used to detect pH used in determining if amniotic fluid is present

NuvaRing:
vaginal contraceptive ring that contains estrogen and progesterone

oligohydramnios:
severely reduced and highly concentrated amniotic fluid

oocyte:
incompletely developed ovum

oogenesis:
formation and development of the ovum

ovum:
conceptus from time of conception until primary villi appear (approximately 4 weeks after the last menstrual period)

perimetrium:
outer serosal layer of the uterus

polyhydramnios:
abnormally large amount (more than 2,000 ml) of amniotic fluid in the uterus

premonitory:
serving as a warning

primordial:
existing in the most primitive form

puerperium:
interval between delivery and 6 weeks after delivery

radiation:
loss of body heat to a solid cold object without direct contact

regional anesthesia:
blockage of large sensory nerve pathways in an organ and its surrounding tissue, producing loss of sensation in that organ and in the surrounding region

ripening:
softening and thinning of the cervix in preparation for active labor

Ritgen maneuver:
manual pressure applied through the perineum to the occiput of the head as the fetus is extending and emerging during birth

rugae:
folds in the vaginal mucosa and scrotum

semen:
white, viscous secretion of the male reproductive organs that consists of spermatozoa and nutrient fluids ejaculated through the penile urethra

smegma:
whitish secretions around the labia minora and under the foreskin of the penis

sperm:
male sex cell

spermatogenesis:
formation and development of spermatozoa

sphingomyelin:
a general membrane phospholipid that isn't directly related to lung maturity but is compared with lecithin to determine fetal lung maturity; levels remain constant during pregnancy

station:
relationship of the presenting part to the ischial spines

strabismus:
condition characterized by imprecise muscular control of ocular movement

subinvolution:
failure of the uterus to return to normal size following delivery

surrogate mothering:
conceiving and carrying a pregnancy to term with the expectation of turning the infant over to contracting, adoptive parents

sutures:
narrow areas of flexible tissue on the fetal scalp that allow for slight adjustment during descent through the birth canal

teratogen:
any drug, virus, irradiation or other nongenetic factor that can cause fetal malformation

tocolytic agent:
medication that stops premature contractions

tocotransducer:
an external mechanical device that translates one physical quantity to another, most often seen in capturing fetal heart rates and transmitting and recording the value onto a fetal monitor

trisomy:
condition where a chromosome exists in triplicate instead of in the normal duplicate pattern

Wharton's jelly:
whitish, gelatinous material that surrounds the umbilical vessels within the cord

X chromosome:
sex chromosome in humans which exist in duplicate in the normal female and singly in the normal male

Y chromosome:
sex chromosome in the human male that's necessary for development of the male sex glands, or gonads

zygote intrafallopian tube transfer:
fertilization of the ovum outside the mother's body, followed by reimplantation of the zygote into the fallopian tube via laparoscope

Selected references

Association of Women's Health, Obstetric, and Neonatal Nurses. *Core Curriculum for Maternal-Newborn Nursing*, 2nd ed. Philadelphia: W.B. Saunders Co., 2000.

Association of Women's Health, Obstetric, and Neonatal Nurses. *Women's Health Nursing: Toward Evidence-Based Practice.* Philadelphia: W.B. Saunders Co., 2003.

Becker, R., et al. "Doppler Sonography of Uterine Arteries at 20-23 Weeks: Risk Assessment of Adverse Pregnancy Outcome by Quantification of Impedance and Notch," *Journal of Perinatal Medicine* 30(5):388-94, 2002.

Berkowitz, J., et al. "Weighing Preterm Infants Before & After Breastfeeding: Does It Increase Maternal Confidence and Competence?" *American Journal of Maternal-Child Nursing* 27(6): 318-26, November-December 2002.

Blackburn, S. *Maternal, Fetal, and Neonatal Physiology: A Clinical Perspective*, 2nd ed. Philadelphia: W.B. Saunders Co., 2003.

Callister, L.C., et al. "First Time Mothers' Views of Breastfeeding Support from Nurses," *American Journal of Maternal-Child Nursing* 28(1):10-15, January-February 2003. Hill, W.C. *Ambulatory Obstetrics.* Philadelphia: Lippincott Williams & Wilkins, 2002.

Lowdermilk, D.L., et al. *Maternity and Women's Health Care*, 8th ed. Philadelphia: W.B. Saunders Co., 2004.

Matteson, P.S. *Women's Health During the Childbearing Years: A Community-Based Approach.* Philadelphia: W.B. Saunders Co., 2001.

Moos, M.K. "Unintended Pregnancies: A Call for Nursing Action," *American Journal of Maternal-Child Nursing* 28(1):24-30, January-February 2003.

Morgan, G., and Hamilton, C. *Practice Guidelines for Obstetrics & Gynecology*, 2nd ed. Philadelphia: Lippincott Williams & Wilkins, 2002.

Murphy, P.A. "New Methods of Hormonal Contraception," *Nurse Practitioner* 28(2):11-21, February 2003.

Murray, S.S., et al. *Foundations of Maternal-Newborn Nursing*, 3rd ed. Philadelphia: W.B. Saunders Co., 2002.

Newman, M.G., et al. "Perinatal Outcomes in Preeclampsia that is Complicated by Massive Proteinuria," *American Journal of Obstetrics & Gynecology* 188(1):264-68, January 2003.

Pillitteri, A. *Maternal and Child Health Nursing: Care of the Childbearing and Childrearing Family*, 4th ed. Philadelphia: Lippincott Williams & Wilkins, 2002.

Schiff, M.A., and Holt, V.L. "The Injury Severity Score in Pregnant Trauma Patients: Predicting Placental Abruption and Fetal Death," *Journal of Trauma* 53(5): 946-49, November 2002.

Scott, J.R., et al. *Danforth's Obstetrics and Gynecology*, 9th ed. Philadelphia: Lippincott Williams & Wilkins, 2003.

Sheiner, E., et al. "Incidence, Obstetric Risk Factors, and Pregnancy Outcome of Preterm Placental Abruption: A Retrospective Analysis," *Journal of Maternal and Fetal Neonatal Medicine* 11(1):34-39, January 2002.

Simpson, K.R., and Creehan, P.A. *AWHONN's Perinatal Nursing*, 2nd ed. Philadelphia: Lippincott Williams & Wilkins, 2001

Speroff, L., and Darney, P. *A Clinical Guide for Contraception*, 3rd ed. Philadelphia: Lippincott Williams & Wilkins, 2000.

Index

A

Abdomen
  effect of pregnancy on, 129, 130i
  neonatal, assessing, 500
Abdominal discomfort, minimizing, 208
Abortion
  as ethical dilemma, 20
  induced, 89, 102
  spontaneous. *See* Spontaneous
    abortion.
Abruptio placentae, 215-219, **C7**
  causes of, 215
  nursing care in, 218
  signs and symptoms of, 216-217, 217i
  testing for, 217
  treatment of, 218-219
Abstinence, 62
Acid phosphatase values, normal
  neonatal, 567t
Acoustic blinking reflex, 502
Acrosome, 45i, 46, **C3**
Acrocyanosis, 486, 495
Activity level, labor onset and, 314
Acupressure, 352
Acupuncture, 352
Adoptive family, 8
Adrenal gland, effect of pregnancy
  on, 118
Age
  and family response to pregnancy,
    19-20
  maternal, 15, 149, 209
    and high-risk pregnancy, 212
Aging, and sexual function, 34
Albumin values, normal neonatal, 567t
Alcohol, during pregnancy, 192

Aldosterone, during pregnancy, 118
Alkaline phosphatase values, normal
  neonatal, 567t
Alpha-fetoprotein testing, 185
Alpha-fetoprotein values, normal
  neonatal, 567t
Ambivalence, trimester of, 139
Amenorrhea, 104, 105t
American Nurses Association's
  Maternal Child Health Nursing
  Practice, 2
Ammonia values, normal neonatal,
  567t
Amniocentesis, 177-178
Amniotic fluid, 52
  analysis of, 178, 179t
  membrane rupture and, 317
  proper handling of, 178
Amniotic fluid embolism, 364-365
Amniotic sac, development of, 52,
  53i, 58
Amniotomy, 308, 309
Amphetamine withdrawal, in neonate,
  522
Ampulla, 30, 39
Amylase values, normal neonatal, 567t
Androgens, 32
Anencephaly, 186
Anesthesia
  local, 357, 359i
  lumbar epidural, 354, 355i, 361
  regional, 354
  spinal, 357
Ankle edema, minimizing, 199t, 203
Anovulation
  and infertility, 94
  medications for, 95-97
Antepartum period, 2, 25

Antibody screening tests, prenatal, 183
Anticoagulation values, therapeutic,
  472
Aorta, fetal, **C8**
Apgar scoring, 484, 485t, 517
Apical pulse, neonatal, 500, 518
Apnea of prematurity, 550
Appetite, during pregnancy, 131
Arab-Americans, childbearing
  practices of, 18t
Areolae, secondary, 115
Arrhythmias
  fetal, 338-340t
  during pregnancy, 121
Arterial blood gas values, normal
  neonatal, 567t
Artificial sweeteners, 192
Asian-Americans, childbearing
  practices of, 17t
Asians, cultural beliefs of, 151
Assessment
  neonatal, 484-504
  postpartum, 424-430
Association of Women's Health, Ob-
  stetric, and Neonatal Nurses, 2
Atria, fetal, **C8**
Attachment, 138
Axillary temperature, neonatal, 491,
  492

B

Babinski's reflex, 502
Baby blues, 422, 423
Back, prenatal assessment of, 163
Backache, minimizing, 199t, 206
Bacterial vaginosis, 283t

---

i refers to an illustration; t refers to a table; boldface refers to full-color pages.

i refers to an illustration; t refers to a table; boldface refers to full-color pages.

i refers to an illustration; t refers to a table; boldface refers to full-color pages.

i refers to an illustration; t refers to a table; boldface refers to full-color pages.

i refers to an illustration; t refers to a table; boldface refers to full-color pages.

i refers to an illustration; t refers to a table; boldface refers to full-color pages.

i refers to an illustration; t refers to a table; boldface refers to full-color pages.

i refers to an illustration; t refers to a table; boldface refers to full-color pages.

i refers to an illustration; t refers to a table; boldface refers to full-color pages.

i refers to an illustration; t refers to a table; boldface refers to full-color pages.

Notes

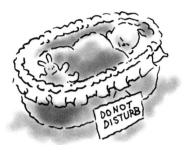

Notes

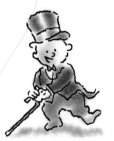

Notes

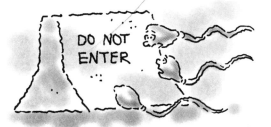

Notes

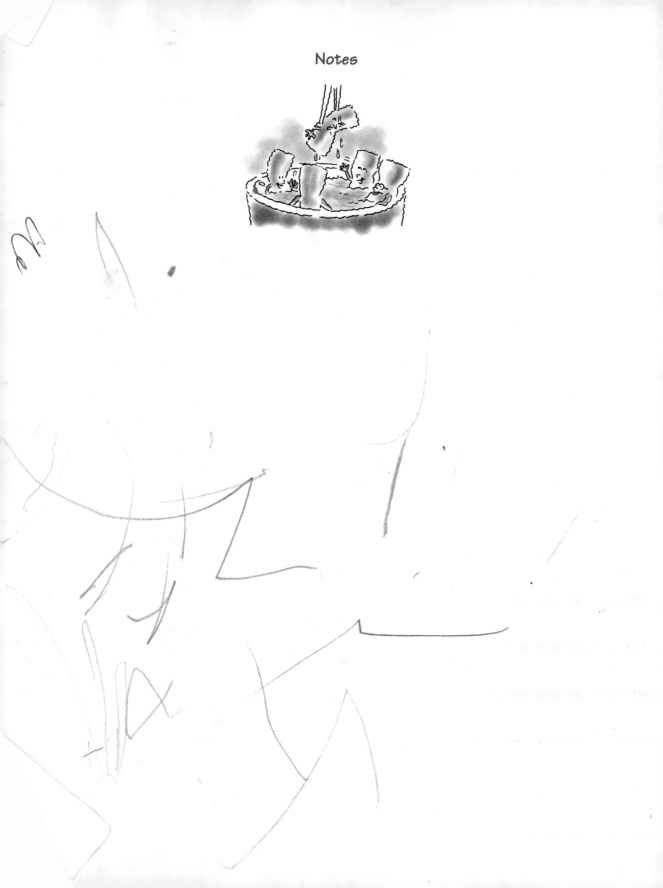

Staff

Publisher
Judith A. Schilling McCann, RN, MSN

Editorial Director
David Moreau

Clinical Director
Joan M. Robinson, RN, MSN

Senior Art Director
Arlene Putterman

Art Director
Mary Ludwicki

Clinical Editors
Beverly Ann Tscheschlog, RN, BS (clinical project manager); Joanne M. Bartelmo, RN, MSN; Maryann Foley, RN, BSN

Senior Editor
Jaime L. Stockslager

Editors
Marylou Ambrose, Kevin Haworth, Brenna H. Mayer, Liz Schaeffer

Copy Editors
Kimberly Bilotta (supervisor), Scotti Cohn, Tom DeZego, Amy Furman, Shana Harrington, Dorothy P. Terry, Pamela Wingrod

Designers
Lynn Foulk, Jacalyn B. Facciolo

Illustrator
Bot Roda, Betty Winnberg

Digital Composition Services
Diane Paluba (manager), Joyce Rossi Biletz, Richard Eng

Manufacturing
Patricia K. Dorshaw (senior manager), Beth Janae Orr

Editorial Assistants
Megan Aldinger, Tara Carter-Bell, Arlene Claffee, Linda Ruhf

Indexer
Karen C. Comerford

The clinical treatments described and recommended in this publication are based on research and consultation with nursing, medical, and legal authorities. To the best of our knowledge, these procedures reflect currently accepted practice. Nevertheless, they can't be considered absolute and universal recommendations. For individual applications, all recommendations must be considered in light of the patient's clinical condition and, before administration of new or infrequently used drugs, in light of the latest package-insert information. The authors and publisher disclaim any responsibility for any adverse effects resulting from the suggested procedures, from any undetected errors, or from the reader's misunderstanding of the text.

© 2004 by Lippincott Williams & Wilkins. All rights reserved. This book is protected by copyright. No part of it may be reproduced, stored in a retrieval system, or transmitted, in any form or by any means — electronic, mechanical, photocopy, recording, or otherwise — without prior written permission of the publisher, except for brief quotations embodied in critical articles and reviews and testing and evaluation materials provided by publisher to instructors whose schools have adopted its accompanying textbook. Printed in the United States of America. For information, write Lippincott Williams & Wilkins, 1111 Bethlehem Pike, P.O. Box 908, Springhouse, PA 19477-0908.

MNIE—D N O S
05 04 03   10 9 8 7 6 5 4 3 2 1

Library of Congress Cataloging-in-Publication Data
Maternal-neonatal nursing made incredibly easy.
    p. ; cm.
    Includes bibliographical references and index.
    1. Maternity nursing. 2. Neonatology.
    [DNLM: 1. Maternal-Child Nursing. WY 157.3 M42555 2004]
  I. Lippincott Williams & Wilkins.

RG951.M3143 2004
610.73'678 — dc21
ISBN 1-58255-268-1 (alk. paper)   2003012896

Maternal-Neonatal Nursing

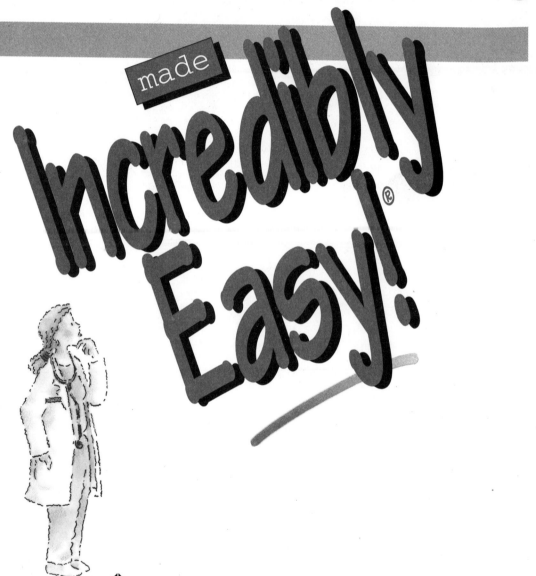

made Incredibly Easy!®

LIPPINCOTT WILLIAMS & WILKINS
A **Wolters Kluwer** Company

Philadelphia • Baltimore • New York • London
Buenos Aires • Hong Kong • Sydney • Tokyo

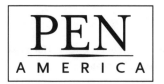

Published by PEN American Center,
an affiliate of International PEN,
the worldwide association of writers
working to advance literature
and defend free expression.

PEN America: A Journal for Writers and Readers
Issue 3 (Volume 2)

PEN American Center
568 Broadway, Suite 401
New York, NY 10012

This issue is made possible in part by the generous funding of The Sol Goldman Charitable Trust and The Kaplen Foundation.

Copyright © 2002 PEN American Center.

All rights reserved. No portion of this journal may be reproduced by any process or technique without the formal written consent of PEN American Center. Authorization to photocopy items for internal, informational, or personal use is granted by PEN American Center. This consent does not extend to other kinds of copying, such as copying for general distribution, for advertising or promotional purposes, for creating collective works, or for resale.

Opinions expressed in *PEN America* are those of the author of each article, and not necessarily those of the editor, the advisory board, or the officers of PEN American Center.

Printed in the United States of America by McNaughton and Gunn.

Postmaster: Send address changes to *PEN America*, c/o PEN American Center, 568 Broadway, Suite 401, New York, NY 10012.

ISBN: 0-934638-19-5

ISSN: 1536-0261

Cover photograph: PEN dinner in honor of Sinclair Lewis, the first American writer to receive the Nobel Prize, Hotel Commodore, November 25, 1930. Photograph by Empire Photographers, N.Y.

Because of limited resources, at present we are unable to review unsolicited submissions of writing except from members of PEN American Center. We do, however, seek color photographs for the cover and black-and-white images (single photos as well as photo essays) for the inside. The theme of issue 4 will be "Fact/Fiction." See *www.pen.org/journal/submit.html* for guidelines. No manuscripts, requests, or artwork will be returned without the inclusion of a self-addressed stamped envelope. We do not accept unsolicited submissions of any kind via e-mail; these will be deleted unopened.

Please see page 228 for text acknowledgments.

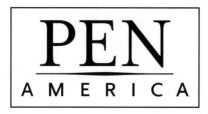

3 | Tribes

EDITOR
M. Mark

MANAGING EDITOR
India Amos

ASSISTANT EDITORS
Jedediah Berry, Sara Crosby, Abbey Dean, Audra Epstein,
Lily Saint, Jeffrey Salane, Nick Torrey

INTERNS
Chelsea Adewunmi, E.T. Bertrando, Jenny Brown, Sarah Buller,
Rania Jawad, Lauren Thogersen, Justine van der Leun

ART DIRECTOR
Adam B. Bohannon

ADVISORY BOARD
Patricia Bosworth, Thulani Davis, Lynn Goldberg, Amy P. Goldman,
Neil Gordon, Jessica Hagedorn, Robert Kelly, Ann Lauterbach,
Phillip Lopate, Albert Mobilio, Honor Moore, Laurie Muchnick,
Geoffrey O'Brien, Grace Paley, Ann Patty, Robert Polito,
Elaine Showalter, William Weaver

CONTENTS

Retorts

E-mail Forum

TRIBUTES

Send for Langston

MEMOIR

ESSAYS

FICTION

LAGNIAPPE

Literary Manifestos

EDITOR'S NOTE

Since the days of clay tablets and papyrus scrolls, writers have been seeking relief from the solitude that's part of our job description. We've left our desks, left our rooms, and joined other writers to celebrate ideas or denigrate them, claim intellectual territory in the company of kindred souls or cast aspersions on those deemed less kindred. Some writers, of course, shun the collective, but even they may find themselves assigned to a group by critics who see the past as a succession of literary movements and the present as a map of stylistic schools.

Half a century ago, Philip Rahv divided American writers into cerebral "palefaces" and earthy "redskins." Though such labels make some of us cringe, tribal allusions persist—in part, perhaps, because the word "tribe" is so elastic that it can encompass literary tradition, genre, style, geography, subculture, identity, ideology, ethnicity, nationality, intellectual or emotional affinity, shared taste, shared quirks, shared prejudices, shared readers, and shared marketing strategies. A literary tribe can be a group of ancestors or a group of friends, a support group, a gang, a club or a fan club, a clan.

The fiction, nonfiction, and poetry in this issue approach the juncture of writers and tribes from angles that suggest more junctures: us/them, insider/outsider, familiar/exotic, dissident/patriotic, East/West, black/white, rooted/rootless, mindful/mindless. In a symposium on tribes, essayists (including two of the stouthearted young editors of this journal) sift through their mixed feelings. Here and there in the issue, you'll find strikingly unambivalent pronouncements, many of them from *Manifesto: A Century of Isms*, edited by Mary Ann Caws and published by the University of Nebraska Press, an illuminating anthology that helped those of us who put together *PEN America* as we tried to organize our own mixed feelings about literary tribes.

—M. Mark

MANIFESTO: 1916

Nunism

Pierre Albert-Birot

Translated by Mary Ann Caws

An "ism" to outlast the others.

Nunism was born with man and will only disappear with him.

All the great philosophers, the great artists, the great poets, the great scientists, all the flamebearers, the creators of all ages have been, are, will be nunists.

All of us who are seeking something, let's be nunists first.

No life outside of nunism.

To be a nunist or not be.

MANIFESTO: 1991

Oulipo

Jacques Roubaud

Translated by Harry Mathews

. . . Periodically, generation after generation, *literary groups* appear (or are invented after the fact by literary historians) that share the following characteristics:

► The groups are formed with a view to renewing and re-establishing a literature that has, according to them, deteriorated to an appallingly low level.
► Their motto is: everything done prior to us is worthless; everything done after us can only exist because of us. . . .
► The group thoroughly despises its contemporaries, particularly rival groups to which the fact of its existence and the claims it makes inevitably give rise.
► The very way the group works leads, through splits, divergences, "deviations," and exclusions, to its fairly rapid destruction. . . .

Raymond Queneau had been a Surrealist; and he had, as we know, taken violent leave of the Bretonian sect. It was unquestionably as a result of his reflections on this unfortunate example that he "invented" the following rules, original, if few in number. . . .

► The Oulipo is not a closed group; it can be enlarged through the co-optation of new members. No one can be expelled from the Oulipo.
► Conversely, no one can resign. . . . The dead continue to belong to the Oulipo.
► One may relinquish membership of the Oulipo under the following circumstances: suicide may be committed in the presence of an officer of the court, who then ascertains that, according to the Oulipian's explicit last wishes, his suicide was intended to release him from the Oulipo and restore him his freedom of maneuver for the rest of eternity. . . .

Oulipian writing—that is, writing with constraints—endeavors to rediscover another way in which to practice artistic freedom, one that is at work in all (or nearly all) literatures and poetic enterprises of the past: the freedom of difficulty mastered. . . . Definition: An Oulipian author is a rat who himself builds the maze from which he sets out to escape.

TRIBES: A SYMPOSIUM

For this issue, we invited several writers to consider their tribal associations. "What is your literary lineage?" we asked. "Who are your tribal elders, the writers from whom you've learned? Who are your contemporaries? your heirs? Does your tribe include your readers? In what ways are tribes useful? Are you ambivalent about them? Is tribal identification merely a label that has little bearing on writers and their work? Do tribes necessarily imply exclusivity? territoriality? Are you a loner? Do loners constitute a tribe?" Here are the responses we received:

UNEASY PEACE | FRANCISCO GOLDMAN

Many years ago, during what would have been my senior year in college if I hadn't left college and moved to New York, I got to attend a writers' conference in Sarasota, Florida—it was organized by Rust Hills, fiction editor of *Esquire*, and included, among others, William Gaddis and William Gass. In New York I had a job removing thorns from rose stems and wiring pine cones to Christmas wreaths in a florist's shop (I belong to the grand tribe of retired de-thorners) and so I was especially grateful for a scholarship to the conference, arranged by the creative-writing teacher I'd had in college, from whom I'd learned, "A fiction writer has to be like a truck driver, he has to get into that cab and drive." This excellent piece of advice, with which I still often futilely cajole myself, is one of two lasting lessons I took away from writing classes; the second, from that Sarasota conference, was spoken by William Gass. Another student had asked him how being a philosophy professor influenced his fiction writing, and William Gass answered that there was no conscious influence at all. "I know I'm smart," I remember him saying, so he knew his writing would also be "smart," but he was busy paying attention to his sentences. (He was probably a little more specific, but I wouldn't dare put words in the maestro's mouth.) He didn't think about philosophy or about himself as a philosophy professor when he wrote; he worked on his sentences.

I don't think about my allegiances to any particular tribes when I am working on a novel, I just pay attention to my sentences, while also trying to divine the eventual shape of the thing—*yo persigo una forma*—and I know that when the book is done it will be as fully expressive of myself as I need it to be . . .

I was going to begin this little essay by saying that I am not a person of tribal feelings, that I don't even like the word "tribal"—it sounds trendy to me—but then why did I so deeply yearn for Mexico to beat the U.S.A. in World Cup soccer? Fashionably anti-gringo? Not at all! Guatemala is the country of my "Latino" heritage, yet if Guatemala had been playing Mexico, I still would have been for Mexico. How disloyal! It's just that I'd never cared much for futbol until Mexico's thrilling if short-lived World Cup adventure of '98—I was living in Mexico at the time, and still do part of each year—and my loyalty is to the team that initiated me into the worldwide tribe of futbol fans. I follow "el Tri." Mexico, situated between my two natural national tribes, Guate and the U.S.A.—I'm in love with the muchacha next door.

And there I was at the long Brooklyn bar, with a group of Mexicans on my right, and a group of white American guys on my left—quite alone, a loner. The woman on my right had a beautiful bare calf, crooked and glowing down there in the lower-barstool region like the moon the cow jumped over, and my attention was pulled in that direction from the disaster on the television screen. I was not in any way being a demonstrative fan. By 3:30 A.M. it was clear that all was lost, and I was just trying to stay awake. The bartender served me a consolation vodka, courtesy of the white American guys on my left, a drink I definitely did not need. The Mexican contingent, sunk into gloom, quietly slipped out of the bar. I left just after, and walked home in a mood of sadness and even despair, mulling the inevitable fates of poor nations (Mexico had lost the game before they even took the field) and feeling like an overwrought, drunken sad sack at the end of an Isaac Babel story.

This whole issue of "tribes" can seem dangerous to me, if I let it. Jewish tribe. Latin American mestizo-Catholic tribe. Well, it's pretty hard to be an observant Jew and an observant Catholic at the same time. There is of course no contradiction between being a New Yorker and ethnically anything else. If belonging to any "tribe" also implies meeting some standard of purity, to hell with it anyway. I do not worry about these things in my walking-around life, and in my writing one, I pay attention to my sentences, and so on . . .

But, *pues si*, the Latin American novel has been especially important to me over the years. A novel as familiar as *One Hundred Years of Solitude* will always have revealing, challenging, even dark things to say to a reader with some intimate relationship to that culture—to "us," whatever I mean by that—no matter what that book's eventual fate elsewhere. Yet García Márquez, Vargas Llosa, Onetti, and others also belong to the "tribe" of Faulkner, and are perhaps truer heirs of his than any subsequent generations of writers in the U.S. Just as the literary heirs to some of the greatest Latin American writers' experimental verve have not been, in this country, for the most part, Latino writers (a tribe of many tribes and also traditions of their own). We all know that literature transcends frontiers. There is no contemporary writer I love more than Murakami.

Then what about Guatemala—what's my "tribal" affiliation there, why do I keep coming back to that small, often terrifying and heartbreaking little country that has also been, in an inescapable way, over the last sixty years, the United States' most sustained and tragically wacky experiment in nation building and social engineering? Though Guatemala may seem small, it's actually enormous, larger than the U.S., and is not only the center of "the universe," but a portal (and look, I can move back and forth, between this "tribe" and that one, the one yankees famously don't want to know about) to the rest of the world, the small poor country that is also all the small poor countries. And isn't that what every fully imagined novel is? A small remote country that—for at least as long as it might hold your attention during the reading of a book—is also the center of the world.

A PLACE IN THE PROCESSION | C. D. WRIGHT

Long long ago I dreamed this: an old soul, mud-colored, thin, ropy-haired, hunkers at a campfire. A line of naked youth has formed on the lip of a cliff. The old one is reciting the history of poetry. And as he intones, the youth dive from the cliff one after another. Presumably there is water below.

I would like to sit around with people I like and people about whom I haven't made up my mind yet and drink wine and eat a crazy salad with my meat, talking straight poetry. It wouldn't matter if anything were written down or not. The words would burn into our brains. I've always preferred the communal aspect of art to the solitary. That is, I feel complete when it is shared, and when it is being made, alone, in the dark, I feel like a spider who has to get that web made because she's hungry. She's always hungry. I have a spidery hand, and I try to get it to transmit to my mind, and then I try to make it attractive enough to draw others in. They say Walt Whitman's beard drew butterflies.

It's harder for me to feel that dreamy about poetry nowadays. The art is thoroughly divorced from the multi-million–dollar spectacles that play to the numbers, and entropically inclined from within. It does hang in there. Poetry will not go quietly. You would have to starve it out, and it can live on very little. Hunger and love move the world, didn't Schiller say.

Poets are mostly voters and taxpayers, but the alienation of the poet is a common theme. Among poets there is also probably a higher-than-average rate of clutch burnout, job turnover, rooting about, sleep apnea, noncompliance, nervous leg syndrome, depression, litigation, black clothing, etc., but this is where we live, or as Leonard Cohen put it, Poetry is the opiate of the poets.

There are other honorable paths, if I may without explanation call this one honorable, but they are not necessarily chosen, and they are not necessarily binding the way poets choose and bind.

The decade-long disturbance over fragmentation and wholeness aside, I would say poetry provides a place in the procession, and in so doing it keeps us intact, one after another. This is an altogether beautiful position from which to leap.

INDEPENDENT STUDIES | MARY GAITSKILL

I don't think the concept of "tribes" applies to writers because writing is an innately solitary activity. It becomes social when people read and respond to it, but, valuable as that response is, it exists as something apart from the work itself. There is a great difference between the book as it exists nested in the mind of the writer, the book out in the world without that organic context, and the book as it's received by the reader and given a home in that reader's mind.

A pop song must be something very different in the mind of the musician than the sound you hear whipping by you on a car radio or coming out of a restaurant sound system. That sound can be powerful for the listener, and it gets associated with feelings and experiences she's having around it—which might have to do with the actual music or not. In a similar way, reader responses, while interesting on their own terms, sometimes don't seem to have much to do with what the writer has actually written. The difference is that responses to music have a tribal feeling because music can be experienced in groups; it penetrates people in such a fluid, emotional way that you can feel everyone is experiencing it as you are. But reading takes place as writing does—alone. It penetrates you less quickly and viscerally than music, and it gets filtered through the brain with more nitty particularity. It's an intense one-on-one interaction between the creative and the intelligent receptive, which brings the book a very individual life. Readers can translate a beautiful book into something ugly and stupid, or they can blithely accomplish the reverse. For better or worse, they make it theirs in a different way than it belongs to the writer, or to other readers. For that reason, I can't imagine a tribe of readers, let alone readers existing as a tribe for a writer.

Because of the individual and private nature of the experience, I don't feel a tribal kinship with any group of writers past or present. I like and admire many writers of all kinds, but I don't feel that kind of affinity. I feel a certain recognition or emotional/perceptual identification on reading a variety of writers: Nabokov, the early Updike, Emily Brontë, Carson McCullers, Charles Dickens, also newcomers Rebecca Godfrey, J. T. Leroy, and Nani Power. But I don't think that makes me like them, nor do I think they are like each other, tribally or otherwise. If I think in terms of species, I would say Updike and Nabokov are the most closely related—to each other, not to me—but I don't think of either as a species that travels in packs!

A DEMURRAL | LYNN FREED

Being asked what tribe one considers oneself a part of is rather like being asked what one is reading. Reading? I go blank. Catalogues? Appliance instructions? I *love* reading appliance instructions, particularly in bed. Keep hands, hair, and clothing away from appliance during operation. Do not reach for an appliance that has fallen into water. Simply hold the nozzle of the vacuum near the cover and the suction will remove any dust particles.

But now comes, "Our topic for this issue of *PEN America* is literary tribes." Tribes? As a child, I had thought that death would come roaring over the hill one day in the form of Zulus dressed for war—men in fur and shells, with spears and shields, and their women ululating after them. I had thought of literary women as spinsters with ample bosoms and bad breath, who lived in tiny rooms with their cats and a kettle and a type-writer. Had it occurred to me that, one day, I would be asked to put myself into a literary tribe, I would have married the first man who promised to carry me away from there. Or become a dentist. Or a vet.

THE SPACE BETWEEN | MARINA BUDHOS

I was never very good at cliques.

In high school, I often found myself peering anxiously at the cool white girls who gathered on the steps every morning, brushed cheeks to say hello, and flicked straight, combed hair from their shoulders while they talked. But the minute I was let into that clique (and allowed to brush cheeks), I began anxiously scanning for escape. I went to a large New York City school where I bounced between groups, ethnically, racially, up and down the academic scale. I hung with the tiny group of Jewish kids bound for careers as lawyers and bankers; the black kids from south Jamaica who knew how to dance and party; the theater arts crew, a motley collection of wannabes who spent their allowances on plays in Manhattan; and the potheads who cut class and went home, mashing cigarettes and joints in tinfoil ashtrays that could be swiftly discarded before their parents arrived. And finally, I was an art-house loner, who stuffed a George Eliot into my thrift-store coat and snuck off to watch double-feature European films at the Bleecker Street Cinema.

Some of this has to do with my own mixed background and my mix-it-up upbringing. My father was a diasporic Indian—raised in the Caribbean and educated at strict British-style missionary schools. My mother came from an Orthodox Jewish home, where her parents barely spoke English. We children were raised in a community built for UN families; our neighbors were from Egypt, Jordan, Japan, South Africa. Americans were the exotics. My father taught in a high school of mostly black kids; we shopped on Jamaica Avenue, where the faces were mostly brown and black, and my father could buy his West Indian rotis and goat curry, and the clothes were cheap.

Years later, I went to a graduate program that emphasized "voice" and "experimentation." One week I wrote a *New Yorker*-style short story about an anorexic graduate student recovering from a failed romance; another week, I was imitating Angela Carter and writing a Gothic tale. Yet another week I was writing semiautobiographical stories about my mixed family. Stylistically, I was all over the map, and the writers I defined myself by were terribly eclectic.

I found kindred spirits in classic short-story writers such as V. S. Pritchett, Flannery O'Connor, Alice Munro. But my stories were bursting at the seams; they were narratives that wanted a more spacious home, like big families ready to break out of their tight little apartments. So I had to look to novelists. I went back to Virginia Woolf, my undergraduate heroine, and took solace in her lovely flights of language, her capacity to write a stylistically different book each time and yet still be, well, so *Virginia*. I began a bracing diet of V. S. Naipaul, since I was starting to discover my material in the Caribbean and Indian milieu of my father.

But just as in high school, I wasn't adept at finding a place for myself. I skittered around and fell between the cracks; I shied away from the MFA world, even though, I suppose, they were my "group." In some way, I still felt like an outsider here in the U.S., the child-of-immigrant, mixed-race, mixed-influence kid who half-belongs to the white girls on the steps and is also in some other cultural zone. I recoiled a bit from the indulgences of the young wordsmiths honing their craft in workshops, for they did not offer, in my mind, much social or cultural insight.

In 1989, after a month at Yaddo, where I'd keenly felt my usual "in-betweenness," I wrote these feelings down in an essay, "From Village to Global Village." Little did I know, I was writing my way to a tribe that hadn't yet arrived. For about the time I began publishing books, a new literary "tribe" was coming to the fore: Asian-American writers. Suddenly I was part of a family tree, and I didn't entirely mind. Some of the concerns were dear to my heart—immigrant, second-generation conflicts. The cadences of those voices, their way of phrasing sentences, the focus on family, felt familiar. I was giving readings and teaching workshops under the banner of Asian-American literature. Then came the next wave: Indian or South Asian writers. Once again, I found myself in a tribe that felt familiar. I was reviewed by the Indian press like a cherished daughter; I saw my photograph stretched across a page like a Bollywood movie poster in *India Today*, the equivalent of *Time* magazine. It felt great to be part of a lively, growing tribe.

This tribe gave me a feeling of home less because I was an "Asian" author or an "Indian" author (which I'm not, really) than because these works (and their authors) carry an awareness of culture that doesn't quite make it into my American peers' work. American minimalism leaves too much out, takes too much for granted. That slight difference in voice—as if the author is broadcasting, "Here I am, on a margin between worlds, and I'm going to explain it to you"—struck a chord in me, and continues to do so.

In my last novel, I was most inspired by Maxine Hong Kingston—her blend of family memoir and fabulous mythmaking. But having attempted my own version of this mix, I am still pulled between two allegiances: wild and magical versus realistic and psychological. I want lush language to take me on its own darkening river, yet I want to document, in fine and intimate detail, the grainy social reality we live in. Most recently, the filmmaker Mira Nair, who fluctuates between documentary and feature filmmaking, has offered a new kind of inspiration.

For the more I write, the more I discover another layer: a social conscience, an interest in political matters. Having grown up in a home where my father passionately followed India's independence movement and studied the Soviet economy, having lived in a community created out of a utopian ideal and lived through an era when civil rights exploded in our faces, I couldn't lose track of those concerns, that way of seeing and interpreting the world. Social realism, however, bores me as a writer. So from fiction I expanded into nonfiction, where I'm drawn to the "narrative journalism" approach—reporting done with a novelist's eye for detail. Suddenly the work of writers such as Jonathan Kozol, Frances FitzGerald, and Anne Fadiman means as much to me as the turbulent, imaginative prose of my favorite novelists.

These days I'm scattered over too many projects. In the back of my mind I hear the beginnings of a sprawling, semimagical multigenerational tale of India, the Caribbean, and turn-of-the century New York. At the same time, I'm working on a nonfiction book about American women and immigrant nannies, a work that has me stretching toward sociology and theorizing and sometimes makes my brain burn, as I climb into new analytic reaches. Along with this I've been scribbling a children's picture book, an Elizabethan screenplay, and some young-adult fiction. Occasionally, out of exhaustion, I just want to cut myself up and feed pieces to each genre and style, so I don't have to hold it all inside.

Still, I think in this haphazard and zig-zagging madness, there lies a kind of logic. I am interested in exchange, both literary and cultural, since this is my core, who I am. My Jewish mother speaks a staccato English, and my mellow Caribbean-Indian father was a real-life To Sir With Love. In high school I belonged as much to the white girls flicking their hair as I did to the black kids who felt considerably less assured about their futures in America. I was something of a voyeur, a noncommittal spy who swam between these and other worlds. It's often a struggle to find the vocabulary to give voice to this half-in, half-out space. This is the very hard lesson I'm trying to learn—that being in between is actually a place of strength.

PEER PLEASURE | LILY SAINT

For many young writers, moving to New York City is like taking an enormous step across the moon. Expectation, wariness, and excitement hover in one gravity-defying moon-booted moment. The writer, who has complained all her life of literary isolation, eagerly anticipates the comrades she will find in the city. She expects that they will be as excited as she is to discuss the latest literary review or revitalize stagnating English departments nationwide. She looks forward to the gossip mill, the cocktail conversations, and the romance; to an ideal intellectual tribe of her peers.

These expectations seem to be shared by most of the young writers I meet. Often, to facilitate the creation of their tribe, they attend MFA programs, where they imagine that their classmates will provide the foundation for a new and impressive literary coterie. On one of my first days in a New York City MFA program, a student from Nebraska bemoaned the absence of "movements" in her life. Where were the twentieth-century versions of the interbreeding Romantics, where the Anaïs Nins and Henry Millers, where for christsake were the *New York* poets? This pressing need to belong to a tribe of writers got me thinking. Having been in New York for several years, did *I* have a tribe?

Part of the difficulty in finding a tribe might lie in my taste for instant gratification. Did I expect to be recognized immediately as a precocious literary genius? Did I *really* want to oust entrenched literary intelligentsia with my iconoclastic ideas, or was I all too easily satisfied with the general peacefulness of my life? Is my inability to find and form these tribes related to an embarrassing political apathy? Indeed, are all literary tribes formed, however obliquely, as a response to social and political upheaval? If so, no wonder the tribes I form with my friends lack direction and instead consist mostly of infighting—bickering about writers we know who write in ways we just don't like. Our tribalism comes down to matters of taste: who still subscribes to *The Paris Review*, who "writes" found poetry, who has bad breath.

What emerges, instead of clearly delineated literary groups, is a cross-over, mutating sort of tribalism, in which writers move fluidly between overlapping circles of peers—circles that lack both ideological and formal centers. A writer featured in a journal espousing nontraditional forms might pop up leading a seminar on the sonnet; a novelist without a poem in her oeuvre might publish a whole book of works which exactly resemble prose poetry but are called fiction. Genres *and* writers are experiencing radical redefinition.

All of the young writers I know are, to one extent or another, cross-breeds. The tribes they form may be confusing and unwieldy, but people still want to surround themselves with others who do similar work. We find each other at readings, in classrooms, in bars, and even on the subway. We give up our late-night lunar dreams, and settle finally for the solid earth.

ONLY CONNECT | SARA CROSBY

I started rereading Graham Greene's novels not long ago, and somewhere in the middle of *The Quiet American* I realized that he is the reason I occasionally use the odd colon. Joseph Mitchell and George Orwell taught me that it's all right to go hang around with overlooked people. Joan Didion encouraged me to fiddle with "nonfiction." James Baldwin showed me that rage should be embraced and drawn upon. And William Maxwell made me want to write simple, vivid sentences. But I don't affiliate my writing with theirs—and would be too sheepish to say so even if I did.

I, like almost everyone, am part of a loose pack of people, and writing—though a large part of my life—is only one of the many threads that connect us. What about food, movies, and baseball? Or fashion, the Midwest, and dogs? What about memories? Obviously there are people in my pack who write. Jon, Tamar, Stephen, and I meet for dinner, we establish that Jon's working on a piece about fishing and just bought a pair of chest waders off eBay or that Stephen finished his essay on being obsessed with W Hotels, and then we order drinks. Or Cramer and I meet at Burger Heaven on our lunch breaks to swap paper-clipped pages and then spend an hour recapping bird sightings on his recent trip to Trinidad. Or I go up to Honor's neighborhood. We walk the dogs, eat something sweet, maybe think about rearranging her furniture. And eventually she slips me slivers of advice ("Darling, have you thought about going to therapy?").

Somewhere in this loose pack (in Cape Cod, actually) is my friend Peter's mother, Carolyn, who has known me since Pete and I were in the same toddler playgroup in St. Louis. She put up with my awkward telephone manners when I would call to ask Pete over for a run in the sprinkler. She poured mugs of hot chocolate for me and Pete while we waited for the sixth-grade bus in front of his house. Once, when I was in college, she gave me a feathery pillow from her linen closet. She also writes children's books and has been reassuring me about writing since she came to play word games with my elementary school class. It's very simple. Every time I see her, she says, "Keep writing, Sara," or "Send me something to read," and I keep writing and knowing that I can send her something, even though I never do. I like the idea of it—sending her something—but really all I need is to know that the connection between my past and Carolyn and writing is there.

NURSERY GUERRILLAS | WENDY GIMBEL

We were the Flashlight Gang. The pajama-clad members of my secret literary tribe went into action as soon as the bedroom lights were out. Night children who couldn't put a book down, we were nursery guerrillas who climbed into bed, rested books on raised knees, pulled up the covers, turned on our flashlights, and vanished into a world of stories.

Because they controlled our behavior, parents were the natural enemies of flashlighters. Cunning, resourceful combatants, they made it clear that during the day we had to play by their rules. With no success, we tried to hide novels under our school desks and bring slim volumes of stories to the dining room table. Alas. (I couldn't even fit my unwieldy copy of *The Count of Monte Cristo* into the narrow space between my lap and the bottom of the desk.) Before sundown, we were prisoners with no recourse but to do what we were told. At night, flashlights in hand, we couldn't be defeated.

Under a faded blue blanket, I delivered myself into the elemental, magical world of Hans Christian Andersen and the Brothers Grimm. I read scores of fairy tales: "Beauty and the Beast," "Rapunzel," "The Fisherman's Wife" . . . The stories, though famously predictable, were set in a landscape that enchanted me. Witches flew about casting evil spells; stepmothers busied themselves with daily acts of cruelty. Restless princes wandered around their kingdoms in search of Cinderella and Sleeping Beauty.

Perhaps Andersen's "Little Mermaid" had the most resonance for me. Didn't the love-struck mermaid convince the witch to replace her glorious fish tail with human "legs"? And didn't these human limbs feel like knives that stabbed her as she danced with her prince? It must have been my first cautionary tale about desire: The price paid for what one wants is often too high.

My earliest years as a flashlighter, the huge amount of reading I did, contributed to my emerging sense of identity. In the printed word created by my favorite writers, I found the world I embraced. Trying to get a fix on my expectations for the future, I used a very literary yardstick. I judged myself as though I were a fictional character in the universe of one of the novels I loved. In these treasured books—so many of which I had read in the clandestine, nocturnal library which was my bedroom—moral values were embedded in the very text: Anna Sewell's *Black Beauty*, Walter Farley's *The Black Stallion*, and Frances Hodgson Burnett's *A Little Princess* weave narratives that make the case for kindness. Dickens's *Great Expectations* condemns snobbery and advocates compassion.

By the time I packed my flashlight and moved out of the nursery, I knew that printed words were the medium through which I made sense of things. Being a successful flashlighter, I must have earned a modest place in the "land of letters." I read everything I could find and I read all the time. Summer nights, in my bunk at a Vermont summer camp, I used my flashlight for hours. If I hadn't finished my book in the morning, I schemed to find the fastest way back to it. ("I can't go to archery practice because I have a sore ankle. I'll just lie on my bed and read.")

Often, the novels I treasured didn't have much of a literary pedigree. I didn't know about scholars who insisted that it was scandalous to mention Margaret Mitchell in the same breath as Henry James. That wasn't how a flashlighter thought about things. To us, a wonderful novel was simply one you couldn't bear to finish. Whether stories came from the pen of a literary aristocrat—a Tolstoy, a Dickens, or a Jane Austen—was unimportant. Great fiction was a book with characters that couldn't be left behind.

The passionate heroines whom I wanted to emulate dominated the books I chose when I was older: *Gone with the Wind*, *Tess of the D'Urbervilles*, *Anna Karenina*, *Rebecca*, and Anya Seton's fabulous *Katherine*, the story of the woman who loved John of Gaunt. These women had a romantic intensity that was hypnotic. And those I loved most had a sense of their own special vividness. They had what the dowager Mrs. de Winter in *Rebecca* called the essential three Bs: beauty, brains, and breeding. (She never mentioned that they might need a heart.)

An indefatigable flashlighter never stops reading. That's the way we learn to tell one sort of writing from another, the good from the bad, the innovative from the merely fashionable. It's also a way to continue to search for that ever elusive reality. Perhaps Virginia Woolf is right when she describes that reality as a "luminous halo, a semitransparent envelope surrounding us from the beginning of consciousness to the end." Through the power of words, at least we have a chance to catch a bit of the glow.

During the '90s, I traveled frequently to Havana. Having spent some of my childhood there, I wanted to see what had happened since Fidel Castro's coup d'état and was eager to write about it. Those were the years of the revolution's so-called special period, with electrical blackouts every night. Nothing brightened the mood of the Cubans who struggled in the darkness. But for me, it was different. Turning on my flashlight, I propped myself on the bed, raised my knees, and settled in to read. Then I began to write my book.

TIMELINE | BOB HOLMAN

Tribe is a word. Last week's *New York Times* "Sunday Styles" investigated "Youth Tribes": take the same drugs, wear the same pants (Phat). I belong to Tribe "Poet" in the way that Khlebnikov declared *everyone* President.

What's *Tribes*? A magazine. *A Gathering of the Tribes*, published by Steve Cannon out of his open house/art gallery/crash pad at 285 East Third Street between C and D. That's what, 2002, the word *Tribes* means to me. Steve is the ur-poet of the Always Open Tribe. When the Icelandic Rock 'n' Roll Poet Laureate, Megas (the Tribe of U.S. R 'n' R Poets Laureate: Capt. Beefheart/Lou Reed/Patti Smith/Jim Carroll/Michael Franti/Ani DiFranco), managed to get a ticket to come to the U.S. for the Bowery Poetry Club's "Viking Hillbilly Review," he slept in the gallery chez *Tribes*.

HISTORY OF MY TRIBES:

1968–71: HEAVUS TUNUS TRIBE (BROOKLYN). When I graduate from Columbia, I write poems for the commune Heavus Tunus and consider that my job. We leave Brooklyn and move back to the land, where we break up. I have to find a new job.

1971–74: BODY POLITIC/YELLOW PRESS (CHICAGO) TRIBE. I'd

never hung out with poets in New York, they seemed so artsy: dedicated radical hippie chafes at cocktail-party apprenticeship program. While working at the Whole Earth Bookstore in Evanston, I come in contact with the Body Politic/Yellow Press scene: Bob Rosenthal, Shelley Kraut, Richard Friedman, Darlene Pearlstein, Peter Kostakis, Al Lange, Rose Lesniak, Neil Hackman (Ravi Singh), Barb Barg, Chassler, Steve Levine. Paul Carroll is éminence grise—his *Young American Poets* is much more our anthology than *The New American Poetry*. (A favorite pastime: counting how many pages poets got in each.) Maxine Chernoff and Paul Hoover are in the mix; Terry Jacobus and Al Simmons, too. Just before Elaine Equi and Jerome Sala. Crossover to Iowa City, Allan and Cinda Kornblum, Dave Morice, the Actualists. But the big presence is Ted Berrigan (I still carry a card, or torch, for the Tribe of Ted). And his then-new bride, Alice Notley. And the true Poet Laureate of the U.S., Bill Knott.

1974–84: SECOND GENERATION ST. MARK'S POETRY PROJECT TRIBE. Many of the Chicago poets move to New York. We gather around Ed Friedman's Monday night series, the precursor of PS 122. Poetry/performance/open mic mix. We attend Alice Notley's workshop. That Tribe: Eileen Myles, Charles Bernstein, Bob and Shelley, Steve Levine, Susie Timmons, Patricia Jones, James Sherry, Greg Masters, Michael Scholnick, Gary Lenhart, Barb Barg, Rose Lesniak. Exciting years at the Project as Ron Padgett sees us through institutionalization processes that include community-elected members of the board. Ted Berrigan is the first voter, and I'm sure the one blank ballot is his.

1977–80: TRIBE OF CETA. Not only poets, but 350 artists from every discipline employed in the largest federally funded artist project since the WPA. The Poets Overland Expeditionary Troop (POET) is born, a gang of performing poets who tour the state: Sandra Esteves, Roland Legiardi-Laura, Barb Barg, Chris Kraus, Rose Lesniak, Diane Burns, Pedro Pietri, Brenda Connor-Bey. This is the first Tribe of Performing Poets I know of (well, after Dada, say). CETA spawns poetry-dance collabs (Yoshiko Chuma, Kenneth King, "taprap" with Jane Goldberg). Marc Levin's film *Slam* wins at Sundance twenty years later, based on dynamics originating at CETA. The understreams of CETA still flow. Bring back federally funded arts projects!

1984–88: NATIONAL POETRY CIRCUIT SCENE. Joe Flaherty at Writers and Books in Rochester, George and Chris Tysh at Detroit Institute of Art, Dennis Cooper et al. at Beyond Baroque. Mike Warr is starting the Guild Complex in Chicago; The Loft and then SASE Minneapolize lit. *River Styx* in St. Louis. I'm circling the country performing "Panic*DJ!" I'm going in circles, but they seem all the right circles till I realize there's nowhere to go, and get the bug to create a place where everyone can feel at home.

1988–96: THE NUYORICAN POETS CAFÉ TRIBE AND THE SLAM TRIBE. Multi-culti in the house of Café via the crazed energy of Slam. Poetry is Speakers Corner meets Olympic Diving. Interactivity (aka "heckling") and democratization, hip-hop and performance, enter the poetry dialectic. Paul Beatty, Maggie Estep, Willie Perdomo, Edwin Torres, Tracie Morris, reg E gaines, Dana Bryant, Dael Orlandersmith, Emily XYZ, Mike Tyler, Saul Williams, Beau Sia, Mumz the Schemer, Sarah Jones all find a place to work. Slam moves across the country, creating a community of controversy and a tribe of vagabond sofa-surfers (see Juliette Torres's *Sofa Surfers Handbook* from Manic D), a controversial community wherever it sets up shop. Spawns record label (Mouth Almighty) and appearances on MTV and PBS.

1996–NOW: THE UNITED STATES OF POETRY/THE WORLD OF POETRY/BOWERY POETRY CLUB. Media, particularly film/video, provide a new book for the poem, one that contains physicality and collaboration. The Bowery Poetry Club (*www.bowerypoetry.com*), just opened, is a for-profit enterprise with a coffee shop, bar, great sound system, available as a nexus for world poetry tribes.

SANGHA POETICS | ANNE WALDMAN

There's a Sanskrit term—*sangha*—that refers to a spiritual community with whom, in effect, one takes a vow of mutual support and commitment. I have found this term useful in getting a sense of my own (now quite large) poetic community, since to some extent this community has had to define and even invent itself outside the norms of academe and the literary establishment—what the poet and critic Charles Bernstein calls "official verse culture."

Although I was very much a student of Howard Nemerov's at Bennington College, I think I declared myself officially a poet at age twenty, in 1965, at the Berkeley Poetry Conference, a gathering of some of the major figures represented in Donald Allen's Grove Press anthology *The New American Poetry*. This collection—while woefully short on women and writers of color—was exciting for its sense of a new "poet-ics" coming on the heels of modernism and the work of Wallace Stevens, Ezra Pound, Marianne Moore, William Carlos Williams, Gertrude Stein, and H. D.

The New American Poetry brought together various postwar strands, including the Beat literary movement, the San Francisco Renaissance, the Black Mountain School, and the New York School, now familiar nexuses of writers that "moved the century a few inches" (Williams's dictum) with pro-jective verse, disruptions of syntax, attention to the line as breath, influence of jazz and other music, playful interventions, cut-up, chance operation, and so on. Principal figures of these new inventions and extensions included Barbara Guest, John Ashbery, Frank O'Hara, Kenneth Koch, James Schuyler (New York School); Charles Olson, Robert Creeley (Black Mountain); Robert Duncan, Jack Spicer, Helen Adam the balladeer, Joanne Kyger (San Francisco Renaissance); and Allen Ginsberg, Jack Kerouac, William Burroughs, Gary Snyder, Diane Di Prima (Beat literary movement).

Amiri Baraka (then LeRoi Jones), also a radical outsider, pushed the envelope with his cultural activism. John Cage was a champion of chance and aleatory practices. And many others were part of this exciting sweep that defined the poem as an experience and found pleasure not in an extrap-olation of meaning and content but rather in the kinetics of the actual writing.

In the mid-'60s, my most intimate tribe was the community I helped create around the Poetry Project at St. Mark's Church in-the-Bowery—usually referred to as the second-and-a-half New York School generation. We were young and active both culturally and politically; rather than waiting to be published, we started our own presses and created a com-munity with a far-reaching sense of "keeping the world safe for poetry."

In 1974, Allen Ginsberg and I founded the Jack Kerouac School of Disembodied Poetics at the Buddhist-inspired Naropa University in Boulder, Colorado, a continuation in many respects of the kind of com-munity begun at St. Mark's. Kerouac was seen as a writer of spontaneity that would propel our project forward. He was also the quintessential mon-grel American—troubled, sensitive, complex, and wildly experimental.

The mission statement we proposed had to do with a sense of literary lineage stretching back to Sappho, Dante, Blake, and Christopher Smart; noncompetitive education of "intellect and intuition"; a serious curriculum that would include scholarly reading and translation, ethnopoetics, and ecopoetics; outreach work in prisons, schools, elderly homes, and "at-risk" communities; a print shop and small desktop publishing operation; performance, collaboration (with dancers, artists, musicians), and activism.

The idea was and is to empower artists, not just feed them into a passive careerist paradigm of tenure-track poetics (I mean, there would never be enough of those jobs around for the number of creative writers coming forward). The Naropa Summer Writing Program has inspired projects and schools in Vienna and in Prague. I have also been active in other parts of the world (Bali, Italy), helping out with new projects that share an old Bohemian idea of person-to-person grassroots activity, benefit a wide range of individuals, and challenge the sorry economics of being an artist in the New World Order.

Writers of younger generations of all ilks who are first heard in these "temporary autonomous zones" (a term from the work of anarchist Hakim Bey), outside the cultural mainstream, continue to create alternatives and fight for human rights, civil rights, freedom of speech and artistic expression. The voices in this huge *sangha* sound prominent and loud.

ANCESTOR WORSHIP | SAMUEL G. FREEDMAN

In a speech eight or nine years ago, I referred to writers like myself, Melissa Fay Greene, Nick Lemann, and Alex Kotlowitz as "the children of Lukas." The Lukas in question, of course, is J. Anthony Lukas, the late and immeasurably missed author of *Common Ground*. And the writers of narrative nonfiction whom I consider my friends, peers, and tribal companions were all affected profoundly by that book, and often by Tony's personal kindness and interest as well.

It no longer surprises me that when I read and admire a work of narrative nonfiction by a writer I'm newly discovering—Cynthia Gorney with *Articles of Faith* or Diane McWhorter with *Carry Me Home*—it turns out that writer had studied up on *Common Ground* and had also enjoyed Tony's personal tutelage.

To a greater or lesser extent, the books by all of us "children" use Tony's model of braided lives, of history-from-below, of novelistic narration combined with scrupulous factuality. In a broader sense, I think we all take inspiration from his example: what a devout Christian might call his witness. In my tribe, our religion is ancestor worship, and it's obvious which ancestor we worship, and mourn, above all others.

ENDGAME | ANNABEL DAVIS-GOFF

Castle Rackrent and *The Last September* are the two great Anglo-Irish novels. Both end with the loss of a house. In Elizabeth Bowen's book the house is burned down during the Irish struggle for independence in 1919, and Maria Edgeworth's eighteenth-century Rackrent estate is pissed away in dissipation, extravagance, fecklessness, and an inability to look the future in the eye.

The Anglo-Irish are a tribe—a little less than a race and somewhat more than a caste—a tribe that is almost extinct. Brendan Behan's definition of an Anglo-Irishman as "a Protestant on a horse" sums it up pretty neatly and excludes not only George Bernard Shaw and the working-class Sean O'Casey, but Oscar Wilde, a product of the cultured urban middle class. Today's Anglo-Irish are what remain of the Protestant landowning gentry.

The population of Ireland, from prehistory until the Reformation, was formed by waves of invaders who embraced the ways of those they conquered while contributing to their culture and bloodlines. Gaels, Celts, Vikings, Normans came, conquered, and conformed; but the sixteenth-century wave of land-grabbing Elizabethans were Protestant, and intermarriage, which had sometimes produced integration in one generation, was no longer possible. Instead, the two-religion, two-race country resulted in today's Northern Ireland tragedy and the development of the Anglo-Irish as the separate landowning Ascendancy of the South. Following the Treaty of 1921, Ireland became the Irish Free State, and the Anglo-Irish dwindled to an isolated and diminished minority in a tiny and poor population.

The population of Ireland, in the wake of our new prosperity, has crept up to four million. Of the four million, a small percentage is Protestant; of that subsection the Anglo-Irish are now an almost invisible minority. About a third left Ireland after the Treaty and in the wake of the Troubles, possibly imagining reprisals and further house-burnings would follow independence and, unless they were among the very few great landowners, certain that there was no future, economic or other, for them in the new Ireland. In the first they were wrong; in the second, of course, absolutely right. Those that remained were the Anglo-Irish among whom I grew up.

The end of my tribe is in sight. Religion no longer holds the power it once did, and in my family the next generation has married, as I did, out of the tiny genetic pool. Those of the new generation who remain in Ireland do not sound different from their—for want of a better term—native Irish contemporaries. And, religion apart, the old order has changed. The new economy has produced a new class of rich people, some of whom now live in the Georgian houses of those Anglo-Irish families who subscribed to a tradition that my brother refers to as "rags to rags in three generations."

Most of the great houses are gone, some burned during the Troubles, more pulled down, left to fall down, or burned accidentally; of those that remain too many are hotels or golf clubs.

My generation is not the last of the Anglo-Irish, but of the next generation there will be only a handful who have failed to become part of the mainstream of Irish life. It is not likely there will be much if any further contribution to literature by the Anglo-Irish. It will not be a huge loss: those who write will become what they always were—part of a country whose very small population have produced a disproportionate amount of the world's literature.

TRIBE, TRIBUTE, TRIBULATION

Meena Alexander

It is not enough to cover the rock with leaves.

—WALLACE STEVENS

1.

Twilight, I stroll through stubble fields,
clouds lift, the hope of a mountain.
What was distinct turns to mist.

What was fitful burns the heart.
When I dream of my tribe gathering
by the red soil of the Pamba river

I feel my writing hand split at the wrist.
Dark tribute or punishment. Who can tell?
You kiss the stump and where the wrist

bone was, you set the stalk of a lotus.
There is a blue lotus in my grandmother's garden,
its petals whirl in moonlight like this mountain.

2.

An altar, a stone cracked down the spine
a shelter, a hovel of straw and sperm
out of which rise a man and a woman

and one is a ghost though I cannot tell which
for the sharpness between them scents
even the orchids, a sharing of things

invisible till the mountain fetches
itself out of water, out of ice, out of sand
and they each take tiny morsels

of the mountain and set it on banana leaves
and as if it were a feast of saints
they cry out to their dead and are satisfied.

3.

I have climbed the mountain and cleared
away the sand and ice using first my bare hands
then a small knife. Underneath I found

the sign of the four-cornered world, *gammadion*,
which stands for migration, for the scattering
of the people. The desolation of the mothers

singing in their rock houses becomes us,
so too the child at the cliff's edge
catching a cloud in her palm

as stocks of blood are gathered on the plain
spread into sheaves, a circlet for bones
and flint burns and the mountain resurrects itself.

4.

Tribe, tribute, tribulation
to purify the tongue and its broken skin
I am learning the language again.

A new speech, for a new tribe.
How did I reach this nervous empire,
sharp store of sense?

Donner un sens plus pur etc etc
does not work so well anymore,
nor calme bloc ici-bas.

Blunt metals blossom.
Children barter small arms.
Ground rules are abolished.

The earth has no capitals.
In my distinct note books
I write things of this sort.

Monsoon clouds from the shore
near my grandmother's house
float through my lines.

I take comfort in sentences.
Who cares what you write?
someone cries.

A hoarse voice, I cannot see the face
He smells like a household ghost
There can be no concord between us.

I search out a bald rock between two trees
ash trees on the riverbank
on an island city where towers blazed.

This is my short
incantation,
my long way home.

William, Rabindranath, Czeslaw,
Mirabai, Anna, Adrienne,
reach out your hands to me.

Now stones have tongues.
Serendipitous scattering,
stormy grace!

SUN: SET

PAST TENSE | AMITAV GHOSH

I have recently learned that my novel *The Glass Palace* has been named the Eurasia regional winner for the 2001 Commonwealth Writers Prize. . . . I have on many occasions publicly stated my objections to the classification of books such as mine under the term "Commonwealth Literature." Principal among these is that this phrase anchors an area of contemporary writing not within the realities of the present day, nor within the possibilities of the future, but rather within a disputed aspect of the past. In this it is completely unlike any other literary term (would it not surprise us, for instance, if that familiar category "English literature" were to be renamed "the literature of the Norman Conquest"?).

As a grouping of nations collected from the remains of the British Empire, the Commonwealth serves as an umbrella forum in global politics. As a literary or cultural grouping, however, it seems to me that "the Commonwealth" can only be a misnomer so long as it excludes the many languages that sustain the cultural and literary lives of these countries (it is surely inconceivable, for example, that athletes would have to be fluent in English in order to qualify for the Commonwealth Games).

So far as I can determine, *The Glass Palace* is eligible for the Commonwealth Prize partly because it was written in English and partly because I happen to belong to a region that was once conquered and ruled by Imperial Britain. Of the many reasons why a book's merits may be recognized, these seem to me to be the least persuasive. That the past engenders the present is of course undeniable; it is equally undeniable that the reasons I write in English are ultimately rooted in my country's history. Yet, the ways in which we remember the past are not determined solely by the brute facts of time: they are also open to choice, reflection, and judgment. The issue of how the past is to be remembered lies at the heart of *The Glass Palace* and I feel that I would be betraying the spirit of my book if I were to allow it to be incorporated within that particular memorialization of Empire that passes under the rubric of "the Commonwealth." I therefore ask that I be permitted to withdraw *The Glass Palace* from your competition. . . .

From a letter to the administrators
of the Commonwealth Writers Prize (2001)

SEEING GREEN | SEAMUS HEANEY

Don't be surprised
If I demur, for, be advised
My passport's green.
No glass of ours was ever raised
To toast *The Queen*.

From "Open Letter," a rebuke to editors of
The Penguin Book of Contemporary British Poetry (1982)
for including Heaney among its authors

MANIFESTO: 1979

L=A=N=G=U=A=G=E
Charles Bernstein

I don't believe in group formation, I don't like group formation, but I am constantly finding myself contending with it, living within it, seeing through it. "Okay, break it up boys." First, there is the isolation of the atom, looking for some place to feel housed by, a part of. . . . But every group as well has the same possibility for insularity as each individual: this new "we" having the same possibility for vacancy or satisfaction, a group potentially as atomized in its separation from the other groups as a person from other persons. This is the problem of family life. Property, territory, domain. But, "for us now," group (family, aesthetic, social, national) is merely another part of our commoditized lives—for we consume these formations, along with most other things, as commodities, & are ourselves consumed in the process. ((Putting aside here the extent to which political groupings and parties would be different from groups of "artists"; also the place of groupings based on class oppression on the one hand and minority oppression—women, gays, mental patients—on the other.)) So we use groups as badges—shields—as much screening us off from the intrusion of outside, others, as sheltering us from the sheer invasiveness of it, them (& so allowing us a place to occupy, inhabit). I don't so much think that such shelter is a fraud, unnecessary, as much as "let's look at it, call the structures into question, understand that we can reshape": a call against paralysis from a sense of boundaries fixed without, or before, our having had a chance to participate in their making. "The danger is that our demands on each other will trample what we really feel." The danger is that we will hide ourselves midst the shuffle to proclaim who we are. . . .

A kind of blinder's vision begins as we look at the world in terms of the configurations being made. "At any given time, we responded to each other's work, were there for each other." "To the permanent removal of everyone else after, simultaneous?" No. These things arise in practice, have a practical value. ((Imagine a world in which people allied along lines of hair color. Or what unified a group of artists was their use of a given shade of blue, or that they live (or grew up in, or went to school in) the same place—the impress of a common environment a constant to facilitate art-historical apprehension. . . .)) But the final cuts have not been—will not be—made. Only cuts for "here" & "there"—

The identification of "younger" poets "coming up" by a group or community can imply the beginning for these people of inclusion within a paternalistic hierarchy—an initiation into it.—Simply, the walls must be stripped down & new ones constantly built as (re)placements—or rather this is always happening, whether we attend to it or not. We see through these structures, which we have made ourselves & cannot do even for a moment without them, yet they are not fixed but provisional. (. . . that poetry gets shaped—informed and transformed—by the social relations of publication, readership, correspondence, readings, etc. (or, historically seen, the "tradition") and, indeed, that the poetry community(ies) are not a secondary phenomenon to writing but a primary one. So it won't do to just "think about the work." But it still needs to be explored what the relation between "normal" and "extraordinary" poetry is—& why both need to be more valued in some respects and devalued in others (snobbery, elitism, cliquishness, historical over-self-consciousness, self-aggrandizement, &c)—especially at a time in which there is an increase in the number of people and the number of people engaging in art activities—not just a few "men" "out there" doing the "heroic" work.—That poetry, with written language as its medium, is, in fact, the exploration and realization of human common ground, of "us," . . .)

HOMEBODY

Tony Kushner

The shape of the map of present-day Afghanistan resembles a left-hand fist with the thumb open.

—NABI MISDAQ, *AHMAD SHAH DURRANI, 1722–1772*

It is more appropriate to consider Afghanistan as a place of enormous complexity that has been subject to a constant state of flux throughout history rather than to view it as somehow caught in a time-warp, with life going on as it has always done.

—PETER MARSDEN, *THE TALIBAN*

Afghanistan lies at the crossroads of South and Central Asia; its northern plains an extension of the steppes to Turkmenistan, the Hindu Kush mountains an adjunct to the Himalayas, its southern deserts a prelude to the Persian Gulf. Linguistically, culturally, and ethnically Afghanistan's northern Uzbeks, Turkmen, and Tajiks look northwards to Central Asia, the centrally located Hazaras look westwards to Iran, and the southern and eastern Pashtuns and Baluch find more resonance in the east in Pakistan. Although distinct from them, each group and region has more in common with its neighbors over the border than with each other.

—CHRIS BOWERS, "A BRIEF HISTORY OF AFGHANISTAN,"
FROM *ESSENTIAL FIELD GUIDE TO AFGHANISTAN*

Tony Kushner received the 2002 PEN/Laura Pels Foundation Award for Drama, given to recognize an American playwright in mid-career.

"Periplum" is Pound's shorthand for a tour which takes you round then back again. And such a tour is by definition profitable, if not in coins then in knowledge.

—HUGH KENNER, *THE ELSEWHERE COMMUNITY*

These examples should teach you the way to treat hearts. . . . The general technique consists in doing the opposite of everything the soul inclines to and craves. God (Exalted is He!) has summed up all these things in His statement: "And whoever fears the standing before his Lord, and forbids his soul its whim, for him Heaven shall be the place of resort."

—AL-GHAZALI, *ON DISCIPLINING THE SOUL
AND BREAKING THE TWO DESIRES*

The world had been destroyed several times before the creation of man.

—LORD BYRON, *CAIN*

In Washington, Pentagon officials said that a U.S. warplane missed a Taliban military target at Kabul airport and that a 2,000-pound bomb the plane was carrying apparently struck a residential neighborhood.

At the scene of the hit, one man sat in his wheelchair, weeping next to a pile of rubble where his house once stood. Other residents wandered about in a daze.

"We lost everything, our house and property," one woman said. "We are so afraid of the attacks we have forgotten our own names and can't even understand what we say to each other."

—*NEW YORK TIMES*, OCTOBER 13, 2001

ACT ONE

SCENE I

A woman is sitting in a comfortable chair, in a pleasant room in her home in London. A table stands nearby, a lamp on the table. On the floor near her chair, a shopping bag. She is reading from a small book:

THE HOMEBODY

"Our story begins at the very dawn of history, circa 3,000 B.C. . . ."

(Interrupting herself:)

I am reading from an outdated guidebook about the city of Kabul. In Afghanistan. In the valleys of the Hindu Kush mountains. A guidebook to a city which as we all know, has . . . undergone change.

My reading, my research is mothlike. Impassioned, fluttery, doomed. A subject strikes my fancy: Kabul—you will see why, that's the tale I'm telling—but then, I can't help myself, it's almost perverse, in libraries, in secondhand bookshops, I invariably seek out not The Source but all that which was dropped by the wayside on the way to The Source, outdated guidebooks—this was published in 1965, and it is now 1998, so the book is a vestige superannuated by some . . . thirty-three years, long enough for Christ to have been born and die on the cross—old magazines, hysterical political treatises written by an advocate of some long-since defeated or abandoned or transmuted cause; and I find these irrelevant and irresistible, ghostly, dreamy, the knowing what *was* known before the more that has since become known overwhelms . . . As we are, many of us, overwhelmed, and succumbing to luxury . . .

(She reads from the guidebook:)

"Our story begins at the very dawn of history, circa 3,000 B.C., when the Aryans, not in armies but in family groups, traveled south from beyond the River Oxus to cross the Hindu Kush mountains on their way to northern India. This crossing must have made a great impression for, nearly two thousand years later, when the Rigveda, the great hymnic epic poem of the Aryan peoples, is written down, several verses retain the memory of the serene beauty of the valleys of the Kabul River."

(She looks up from the guidebook)

Several months ago I was feeling low and decided to throw a party, and a party needs festive hats. So I took the tube to _____, *(She gestures)* where there are shops full of merchandise from exotic locales, wonderful things made by people who believe, as I do not, as *we* do not, in magic; or who used to believe in magic, and not so long ago, whose grandparents believed in magic, believed that some combination of piety, joy, ecstasy, industry, brought to bear on the proper raw materials, wood for instance known to be the favored nesting place of a certain animus or anima possessed of powers released, enlisted in beneficent ways towards

beneficent ends when carved, adorned, adored just so . . . Before coloniza-
tion and the savage stripping away of such beliefs. For magic beliefs are
immensely strong, I think, only if their essential fragility is respected. It's
a paradox. If such beliefs, magic beliefs, are untouched, they endure. And
who knows? Work magic, perhaps. If they are untouched; and that is hard,
for such is the expansive nature of these times that every animate and
inanimate thing, corporeal or incorporeal, actual or ideational, real or
imagined, every, every discrete unit of . . . of *being*: if a thing can be said to
be, to *exist*, then such is the nature of these expansive times that this thing
which is must suffer to be *touched*. Ours is a time of connection; the private, and we must accept this, and it's a hard thing to accept, the private is
gone. All must be touched. All touch corrupts. All must be corrupted. And
if you're thinking how awful these sentiments are, you are perfectly correct,
these are awful times, but you must remember as well that *this* has always
been the chiefest characteristic of The Present, to everyone living through
it; always, throughout history, and so far as I can see for all the days and
years to come until the sun and the stars fall down and the clocks have all
ground themselves to expiry and the future has long long shaded away into
Time Immemorial: The Present is *always* an awful place to be. And it
remains awful to us, the scene of our crime, the place of our shame, for at
least, oh, let's say three full decades of recession—by which word, *recession*,
I am to be taken to mean *recedence*, not *recession* as in *two consecutive quarters of negative growth in gross domestic product*. For a three-decades regnum
of imperceptible but mercifully implacable recedency we shudder to recall
the times through which we have lived, the Recent Past, about which no
one wants to think; and then, have you noticed? Even the most notorious
decade three or four decades later is illumined from within. Some light
inside is switched on. The scenery becomes translucent, beautifully lit; features of the landscape glow; the shadows are full of agreeable color. Cynics
will attribute this transformation to senescence and nostalgia; I who am
optimistic, have you noticed? attribute this inner illumination to understanding. It is wisdom's hand which switches on the light within. Ah, now
I see what that was all about. Ah, now, now I see why we suffered so back
then, now I see what we went through. I understand.

(She reads from the guidebook:)

"Nothing is known of the Aryan passage through the valleys of the
Hindu Kush, no writing or significant structure remains from the Aryan
settlements which undoubtedly existed on the banks of the Kabul River,
one of which would eventually grow into the city of Kabul. The first

contemporaneous account to mention the city is recorded circa 520 B.C., when Darius the Great, Achaemenid Persian conqueror and builder of Persepolis, annexed twenty-nine countries to the Persian empire, parts of India, all of what we now know as Afghanistan, including the Kabul Valley. In the summer of 329 B.C., Alexander the Macedonian, having trampled the Achaemenid imperium in his victorious march through Persia, makes camp in the Hindu Kush city of Khandahar, and orders the building of the city of Alexandria-ad-Caucasum."

(She looks up from the guidebook)

Oh I love the world! I love love love love the world! Having said so much, may I assume most of you will have dismissed me as a simpleton? I cannot hope to contravene your peremptory low estimation, which may for all its peremptoriness nevertheless be exactly appropriate. I live with the world's mild censure, or would do were it the case that I ever strayed far enough from my modesty, or should I say my essential surfeit of inconsequence, to so far attract the world's attention as to provoke from it its mild censure; but I have never strayed so far from the unlit to the spotlight, and so should say rather that I live with the world's utter indifference, which I have always taken to be a form of censure-in-potentia.

I speak . . . I can't help myself. Elliptically. Discursively. I've read too many books, and that's not boasting, for I haven't read *many* books, but I've read too many, exceeding I think my capacity for syncresis—is that a word?—straying rather into synchisis, which is a word. So my diction, my syntax, well, it's so *irritating*, I apologize, I do, it's very hard, I know. To listen. I blame it on the books, how else to explain it? My parents don't speak like this; no one I know does; no one does. It's an *alien influence*, and my borders have only ever been broached by books. Sad to say.

Only ever been broached by books. Except once, briefly. Which is I suppose the tale I'm telling, or rather, trying to tell.

You must be patient. There is an old Afghan saying, which, in rough translation from the Farsi, goes: *"The man who has patience has roses. The man who has no patience has no trousers."* I am not fluent in Farsi, of course—I read this, and as I say it must be a rough translation.

(She reads from the guidebook:)

"Alexander the Great summoned to the Kabul Valley a mighty army comprising tens of thousands of soldiers from Egypt, Persia, and Central Asia and went on to conquer India. When Alexander's own troops grew weary of battle, in 325 B.C., they forced their commander to desist from further conquest. Alexander died in 323 B.C., just as he was planning a

return to the Hindu Kush to oversee the Grecianization of this most
remarkable land."

(She pauses her reading)

My husband cannot bear my . . . the sound of me and has threatened
to leave on this account and so I rarely speak to him anymore. We both
take powerful antidepressants. His pills have one name and mine another.
I frequently take his pills instead of mine so I can know what he's feeling.
I keep mine in a glass bowl next to the bathroom sink, a nice wide-
mouthed bowl, very wide, wide open, like an epergne, but so far as I know
he never takes my pills but ingests only his own, which are yellow and red,
while mine are green and creamy-white; and I find his refusal to sample
dull. A little dull.

(She resumes, from the guidebook:)

"By 322 B.C., only a year after Alexander's death, his vast Macedonian
empire had disassembled. Herodotus tells us that the hill tribes of the
Kabul Valley were among the first and the most ferocious in rejecting
Macedonian authority. Seleucus Nicator, Alexander's successor in the east,
attempted to regain the Hindu Kush but was daunted when he encountered, in 305 B.C., in the passes of the Hindu Kush, the armed forces of
the Maurya Dynasty which had come to rule India. In exchange for the
hand of the daughter of the Maurya emperor, Chandragupta, and for five
hundred elephants, the Kabul Valley passed for the first time under Indian
suzerainty."

(She puts the guidebook down)

A party needs hats. I had no hope that this would be a good party. My
parties are never good parties. This party was intended to celebrate my
husband's having completed some joyless task at his place of business,
which has something to do with the routing of multiple-y expressive electronic tone signals at extraordinary speeds across millions upon millions
of kilometers of wire and cable and fiber and space; I understand none of
it and indeed it's quite impossible imagining my husband having to do in
any real way with processes so . . . speedy, myriad, nervous, miraculous.
But that parti-colored cloud of gas there, in that galaxy there so far away,
that cloud there so hot and blistered by clustering stars, exhaling protean
scads of infinitely irreducible fiery data in the form of energy pulses and
streams of slicing, shearing, unseeable light—does that nebula know it
nebulates? Most likely not. So my husband. It knows nothing, its *nature*
is to stellate and constellate and nebulate and add its heft and vortices and
frequencies to the Universal Drift, unself-consciously effusing, effusing,

gaseously effusing, and so my husband, and so not I, who seem forever to be imploding and collapsing and am incapable it would seem of lending even this simple tale to the Universal Drift, of telling this simple tale without supersaturating my narrative with maddeningly infuriating or more probably irritating synchitic expegeses.

Synchitic expegeses. Jesus.

A party needs hats and in my mind's eye I remembered quite remarkable hats, not as tall as fezzes nor yet as closely cleaving to the curve of the skull as a skullcap, but really rather pillboxy as ladies wore hats in the early '60s; but these mind's-eye hats were made of tough brilliant dyed wools and scraps of elaborate geometrically arabesqued carpet into which sequins and diamantines and carbuncles and glassine beading had been sewn to dazzling, charming premodern effect. I could see these hats perched on top of the heads of the family members and friends who usually appear at my parties, lovely lovely people all of them but when we assemble we rather . . . affect one another, one might even say *afflict* one another, in baleful ways and tend to dampen one another's festive spirits, there's no . . . I suppose one would like something combustible at a party, something catalytic, some fizz, each element triggering transformation in all the other elements till all elements, which is to say, *guests*, are . . . surprising to themselves and return home feeling less . . . less certain of . . . those certainties which . . . *Because* of which, for example, powerful antidepressants are consumed.

(She reads from the guidebook:)

"The third century B.C. was a prosperous time for the Kabul Valley, situated midway between the empires of the Seleucids and the Mauryas, profiting thusly from an extensive trade with both which must have included furs from Central Asia and a recent discovery of the Chinese, silk. By the end of the third century the far-flung Mauryan empire had disappeared and a period of disorder, migration, and tribal unrest followed, for which the records are clouded and confused."

(She looks up from the guidebook)

My antidepressant is called . . . something, a made-up word, a portmanteau chemical cocktail word confected by punning psychopharmacologists but I can never remember precisely what to ask for when I . . . My husband explains to me with bitter impacted patience each time I request it of him the workings of . . . Ameliorate-za-pozulac, its workings upon my brain; I cannot retain his bitter impacted explanation, but I believe it's all to do with salt somehow. I believe in fact this drug is a kind of talented salt. And so I imagine my brain floating in a salt bath, frosted with a rime of salt, a pickle-brine brain, pink-beige walnut-wrinkled nutmeat within a crystalliform quartzoid ice-white hoarfrost casing, a gemmy shell, gemmiparous: budding. How any of this is meant to counteract depression is more than I can say.

Perhaps it is the sufficient pleasing image which cheers one and makes life's burdens less difficult to bear.

(She reads from the guidebook:)

"In the middle of the second century B.C., during the Greco-Bactrian Confusion, a Chinese tribe, the Hsiung-Nu, attacked a rival tribe, the Yueh-Chih, and drove them from their homes to what is now southern Afghanistan. Then the Hsiung-Nu, displaced from their new homes by another Chinese tribe, also migrated to Afghanistan and once again displaced the Yueh-Chih, who emigrated to the Kabul Valley. As the first century B.C. dawns, the Valley, populated by Indo-Greeks, Mauryas, and Macedonians, is now surrounded by the restless nomadic kingdoms of the Yueh-Chih.

"By 48 B.C. the Chinese tribes are united under the banner of their largest clan, the Kushans. From the city of Kapisa, the Kushan court came to rival the Caesars in Rome." And I'd never *heard* of the Kushans, have you? Nor for that matter the Greco-Bactrian Confusion! Though it *feels* familiar, does it not, the Greco-Bactrian Confusion? When did it end? The guidebook does not relate. *Did* it end? Are we perhaps still in it? Still *in* the Greco-Bactrian Confusion? Would it surprise you, really, to learn that we are? Don't you feel it would, I don't know, *explain* certain things? "Ah yes, it is hard, I know, to *understand* but you see it's the Greco-Bactrian Confusion, which no one ever actually bothered clearing up, and, well here we are."

But let us return to the Kushans:

"From the city of Kapisa, the Kushan court came to rival the Caesars in Rome. Buddhism, Hinduism, Grecian, and Persian deities are gathered into the valleys of the Hindu Kush, where a remarkable cross-fertilization takes place."

(She puts the guidebook down)

In my mind's eye, yet from memory: I had seen these abbreviated fez-like pillboxy attenuated yarmulkite millinarisms, um, *hats*, I'm sorry I *will* try to stop, *hats*, yes, in a crowded shop on _____ *(Gesture)* which I must have passed and mentally noted on my way towards God knows what, who cares, a dusty shop crowded with artifacts, relics, remnants, little . . .

doodahs of a culture once aswarm with spirit matter, radiant with potent magic the disenchanted dull detritus of which has washed up upon our culpable shores, its magic now shriveled into the safe container of *aesthetic*, which is to say, *consumer* appeal. You know, Third World junk. As I remember, as my mind's eye saw, through its salt crust, Afghan junk. That which was once Afghan, which we, having waved our credit cards in its general direction, have made into junk. I remembered the shop, where I thought it was, what its windows were like, sure I'd never find it again and yet there it was in my mind's eye and I traveled to the spot my mind's eye had fixed upon and I was correct! Took the tube, chewed my nails, there was the shop! Precisely as my salt-wounded mind's eye's corneal rotogravured sorry sorry. I found the shop. It was run by Afghan refugees.

And here are the hats. There are ten. They cost three ninety-nine each.

(She displays the hats, removing them one by one from the shopping bag and putting them on the table)

Looking at the hat we imagine not bygone days of magic belief but the suffering behind the craft, this century has taught us to direct our imagination however fleetingly toward the hidden suffering: evil consequence of evil action taken long ago, conjoining with relatively recent wickedness and wickedness perpetuated now, in August 1998, now now now even as I speak and speak and speak . . . But whether the product of starveling-manned sweatshop or remote not-on-the-grid village, poor yet still resisting the onslaught of modernity, touched, of course, yet not, though it is only a matter of time, isn't it? not corrupted; whether removed from the maker by the middleman to the merchant by filch or swindle or gunpoint or even murder; whether, for that matter, even Afghan in origin; and not Pakistani; or Peruvian; if not in point of fact made in London by children, aunts, and elderly uncles in the third-floor flat above the shop on _____ *(Gesture)*: the hats are beautiful; relatively inexpensive; sinister if you've a mind to see them that way; and sad. As dislocations are. And marvelous, as dislocations are. Always bloody.

This one is particularly nice.

(She puts a hat on her head, and reads from the guidebook:)

"Severe economic crises throughout the region in the second century A.D. made it easy for the Sassanians, a purely Iranian Persian dynasty, to claim the Hindu Kush Valley as a semi-independent satrapy. The inhabitants of Kabul from the Kushano-Sassanian period appear to have remained Buddhist, while their Sassanian overlords were obstreperous worshipers of Zoroaster." *(She looks up from the book)* "Obstreperous worshipers of Zoroaster"! For that phrase alone I deem this book a worthy addition to my pickpenny library of remaindered antilegomenoi. *(Back to the book)* "Sassanian hegemony—" *(Up from the book)* Antilegomenoi are volumes of cast-off or forgotten knowledge, in case you were wondering. *(Back to the book)* "Sassanian hegemony was toppled by the Hephthalites, or white Huns, who commenced a reign of legendary destructiveness around 400 A.D., savagely persecuting the indigenous worship of Buddha—Buddhism having found many adherents among Hindu Kush peoples as its monks carried news of the Buddha from India through Afghanistan to China. Apart from their fabled viciousness, almost nothing is known about the Hephthalites."

(She looks up from the guidebook)

Nothing when this book was written, and it is rather old. Perhaps more is known now though archaeology in the area has been interrupted. Very little digging, except recently, did you read this, the bodies of two thousand Taliban soldiers were found in a mass grave in northern Afghanistan, prisoners who were executed, apparently by soldiers loyal to the overthrown government of Burhanuddin Rabbani. So someone is digging, and perhaps more now is known about the Hephthalites.

(She reads from the guidebook:)

"Hephthalite rule ended in 531 A.D., after which a state of anarchy prevailed over the entire region, each town protected by an independent chieftain, and the remaining Hephthalite princes"—who, you will remember, made their appearance just one paragraph previous, razing Buddhist temples—"the remaining Hephthalite princes having by this time *converted to Buddhism.*"

And made a great vulgar noise about it, I shouldn't wonder. I find myself disliking intensely the Hephthalites.

"Meanwhile, in 642, the banner of Islam"—Islam at last!—"carried forth from the deserts of Arabia, halted its eastern progress when its armies tried to penetrate the heart of what is now Afghanistan; for every hill and town was defended by fierce tribal warriors. Several hundred years were to pass before Kabul would fully surrender to Islam."

(Turning pages, summarizing:)

This brings us to the end of the millennium, 1023. Kabul over the next three or four hundred years will be conquered by first this empire builder and then that one. Genghis Khan swam through the area on a river of blood. The Great Tamurlaine, a Timurid, wounded his foot during a battle near Kabul, says the guidebook, and whatever it was he was named before (the book is not helpful on this) he was henceforth and forevermore known as Timur-I-Lang, Timur Who Limps. Timur-I-Lang, Tamurlaine. Kabul rebaptized him.

(She puts the guidebook down)

And this is what happened, and it's all there is to my little tale, really: the hats were in a barrel which could be seen through the window; puppets hung from the ceiling, carved freestanding figurines, demiurges, attributes, symbols, carven abstractions representing metaphysical principles critical to the governance of perfect cosmologies now lost to all or almost all human memory; amber beads big as your baby's fists, armor plates like pangolin scales strung on thick ropy catgut cordage meant to be worn by rather large, rather ferocious men, one would imagine, or who knows; hideous masks with great tusks and lolling tongues and more eyes than are usual, mind's eyes, I suppose, and revolving wire racks filled with postcards depicting the severed heads of the Queen and Tony Blair, well not *severed* necessarily but with no body appended; Glaswegian *A to Zed Guides* and newspapers in Arabic, in Urdu, in Pushtu, videocassettes of rock balladeers from Benares: well why go on and on, sorry I'm sorry, we've all been in these sorts of shops, no bigger than from here to there, haven't we? As if a many-cameled caravan, having roamed across the entire postcolonial not-yet-developed world, crossing the borders of the rainforested kingdoms of Kwashiorkor and Rickets and Untreated Gum Disease and High Infant Mortality Rates, gathering with desperate indiscriminateness—is that the word?—on the mudpitted unpaved trade route its bits and boodle, had finally beached its great heavy no longer portable self in a narrow coal-scuttle of a shop on _____ *(Gesture)*, *here*, here, caravanseraied here, in the developed and overdeveloped and over-overdeveloped paved wasted now deliquescent post-First World postmodern city of London; all the camels having flopped and toppled and fallen here and died of exhaustion, of shock, of the heartache of refugees, the goods simply piled high upon their dromedary bones, just where they came to rest, and set up shop atop the carcasses, and so on.

I select ten hats, thread my way through the musty heaps of swag and thrownaway and offcast and godforsaken sorry sorry through the merchandise to the counter where a man, an Afghan man, my age I think, perhaps a bit older, stands smiling eager to ring up my purchases and make an imprint of my credit card, and as I hand the card to him I see that three fingers on his right hand have been hacked off, following the line of a perfect clean diagonal from middle to ring to little finger, which, the last of the three fingers in the diagonal cut's descent, by, um, hatchet blade? was hewn off almost completely—like this, you see?

(She demonstrates)

But a clean line, you see, not an accident, a measured surgical cut, but not surgery as we know it for what possible medicinal purpose might be served? I tried, as one does, not to register shock, or morbid fascination, as one does my eyes unfocused my senses fled startled to the roof of my skull and then off into the ether like a rapid vapor indifferent to the obstacle of my cranium WHOOSH, clean slate, tabula rasa, terra incognita, where am I yet still my mind's eye somehow continuing to record and detail that poor ruined hand slipping my MasterCard into the . . . you know, that thing, that roller-press thing which is used to . . . Never mind. Here, in London, that poor ruined hand.

Imagine.

I know nothing of this hand, its history, of course, nothing.

I did know, well I have learnt since through research that Kabul, which is the ancient capital of Afghanistan, and where once the summer pavilion of Amir Abdur Rahman stood shaded beneath two splendid old chinar trees, beloved of the Moghuls, Kabul, substantial portions of which are now great heaps of rubble, was, it was claimed by the Moghul Emperor Babur, founded by none other than Cain himself. Biblical Cain. Who is said to be buried in Kabul, in the gardens south of Bala-Hissar in the cemetery known as Shohada-I-Salehin.

I should like to see that. The Grave of Cain. Murder's Grave. Would you eat a potato plucked from *that* soil?

(She reads from the guidebook:)

"The mighty Moghul emperors, who came to rule the Hindu Kush and all of India, adored Kabul and magnified and exalted it. By the eighteenth century the Moghuls, ruling from Delhi and Agra, succumbed to luxury"—that's what it says, they succumbed to luxury. "Modern Afghanistan is born when, in 1747, heretofore warring Afghan tribal chiefs forge for themselves a state, proclaiming Ahmed Shah Durrani, age twenty-five, King of the Afghans."

(She looks up from the guidebook)

And so the Great Game begins. The Russians seize Khazakhstan, the British seize India, Persia caves in to the Russians, the first Anglo-Afghan war is fought, the bazaar in Kabul is burnt and many many people die, Russia seizes Bokhara, the second Anglo-Afghan war, the First World War, the October Revolution, the third Anglo-Afghan war, also known as the Afghanistan War of Independence, Afghanistan sovereignty first recognized by the Soviet Union in 1921, followed by aid received from the Soviet Union, followed by much of the rest of the twentieth century, Afghanistan is armed by the USSR against the Pakistanis, the U.S. refuses assistance, militant Islamic movements form the seed of what will become the Mujahideen, the U.S. begins sending money, much civil strife, approaching at times a state of civil war, over liberal reforms such as the unveiling of and equal rights for women, democratic elections held, martial law imposed, the Soviet Union invades, the Mujahideen are armed, at first insufficiently, then rather handsomely by the U.S., staggering amounts of firepower, some captured from the Soviets, some purchased, some given by the West, missiles and antiaircraft cannon and etc. etc., the Soviets for ten years do their best to outdo the Hephthalites in savagery, in barbarism, then like so many other empires traversing the Hindu Kush the USSR is swept away, and now the Taliban, and . . .

Well.

(She closes the guidebook and puts it down)

Afghanistan is one of the poorest countries in the world. With one of the world's most decimated infrastructures. No tourism. Who in the world would wish to travel there? In Afghanistan today I would be shrouded entirely in a *burqa*, I should be subject to *hejab*, I should live in terror of the *sharia hudud*, or more probably dead, unregenerate chatterer that I am.

While I am signing the credit card receipt I realize all of a sudden I am able to speak perfect Pushtu, and I ask the man, who I now notice is very beautiful, not on account of regularity of features or smoothness of the skin, no, his skin is broken by webs of lines inscribed by hardships, siroccos, and strife, battle scars, perhaps, well certainly the marks of some battle, some life unimaginably more difficult than my own; I ask him to tell me what had happened to his hand. And he says: I was with the Mujahideen, and the Russians did this. I was with the Mujahideen, and an enemy faction of Mujahideen did this. I was with the Russians, I was known to have assisted the Russians, I did informer's work for Babrak Karmal, my name is in the files if they haven't been destroyed, the names I gave are in the files, there are no more files, I stole bread for my starving family, I stole bread *from* a starving family, I profaned, betrayed, according to some stricture I erred and they chopped off the fingers of my hand. *Look, look at my country, look at my Kabul, my city, what is left of my city? The streets are as bare as the mountains now, the buildings are as ragged as mountains and as bare and empty of life, there is no life here only fear, we do not live in the buildings now, we live in terror in the cellars in the caves in the mountains, only God can save us now, only order can save us now, only God's Law harsh and strictly administered can save us now, only The Department for the Promotion of Virtue and the Prevention of Vice can save us now, only terror can save us from ruin, only never-ending war, save us from terror and never-ending war, save my wife they are stoning my wife, they are chasing her with sticks, save my wife save my daughter from punishment by God, save us from God, from war from exile, from oil exploration, from no oil exploration, from the West, from the children with rifles, carrying stones, only children with rifles, carrying stones, can save us now.* You will never understand. It is hard, it was hard work to get into the U.K. I am happy here in the U.K. I am terrified I will be made to leave the U.K. I cannot wait to leave the U.K. I despise the U.K. I voted for John Major. I voted for Tony Blair. I did not, I cannot vote, I do not believe in voting, the people who ruined my hand were right to do so, they were wrong to do so, my hand is most certainly ruined, *you will never understand*, why are you buying so many hats?

(Little pause)

We all romp about, grieving, wondering, but with rare exception we mostly remain suspended in the Rhetorical Colloidal Forever that agglutinates between Might and Do. "Might do, might do." I have a friend who says that. "Off to the cinema, care to come?" "Might do." "Would you eat a potato plucked from that soil?" "Might do." Jesus wants you hot or cold but she will hedge her every bet, and why should she not? What has this century taught the civilized if not contempt for those who merely contemplate; the lockup and the lethal injection for those who Do. Awful times, as I have said, our individual degrees of culpability for said awfulness being entirely bound up in our correspondent degrees of action, malevolent or not, or in our correspondent degrees of inertia, which can be taken as a form of malevolent action if you've a mind to see it that way. I do. I've such a mind. My husband . . . Never mind. We shall most of us be adjudged guilty when we are summoned before the Judgment Seat. But guilt? Personal guilt? *(Wringing hands)* Oh, oh . . . No more morally useful or impressive than adult nappy rash, and nearly as unsightly, and ought to be kept as private, ought guilt, as any other useless unimpressive unsightly inflammation. Not suitable for public exchange. And all conversation such as we are having, and though you've said nothing whatsoever we are still conversing, I think, since what I say is driven by fear of you, sitting there before me, by absolute terror of your censure and disdain, and so you need say nothing, you would only weaken your position, whatever it may be, whatever you may be making of this, by speaking, I mean, look at me, look at what I am doing, to myself, to what you must think of me, if ever you chance upon me on _____ *(Gesture)*, out shopping, what will you think? Avoid! Her! All conversation constitutes public exchange was my point, and there are rules of engagement, and skin rash should be displayed in public only for medicinal restorative purposes, inviting the healing rays of the sun and the drying authority of the fresh crisp breeze, and not for the garnering of admiration and the harvesting of sympathy. For most of us deserve neither, and I include myself in that harsh judgment, no matter how guilty we are or feel ourselves to be, my optimism notwithstanding.

I watch as he puts the ten hats in a carrier-bag and feel no surprise when he informs someone in the back of the shop, in Pushto, in which language as I mentioned I now find myself fluent, he's taking the rest of the afternoon off, and he offers me his right hand. I take it and we go out of the shop but no longer on _____ *(Gesture)*, we are standing on a road, a road in Kabul. I hold on tight to his ruined right hand, and he leads me on a guided tour through his city. There are the mountains, unreal as clouds; it is shamelessly sweet, the wreckage rack and ruination all there of course, it's ineffaceable now, this holocaustal effacement, but the gardens of Babur Shah are there too, just like the outdated guidebook promises, and the room in which handsome Shah Shujah, about thirty years of age, of olive complexion and thick black beard, puppet monarch of the British Mission, detested and soon to be murdered by his own insurgent people, displays himself to breathtaking effect, his visitors imagining him at first to be dressed in an armor of jewels, how impractical *that* would be, but actually he wears a green tunic over which are worked flowers of gold and a breast plate of diamonds, shaped like flattened fleurs-de-lis, ornaments of the same kind on each thigh, emeralds above the elbows, diamonds on each wrist, strings of pearls like cross belts but loose, a crown not encrusted with jewels but apparently entirely formed of those precious materials, the whole so complicated and dazzling it is difficult to understand and impossible to describe, and the throne is covered with a cloth adorned with pearls . . .

(She cries softly)

And the scent of the hat merchant takes me by surprise, toasted almonds, and he smiles a broader shy smile which shatters his face into a thousand shards and near a place called Bemaru, thought to be the grave of Bibi Mahru, the Moon-Faced Lady, who died of grief when her betrothed was reported slain on the battlefield, but he wasn't slain, he'd only lost his hand, near her grave, visited by mothers with ailing children, even today, *especially today* when there are many many such cases, many ailing children—demurely hidden from the sight of the ailing and the destitute and war-ravaged we, the hat merchant and I, make love beneath a chinar tree, which is it is my guess a kind of plane tree, beloved of the Moghuls. We kiss, his breath is very bitter, he places his hand inside me, it seems to me his whole hand inside me, and it seems to me a whole hand. And there are flocks of pigeons the nearby villagers keep banded with bronze rings about their legs, and they are released each afternoon for flight, and there is frequently, in the warmer months, kite flying to be seen on the heights of Bemaru.

(Pause)

I sign the receipt, I have paid, he hands me the carrier-bag stuffed with my purchase and with his smile indicates we are done and I should depart. And a chill wind blows up my bones and I long to be back in the safety of my kitchen and I leave the shop pondering the possibility that my prescribed dosage of . . . Mealy-aza-opzamene is too strong, or that sampling my husband's pills . . . perhaps these two chemicals are immiscible.

And yes in fact I do have children, well, *one*. A child. For whom alas nothing ever seems to go well. The older she gets. My fault entirely I'm sure or at least so I am told by my husband the near-mute purveyor of reproachful lids-lowered glances. But this is neither here nor there. We all loved one another, once, but today it simply isn't so or isn't what it used to be, it's . . . well, love.

I love the world. I know how that sounds, inexcusable and vague, but it's all I can say for myself, I love the world, really I do . . . *Love*. Not the vast and unembraceable and orbicular world, this is no gigantine rhapsodic— for all that one might suspect a person who uses words like gigantine— God!—of narcissism, my love is not that overstretched self-aggrandizing hyperinflated sort of adulation which seeks in the outsized and the impossible-to-clearly-comprehend a reflection commensurate with its own oceanic . . . of, well, I suppose of the extent to which the soul excuse me I mean the self is always an insoluble mystery to the narcissist who flatters herself that feeling of vagueness always hanging about her which not a salt in the world can cure is something grand, oceanic, titanically erotic while of course what it really is is nothing more than an inadequately shaped unsteady incoherent . . . quaggy sort of bubble where the solid core ought to be.

I love . . . this guidebook. Its foxed unfingered pages, forgotten words: "Quizilbash." Its sorrowing supercessional displacement by all that has since occurred. So lost; and also so familiar. The home *(She makes the gesture)* away from home. *Recognizable*: not how vast but how *crowded* the world is, consequences to *everything*: the Macedonians, marching east; one tribe displacing another; or one moment in which the heart strays from itself and love is . . . gone?

What after all is a child but the history of all that has befallen her, a succession of displacements, bloody, beautiful? How could any mother not love the world? What else is love but recognition? Love's nothing to do with happiness. Power has to do with happiness. Love has only to do with home.

(Little pause)

Where stands the homebody, safe in her kitchen, on her culpable shore, suffering uselessly watching others perishing in the sea, wringing her plump little maternal hands, oh, oh. Never *joining* the drowning. Her feet, neither rooted nor moving. The ocean is deep and cold and erasing. But how dreadful, really unpardonable, to remain dry.

Look at her, look at her, she is so unforgivably dry. Neither here nor there. She does not drown, she . . . succumbs. To Luxury. She sinks. Terror-struck, down, down into . . . um, the dangerous silent spaces, or rather places, with gravity and ground, down into the terrible silent gardens of the private, in the frightening echoing silence of which a grieving voice might be heard, chattering away, keening, rocking, shrouded, trying to express that which she lacks all power to express but which she knows must be expressed or else . . . death. And she would sound I suppose rather like what I sound like now:

(Whispers:)

Avoid! Her!

And now my daughter. Come home as one does. She must have and may not budge, and I understand, I am her mother, she is . . . starving. I . . . withhold my touch.

The touch which does not understand is the touch which corrupts, the touch which does not understand that which it touches is the touch which corrupts that which it touches, and which corrupts itself.

And so yes, when unexpectedly a curtain I'd not noticed before is parted by a ruined hand, which then beckons, I find myself improbably considering . . .

(Pause)

The hats at the party are a brilliant success. My guests adore them. They are hard to keep on the head, made for smaller people than the people we are and so they slip off, which generates amusement, and the guests exchange them while dancing, kaleidoscopic and self-effacing and I think perhaps to our surprise in some small way meltingly intimate, someone else's hat atop your head, making your scalp stiffen at the imagined strangeness; and to a select group in the kitchen I tell about the merchant who sold them to me, and a friend wisely asks, how do you even know he's Afghan, and of course that's a good question, and the fact is I don't. And I wonder for an instant that I didn't ask. "Would you make love to a stranger with a mutilated hand if the opportunity was offered you?" "Might do," she says. Frank Sinatra is playing: such an awful awful man, such perfect perfect music! A paradox!

(Frank Sinatra starts to sing "It's Nice to Go Trav'ling." She sings the first two verses with him, putting the hats back in the shopping bag, one by one:)

It's very nice to go trav'ling
To Paris, London, and Rome
It's oh so nice to go trav'ling,
But it's so much nicer yes it's so much nicer
To come home.
It's very nice to just wander
The camel route to Iraq,
It's oh so nice to just wander
But it's so much nicer yes it's oh so nice
To wander back . . .

(The music fades. The Homebody stands, takes the coat draped over the back of the empty chair, and puts it on. Buttoning the coat, she says:)

In the seventeenth century the Persian poet Sa'ib-I-Tabrizi was summoned to the court of the Moghul emperors in Agra, and on his way he passed, as one does, Kabul, the city in the Hindu Kush, and he wrote a poem, for he had been touched by its strangeness and beauty, moved only as one may be moved through an encounter with the beautiful and strange; and he declared he would never be the same again:

(She picks up the guidebook, but does not open it)
Oh the beautiful city of Kabul wears a rugged mountain skirt,
And the rose is jealous of its lash-like thorns.
The dust of Kabul's blowing soil smarts lightly in my eyes,
But I love her, for knowledge and love both come from her dust.
I sing bright praises to her colorful tulips,
The beauty of her trees makes me blush.
Every street in Kabul fascinates the eye.
In the bazaars, Egypt's caravans pass by.
No one can count the beauteous moons on her rooftops,
And hundreds of lovely suns hide behind her walls.
Her morning laugh is as gay as flowers,
Her dark nights shine like beautiful hair.
Her tuneful nightingales sing with flame in their throats,
Their fiery songs fall like burning leaves.
I sing to the gardens of Kabul;
Even Paradise is jealous of their greenery.

From *Homebody/Kabul*

AN AFTERWORD | TONY KUSHNER

When the Twin Towers collapsed I was standing on a rainy beach on the Dingle Peninsula in Ireland, watching my four-year-old niece and her newfound playmate, a little British girl, splashing about in a tidal pool. I noticed a crowd gathering around a nearby car radio; I joined it just as the second tower came down. Minutes later, the beach was abandoned. Everyone went home to wait for what seemed like the end of the world.

The next day, as my sister and I tried to get back to New York (it took five days), I received e-mails from a few newspapers asking for an article about the attack. I imagine everyone who'd ever written anything was asked to write about the attack. I refused. I've never been shy about offering opinions, but opining felt hasty, unseemly, and unwise. One of the papers was gathering short essay responses to the question: "What is the meaning of 9/11?" This on 9/12. I thought about the wisdom of Jewish laws of *shiva*, the weeklong period of silence, retirement, prayer mandated as one begins mourning. I didn't write.

A month later, as the cast of *Homebody/Kabul* was beginning rehearsals at New York Theatre Workshop and letters containing anthrax spores were arriving in newsrooms all over the city, I was asked to prepare a statement for the press, since it was assumed that, given the subject of the play, there might be controversy. This is what I wrote:

> *Homebody/Kabul* is a play about Afghanistan and the West's historic and contemporary relationship to that country. It is also a play about travel, about knowledge and learning through seeking out strangeness, about trying to escape the unhappiness of one's life through an encounter with Otherness, about narcissism and self-referentiality as inescapable booby traps in any such encounter; and it's about a human catastrophe, a political problem of global dimensions. It's also about grief. I hate having to write what a play is *about*, but I suppose these are some of the themes of this play.
>
> I didn't imagine, when I was working on the play, that by the time we produced it the United States would be at war with Afghanistan. My play is not a polemic; it was written before September 11, before we began bombing, and I haven't changed anything in the play to make it more or less relevant to current events. It was my feeling when writing the play that more arrogance, more aggression, more chaos, and more bloodshed were the last things needed in addressing the desperate situation in which the Afghan people find themselves. . . .

I'm not psychic. . . . If lines in *Homebody/Kabul* seem "eerily prescient" (a phrase repeated so often that my boyfriend Mark suggested I adopt it as a drag name: Eara Lee Prescient), we ought to consider that the information required to foresee, long before 9/11, at least the broad outline of serious trouble ahead was so abundant and easy of access that even a playwright could avail himself of it; and we ought to wonder about the policy, so recently popular with the American right, that whole countries or regions can be cordoned off and summarily tossed out of the international community's considerations, subjected to sanction, and refused assistance by the world's powers, a policy that helped blind our government to geopolitical reality, to say nothing of ethical accountability and moral responsibility. . . .

What time in human history is comparable to this? It's nearly impossible to locate plausible occasions for hope. Foulness, corruption, meanness of spirit carry the day. I think a lot about 1939, of the time the Russian writer Victor Serge called "the midnight of the century," when women and men of good conscience, having witnessed the horrors of World War I, watched helplessly, overwhelmed by despair, as fascism and war made their inexorable approaches; as Leninism transformed into Stalinism; a time like this one, when, in Brecht's immortal phrase, "there is injustice everywhere / and no rebellion."

Great historical crimes reproduce themselves. One injustice breeds new generations of injustice. Suffering rolls on down through the years, becomes a bleak patrimony, the only inheritance for the disinherited, the key to history, the only certain meaning of life. Sorrow proliferates, evil endures, the only God is the God of Vengeance. Hope dies, the imagination withers and with it the human heart. We no longer dream, not as a people; we are instead demonically possessed. Confronted with the massacre of innocent people, we quibble rather than act; the death of children becomes a regular feature of our daily entertainment. Technology offers oppressor and oppressed alike efficient and cost-effective means of mass murder, and even acts expressive of dissent, defiance, and liberation are changed by the appalling progress of weapons development and the global arms market into suicide bombings, into brutal expressions of indiscriminate nihilistic mayhem. . . .

April 2002

MANIFESTO: 1959

Personism
Frank O'Hara

. . . I don't believe in god, so I don't have to make elaborately sounded structures. I hate Vachel Lindsay, always have, I don't even like rhythm, assonance, all that stuff. You just go on your nerve. If someone's chasing you down the street with a knife you just run, you don't turn around and shout, "Give it up! I was a track star for Mineola Prep."

That's for the writing poems part. As for their reception, suppose you're in love and someone's mistreating (*mal aimé*) you, you don't say, "Hey, you can't hurt me this way, I *care*!" you just let all the different bodies fall where they may, and they always do may after a few months. But that's not why you fell in love in the first place, just to hang onto life, so you have to take your chances and try to avoid being logical. Pain always produces logic, which is very bad for you.

I'm not saying that I don't have practically the most lofty ideas of anyone writing today, but what difference does that make? they're just ideas. The only good thing about it is that when I get lofty enough I've stopped thinking and that's when refreshment arrives.

But how can you really care if anybody gets it, or gets what it means, or if it improves them. Improves them for what? For death? Why hurry them along? Too many poets act like a middle-aged mother trying to get her kids to eat too much cooked meat, and potatoes with drippings (tears). I don't give a damn whether they eat or not. Forced feeding leads to excessive thinness (effete). Nobody should experience anything they don't need to, if they don't need poetry bully for them, I like the movies too. And after all, only Whitman and Crane and Williams, of the American poets, are better than the movies. As for measure and other technical apparatus, that's just common sense: if you're going to buy a pair of pants you want them to be tight enough so that everyone will want to go to bed with you. There's nothing metaphysical about it. Unless, of course, you flatter yourself into thinking that what you're experiencing is "yearning." . . .

FOUR POEMS

Frederick Seidel

BALI

Is there intelligent life in the universe?
No glass
In the windows of the bus
In from the airport, only air and perfume.

Every porch in the darkness was lighted
With twinkling oil lamps
And there was music
At 2 A.M., the gamelan.

I hear the cosmos
And smell the Asian flowers
And there were candles
Mental as wind chimes in the soft night.

Translucency the flames showed through,
The heavy makeup the little dancers wore,
The scented sudden and the nubile slow
Lava flow of the temple troupe performing for the hotel guests.

Frederick Seidel won the 2002 PEN/Voelcker Award for Poetry.

Her middle finger touches her thumb in the *vitarkamudra*,
While her heavily made-up eyes shift wildly,
Facial contortions silently acting out the drama,
And the thin neck yin-yangs back and forth to the music.

Announcing the gods,
The room jerked and the shower curtain swayed.
All the water in the swimming pool
Trampolined out, and in the mountains hundreds died.

The generals wanted to replace Sukarno.
Because of his syphilis he was losing touch
With the Communist threat and getting rather crazy.
So they slaughtered the Communists and the rich Chinese.

Gentle Balinese murdered gentle Balinese,
And, in the usual pogrom, killed
The smart hardworking Chinese,
Merchants to the poor, Jews in paradise.

FRENCH POLYNESIA

Drinking and incest and endless ease
Is paradise and child abuse
And battered wives.
There are no other jobs.

Everything else is either
Food or bulimia.
The melon drips with this.
It opens and hisses happiness.

A riderless horse sticks out,
Pink as an earthworm, standing on the beach.
Fish, fish, fish,
I feel fishish.

I develop
When I get below my depth.
I splinter into jewels, Cadillac-finned balls,
Chromed mercury no one can grab.

I care below the surface.
Veils in
Colors I haven't seen in fifty years nibble
Coral.

Easter Sunday in Papeete.
Launched and dined at L'Acajou.
The Polynesians set off for outer space
In order to be born, steering by the stars.

Specialists in the canoes chant
The navigation vectors.
Across the universe,
A thousand candles are lighted

In the spaceships and the light roars
And the choir soars. A profusion
Of fruit and flowers in tubs being offered
Forms foam and stars.

THE OPPOSITE OF A DARK DUNGEON

Three hundred steps down
From the top
Pilgrims are
Looking up.

The temple is above
In a cave.
The stairs to it start next
To the standard frantic street.

Monkeys beg on
The stairs
All the way
Up to the entrance.

Vendors sell treats
To the pilgrims to feed to them.
Some people are afraid of monkeys
Because they think they might get bitten.

When you finally reach the top, somewhat
Out of breath, you enter
The heavy cold darkness
And buy a ticket.

The twenty-foot gilded figures recline.
There are trinkets you can buy to lay at their smiling feet.
They use up the universe with their size.
Their energy is balm and complete.

Everything in the cosmos
Is in the cave, including the monkeys
Outside. Everything is
The opposite of a dark dungeon. And so

A messenger from light arrived.
Of course they never know that they're a messenger.
Don't know they carry a message.
And then they stay a while and then they leave.

STAR BRIGHT

The story goes one day
A messenger from light arrived.
Of course they never know that they're a messenger.
Don't know they carry a message.

The submarine stayed just
Below the surface with its engines off near the shore observing.
One day the world took off its shoes and disappeared
Inside the central mosque

And never came back out. Outside the periscope the rain
Had stopped, the fires on shore were
Out. Outside the mosque
The vast empty plaza was the city's outdoor market till

The satellite observed the changing
Colors of the planet
And reported to the submarine that
No one was alive.

A messenger from light arrived.
Of course they never know that they're a messenger.
Don't know they carry a message.
And then they stay a while and then they leave.

Arrived, was ushered in,
Got in a waiting car and drove away.
Was ushered in,
Kowtowed to the Sacred Presence the required ten times

And backed away from the Sacred Presence blind,
And turned back into light.
Good night,
Blind light.

Far star, star bright.
And though they never know that they're a messenger,
Never know they carry a message,
At least they stay a while before they leave.

From *Life on Earth*

MANIFESTO: 1959

Poetry, Violence, and the Trembling Lambs; or, Independence Day Manifesto
Allen Ginsberg

. . . The suppression of contemplative individuality is nearly complete.

The only immediate historical data that we can know and act on are those fed to our senses through systems of mass communication.

These media are exactly the places where the deepest and most personal sensitivities and confessions of reality are most prohibited, mocked, suppressed. . . .

Because systems of mass communication can communicate only officially acceptable levels of reality, no one can know the extent of the secret unconscious life. No one in America can know what will happen. No one is in real control. America is having a nervous breakdown. Poetry is the record of individual insights into the secret soul of the individual and because all individuals are one in the eyes of their creator, into the soul of the world. The world has a soul. America is having a nervous breakdown. San Francisco is one of many places where a few individuals, poets, have had the luck and courage and fate to glimpse something new through the crack in mass consciousness; they have been exposed to some insight into their own nature, the nature of the governments, and the nature of God.

Therefore there has been great exaltation, despair, prophecy, strain, suicide, secrecy, and public gaiety among the poets of the city. Those of the general populace whose individual perception is sufficiently weak to be formed by stereotypes of mass communication disapprove and deny the insight. The police and newspapers have moved in; mad movie manufacturers from Hollywood are at this moment preparing bestial stereotypes of the scene.

The poets and those who share their activities or exhibit some sign of dress, hair, or demeanor of understanding, or hipness, are ridiculed. Those of us who have used certain benevolent drugs (marijuana) to alter our consciousness in order to gain insight are hunted down in the street by police. Peyote, a historic vision-producing agent, is prohibited on pain of arrest. . . . Deviants from the mass sexual stereotype, quietists, those who will not work for money, or fib and make arms for hire, or join armies in murder and threat, those who wish to loaf, think, rest in visions, act beautifully on their own, speak truthfully in public, inspired by Democracy—what is their psychic fate now in America? An America the greater portion of whose economy is yoked to mental and mechanical preparations for war?

Literature expressing these insights has been mocked, misinterpreted, and suppressed by a horde of middlemen whose fearful allegiance to the organization of mass stereotype communication prevents them from sympathy (not only with their own inner nature but) with any manifestation of unconditioned individuality. I mean journalists, commercial publishers, book-review fellows, multitudes of professors of literature, etc., etc. Poetry is hated. Whole schools of academic criticism have risen to prove that human consciousness of unconditioned spirit is a myth. A poetic renaissance glimpsed in San Francisco has been responded to with ugliness, anger, jealousy, vitriol, sullen protestations of superiority.

And violence. By police, by customs officials, post office employees, by trustees of great universities. By anyone whose love of power has led him to a position where he can push other people around over a difference of opinion—or vision. The stakes are too great—an America gone mad with materialism, a police state America, a sexless and soulless America prepared to battle the world in defense of a false image of its authority. Not the wild and beautiful America of the comrades of Walt Whitman, not the historic America of William Blake and Henry David Thoreau where the spiritual independence of each individual was an America, a universe, more huge and awesome than all the abstract bureaucracies and authoritative officialdoms of the world combined. . . .

© 1955 ALLEN GINSBERG TRUST

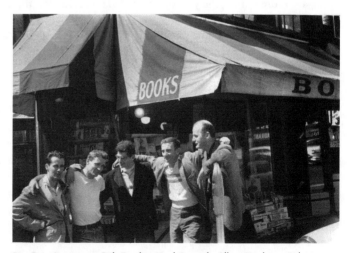

San Francisco, 1955: Bob Donlin, Neal Cassady, Allen Ginsberg, Robert Lavigne, and Lawrence Ferlinghetti.

DEPARTURES

Edward Said

All families invent their parents and children, give each of them a history, character, fate, and even a language. There was always something wrong with how I was invented and meant to fit in with the world of my parents and four sisters. Whether this was because I constantly misread my part or because of some deep flaw in my being I could not tell for most of my early life. Sometimes I was intransigent, and proud of it. At other times I seemed to myself to be nearly devoid of character, timid, uncertain, without will. Yet the overriding sensation I had was of never being quite right. As I have said before, it took me about fifty years to become accustomed to, or more exactly to feel less uncomfortable with, "Edward," a foolishly English name yoked to the unmistakably Arabic family name "Said." True, "Edward" was for the Prince of Wales who cut so fine a figure in 1935, the year of my birth, and "Said" was the name of various uncles and cousins. But the rationale of my name broke down when I discovered no grandparents called "Said," and when I tried to connect my fancy English name with its Arabic partner. For years, I would rush past "Edward" and emphasize "Said," or do the reverse, or connect the two to each other so quickly that neither would be clear. The one thing I could not tolerate, but very often would have to endure, was the disbelieving, and hence undermining, reaction: Edward? Said?

The travails of bearing such a name were compounded by an equally unsettling quandary when it came to language. I have never known what language I spoke first, Arabic or English, or which one was mine beyond any doubt. What I do know, however, is that the two have always been together in my life, one resonating in the other, sometimes ironically, sometimes nostalgically, or, more often, one correcting and commenting on the other. Each can seem like my absolutely first language, but neither is. I trace this primal instability to my mother, whom I remember speaking to me both in English and Arabic, although she always wrote to me in English—once a week, all her life, as did I, all of hers. Certain spoken phrases of hers, like *tislamli* or *Mish 'arfa shu biddi 'amal?* or *rouh'ha*—dozens of them—were Arabic, and I was never conscious of having to translate them or, even in cases like *tislamli*, of knowing exactly what they meant. They were a part of her infinitely maternal atmosphere, for which in moments of stress I found myself yearning in the softly uttered phrase *ya mama*, always dreamily seductive then suddenly snatched away, with the promise of something in the end never given.

But woven into her Arabic speech were English words like *naughty boy* and of course my name, pronounced *Edwaad*. I am still haunted by the sound, at exactly the same time and place, of her voice calling me *Edwaad*, the word wafting through the dusk air at the Fish Garden's closing time, and me, undecided whether to answer or to remain in hiding for just a while longer, enjoying the pleasure of being called, being wanted, the non-Edward part of myself finding luxurious respite in not answering until the silence of my being became unendurable. Her English deployed a rhetoric of statement and norms that has never left me. Once my mother left Arabic and spoke English there was a more objective and serious tone that mostly banished the forgiving and musical intimacy of *her* first language, Arabic. At age five or six I knew that I was irremediably *naughty* and at school all manner of comparably disapproved-of things like *fibber* and *loiterer*. By the time I was fully conscious of speaking English fluently, if not always correctly, I regularly referred to myself not as *me* but as *you*. "Mummy doesn't love you, naughty boy," she would say, and I would respond, half plaintive echoing, half defiant assertion: "Mummy doesn't love you, but Auntie Melia loves you." Auntie Melia was her elderly maiden aunt who doted on me when I was a very young child. "No she doesn't," my mother persisted. "All right. Saleh loves you," I would conclude—Saleh was Auntie Melia's driver—rescuing something from the enveloping gloom.

I hadn't then any idea where my mother's English came from or who, in the national sense of the phrase, she was: this strange state of ignorance continued until relatively late in my life, when I was in graduate school. In Cairo, one of the places where I grew up, her spoken Arabic was fluent

Egyptian, but to my keener ear, and to the many Egyptians she knew, it was, if not outright *Shami*, then perceptibly inflected by it. *Shami* (Damascene) is the collective adjective and noun used by Egyptians to describe both an Arabic-speaker who is not Egyptian and someone who is from Greater Syria, i.e., Syria itself, Lebanon, Palestine, Jordan; but *Shami* is also used to designate the Arabic dialect spoken by a *Shami*. Much more than my father, whose linguistic ability was primitive compared to hers, my mother had an excellent command of the classical language as well as the demotic. Not enough of the latter to disguise her as Egyptian, however, which of course she was not. Born in Nazareth, then sent to boarding school and junior college in Beirut, she was Palestinian, even though her mother, Munira, was Lebanese. I never knew her father, but he, I discovered, was the Baptist minister in Nazareth, although he originally came from Safad, via a sojourn in Texas.

I couldn't absorb, much less master, all the meanderings and interruptions of these details as they broke up a simple dynastic sequence; nor could I grasp why she was not a straight English mummy. I have retained this unsettled sense of many identities—mostly in conflict with each other—all my life, together with an acute memory of the despairing wish that we could have been all-Arab, or all-European and American, or all-Christian, or all-Muslim, or all-Egyptian, and on and on. I found I had two alternatives with which to counter the process of challenge, recognition, and exposure to which I felt subject, questions and remarks like: "What are you?" "But Said is an Arab name." "You're American?" "You're an American without an American name, and you've never been to America." "You don't look American!" "How come you were born in Jerusalem and you live *here*?" "You're an Arab after all, but what kind are you?"

I do not remember that any of the answers I gave out loud to such probings were satisfactory, or even memorable. My alternatives were hatched entirely on my own: one might work, say, in school, but would not work in church or on the street with my friends. My first approach was to adopt my father's brashly assertive tone and say to myself: "I'm an American citizen, and that's it." He was American by dint of having lived in the United States followed by service in the Army during World War I. Partly because this alternative was not only implausible but imposed on me, I found it far from convincing. To say "I am an American citizen" in the setting of an English school, with wartime Cairo dominated by British troops and what seemed to me a totally homogeneous Egyptian populace, was foolhardy, something to be risked in public only when I was challenged officially to name my citizenship; in private I could not maintain it for long, so quickly did the affirmation wither under existential scrutiny.

The second of my alternatives was even less successful. It was to open myself to the deeply disorganized state of my real history and origins as I had gleaned them and then try to make some sort of sense of them. But I never had enough information; there was never the right number of functioning connectives between the parts I knew about or was able to excavate; the total picture was never quite right. The trouble seemed to begin with my parents, their pasts and names. My father, Wadie, was later called "William" (an early discrepancy that I assumed for a long time was only an Anglicization of his Arabic name, but soon it appeared to me suspiciously like a case of assumed identity, with the name "Wadie" cast aside, for not very creditable reasons, except by his wife and sister). Born in Jerusalem in 1895 (my mother said it was more likely 1893), he never told me more than ten or eleven things about his past, none of which ever changed and which hardly conveyed anything except a series of portable words. He was at least forty at the time of my birth.

He hated Jerusalem, and although I was born there and we spent long periods of time there, the only thing he ever said about it was that it reminded him of death. At some point in his life his father was a dragoman and because he knew German was said to have shown Palestine to Kaiser Wilhelm. Never referred to by name except when my mother, who never knew him, called him "Abu Assad," my grandfather bore the surname "Ibrahim." In school, therefore, my father was known as Wadie Ibrahim. I still do not know where "Said" came from, and no one seems able to explain it. The only relevant detail about his father that my father thought fit to convey to me was that Abu Assad's whippings of him were much more severe than his of me. "How did you endure it?" I asked, to which he replied with a chuckle, "Most of the time I ran away." I was never able to, and never even considered it.

One day my mother announced that John Gielgud was coming to Cairo to perform *Hamlet* at the Opera House. "We must go," she said with infectious resolve, and indeed the visit was duly set up, although of course I had no idea who John Gielgud was. I was nine at the time and had just learned a bit about the play in the volume of Shakespeare stories by Charles and Mary Lamb I had been given for Christmas a few months earlier. Mother's idea was that she and I should gradually read through the play together.

For that purpose a beautiful one-volume Shakespeare was brought down from the shelf, its handsome red morocco-leather binding and its delicate onionskin paper embodying for me all that was luxurious and exciting in a book. Its opulence was heightened by the pencil or charcoal drawings illustrating the dramas, *Hamlet*'s being an exceptionally taut tableau by Henry Fuseli of the Prince of Denmark, Horatio, and the Ghost seeming to struggle against each other as the announcement of murder and the agitated response to it gripped them.

The two of us sat in the front reception room, she in a big armchair, I on a stool next to her, with a smoky half-lit fire in the fireplace on her left, and we read *Hamlet* together. She was Gertrude and Ophelia, I Hamlet, Horatio, and Claudius. She also played Polonius, as if in solidarity with my father, who often quoted "neither a borrower nor a lender be" as a reminder of how risky it was for me to be given money to spend on my own. We skipped the whole play-within-a-play sequence as it was too bewilderingly ornate and complicated for the two of us.

There must have been at least four, and perhaps even five or six sessions when, sharing the book, we read and tried to make sense of the play, the two of us completely alone and together, with Cairo, my sisters, and father shut out.

I did not understand many of the lines, though Hamlet's basic situation, his outrage at his father's murder and his mother's remarriage, his endless wordy vacillation, did come through half-consciously. I had no idea what incest and adultery were but could not ask my mother, whose concentration on the play seemed to have drawn her in and away from me. What I remember above all was the change from her normal voice to a new stage voice as Gertrude: it went up in pitch, smoothed out, became exceptionally fluent and, most of all, acquired a bewitchingly flirtatious and calming tone. "Good Hamlet," I remember her clearly saying to me, not to Hamlet, "cast thy nighted colour off, / And let thine eye look like a friend on Denmark." I felt that she was speaking to my better, less disabled, and still fresh self, hoping perhaps to lift me out of the sodden delinquency of my life, already burdened with worries and anxieties that I was now sure were to threaten my future.

Reading *Hamlet* as an affirmation of my status in her eyes, not as someone devalued, as in mine I had become, was one of the great moments in my childhood. We were two voices to each other, two happily allied spirits in language. I knew nothing consciously of the inner dynamics that link desperate prince and adulterous queen at the play's interior, nor did I really understand the fury of the scene between them when Polonius is killed and Gertrude verbally flayed by Hamlet. We read together through all that, since what mattered to me was that in a curiously un-Hamlet-like way, I could count on her to be someone whose emotions and affections engaged mine without really being more than an exquisitely maternal, protective, and reassuring person. Far from feeling that she had tampered with her obligations to her son, I felt that these readings confirmed the deepness of our connection to each other; for years I kept in my mind the higher than usual pitch of her voice, the unagitated poise of her manner, the soothing, conclusively patient outline of her presence, as goods to be held onto at all costs, but rarer and rarer as my delinquencies increased in number, and her destructive and dislocating capacities threatened me more.

When I saw the play at the Opera House I was jolted out of my seat by Gielgud's declaiming "Angels and ministers of grace defend us," and the sense it conveyed of being a miraculous confirmation of what I had read privately with Mother. The trembling resonance of his voice, the darkened, windy stage, the distantly shining figure of the ghost, all seemed to have brought to life the Fuseli drawing that I had long studied, and it raised my sensuous apprehension to a pitch I do not think I have ever again experienced. But I was also disheartened by the physical incongruities between me and the men whose green and crimson tights set off fully rounded, perfectly shaped legs that seemed to mock my awkward carriage, my unskilled movements, my spindly, shapeless legs. Everything about Gielgud and the blond man who played Laertes communicated an ease and confidence of being—they were English heroes after all—that reduced me to buglike status, curtailing my capacity to enjoy the play. A few days later, when an Anglo-American classmate called Tony Howard invited me to meet Gielgud at his house, it was all I could do to manage a feeble, silent handshake. Gielgud was in a gray suit but said nothing; he pressed my small hand with an Olympian half-smile.

It must have been the memory of those long-ago *Hamlet* afternoons in Cairo that made my mother, during the last two or three years of her life, enthusiastic once again about us going to the theater together. The most memorable time was when—her cancer afflictions already pronounced—she arrived in London from Beirut on her way to the United States to consult a specialist; I met her at the airport and brought her to Brown's Hotel for the one night she had to spend there. With barely two hours to get ready and have an early supper, she nevertheless gave an unhesitating "yes" to my suggestion that we see Vanessa Redgrave and Timothy Dalton as Antony and Cleopatra at the Haymarket. It was an understated, unopulent production, and the long play transfixed her in a way that surprised me. After years of Lebanese war and Israeli invasion she had become distracted, often querulous, worried about her health and what she should do with herself. All of this, however, went into abeyance as we watched and heard Shakespeare's lines ("Eternity was in our lips and eyes, / Bliss in our brows' bent"), as if speaking to us in the accents of wartime Cairo, back in our little cocoon, the two of us very quiet and concentrated, savoring the language and communion with each other—despite the disparity in our ages and the fact that we were mother and son—for the very last time. Eight months later she had begun her final descent into the disease that killed her, her mind ravaged by metastases which, before striking her completely silent for the two months before she died, caused her to speak fearsomely of plots around her. The last lucidly intimate thing she ever said to me was "my poor little child," pronounced with such sad resignation, a mother taking final leave of her son. Eighteen months later I was diagnosed with the leukemia that must have already been in me when she died. . . .

In early September 1991, on the eve of the Madrid Peace Conference and forty years after I left the Middle East for the United States, I was in London for a seminar I had convened of Palestinian intellectuals and activists. After the Gulf War and the Palestinian leadership's fatal stand alongside Saddam Hussein, we were in a very weak negotiating position. The idea of the conference was to try to articulate a common set of themes that would assist our progress towards self-determination. We came from all over the dispersed Palestinian world—the West Bank and Gaza, the Palestinian diaspora in various Arab countries, Europe, and North America. What transpired during the seminar was a terrible disappointment: the endless repetition of well-known arguments, our inability to fix on a collective goal, the apparent desire to listen only to ourselves. In short, nothing came of it except an eerie premonition of the Palestinian failure at Oslo.

Midway through the debate, during one of the scheduled breaks, I phoned Mariam, my wife, in New York to ask her if the results of the blood test I had taken for my annual physical had been satisfactory. Cholesterol was what had concerned me and no, she said, everything was fine on that front but added with some hesitation: "Charles Hazzi"—our doctor—"would like to speak to you when you get back." Something in her voice suggested to me that all was not well, so I immediately rang Charles at his office. "Nothing to get excited about," he said, "we'll talk in New York." His repeated refusals to tell me what was wrong finally provoked me to impatience. "You must tell me, Charles. I'm not a child, and I have a right to know." With a whole set of demurrals—it's not serious, a hematologist can very easily take care of you, it's chronic after all—he told me that I had chronic lymphocytic leukemia (CLL), although it took me a week to absorb the initial impact of my diagnosis. I was asymptomatic and sophisticated diagnostic techniques were needed to confirm the original finding. It was another month before I understood how thoroughly shaken I was by this "sword of Damocles," as one doctor called it, hanging over me, and a further six months before I found the extraordinary doctor, Kanti Rai, under whose care I have been since June 1992.

A month after I was diagnosed I discovered myself in the middle of a letter to my mother, who had been dead for a year and a half. Somehow the urge to communicate with her overcame the factual reality of her death, which in mid-sentence stopped my fanciful urge, leaving me slightly disoriented, even embarrassed. A vague narrative urge seemed to be stirring inside me, but I was too caught up in the anxieties and nervousness of my life with CLL to pay it much attention. During that period in 1993 I contemplated several changes in my life which I realized without any fear would be shorter and more difficult now. I thought about moving to Boston to return to a place I had lived in and enjoyed when I was a student, but soon admitted to myself that because it was a quiet town relative to New York I had been thinking regressively about finding a place to die in. I gave up the idea.

So many returns, attempts to go back to bits of life, or people who were no longer there: these constituted a steady response to the increasing rigors of my illness. In 1992 I went with my wife and children to Palestine for the first time in forty-five years. In July 1993 I went on my own to Cairo, making it a point in the middle of a journalistic mission to visit old haunts. All this time I was being monitored, without treatment, by Dr. Rai, who occasionally reminded me that I would at some point require chemotherapy. By the time I began treatment in March 1994 I realized that I had at least entered, if not the final phase of my life, then the period—like Adam and Eve leaving the Garden—from which there would be no return to my old life. In May 1994 I began work on the memoir I am writing.

These details are important as a way of explaining to myself and to my reader how the time of the memoir is intimately tied to the time, phases, ups and downs, variations in my illness. As I grew weaker, the more the number of infections and bouts of side effects increased, the more the memoir was my way of constructing something in prose while in my physical and emotional life I grappled with the anxieties and pains of degeneration. Both tasks resolved themselves into details: to write is to get from word to word, to suffer illness is to go through the infinitesimal steps that take you from one state to another. With other sorts of work that I did, essays, lectures, teaching, journalism, I was going across the illness, punctuating it almost forcibly with deadlines and cycles of beginning, middle, and end: with this memoir I was borne along by the episodes of treatment, hospital stay, physical pain and mental anguish, letting those dictate how and when I could write, for how long and where. Periods of travel were often productive since I carried my handwritten manuscript with me wherever I went and took advantage of every hotel room or friend's house I stayed in. I was therefore rarely in a hurry to get a section done, though I had a precise idea of what I planned to put in it. Curiously the memoir and the phases of my illness share exactly the same time, although most traces of the latter have been effaced in the story of my early life. This record of a life and the ongoing course of a disease are one and the same, it could be said; the same but deliberately different.

And the more this relationship developed the more important it became to me, the more also my memory—unaided by anything except concentrated reflection on and archaeological prying into a very distant and essentially irrecoverable past—seemed hospitable and generous to my often importunate forays. Despite the travail of disease and the restrictions imposed on me by my having left the places of my youth, I can say with the poet: "nor in this bower, / This little lime-tree bower, have I not mark'd / Much that has soothed me." There had been a time when I could not bear to think about my past, especially Cairo and Jerusalem, which for two sets of different reasons were no longer accessible. The latter had been replaced by Israel, the former, by one of those cruel coincidences, was closed to me for legal reasons. Unable to visit Egypt for the fifteen years between 1960 and 1975, I rationed early memories of my life there (considerably chopped up, full of atmospherics that conveyed a sense of warmth and comfort by contrast with the harsh alienation I felt in my New York life) as a way of falling asleep, an activity that has grown more difficult with time, time that has also dissolved the aura of happiness around my early life and let it emerge as a more complicated and difficult period. To grasp it, I realized, I would have to be sharply alert, awake, avoiding dreamy somnolence. I've thought in fact that the memoir in some fundamental way is all about sleeplessness, all about the silence of wakefulness and, in my case, the need for conscious recollection and articulation as a substitute for sleep. Not just for sleep but for holidays and relaxation, all that passes for middle- and upper-class "leisure," on which, about ten years ago, I unconsciously turned my back. As one of the main responses to my illness I found in the memoir a new kind of challenge: not just a new kind of wakefulness but a project about as far from my professional and political life as it was possible for me to go.

The underlying motifs for me have been, on the one hand, the emergence of a second self buried for a very long time beneath a surface of often expertly acquired and wielded social characteristics belonging to the self my parents tried to construct, the "Edward" I speak of intermittently, and, on the other, an understanding of the way an extraordinary number of departures have unsettled my life from its earliest beginnings. To me, nothing more painful and paradoxically sought after characterizes my life than the many displacements from countries, cities, abodes, languages, environments that have kept me in motion all these years. Twelve years ago I wrote in *After the Last Sky* that when I travel I always take too much with me, and that even a trip downtown requires the packing of a briefcase stocked with items disproportionately larger in size and number than the actual period of the trip. Analyzing that, I concluded that I had a secret but ineradicable fear of not returning. What I've since discovered is that despite this fear I fabricate occasions for departure, thus giving rise to the fear voluntarily. The two seem absolutely necessary to my rhythm of life and have intensified dramatically during the period of my illness. I say to myself: if you don't take this trip, don't prove your mobility and indulge your fear of being lost, don't override the normal rhythms of domestic life now, you certainly will not be able to do so in the near future. I also experience the anxious moodiness of travel (*la mélancholie des paquebots*, as Flaubert calls it; *bahnhofstimmung* in German), along with envy for those who stay behind, whom I see on my return, their faces unshadowed by dislocation or what seems to be enforced mobility, happy with their families, draped in a comfortable suit and raincoat, there for all to see. Something about the invisibility of the departed, being missing and perhaps missed, in addition to the intense, repetitive, and predictable sense of banishment that takes you away from all you know and can take comfort in, makes you feel the need to leave out of some prior but self-created logic, and a sense of rapture. In all cases, though, the great fear is that departure is the state of being abandoned, even though it is you who leave.

During the last few months of my mother's life she would tell me plaintively and frequently about the misery of trying to fall asleep. She was in Washington, I in New York, we would speak constantly, see each other about once a month. Her cancer was spreading, I knew. She refused to have chemotherapy: "Ma biddee at'adthab," she would say: "I don't want the torture of it." Years later I was to have four years of it with no success; she never buckled, never gave in even to her doctor's importunings, never had chemotherapy. But she could not sleep at night. Sedatives, sleeping pills, soothing drinks, the counsel of friends and relatives, reading, praying: none, she said, did any good. "Help me to sleep, Edward," she once said to me with a piteous trembling in her voice that I can still hear as I write. But then the disease spread to her brain, and for the last six weeks she slept all the time. Sitting by her bed with my sister Grace, waiting for her to awaken, was, for me, the most anguished and paradoxical of my experiences with her.

Now I have divined that my own inability to sleep may be her last legacy to me, a counter to her struggle for sleep. For me sleep is something to get over as quickly as possible. I can only go to bed very late, but I am up, literally, at dawn. Like her, I don't possess the secret of long sleep, though unlike her I have reached the point where I do not want it. For me, sleep is death, as is any diminishment in awareness. During my last treatment— a twelve-week ordeal—I was most upset by the drugs I was given to ward off fever and shaking chills, and manifestly upset by the sense of being infantilized, the helplessness that many years ago I had conceded as that of a child to my mother and, differently, to my father. I fought the medical soporifics bitterly, as if my identity depended on that resistance.

Sleeplessness for me is a cherished state, to be desired at almost any cost; there is nothing for me as invigorating as the early-morning shedding of the shadowy half-consciousness of a night's loss, reacquainting myself with what I might have lost completely a few hours earlier. I occasionally experience myself as a cluster of flowing currents. I prefer this to the idea of a solid self, the identity to which so many attach so much significance. These currents, like the themes of one's life, are borne along during the waking hours, and at their best they require no reconciling, no harmonizing. They may be not quite right, but at least they are always in motion, in time, in place, in the form of strange combinations moving about, not necessarily forward, against each other, contrapuntally yet without one central theme. A form of freedom, I'd like to think, even if I am far from being totally convinced that it is. That skepticism, too, is something I particularly want to hold onto. With so many dissonances in my life I have learned to prefer being not quite right, out of place.

From *Out of Place*

LACRIMAE RERUM

Ann Snitow

I confess I like things in themselves. I'm not a connoisseur, there's no way to dress this up. Though classical objects can impress me—a perfect eighteenth century chair in a shop window—I'm quite the lowbrow about things. I like bazaars. Joyce's Araby would have been no disappointment to me, as long as there was anything at all left to look at. If this brushes mere shopping, so be it.

In Pristina just before the war, a place which certainly offered one of the poorest opportunities to shop imaginable, I managed to buy a set of tiny wooden pegs with adhesive backs. Pot holders are hanging from them on my kitchen wall in New York, a jolly man with a hat, a toadstool, a pig face, each a quarter of an inch across. Their charm is that they come from somewhere else—not to be naïve about this, probably, originally, from a sweatshop in China. But quite by chance, they are also something *far niente* left over from my pained trip to Kosova. Though I forget so much of my experience, I remember that walk alone in Pristina on a gray day, the broken tiles and crumbling curbstones, the minimal shops where, for fifty cents, I glued that afternoon to my faithless memory.

When I was living in Vienna for a few months, I missed my father. It was obvious, since he was ninety-two at the time, that his days were numbered, in spite of his continuing vitality and wit. In the *Naschmarkt* I bought a cheap, white antique cup. It had—and has—four roses painted on it, and, in the center, the single word "Papa."

That I miss my father now that he's dead is a constant, but the cup objectifies him. I visit him in his cup and he visits me. When it breaks—

and everything does—I'll let this stage go. That moment will break my tie to a time when my father was still alive and I had the luxury of missing him before he had actually left.

I've always looked down on religion as a refusal to face the facts; my father's death didn't change that. There he lies, in the ground, and his absence matters only to a small and dwindling group of people who could (and sometimes do) arrange themselves easily around a dinner table. But Pop's sudden, at that moment unexpected, death has made me understand religion better. "This is my body and this is my blood." I took a long time over finishing a box of crackers he had started. Things he had been using the day before seemed to hold onto something of him, like reliquaries, and I hung onto them. At the same time, their presence felt insulting. They were still here while he was being thrust into the past.

The things—quite many, from the precious to the banal—which he has left make me miss him more, with their little stabs, bids for attention in my busy life. But they also assuage the grief. My father was a generous man and the things littered around in all his many haunts were meant to be there for my brother and me to find.

This spiritual materialism, this luminous love of things comes down to me from my father and his whole family, people who were poor and then had the luck to make good from hard work in the hardware business. At the high holy days, we sat with aunts and uncles and cousins at a long mahogany table covered with a damask cloth embroidered with the family initials. The table was Aunt Lil's and Uncle Abe's. (She, a diamond pin, the import duty paid at the airport because America is great and must never be cheated; he, a thick cotton white shirt, starched and perfectly ironed, of a fineness that was the whole simple truth about him.) The silver was heavy and on the dark wooden sideboard sat an impressive humidor. ("Have a cigar, Charlie," my Uncle Abe would say to my father at the end of the elaborate meal.) The empire of things was solid, worldly, decent, humorous.

After Uncle Abe and Aunt Lil died, their things were saturated with the hard-earned pride of having, and of giving, with their unfussy delight in the world as they had found it, and as they had helped make it in an older, manufacturing New York:

I make 2-in-1 holders
To hang on your wall.

They'll hold all your brooms,
So they won't fall.

The empire of things came down to their universally loved daughter, my father's niece Dorothy, in an unbroken stewardship. The things grounded us—in all senses of the word.

Then Dorothy, too, died. This was unlooked for. She was decades younger than my father. The objects she left behind—silk nightgowns, pearl earrings, fine suits hanging in vinyl sheaves in the closet—weren't ready to circulate. They, too, were in the middle of their lives.

Dorothy's last two Passovers were at my table, a flimsy board by family standards, in fact, rented, and tricked out with unmatched little vases, a variety of plates—call them kitsch or ephemera, depending on how you see the descent in the generations from a taste for permanence to a taste for objects that announce more openly that they are fleeting.

Everyone brought food to this new kind of fly-by-night Passover. The first time, Dorothy, already sick, brought a few light hors d'oeuvres and the small, fluted glass bowls to serve them in. Late that night, I found one of the lovely little bowls left behind among the dirty dishes. In the morning I called Dorothy but she said, "I'll collect it next year."

And the next year came, and she was still there, but now so frail. The signs were unavoidable. I reminded her about the bowl and offered it to her. She made a gesture towards taking it, then drew back. "You keep it, dear. I'll get it next year." Her eyes caressed it, part of a set. She was saying farewell to it, and giving me a gift, a visible sign. At that moment I could see her face—so dear to me—register emotions I completely understood, a family language. She imagined me using the bowl after she was dead. She knew I could never use the bowl, not in the most hasty or casual moment, without thinking of her. She wanted me to think of her, and she knew that in that moment she would be loved.

A few years later, when my partner, Daniel, dropped the bowl, I felt a terrible grief. I was, with all the literalness of my father's family, shattered. But only for a moment. Things and people enter and leave the world, but not usually together. In a lifetime we go through many generations of objects, from teething rings, to shiny leather purses, to keys (on charming key rings) to doors we no longer go through. But at the same time that objects come and go, they can also, sometimes, endure so much longer than we—Shakespeare's house sits in Stratford, Aunt Lil and Uncle Abe's table sits just where it used to in what is now Cousin Gerry's apartment in New York. The art my father bought is precious and such things are only on loan to individuals. They will travel on. But a pastel by Whistler is too damaged; I may well be the last to own it. The museum curator rejected it and told me its decay is called the "inherent vice" in art. The phrase, he said, always reminded him of original sin. Capable of sin or not, we and our objects are both of us not long for this world.

Recently, my friend Sonja brought me a brilliantly colored ceramic Russian doll, a wide-skirted teacher surrounded by a flock of children singing and madly gesturing. This delicate piece of folk nonsense she had carried by hand from Moscow, to her home in Belgrade, and then to New York, assuring jumpy customs officers of its harmlessness, its uselessness, its unimportance, at border after border. By journey's end, one of the funny little kids did lose a leg, but Daniel glued him back together again.

This gift is unlikely to have a long life, but for now it's in good hands. I take care of the silly thing, and the attenuated reality, that I love and am loved by someone who lives so far away, solidifies in my otherwise forgetful and untrusting heart.

On Halloween night I was having dinner with my friend Henry. The restaurant window was huge, floor to ceiling, right on a corner where people rushed past to join the costume parade. One was dressed as a lampshade, one a teapot, one a skeleton. I kept exclaiming as the strange creatures streamed by us. Henry was uninterested. "But Henry, these are people pretending to be things or spirits. We're seeing the soul of all human invention." Several drifted by waving long bamboo stalks with bits of cloth at the end—which gave an illusion of life to a few tatters. We are constantly investing things with life, or, on the other hand, trying to turn ourselves into things, inert, unchanging.

The Czech Pinocchio puppet I saw once at the theater is nothing but a stick, forked at the bottom for legs, with one crossbar for arms. Yet, by some trick of the puppet master, this creature brought me to tears—the wood we are, and yet alive—when it claimed to be enraptured by the cheap phosphorescent decals pasted on the ceiling to represent stars.

To the cousins of the Rosenberg clan: Gerry, Kim, Linda, Martin, Mary, Peter, Ralph, Teresa.

NATIVE TONGUES

TRIBES ON TAPE | LOUISE ERDRICH

For years now I have been in love with a language other than the English in which I write, and it is a rough affair. Every day I try to learn a little more Ojibwe. I have taken to carrying verb conjugation charts in my purse, along with the tiny notebook I've always kept for jotting down book ideas, overheard conversations, language detritus, phrases that pop into my head. Now that little notebook includes an increasing volume of Ojibwe words. My English is jealous, my Ojibwe elusive. Like a besieged unfaithful lover, I'm trying to appease them both.

Ojibwemowin, or Anishinabemowin, the Chippewa language, was last spoken in our family by Patrick Gourneau, my maternal grandfather, a Turtle Mountain Ojibwe who used it mainly in his prayers. Growing up off reservation, I thought Ojibwemowin was a language for prayers, like Latin in the Catholic liturgy. I was unaware for many years that Ojibwemowin was spoken in Canada, Minnesota, and Wisconsin, though by a dwindling number of people. By the time I began to study the language, I was living in New Hampshire, so for the first few years I used language tapes.

I never learned more than a few polite phrases that way, but the sound of the language in the author Basil Johnson's calm and dignified Anishinabe voice sustained me through bouts of homesickness. I spoke basic Ojibwe in the isolation of my car, traveling here and there on twisting New England roads. Back then, as now, I carried my language tapes everywhere . . .

From "Two Languages in Mind, but Just One in Heart"

DIVIDED HIGHWAY | SHERMAN ALEXIE

Being a Spokane Indian, I only pick up Indian hitchhikers. I learned this particular ceremony from my father, a Coeur d'Alene, who always stopped for those twentieth-century aboriginal nomads who refused to believe the salmon were gone. I don't know what they believed in exactly, but they wore hope like a bright shirt.

My father never taught me about hope. Instead, he continually told me that our salmon—our hope—would never come back, and though such lessons may seem cruel, I know enough to cover my heart in any crowd of white people.

"They'll kill you if they get the chance," my father said. "Love you or hate you, white people will shoot you in the heart. Even after all these years, they'll still smell the salmon on you, the dead salmon, and that will make white people dangerous."

All of us, Indian or white, are haunted by salmon.

When I was a boy, I leaned over the edge of one dam or another—perhaps Long Lake or Little Falls or the great gray dragon known as the Grand Coulee—and watched the ghosts of the salmon rise from the water to the sky and become constellations.

For most Indians, stars are nothing more than white tombstones scattered across a dark graveyard.

But the Indian hitchhikers my father picked up refused to admit the existence of sky, let alone the possibility that salmon might be stars. They were common people who believed only in the thumb and the foot. My father envied those simple Indian hitchhikers. He wanted to change their minds about salmon; he wanted to break open their hearts and see the future in their blood. He loved them. . . .

From *The Toughest Indian in the World*

MANIFESTO: 1965

An African Tradition of the Surreal
Léopold Sédar Senghor
Translated by John Reed and Clive Wake

Speech seems to us the main instrument of thought, emotion, and action. There is no thought or emotion without a verbal image, no free action without first a project in thought. This is even more true among peoples who disdained the written word. This explains the power of speech in Africa. The word, the spoken word, is the expression par excellence of the life force, of being in its fullness. . . .

The African languages are characterized first of all by the richness of their vocabulary. There are sometimes twenty different words for an object according to its form, weight, volume, and color, and as many for an action according to whether it is single or repeated, weakly or intensely performed, just beginning or coming to an end. In Fulani, nouns are divided into twenty-one genders, which are not related to sex. The classification is based sometimes on the meaning of the words or the phonetic qualities and sometimes on the grammatical category to which they belong. Most significant in this respect is the verb. On the same root in Wolof can be constructed more than twenty verbs expressing different shades of meaning, and at least as many derivative nouns. While modern Indo-European languages emphasize the abstract notion of time, African languages emphasize the *aspect*, the concrete way in which the action of the verb takes place. These are essentially *concrete* languages. In them words are always pregnant with images. Under their value as signs, their sense value shows through.

The African image is not then an image by equation but an image by *analogy*, a surrealist image. Africans do not like straight lines and false *mots justes*. Two and two do not make four, but five, as Aimé Césaire has told us. The object does not mean what it represents but what it suggests, what it creates. The Elephant is Strength, the Spider is Prudence; Horns are Moon and the Moon is Fecundity. Every representation is an image, and the image, I repeat, is not an equation but a *symbol*, an ideogram. Not only the figuration of the image but also its material . . . stone, earth, copper, gold, fiber— and also its line and color. . . .

MANIFESTO: 1942

Négritude

Aimé Césaire

Translated by Mary Ann Caws

No use stiffening up when we go by, those faces of yours like pale treponema, more buttery than the moon,

No use wasting your pity on us, those indecent smiles like cysts full of pus.

Cops and coppers
Verbalize the great half-baked treason, the great crackpot challenge and the satanic impulse, the insolent nostalgic flow of April moons, green lights, yellow fever . . .

Because we hate you, you and your reasonableness, we stick to our precocious dementia, our flaming folly, our stubborn cannibalism. . . .

Who and what are we? What a fine question!
Haters. Builders. Traitors. Voodoo priests. Especially. For we want all the devils
Yesterday's today's
The iron-collared, the ones with a hoe
Indicted, prohibited, escaped like slaves

not to forget the ones from the slave ship . . .
So we're singing.

We're singing the poisonous flowers springing up in the crazed prairies; the skies of love streaked with embolisms, the epileptic mornings; the white blaze of the abysmal sands, the wreckage floating down the nights stricken with the lightning of savage smells. . . .

The slow mill crushes the cane
The tardy ox doesn't swallow the mill

Is that absurd enough for you?

SEND FOR LANGSTON

THE NEGRO SPEAKS OF RIVERS | LANGSTON HUGHES

I've known rivers:
I've known rivers ancient as the world and older than the
    flow of human blood in human veins.

My soul has grown deep like the rivers.

I bathed in the Euphrates when dawns were young.
I built my hut near the Congo and it lulled me to sleep.
I looked upon the Nile and raised the pyramids above it.
I heard the singing of the Mississippi when Abe Lincoln
    went down to New Orleans, and I've seen its muddy
    bosom turn all golden in the sunset.

I've known rivers:
Ancient, dusky rivers.

My soul has grown deep like the rivers.

UNWEARIED BLUES | ARNOLD RAMPERSAD

Langston Hughes wrote "The Negro Speaks of Rivers" when he was
eighteen years of age and published it when he was nineteen—in 1921, in
W. E. B. Du Bois's magazine, *The Crisis*. And here we are eighty-one
years later, celebrating the centennial of Hughes's birth. And we *are* celebrating. The post office has issued a Langston Hughes stamp; confer-

---

These talks were presented at a PEN Twentieth Century Masters Tribute.

ences have been held in Joplin, Missouri, where he was born; Lawrence, Kansas, where he spent his childhood; Cleveland, where he went to high school; and in New Haven, at Yale, where his wonderful papers are to be found. And according to the folks at the Academy of American Poets, more people visit Langston Hughes's page on the Web site there than that of any other of its more than four hundred poets.

Why is Hughes so popular? More important, why do so many people *love* Langston Hughes? We respect many writers, but I think we love only a few, and he is one of those some of us really *love*. In part, I think, because often we first encounter his poetry early in school and never outgrow him. In part, I also think, because of the way he speaks to our heartbreaking national problem of race. His poetry reflects not only the wrongs and the pain of racism, but also the humanity of those who suffer most at its hands. We respect Langston's conscience, his imagination, his lyric gift, his passion, not only for black America but for America itself. We respect the dedication that kept him writing through years of poverty and political persecution. We respect the sheer variety of his work: the many books of poems, the dozen or more books for children, the dozen or more plays written and produced, two volumes of autobiography, a history of the NAACP, four books of translations from French and Spanish, several anthologies of African-American and African writing, various opera libretti, countless song lyrics, twenty years of weekly newspaper columns, and five volumes of "Simple" stories from those columns.

Langston Hughes loved books. During his lonely childhood, while he was living with his aged grandmother, books comforted him. "Then it was," he confessed, "that books began to *happen* to me, and I began to believe in nothing but books and the wonderful world in books, where, if people suffered, they suffered in beautiful language—not in monosyllables as we did in Kansas." He also grew up with a sense of obligation. In 1859 his grandmother's first husband had died at Harper's Ferry, as a member of John Brown's band of rebels against slavery. Mary Langston made sure that her grandson grew up with a sense of responsibility to the cause of social justice, especially for his fellow blacks facing Jim Crow everywhere. That dedication would drive Langston Hughes for the rest of his days.

He'd lived in many places before he settled down in his beloved Harlem—places such as Lincoln, Illinois, where he wrote his first poem; Cleveland, Ohio, where he attended high school; Mexico, where his father lived; Columbia University, from which he withdrew after one

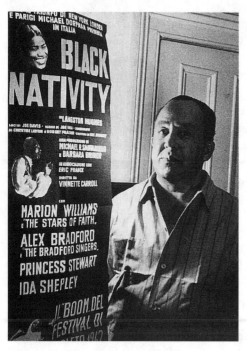

Langston Hughes, 1963.

LOUIS DRAPER

unhappy year. By the age of twenty-two, he had been to Africa; by twenty-three, Europe. By thirty-two, he had spent a year in the Soviet Union and traveled, literally, around the globe. In high school, most of his classmates were the kids of Eastern European immigrants. From them, especially, he learned about radical socialism, and about the dream of interracial and international unity. In English class, he met writers whose work would deliver him from the conventional—particularly Walt Whitman, and Whitman's modern disciple Carl Sandburg ("my guiding star," Hughes called him). Their poems grounded in him a sense of the dynamic relationship between art and democracy in America. But race was central to his consciousness, and thus black writers were also crucial—above all, perhaps, Paul Laurence Dunbar, W. E. B. Du Bois, and Claude McKay. From the start, in poems such as "The South" ("The lazy, laughing South / With blood on its mouth") or "The White Ones" ("I do not hate you, / For your faces are beautiful, too"), Hughes courageously spoke poetical truth to secular power. Many of his lyric poems have nothing to do with the matter of justice, but he never ceased to challenge Jim Crow or to champion the poor. Above all, he saw the beauty of human blackness long before almost any other artist had done so. In 1926, writing in *The Nation*, Hughes deplored the urge in many blacks "toward whiteness, the desire to pour racial individuality into the mold of American standardization, and to be as little Negro and as much American as possible." His poetry embraced blacks: "I am a Negro: / Black as the night is black, / Black like the depths of my Africa." In a world that worshipped whiteness, Hughes dared to say, "The night is beautiful, / So the faces of my people. / The stars are beautiful, / So the eyes of my people. / Beautiful, also, is the sun. / Beautiful, also, are the souls of my people."

In Washington, DC, where he lived in 1925, he learned much from the poorest blacks there, who struggled to live, but who also sang and danced and laughed out loud. "I try to write poems," Hughes said, "like the songs they sang on Seventh Street; gay songs, because you have to be gay or die; sad songs, because you couldn't help being sad sometimes. But gay or sad, you kept on living and you kept on going." For him, the metronome of black racial grace was its music. "Like the waves of the sea coming one after another, always one after another; like the earth moving around the sun: night, day night, day, and night day, forever, so is the undertow of black music—with its rhythm that never betrays you, its strength, like the beat of a human heart, its humor, and its rooted power." Many of Hughes's blues poems enraged critics in the black press, but he had unbreakable confidence in himself and in the masses of his people. It took a personal crisis combined with the onset of the Great Depression to make Hughes shift his focus. In the 1930s he turned to radical socialism, instead of blues and jazz. He penned some of the most radical verse ever written in America—pieces such as "Good Morning Revolution," "Goodbye Christ," "Put one more s in the U.S.A. / to make it Soviet," "Letter to the Academy," and "Revolution": "Great mob that knows no fear— / come here."

With the start of World War II, however, Langston returned to more familiar ground. He returned to jazz and blues. His political energy flowed mainly into the struggling civil rights movement, and his artistic energy into his amazing range of literary forms. By the 1950s he was taking on so many poorly paid writing jobs that he laughed at himself as "a literary sharecropper." But diligently, lovingly, Hughes continued to till that black soil he had first broken in 1921. The black masses loved him, but the critics, black as well as white, often did not. His work was, and is, often seen as too simple, or stale and inconsequential. For example, the *New York Times Book Review* jeered at Hughes's *Selected Poems* when it came out in 1959. "Every time I read Langston Hughes," according to its reviewer, "I am amazed all over again by his genuine gifts—and depressed that he has done so little with them." The reviewer was James Baldwin, who lived long enough to change his mind. Many people have had to change their minds about the art of Langston Hughes. The truth is that he possessed the power to see, more clearly than others, what was reality in the African-American world, and what was only prejudice and illusion. He also possessed the skills to convert this vision into its appropriate art. To my mind, Langston Hughes created a body of writing that, like jazz and the blues, speaks in a priceless way both of and to America.

He belongs with a small but heroic circle of artists and leaders of color, including Diego Rivera, Mahatma Gandhi, Nelson Mandela, and Martin Luther King Jr. In the twentieth century, in stubborn but principled and imaginative ways, these leaders resisted political and cultural colonialism. In so doing, they led all of us to a transformed sense of ourselves, and a transformed sense of the world we live in.

LAYING IT DOWN | WILLIE PERDOMO

This Langston riff is for that cardigan-sweater-wear
in' blues poet Raymond R. Patterson, Professor Emeritus, CCNY, author of
26 Ways of Looking at a Black Man and *Elemental Blues*.

I found Langston behind his typewriter the year after Ed Randolph, my first mentor, gave me poetry so I could stop fighting in a Quaker school. Freshman year Joyce and Piri Thomas were required reading in Mr. Byrne's lit class, but I took the liberty of putting Langston on my financial-aid voucher. That night, taking breaks from algebra, I heard the dogs in the street bark, couples argued, kids were being called in for dinner, and I went through those selected poems like I was stranded in a desert and a chilled bottle of Poland Spring water fell from the sky. I had a pop-up book in my hand, complete with the language to get around Lenox Avenue, to talk with the Madam, to play bop rim shots, to get inside the revolution, and to fall in love. Here I was, walking down the block with brand new ears, big as they were. Langston gave me the first song that I recited to my Sugar Hill thrill, that sweetie I made the "Harlem Love Poem" with, the poem I tried to memorize so that I could recite to her when we had all of Harlem in our hands from her project rooftop.

I could take the Harlem night
and wrap around you,
Take the neon lights and make a crown,
Take the Lenox Avenue busses,
Taxis, subways,
And for your love song tumble their rumble down.
Take Harlem's heartbeat,
Make a drumbeat,

Put it on a record, let it whirl,
And while we listen to it play,
Dance with you till day—
Dance with you, my sweet brown Harlem girl.

Some years later, I started laying it down like Langston, Ntozake, Miky Pinero, Amiri, William Carlos, Nikki, and Sonia, and I got caught between the page and the stage. Everybody said it sounded different when you heard it than when you read it and I was like, *yeah, no doubt, we can't always use the same beat.* I just want to sing, man. I could take you to the racial mountain if you want. If you like it, it don't matter. If you don't like it, that don't matter either. We stay true. Ask Rilke. If you need to write it, then write it. That's all. I've been a street poet, spoken-word artist, performance poet, hip-hop poet; see "Spotlight at the Nuyorican Poets Café"; shit, they even called me Word Perfect on occasion.

My first set was blessed by Langston's "Prime," you know that line at the end, where the brother says he found himself coming to his "prime / In the section of the niggers / Where a nickel costs a dime," yeah, that was it, my first set, and that original manchild from the promised land, Claude Brown, said I had arrived, born again, but this time I was coming with some *coquito* and some *lechon*, some *oye como va* down Lexington Avenue, some straight boogie-woogie rumba, getting on the 6 train to Loisaida, watching Puerto Rican flags fall into the East River, one by one, and kicking it at the Nuyorican Poets Café with Langston riffs like:

WARNING

Daddy
don't let your dog
curb you!

except I liked to catch junkies in the middle of their catch-22s like

in case
of an
emergency

call a
cop

but make
sure

you cop
your cure

before you
call—

quick!

Langston put it down for all of us, and like Miky, he was good when he
was doing bad, when he had to testify but really wanted us to listen to that
tom-tom of those beating feet, marching for the right to live. Singers of
self, those who know that things ain't right, that the avenues need a voice,
that sugar cane workers found dominoes on the curb, that it was time for
Susanna Jones to wear red and get Simple when we needed to, that the
weary blues are color blind . . . that when we stop laughing, stop loving,
and stop living, we stand and tell the world we're here, singing in the face
of what we remember.

Here's a letter Langston wrote to what the kids on my mother's block
call *the haters*:

LETTER TO THE ACADEMY

The gentlemen who have got to be classics and are
    now old with beards (or dead and in their graves)
    will kindly come forward and speak upon the
    subject

Of the Revolution. I mean the gentlemen who wrote
    lovely books about the defeat of the flesh and the
    triumph of the spirit that sold in the hundreds of
    thousands and are studied in the high schools and
    read by the best people will kindly come forward
    and

Speak about the Revolution—where the flesh
    triumphs (as well as the spirit) and the hungry

belly eats, and there are no best people, and the poor
are mighty and no longer poor, and the young by
the hundreds of thousands are free from hunger to
grow and study and love and propagate, bodies and
souls unchained without My Lord saying a
commoner shall never marry my daughter or the
Rabbi crying cursed be the mating of Jews and
Gentiles or Kipling writing never the twain shall
meet—

For the twain have met. But please—all you
gentlemen with beards who are so wise and old
and who write better than we do and whose souls
have triumphed (in spite of hungers and wars and
the evils about you) and whose books have soared in
calmness and beauty aloof from the struggle to the
library shelves and the desks of students and who
are now classics—come forward and speak upon

The subject of the Revolution.

We want to know what in the hell you'd say?

CONGREGATION | LANGSTON HUGHES

The American Writers' Congress was organized in early 1935 with the sup-
port of more than two hundred authors, including Langston Hughes, Nelson
Algren, Van Wyck Brooks, Erskine Caldwell, Malcolm Cowley, Theodore
Dreiser, James Farrell, Waldo Frank, Josephine Herbst, Granville Hicks, James
Weldon Johnson, Lincoln Steffens, and Richard Wright. The first Congress
established the League of American Writers, "a voluntary association of writ-
ers dedicated to the preservation and extension of a truly democratic culture."
The League was an affiliate of the International Association of Writers for the
Defense of Culture, which met in London (1936), Madrid (1937), and Paris
(1938). Hughes, elected a vice president of the League in 1937, remained one
of its most active supporters until the organization was dissolved in 1942.
Here is his speech to the first national session of the American Writers'
Congress:

TO NEGRO WRITERS:

There are certain practical things American Negro writers can do through their work.

We can reveal to the Negro masses from which we come our potential power to transform the now ugly face of the Southland into a region of peace and plenty.

We can reveal to the white masses those Negro qualities which go beyond the mere ability to laugh and sing and dance and make music, and which are a part of the useful heritage that we place at the disposal of a future free America.

Negro writers can seek to unite blacks and whites in our country, not on the nebulous basis of an interracial meeting, or the shifting sands of religious brotherhood, but on the *solid* ground of the daily working-class struggle to wipe out, now and forever, all the old inequalities of the past.

Furthermore, by way of exposure, Negro writers can reveal in their novels, stories, poems, and articles:

The lovely grinning face of Philanthropy—which gives a million dollars to a Jim Crow school, but not one job to a graduate of that school; which builds a Negro hospital with second-rate equipment, then commands black patients and student doctors to go there whether they will or no; or which, out of the kindness of its heart, erects yet another separate, segregated, shut-off, Jim Crow YMCA.

Negro writers can expose those white labor leaders who keep their unions closed against Negro workers and prevent the betterment of all workers.

We can expose, too, the sick-sweet smile of organized religion—which lies about what it doesn't know, and about what it *does* know. And the half-voodoo, half-clown, face of revivalism, dulling the mind with the clap of its empty hands.

Expose, also, the false leadership that besets the Negro people— bought and paid-for leadership, owned by capital, afraid to open its mouth except in the old conciliatory way so advantageous to the exploiters.

And all the economic roots of race hatred and race fear.

And the Contentment Tradition of the O-lovely-Negroes school of American fiction, which makes an ignorant black face and a Carolina head filled with superstition appear more desirable than a crown of gold; the jazz band; and the O-so-gay writers who make of the Negro's poverty and misery a dusky funny paper.

And expose war. And the old My-Country-'Tis-of-Thee lie. And the colored American Legion posts strutting around talking about the privilege of dying for the noble Red, White, and Blue, when they aren't even permitted the privilege of living for it. Or voting for it in Texas. Or working for it in the diplomatic service. Or even rising, like every other good little boy, from the log cabin to the White House.

White House is right.

Dear colored American Legion, you can swing from a lynching tree, uniform and all, with pleasure—and nobody'll fight for you. Don't you know that? Nobody even salutes you down South, dead or alive, medals or no medals, chevrons or not, no matter how many wars you've fought in.

Let Negro writers write about the irony and pathos of the *colored* American Legion.

"Salute, Mr. White Man!"

"Salute, hell! . . . You're a nigger."

Or would you rather write about the moon?

Sure, the moon still shines over Harlem. Shines over Scottsboro. Shines over Birmingham, too, I reckon. Shines over Cordie Cheek's grave, down South.

Write about the moon if you want to. Go ahead. This is a free country.

But there are certain very practical things American Negro writers can do. And must do. There's a song that says, "the time ain't long." That song is right. Something has got to change in America—and change soon. We must help that change to come.

The moon's still shining as poetically as ever, but all the stars on the flag are dull. (And the stripes, too.)

We want a new and better America, where there won't be any poor, where there won't be any more Jim Crow, where there won't be any lynchings, where there won't be any munition makers, where we won't need philanthropy, nor charity, nor the New Deal, nor Home Relief.

We want an America that will be ours, a world that will be ours—we Negro workers and white workers! Black writers and white!

We'll make that world!

SOMETHING RADICAL | SONIA SANCHEZ

In the 1970s I traveled to Cuba for an international writers' conference. After I had read a paper to an appreciative audience, some of the organizers asked me if I wanted anything. I said, "Yes. I'd like to meet Nicolás Guillén." They hesitated, said he wasn't feeling well, told me they would attempt to arrange the meeting. Two hours later, they gathered me up to visit him and as I entered his office he was standing in the middle of the room, feet planted on Cuban earth, legs no longer strong, but arms strong like Elizabeth Catlett's black women's arms. He said, "Sonia Sanchez. Sonia Sanchez. Como Langston Hughes. Como Langston Hughes."

And I smiled a smile of recognition, folded myself into his arms, and he hugged me so hard that I felt I couldn't breathe and I thought, hold it, I didn't come all this way to die in Cuba. Then I realized that if I just stopped struggling, leaned into his breath, I would be okay. We would be okay. And I leaned into his breath and we began to breathe as one. That is what Langston Hughes's poetry/plays/short stories told us. The necessity to learn how to lean into each other's breath and breathe as one.

So listen. Listen, Gentlepersons. I come to you this night with two voices. I come to praise this man. This brother. This genius. This holy man.

This weaver of words threading silver
And gold into our veins.
I come with the voice of the praiser.
I come with the voice of the poet.
I come to you to praise this man who
gave us his eyes and we shone, became perennial,
Who piloted us into the slow bloodstream of America
And we tagged behind, walking on
tiptoes, heard his words, like jazz
like blues, like seculars agitating
Keeping us on the edge of ourselves. Breathing
in our own noise and we became
small miracles . . .

Something underneath your hands, Langston man

Something mighty, something human, something

radical in your hands
accenting our blue flesh
observing us in a familiar city called Harlem
New York, the world.

Where we returned as birth. Blood. Water.
Death.
Where we became traveling men and women
turning corners
Moving like black trains across the country
Landless men and women immortal in our
moving,
Living with nothing.
Dying from everything.

And when you said, ask yo mama and
we attempted to do so,
The country turned over in its blood
Said What Mama, Mammy, Sapphire,
Aunt Jemima you talking bout.
Said Who yo mama is my mammy
and all of our mamas stood still
blowing black in the wind . . .

And you gave us early morning names.

Madame Alberta K. Johnson. Jess B. Simple.
Susanna Jones. Scottsboro Boys. Guillén.

Lorca. Lumumba. Nkrumah. Nasser. Fidel.
Bebopmen imploding spaces. And how to resist
in the "quarter of the negroes."

You gave us the still Harlem air.
The darker brother star
The Christ in Alabama sky.
The knowledge that we were
two nations under one America.

So much life coursing through your pages, man.
So many vacancies filled by your eyes, man.

You made us figure out the humor in tragedy,
the tragedy in humor. Taught us what

we were really missing in our lives
while we lived "20 years in ten."
You knew already "that we make our
history, but only so much of it as
we are allowed to make."

So listen. Gentlemen. Gentlewomen.
Pull your hearts out of your armpits.
Get your tuxedos out of mothballs.
Put your long red dress on girl
and snap your breasts into place,
As we go sailing on Langston Hughes's tongue
Living. Speaking without a crutch.
This is his centennial. His birthday.
Tonight is a political act.

"Hoy es. Hoy ha llegado."
It is today. Today has arrived.

"Hoy es hoy. Ha llegado este mañana."

Today is today. Tomorrow has arrived.

Woke up this morning with my eyes on Langston.
I say, woke up this morning with my eyes on Langston.
Woke up this morning with my eyes on Langston.

Gonna live. Gonna love. Gonna resist just like he did.

And you can't ask yo mama bout that.
You got to do it yo self. Ask yo self. Can
I resist, can I resist for Langston,
for our children, for humankind?

Woke up this morning with my eyes on Langston.
I say, woke up this morning with my eyes on Langston.
Woke up this morning with my eyes on Langston.

Gonna live. Gonna love. Gonna resist, resist,
Resist—just like himmmmm—

And here's one of his poems:

LET AMERICA BE AMERICA AGAIN | LANGSTON HUGHES

Let America be America again.
Let it be the dream it used to be.
Let it be the pioneer on the plain
Seeking a home where he himself is free.

(America never was America to me.)

Let America be the dream the dreamers dreamed—
Let it be that great strong land of love
Where never kings connive nor tyrants scheme
That any man be crushed by one above.

(It never was America to me.)

O, let my land be a land where Liberty
Is crowned with no false patriotic wreath,
But opportunity is real, and life is free,
Equality is in the air we breathe.

(There's never been equality for me,
Nor freedom in this "homeland of the free.")

Say, who are you that mumbles in the dark?
And who are you that draws your veil across the stars?

I am the poor white, fooled and pushed apart,
I am the Negro bearing slavery's scars.
I am the red man driven from the land,
I am the immigrant clutching the hope I seek—
And finding only the same old stupid plan
Of dog eat dog, of mighty crush the weak.

I am the young man, full of strength and hope,
Tangled in that ancient endless chain
Of profit, power, gain, of grab the land!
Of grab the gold! Of grab the ways of satisfying need!
Of work the men! Of take the pay!
Of owning everything for one's own greed!

I am the farmer, bondsman to the soil.
I am the worker sold to the machine.
I am the Negro, servant to you all.
I am the people, humble, hungry, mean—
Hungry yet today despite the dream.
Beaten yet today—O, Pioneers!
I am the man who never got ahead,
The poorest worker bartered through the years.

Yet I'm the one who dreamt our basic dream
In the Old World while still a serf of kings,
Who dreamt a dream so strong, so brave, so true,
That even yet its mighty daring sings
In every brick and stone, in every furrow turned
That's made America the land it has become.
O, I'm the man who sailed those early seas
In search of what I meant to be my home—
For I'm the one who left dark Ireland's shore,
And Poland's plain, and England's grassy lea,
And torn from Black Africa's strand I came
To build a "homeland of the free."

The free?

Who said the free? Not me?
Surely not me? The millions on relief today?
The millions shot down when we strike?
The millions who have nothing for our pay?
For all the dreams we've dreamed
And all the songs we've sung
And all the hopes we've held
And all the flags we've hung,

The millions who have nothing for our pay—
Except the dream that's almost dead today.

O, let America be America again—
The land that never has been yet—
And yet must be—the land where *every* man is free.
The land that's mine—the poor man's, Indian's, Negro's, ME—
Who made America,
Whose sweat and blood, whose faith and pain,
Whose hand at the foundry, whose plow in the rain,
Must bring back our mighty dream again.

Sure, call me any ugly name you choose—
The steel of freedom does not stain.
From those who live like leeches on the people's lives,
We must take back our land again,
America!

O, yes,
I say it plain,
America never was America to me,
And yet I swear this oath—
America will be!

Out of the rack and ruin of our gangster death,
The rape and rot of graft, and stealth, and lies,
We, the people, must redeem
The land, the mines, the plants, the rivers.
The mountains and the endless plain—
All, all the stretch of these great green states—
And make America again!

ROCK, CHURCH | LANGSTON HUGHES

Elder William Jones was one of them rock-church preachers who know how to make the spirit rise and the soul get right. Sometimes in the pulpit he used to start talking real slow, and you'd think his sermon warn't gonna be nothing; but by the time he got through, the walls of the temple would be almost rent, the doors busted open, and the benches turned over from pure shouting on the part of the brothers and sisters.

He were a great preacher, was Reverend William Jones. But he warn't satisfied—he wanted to be greater than he was. He wanted to be another Billy Graham or Elmer Gantry or a resurrected Daddy Grace. And that's what brought about his downfall—ambition!

Now, Reverend Jones had been for nearly a year the pastor of one of them little colored churches in the back alleys of St. Louis that are open every night in the week for preaching, singing, and praying, where sisters come to shake tambourines, shout, swing gospel songs, and get happy while the Reverend presents the Word.

Elder Jones always opened his part of the services with "In His Hand," his theme song, and he always closed his services with the same. Now, the rhythm of "In His Hand" was such that once it got to swinging, you couldn't help but move your arms or feet or both, and since the Reverend always took up collection at the beginning and ending of his sermons, the dancing movement of the crowd at such times was always toward the collection table—which was exactly where the Elder wanted it to be.

In His hand!
In His hand!
I'm safe and sound
I'll be bound—
Settin' in Jesus' hand!

"Come one! Come all! Come, my Lambs," Elder Jones would shout, "and put it down for Jesus!"

Poor old washer-ladies, big fat cooks, long lean truck drivers, and heavyset roustabouts would come up and lay their money down, two times every evening for Elder Jones.

That minister was getting rich right there in that St. Louis alley.

In His hand!
In His hand!
I'll have you know
I'm white as snow—
Settin' in Jesus' hand!

With the piano just a-going, tambourines a-flying, and people shouting right on up to the altar.

"Rock, church, rock!" Elder Jones would cry at such intensely lucrative moments.

But he were too ambitious. He wouldn't let well enough alone. He wanted to be a big shot and panic Harlem, gas Detroit, sew up Chicago, then move on to Hollywood. He warn't satisfied with just St. Louis.

So he got to thinking, "Now, what can I do to get everybody excited, to get everybody talking about my church, to get the streets outside crowded and my name known all over, even unto the far reaches of the nation? Now, what can I do?"

Billy Sunday had a sawdust trail, so he had heard. Reverend Becton had two valets in the pulpit with him as he cast off garment after garment in the heat of preaching, and used up dozens of white handkerchiefs every evening wiping his brow while calling on the Lord to come. Meanwhile, the Angel of Angelus Temple had just kept on getting married and divorced and making the front pages of everybody's newspapers.

"I got to be news, too, in my day and time," mused Elder Jones.

"This town's too small for me! I want the world to hear my name!"

Now, as I've said before, Elder Jones was a good preacher—and a good-looking preacher, too. He could cry real loud and moan real deep, and he could move the sisters as no other black preacher on this side of town had ever moved them before. Besides, in his youth, as a sinner, he had done a little light hustling around Memphis and Vicksburg—so he knew just how to appeal to the feminine nature.

Since his recent sojourn in St. Louis, Elder Jones had been looking for a special female Lamb to shelter in his private fold. Out of all the sisters in his church, he had finally chosen Sister Maggie Bradford. Not that Sister Maggie was pretty. No, far from it. But Sister Maggie was well fed, brownskin, good-natured, fat, and *prosperous*. She owned four two-family houses that she rented out, upstairs and down, so she made a good living. Besides, she had sweet and loving ways as well as the interest of her pastor at heart.

Elder Jones confided his personal ambitions to said Sister Bradford one morning when he woke up to find her by his side.

"I want to branch out, Maggie," he said. "I want to be a really big man! Now, what can I do to get the 'tention of the world on me? I mean, in a religious way?"

They thought and they thought. Since it was a Fourth of July morning, and Sister Maggie didn't have to go collect rents, they just lay there and thought.

Finally, Sister Maggie said, "Bill Jones, you know something I ain't never forgot that I seed as a child? There was a preacher down in Mississippi named old man Eubanks who one time got himself dead and buried and then rose from the dead. Now, I ain't never forgot that. Neither has nobody else in that part of the Delta. That's something mem'rable. Why don't you do something like that?"

"How did he do it, Sister Maggie?"

"He ain't never told nobody how he do it, Brother Bill. He say it were the Grace of God, that's all."

"It might a-been," said Elder Jones. "It might a-been."

He lay there and thought a while longer. By and by he said, "But, honey, I'm gonna do something better'n that. I'm gonna be nailed on a cross."

"Do, Jesus!" said Sister Maggie Bradford. "Jones, you's a mess!"

Now, the Elder, in order to pull off his intended miracle, had, of necessity, to take somebody else into his confidence, so he picked out Brother Hicks, his chief deacon, one of the main pillars of the church long before Jones came as pastor.

It was too bad, though, that Jones never knew that Brother Hicks (more familiarly known as Bulldog) used to be in love with Sister Bradford. Sister Bradford neglected to tell the new reverend about any of her former sweethearts. So how was Elder Jones to know that some of them still coveted her, and were envious of him in their hearts?

"Hicks," whispered Elder Jones in telling his chief deacon of his plan to die on the cross and then come back to life, "that miracle will make me the greatest minister in the world. No doubt about it! When I get to be world-renowned, Bulldog, and go traveling about the firmament, I'll take you with me as my chief deacon. You shall be my right hand, and Sister Maggie Bradford shall be my left. Amen!"

"I hear you," said Brother Hicks. "I hope it comes true."

But if Elder Jones had looked closely, he would have seen an evil light in his deacon's eyes.

"It will come true," said Elder Jones, "if you keep your mouth shut and follow out my instructions—exactly as I lay 'em down to you. I trust you, so listen! You know and I know that I ain't gonna *really* die. Neither is I *really* gonna be nailed. That's why I wants you to help me. I wants you to have me a great big cross made, higher than the altar—so high I has to have a stepladder to get up to it to be nailed thereon, and you to nail me. The higher the better, so's they won't see the straps—'cause I'm gonna be tied on by straps, you hear. The light'll be rose-colored so they can't see the straps. Now, here you come and do the nailin'—nobody else but you. Put them nails *between* my fingers and toes, not through 'em—*between*—and don't nail too deep. Leave the heads kinder stickin' out. You get the jibe?"

"I get the jibe," said Brother Bulldog Hicks.

"Then you and me'll stay right on there in the church all night and all day till the next night when the people come back to see me rise. Ever so often, you can let me down to rest a little bit. But as long as I'm on the cross, I play off like I'm dead, particularly when reporters come around. On Monday night, hallelujah! I will rise, and take up collection!"

"Amen!" said Brother Hicks.

Well, you couldn't get a-near the church on the night that Reverend Jones had had it announced by press, by radio, and by word of mouth that he would be crucified *dead*, stay dead, and rise. Negroes came from all over St. Louis, East St. Louis, and mighty nigh everywhere else to be present at the witnessing of the miracle. Lots of 'em didn't believe in Reverend Jones, but lots of 'em *did*. Sometimes false prophets can bamboozle you so you can't tell yonder from whither—and that's the way Jones had the crowd.

The church was packed and jammed. Not a seat to be found, and tears were flowing (from sorrowing sisters' eyes) long before the Elder even approached the cross which, made out of new lumber right straight from the sawmill, loomed up behind the pulpit. In the rose-colored lights, with big paper lilies that Sister Bradford had made decorating its head and foot, the cross looked mighty pretty.

Elder Jones preached a mighty sermon that night, and hot as it was, there was plenty of leaping and jumping and shouting in that crowded church. It looked like the walls would fall. Then when he got through preaching, Elder Jones made a solemn announcement. As he termed it, for a night and a day, his last pronouncement.

"Church! Tonight, as I have told the world, I'm gonna die. I'm gonna be nailed to this cross and let the breath pass from me. But tomorrow, Monday night, August the twenty-first, at twelve PM, I am coming back to life. Amen! After twenty-four hours on the cross, hallelujah! And all the city of St. Louis can be saved—if they will just come out to see me. Now, before I mounts the steps to the cross, let us sing for the last time 'In His Hand'—'cause I tell you, that's where I am! As we sing, let everybody come forward to the collection table and help this church before I go. Give largely!"

The piano tinkled, the tambourines rang, hands clapped. Elder Jones and his children sang:

In His hand!
In His hand!
You'll never stray
Down the Devil's way—
Settin' in Jesus' hand!

Oh, in His hand!
In His hand!
Though I may die
I'll mount on high—
Settin' in Jesus' hand!

"Let us pray." And while every back was bowed in prayer, the Elder went up the stepladder to the cross. Brother Hicks followed with the hammer and nails. Sister Bradford wailed at the top of her voice. Woe filled the amen corner. Emotion rocked the church.

Folks outside was saying all up and down the street, "Lawd, I wish we could have got in. Listen yonder at that noise! I wonder what *is* going on!"

Elder Jones was about to make himself famous—that's what was going on. And all would have went well had it not been for Brother Hicks—a two-faced rascal. Somehow that night the Devil got into Bulldog Hicks and took full possession.

The truth of the matter is that Hicks got to thinking about Sister Maggie Bradford, and how Reverend Jones had worked up to be her Number-One Man. That made him mad. The old green snake of jealousy began to coil around his heart, right there in the meeting, right there on the steps of the cross. Lord, have mercy! At the very high point of the ceremonies!

Hicks had the hammer in one hand and his other hand was full of nails as he mounted the ladder behind his pastor. He was going up to nail Elder Jones on that sawmill cross.

"While I'm nailin', I might as well nail him right," Hicks thought. "A low-down klinker—comin' here out of Mississippi to take my woman away from me! He'll never know the pleasure of my help in none o' his schemes to out-Divine Father! No, sir!"

Elder Jones had himself all fixed up with a system of straps round his waist, round his shoulder blades, and round his wrists and ankles, hidden under his long black coat. These straps fastened in hooks on the back of the cross, out of sight of the audience, so he could just hang up there all sad and sorrowful-looking and make out like he was being nailed. Brother

Bulldog Hicks was to plant the nails *between* his fingers and toes. Hallelujah! Rock, church, rock!

Excitement was intense.

All went well until the nailing began. Elder Jones removed his shoes and socks and, in his bare black feet, bade farewell to his weeping congregation. As he leaned back against the cross and allowed Brother Hicks to compose him there, the crowd began to moan. But it was when Hicks placed the first nail between Elder Jones's toes that they became hysterical. Sister Bradford outyelled them all.

Hicks placed that first nail between the big toe and the next toe of the left foot and began to hammer. The foot was well strapped down, so the Elder couldn't move it. The closer the head of the nail got to his toes, the harder Hicks struck it. Finally the hammer collided with Elder Jones's foot, *bam* against his big toe.

"Aw-oh!" he moaned under his breath. "Go easy, man!"

"Have mercy," shouted the brothers and sisters of the church. "Have mercy on our Elder!"

Once more the hammer struck his toe. But the all too human sound of his surprised and agonized "Ouch!" was lost in the tumult of the shouting church.

"Bulldog, I say, go easy," hissed the Elder. "This *ain't* real."

Brother Hicks desisted, a grim smile on his face. Then he turned his attention to the right foot. There he placed another nail between the toes and began to hammer. Again, as the nail went into the wood, he showed no signs of stopping when the hammer reached the foot. He just kept on landing cruel metallic blows on the Elder's bare toenails until the preacher howled with pain, no longer able to keep back a sudden hair-raising cry. The sweat popped out on his forehead and dripped down on his shirt.

At first the Elder thought, naturally, that it was just a slip of the hammer on the deacon's part. Then he thought the man must have gone crazy—like the rest of the audience. Then it hurt him so bad, he didn't know what he thought—so he just hollered, "Aw-ooo-oo-o!"

It was a good thing the church was full of noise, or they would have heard a strange dialogue.

"My God, Hicks, what are you doing?" the Elder cried, staring wildly at his deacon on the ladder.

"I'm nailin' you to the cross, Jones! And man, I'm *really* nailin'."

"Aw-oow-ow! Don't you know you're hurting me? I told you not to nail so hard!"

But the deacon was unruffled.

"Who'd you say's gonna be your right hand when you get down from here and start your travelings?" Hicks asked.

"You, brother," the sweating Elder cried.

"And who'd you say was gonna be your left hand?"

"Sister Maggie Bradford," moaned Elder Jones from the cross.

"Naw she ain't," said Brother Hicks, whereupon he struck the Reverend's toe a really righteous blow.

"Lord, help me!" cried the tortured minister. The weeping congregation echoed his cry. It was certainly real. The Elder *was* being crucified!

Brother Bulldog Hicks took two more steps up the ladder, preparing to nail the hands. With his evil face right in front of Elder Jones, he hissed: "I'll teach you nappy-headed jackleg ministers to come to St. Louis and think you-all can walk away with any woman you's a mind to. I'm gonna teach you to leave my women alone. Here—here's a nail!"

Brother Hicks placed a great big spike right in the palm of Elder Jones's left hand. He was just about to drive it in when the frightened Reverend let out a scream that could be heard two blocks away. At the same time he began to struggle to get down. Jones tried to bust the straps, but they was too strong for him.

If he could just get one foot loose to kick Brother Bulldog Hicks!

Hicks lifted the hammer to let go when the Reverend's second yell, this time, was loud enough to be heard in East St. Louis. It burst like a bomb above the shouts of the crowd—and it had its effect. Suddenly the congregation was quiet. Everybody knew that was no way for a dying man to yell.

Sister Bradford realized that something had gone wrong, so she began to chant the song her beloved pastor had told her to chant at the propitious moment after the nailing was done. Now, even though the nailing was not done, Sister Bradford thought she had better sing:

Elder Jones will rise again,
Elder Jones will rise again,
Rise again, rise again!
Elder Jones will rise again,
Yes, my Lawd!

But nobody took up the refrain to help her carry it on. Everybody was too interested in what was happening in front of them, so Sister Bradford's voice just died out.

Meanwhile Brother Hicks lifted the hammer again, but Elder Jones spat right in his face. He not only spat, but suddenly called his deacon a name unworthy of man or beast. Then he let out another frightful yell and, in mortal anguish, called, "Sister Maggie Bradford, lemme down from here! I say, come and get . . . me . . . down . . . *from here!*"

Those in the church that had not already stopped moaning and shouting did so at once. You could have heard a pin drop. Folks were petrified.

Brother Hicks stood on the ladder, glaring with satisfaction at Reverend Jones, his hammer still raised. Under his breath the panting Elder dared him to nail another nail, and threatened to kill him stone-dead with a .44 if he did.

"Just lemme get loost from here, and I'll fight you like a natural man," he gasped, twisting and turning like a tree in a storm.

"Come down, then," yelled Hicks, right out loud from the ladder. "Come on down! As sure as water runs, Jones, I'll show you up for what you is—a woman-chasing no-good low-down faker! I'll beat you to a batter with my bare hands!"

"Lawd, have mercy!" cried the church.

Jones almost broke a blood vessel trying to get loose from his cross. "Sister Maggie, come and lemme down," he pleaded, sweat streaming from his face.

But Sister Bradford was covered with confusion. In fact, she was petrified. What could have gone wrong for the Elder to call on her like this in public in the very midst of the thing that was to bring him famous-glory and make them all rich, preaching throughout the land with her at his side? Sister Bradford's head was in a whirl, her heart was in her mouth.

"Elder Jones, you means you really wants to get down?" she asked weakly from her seat in the amen corner.

"Yes," cried the Elder, "can't you hear? I done called on you twenty times to let me down!"

At this point Brother Hicks gave the foot nails one more good hammering. The words that came from the cross were not to be found in the Bible.

In a twinkling, Sister Bradford was at Jones's side. Realizing at last that the Devil must've done got into Hicks (like it used to sometimes in the days when she knowed him), she went to the aid of her battered Elder, grabbed the foot of the ladder, and sent Hicks sprawling across the pulpit.

"You'll never crucify my Elder," she cried, "not for real." Energetically she began to cut the straps away that bound the Reverend. Soon poor

Jones slid to the floor, his feet too sore from the hammer's blows to even stand on them without help.

"Just lemme get at Hicks," was all Reverend Jones could gasp. "He knowed I didn't want them nails that close." In the dead silence that took possession of the church, everybody heard him moan, "Lawd, lemme get at Hicks," as he hobbled away on the protecting arm of Sister Maggie.

"Stand back, Bulldog," Sister Maggie said to the deacon, "and let your pastor pass. Soon as he's able, he'll flatten you out like a shadow—but now, I'm in charge. Stand back, I say, and let him pass!"

Hicks stood back. The crowd murmured. The minister made his exit. Thus ended the ambitious career of Elder William Jones. He never did pastor in St. Louis any more. Neither did he fight Hicks. He just snuck away for parts unknown.

DIFFERENT HUGHES | MARGO JEFFERSON

Langston Hughes was a performer, and he made being Langston Hughes look triumphantly easy. What was difficult about being Langston Hughes interests me right now. He was the child who kept being lost and found by his perpetually discontented mother, and the boy who was psychically man-handled by an angry, selfish father—when Father had time to be involved at all. Langston Hughes was easy to love, as a poet and a man. And he must have enjoyed being easy to love; people always do. He did not enjoy the intrusiveness of intimacy, and at some point, intimacy always becomes intrusive. It's very complicated to be *the* voice, even the many voices of a people. Your people. We know what boundaries the white world placed on Langston Hughes, but *our* love and judgments made other kinds of demands and imposed other boundaries on him. Our intimacy with him must have been intrusive sometimes, too. He was restless, I think, and independent—something of a chameleon, full of mixed moods. Maybe that's one reason, a temperamental reason, he was drawn to the blues. They're the least self-conscious poems about consciousness—all those warring states of mind and changes of heart, narrative and lyric at the same time. And it must have been why he was drawn to Walt Whitman and Carl Sandburg, because in their work, as in Hughes's, the private merges into the public, and the public voice becomes achingly confessional, or joyously confessional, and unstoppably rhythmic, and if you think of those jazz poems—"Montage of a Dream Deferred," "YARDBIRD! / HELP ME!"—that's the voice you hear.

Langston Hughes came to speak at my college once, and our Black Student Organization had invited him to go out with us afterwards. We gathered around him possessively, but one white student was there, too. She seemed not to know about our plans, and she wanted to talk to Langston Hughes briefly. And since it was 1966 or maybe '67, we wanted him to snub her mercilessly. But he talked amiably with her for just a few minutes. We indicated it was time to get started, to go away. He began to ask her if she wanted to join us, and we managed to convey without being brutally frank that, you know, no: he was with us, and she was to go her own way. He said goodbye to her pleasantly and he went off with us. So he had assuaged everyone, and maybe he had assuaged no one. I remember feeling very snippy and undergraduate-irritated and I thought, "Oh God, he's just too old—he really doesn't get it." I do not know what he thought. He had probably been through something like this many times, and maybe no one in that little scene pleased him either.

Bearing all of these Langstons in mind, I'm going to read "Final Call."

FINAL CALL | LANGSTON HUGHES

SEND FOR THE PIED PIPER AND LET HIM PIPE THE RATS AWAY.
SEND FOR ROBIN HOOD TO CLINCH THE ANTI-POVERTY CAMPAIGN.
SEND FOR THE FAIRY QUEEN WITH A WAVE OF THE WAND
TO MAKE US ALL INTO PRINCES AND PRINCESSES.
SEND FOR KING ARTHUR TO BRING THE HOLY GRAIL.
SEND FOR OLD MAN MOSES TO LAY DOWN THE LAW.
SEND FOR JESUS TO PREACH THE SERMON ON THE MOUNT.
SEND FOR DREYFUS TO CRY, "J'ACCUSE!"
SEND FOR DEAD BLIND LEMON TO SING THE B FLAT BLUES.
SEND FOR ROBESPIERRE TO SCREAM, "ÇA IRA! ÇA IRA! ÇA IRA!"
SEND (GOD FORBID—HE'S NOT DEAD LONG ENOUGH!)
FOR LUMUMBA TO CRY "FREEDOM NOW!"
SEND FOR LAFAYETTE AND TELL HIM, "HELP! HELP ME!"
SEND FOR DENMARK VESEY CRYING, "FREE!"
FOR CINQUE SAYING, "RUN A NEW FLAG UP THE MAST."
FOR OLD JOHN BROWN WHO KNEW SLAVERY COULDN'T LAST.
SEND FOR LENIN! (DON'T YOU DARE!—HE CAN'T COME HERE!)
SEND FOR TROTSKY! (WHAT? DON'T CONFUSE THE ISSUE, PLEASE!)
SEND FOR UNCLE TOM ON HIS MIGHTY KNEES.

SEND FOR LINCOLN, SEND FOR GRANT.
SEND FOR FREDERICK DOUGLASS, GARRISON, BEECHER, LOWELL.
SEND FOR HARRIET TUBMAN, OLD SOJOURNER TRUTH.
SEND FOR MARCUS GARVEY (WHAT?) SUFI (WHO?) FATHER DIVINE (WHERE?)
DU BOIS (WHEN?) MALCOLM (OH!) SEND FOR STOKELY. (NO?) THEN
SEND FOR ADAM POWELL ON A NON-SUBPOENA DAY.
SEND FOR THE PIED PIPER TO PIPE OUR RATS AWAY.

(And if nobody comes, send for me.)

GRACE NOTES | ARNOLD RAMPERSAD

Before Langston died—long before he died—he prepared the order of his funeral service; no minister, no prayers, not even an MC. The folks invited got there, and a jazz band, Randy Weston's trio, played. And all Hughes asked, the only thing that he requested, was that the last tune be Duke Ellington's "Do Nothin' Till You Hear from Me."

In June of 1960 the NAACP gave Langston Hughes its highest honor, the Spingarn Medal. Hughes was moved, but he gave credit where he believed credit was due. It would have been, he said, "of the utmost conceit" for him to accept the medal in his name alone. "I can accept it only," he insisted, "in the name of the Negro people who have given me the materials out of which my poems and stories, plays and songs have come, and who, over the years, have given me as well their love and understanding and support. Without them on my part there would have been no poems, without their hopes and fears and dreams, no stories. Without their struggles, no dramas; without their music, no songs. Had I not heard as a child in the little churches of Kansas and Missouri 'Deep river, my home is over Jordan' or 'My Lord what a mornin' / When the stars begin to fall,' I might not have come to realize the lyric beauty of living poetry."

THE WEARY BLUES | LANGSTON HUGHES

Droning a drowsy syncopated tune,
Rocking back and forth to a mellow croon,
   I heard a Negro play.
Down on Lenox Avenue the other night

By the pale dull pallor of an old gas light
    He did a lazy sway . . .
    He did a lazy sway . . .
To the tune o' those Weary Blues.
With his ebony hands on each ivory key
He made that poor piano moan with melody.
    O Blues!
Swaying to and fro on his rickety stool
He played that sad raggy tune like a musical fool.
    Sweet Blues!
Coming from a black man's soul.
    O Blues!
In a deep song voice with a melancholy tone
I heard that Negro sing, that old piano moan—
    "Ain't got nobody in all this world,
        Ain't got nobody but ma self.
        I's gwine to quit ma frownin'
        And put ma troubles on the shelf."

Thump, thump, thump, went his foot on the floor.
He played a few chords then he sang some more—
    "I got the Weary Blues
        And I can't be satisfied.
        Got the Weary Blues
        And can't be satisfied—
        I ain't happy no mo'
        And I wish that I had died."
And far into the night he crooned that tune.
The stars went out and so did the moon.
The singer stopped playing and went to bed
While the Weary Blues echoed through his head.
He slept like a rock or a man that's dead.

Harlem Renaissance

ALAIN LOCKE

The younger generation comes, bringing its gifts. They are the first fruits of the Negro Renaissance. Youth speaks, and the voice of the New Negro is heard. . . . Here we have Negro young, with arresting visions and vibrating prophecies; forecasting in the mirror of art what we must see and recognize in the streets of reality tomorrow, foretelling in new notes and accents the maturing speech of full racial utterance.

CLAUDE McKAY

The Harlem Renaissance movement of the antic 1920s was really inspired and kept alive by the interest and presence of white bohemians. It faded out when they became tired of the new plaything.

LANGSTON HUGHES

The ordinary Negroes hadn't heard of the Negro Renaissance. And if they had, it hadn't raised their wages any.

THE COLORS OF FEAR

WHITE FRIGHT | MICHAEL MOORE

I don't know what it is, but every time I see a white guy walking towards me, I tense up. My heart starts racing, and I immediately begin to look for an escape route and a means to defend myself. I kick myself for even being in this part of town after dark. Didn't I notice the suspicious gangs of white people lurking on every street corner, drinking Starbucks and wearing their gang colors of Gap turquoise or J. Crew mauve? What an idiot! Now the white person is coming closer, closer—and then—whew! He walks by without harming me, and I breathe a sigh of relief.

White people scare the crap out of me. This may be hard for you to understand—considering that I am white—but then again, my color gives me a certain insight. For instance, I find myself pretty scary a lot of the time, so I know what I'm talking about. You can take my word for it: if you find yourself suddenly surrounded by white people, you better watch out. Anything can happen. As white people, we've been lulled into thinking it's safe to be around other white people. We've been taught since birth that it's the people of that other color we need to fear. They're the ones who'll slit your throat!

Yet as I look back on my life, a strange but unmistakable pattern seems to emerge. Every person who has ever harmed me in my lifetime—the boss who fired me, the teacher who flunked me, the principal who punished me, the kid who hit me in the eye with a rock, the executive who didn't renew *TV Nation*, the guy who was stalking me for three years, the accountant who double-paid my taxes, the drunk who smashed into me, the burglar who stole my stereo, the contractor who overcharged me, the girlfriend who left me, the next girlfriend who left even sooner, the person in the office who stole checks from my checkbook and wrote them out to himself for a total of sixteen thousand dollars—every one of these individuals has been a white person. Coincidence? I think not.

I have never been attacked by a black person, never been evicted by a black person, never had my security deposit ripped off by a black landlord, never had a black landlord, never had a meeting at a Hollywood studio with a black executive in charge, never had a black person deny my child the college of her choice, never been puked on by a black teenager at a Mötley Crüe concert, never been pulled over by a black cop, never been sold a lemon by a black car salesman, never seen a black car salesman, never had a black person deny me a bank loan, and I've never heard a black person say, "We're going to eliminate ten thousand jobs here—have a nice day!"

I don't think that I'm the only white guy who can make these claims. Every mean word, every cruel act, every bit of pain and suffering in my life has had a Caucasian face attached to it.

So, um, why is it exactly that I should be afraid of black people?

From *Dead White Men*

THOSE WHO DON'T | SANDRA CISNEROS

Those who don't know any better come into our neighborhood scared. They think we're dangerous. They think we will attack them with shiny knives. They are stupid people who are lost and got here by mistake.

But we aren't afraid. We know the guy with the crooked eye is Davey the Baby's brother, and the tall one next to him in the straw brim, that's Rosa's Eddie V., and the big one that looks like a dumb grown man, he's Fat Boy, though he's not fat anymore nor a boy.

All brown all around, we are safe. But watch us drive into a neighborhood of another color and our knees go shakity-shake and our car windows get rolled up tight and our eyes look straight. Yeah. That is how it goes and goes.

From *The House on Mango Street*

TWO ESSAYS

John D'Agata

LIVING HISTORY HALL OF FAME, II

9TH MASSACHUSETTS LIGHT ARTILLERY CAMP, VERMONT

Marching through the cold, green, tent-pitched mountains of old Vermont at 6 A.M. while clumps of wind go hurling against the birch-stalk stands, go bouncing and pelting the Hogback River, flinging us both toward dawn, I have been thinking about what makes him tick, about what ticks.

Let us cross over the river, he says, and rest under the shade of the trees.

Father, lying under the bough of a dark holm-oak—clicking and clicking and nailing down the day—has come to watch me write about a war.

"The war," say sandwich boards strewn across the battlefield, "that everyone fought, all of us won, here, on this day, on hallowed ground, where brother v. brother v. father v. son . . . "

What is it that comes after a long civil war?

John D'Agata's *Halls of Fame* was a nominee for the 2002 PEN/Martha Albrand Award for First Nonfiction.

Where we are, it is summer.

There is hanging around his neck a small black camera, and it ticks.

Want to make some money off of this? my father says. You just find a few good anecdotes. Click.

And it's summer.

First time together in fifteen years.

Click.

There are rifle fires, and we hear them.

Troops advance, and we point.

Smoke from cannons curls a quick bow over the valley—but blows away, soon.

Blowing a long sigh out from under the shade of some trees.

Blowing a few hoopskirts like bells across the river.

Blowing off hats, blowing down tents.

Blowing past the rubber banner PEPSI CIVIL WAR EVENT HERE.

Then blowing onto cars slowed down for HAIRPIN TURN.

USE HORN.

But up, over the valley, under the low-roofed pitch of Exhibit Hall A, I can see no smoke.

See: only the flags folded, and the wagon hitched, and the two dozen coffee urns, and the old vendor selling glass she cut from the greenhouse panes of an old Victorian.

Glass, the vendor claims, which someone, long ago, after the war was done, purchased in bulk from the bankrupt Mathew Brady.

Whose six thousand negatives of soldiers who survived the war were no longer necessary, no longer "right."

They were leaded instead into windows in New England.

Then made positive again.

Then bleached clear by the weather.

MUSEUM OF AMERICAN FRONTIER CULTURE AND HALL OF FAME

STAUNTON, VIRGINIA

But what you should concentrate on is my homesickness.

All these road maps, tickets, things-in-a-glass case—

What could make you homesick? For what drive until you glimpsed an end?

Look: here they have a little Pilgrim village, a little farming lot, a small extravaganza of skirmishes.

EVERY HOUR, WEATHER WILLING, the Indians appear, run around, yell, set fire, raid, pretend to kill a young lady, leave.

Every evening with flax the young lady attaches whatever she wants to happen next onto the soaked-blank flour sacks, then waits.

The Indians appear. The Indians leave.

Flax, and now the gown taking shape there, where the collar soon, the insinuation of a sleeve . . .

The Indians there, not there.

The sacks soaked free of their stamped-on trademarks.

The flax soaked up by the gown as it stretches.

The sacks undone into windows of flowers.

Or maybe filigree.

Or are they fringes?

(The Indians continuing to visit her.)

Stop here and it is *wedding dress*. Stop here and it is *tablecloth*.

What do you want to see? Say where you want to go.

I want to come to a full-stop place eventually.

Want to see you looking here, and catch myself looking back, and find between us a distance, after all, that is not so great.

And not so insignificant.

WOMAN FROM AMERICA

Bessie Head

This woman from America married a man of our village and left her country to come and live with him here. She descended on us like an avalanche. People are divided into two camps: those who feel a fascinated love and those who fear a new thing.

Some people keep hoping she will go away one day, but already her big strong stride has worn the pathways of the village flat. She is everywhere about because she is a woman, resolved and unshakable in herself. To make matters worse or more disturbing she comes from the west side of America, somewhere near California. I gather from her conversation that people from the West are stranger than most people.

People of the West of America must be the most oddly beautiful people in the world; at least this woman from the West is the most oddly beautiful person I have ever seen. Every crosscurrent of the earth seems to have stopped in her and blended into an amazing harmony. She has a big dash of Africa, a dash of Germany, some Cherokee, and heaven knows what else. Her feet are big and her body is as tall and straight and strong as a mountain tree. Her neck curves up high and her thick black hair cascades down her back like a wild and tormented stream. I cannot understand her eyes though, except that they are big, black, and startled like those of a wild free buck racing against the wind. Often they cloud over with a deep, intense, brooding look.

It takes a great deal of courage to become friends with a woman like that. Like everyone here, I am timid and subdued. Authority, everything can subdue me; not because I like it that way but because authority carries the weight of an age pressing down on life. It is terrible then to associate with a person who can shout authority down. Her shouting matches with authority are the terror and sensation of the village. It has come down to this. Either the woman is unreasonable or authority is unreasonable, and everyone in his heart would like to admit that authority is unreasonable. In reality, the rule is: if authority does not like you, then you are the outcast and humanity associates with you at their peril. So try always to be on the right side of authority, for the sake of peace, and please avoid the outcast. I do not say it will be like this forever. The whole world is crashing and interchanging itself and even remote bush villages in Africa are not to be left out!

It was inevitable though that this woman and I should be friends. I have an overwhelming curiosity that I cannot keep within bounds. I passed by the house for almost a month, but one cannot crash in on people. Then one day a dog they own had puppies, and my small son chased one of the puppies into the yard and I chased after him. Then one of the puppies became his and there had to be discussions about the puppy, the desert heat, and the state of the world, and as a result of curiosity an avalanche of wealth has descended on my life. My small hut-house is full of short notes written in a wide sprawling hand. I have kept them all because they are a statement of human generosity and the wild carefree laugh of a woman who is as busy as women the world over about things women always entangle themselves in—a man, a home . . . Like this . . .

"Have you an onion to spare? It's very quiet here this morning and I'm all tired out from sweeping and cleaning the yard, shaking blankets, cooking, fetching water, bathing children, and there's still the floor inside to sweep and dishes to wash . . . it's endless!"

Sometimes too, conversations get all tangled up and the African night creeps all about and the candles are not lit and the conversation gets more entangled, intense; and the children fall asleep on the floor dazed by it all.

She is a new kind of American or even maybe will be a new kind of African. There isn't anyone here who does not admire her. To come from a world of chicken, hamburgers, TV, escalators, and whatnot to a village mud hut and a life so tough, where the most you can afford to eat is ground millet and boiled meat. Sometimes you cannot afford to eat at all. Always you have to trudge miles for a bucket of water and carry it home on your head. And to do all this with loud, ringing, sprawling laughter?

Black people in America care about Africa, and she has come here on her own as an expression of that love and concern. Through her, too, one is filled with wonder for a country that breeds individuals about whom, without and within, rushes the wind of freedom. I have to make myself clear, though. She is a different person who has taken by force what America will not give black people.

The woman from America loves both Africa and America, independently. She can take what she wants from both and say, "Dammit." It is a most strenuous and difficult thing to do.

MANIFESTO: 1928

The Revolution of the Word

PROCLAMATION

TIRED OF THE SPECTACLE OF SHORT STORIES, NOVELS, POEMS, AND PLAYS STILL UNDER THE HEGEMONY OF THE BANAL WORD, MONOTONOUS SYNTAX, STATIC PSYCHOLOGY, DESCRIPTIVE NATURALISM, AND DESIROUS OF CRYSTALLIZING A VIEWPOINT. . . .

WE HEREBY DECLARE THAT:

1. THE REVOLUTION IN THE ENGLISH LANGUAGE IS AN ACCOMPLISHED FACT.

2. THE IMAGINATION IN SEARCH OF A FABULOUS WORLD IS AUTONOMOUS AND UNCONFINED.
   (Prudence is a rich, ugly old maid courted by Incapacity . . . Blake)

3. PURE POETRY IS A LYRICAL ABSOLUTE THAT SEEKS AN A PRIORI REALITY WITHIN OURSELVES ALONE.
   (Bring out number, weight, and measure in a year of dearth . . . Blake)

4. NARRATIVE IS NOT MERE ANECDOTE, BUT THE PROJECTION OF A METAMORPHOSIS OF REALITY.
   (Enough! Or Too Much! . . . Blake)

5. THE EXPRESSION OF THESE CONCEPTS CAN BE ACHIEVED ONLY THROUGH THE RHYTHMIC "HALLUCINATION OF THE WORD."
   (Rimbaud)

6. THE LITERARY CREATOR HAS THE RIGHT TO DISINTEGRATE THE PRIMAL MATTER OF WORDS IMPOSED ON HIM BY TEXTBOOKS AND DICTIONARIES.
   (The road of excess leads to the palace of Wisdom . . . Blake)

7. HE HAS THE RIGHT TO USE WORDS FOR HIS OWN FASHIONING AND TO DISREGARD EXISTING GRAMMATICAL AND SYNTACTICAL LAWS.

   (The tigers of wrath are wiser than the horses of instruction . . . Blake)

8. THE "LITANY OF WORDS" IS ADMITTED AS AN INDEPENDENT UNIT.

9. WE ARE NOT CONCERNED WITH THE PROPAGATION OF SOCIOLOGICAL IDEAS, EXCEPT TO EMANCIPATE THE CREATIVE ELEMENTS FROM THE PRESENT IDEOLOGY.

10. TIME IS A TYRANNY TO BE ABOLISHED.

11. THE WRITER EXPRESSES. HE DOES NOT COMMUNICATE.

12. THE PLAIN READER BE DAMNED.

    (Damn braces! Bless relaxes! . . . Blake)

—KAY BOYLE, WHIT BURNETT, HART CRANE, CARESSE CROSBY, HARRY CROSBY, MARTHA FOLEY, STUART GILBERT, A. L. GILLESPIE, LEIGH HOFFMAN, EUGÈNE JOLAS, ELLIOT PAUL, DOUGLAS RIGBY, THEO RUTRA, ROBERT SAGE, HAROLD J. SALEMSON, LAURENCE VAIL

LOVING YOU

Denis Johnson

It felt like the International had one last trip left in it. Two shocks had blown and the frame was cracked and quite a bit of the electrical system had gone dark. This thing's from 1970 and it's been a while since it went on a ride. But you could feel that last trip coming. And Joey said these people he knew from Austin intended to pick him up in Long Beach on their way to the Rainbow Gathering in the national forest over in north-central Oregon. The Gathering of the Tribes it used to be called, tens of thousands of hippies in the woods, seven days of Peace and Love. Four hundred miles to over there where it is—a distance the International could surely make and even possibly manage to retrace back home. You could feel that one last trip coming.

Peace and Love! This tall skinny mean guy in Iowa City in the '70s had a poster on his wall of a peace sign, the upside-down Y symbolizing peace, which he'd altered with a Magic Marker into a lopsided swastika, and he'd added words so that the Peace-and-Love slogan beneath it read PEACE OF THE ACTION/LOVE OF MONEY. I never forgot it. . . . I who have had so much of peace and so much of love, I have never really believed in either one.

The Magical Mystery Message to see the Rainbow was coming from a couple of directions, wasn't just coming from Joey and the teenage past.

Denis Johnson's *Seek: Reports from the Edges of America and Beyond* was nominated for the 2002 PEN/Martha Albrand Award for First Nonfiction.

All spring Mike O, a friend of mine from North Idaho, had been bothering me I should go. Mike O, a regular Mr. Natural: Barefoot Mike, Underground Mike, one of the originals, close to sixty years old now; his white hair hasn't been cut or combed since youth and his white beard looks inhabited. How did we all get so old? Sitting around laughing at old people probably caused it.

How long since I'd seen Joey? We'd taken our first acid trip together, Carter B and him and me and Bobby Z. Hadn't seen Carter in nearly thirty years. Joey since—wow, since '74. That summer I was with Miss X. Bobby Z and Joey came to see us on the second floor where we lived in this place like a box of heat. They owed me a disruption—Joey did anyway, because Bobby and I had invaded him two years before, when he'd been living on the side of this mountain in Hollywood and studying to be, or actually working as, some kind of hairdresser. "What do you want?" I said when I answered the door. "You're not gonna stay here." The place had only one room to sleep in, and a kitchen the size of a bathroom, a bathroom the size of a closet. There weren't any closets.

Miss X and I were always fighting. Every time a knock came on the door we had to stop screaming and collect our wits.

"We're economizing on space," I said when I saw who it was this time.

"Obviously," Bobby said.

Joey had his guitar case leaning up against him and his arm draped around it like a little sibling. Miss X stood behind me breathing hard with the mascara streaking her cheeks, radiant with tears and anger and her wet eyelashes like starbursts.

In short, three weeks or two weeks or one week later I made loud vague accusations in a scene, basically the result of the August heat, that ended with Bobby Z and Joey heading north for Minnesota, taking Miss X.

I was stabbing through the window screen with a pair of scissors as they headed down the back stairs, and I didn't see Bobby again until he was sick on his deathbed five years ago in Virginia, and Joey never since.

It's funny, but Joey called me from Huntington Beach just last night— two years after this trip to the hippies I'm describing—just to say hello, partly, and partly because his band broke up and he's just started AA and begun a program of meds for his depression and needs a place to lay back, because he's homeless. He mentioned he'd heard from Carter B. Carter said he's got hepatitis C and thinks I probably have it, too, because he must have picked it up way back during the era we were sharing needles when we were kids. I feel all right. I don't feel sick. But it's funny. Thirty years go by, and the moves we made just keep bringing this old stuff rolling over us.

The International throws a tire down in the Tri-City area of Hanford, Washington. It's so hot on the tarmac I get confused in my head and forget to put the nuts back on when I change the flat, and the loose rim tears up the wheel a good bit before I figure out what's happening and pull over, and I have to roll the thing in front of me a half mile to a garage and get the whole business straightened out. But the truck still works when all is said and done. After I'm in the mountains I start getting glad I agreed to go. Our vehicles, our hamlets and commerce miniaturized in the shadow of these mountains ... RU FREE—Minnesota plates on a VW bus in the one-street town of Mitchell not far from the beginning of the Ochoco National Forest. Five youngsters all around twenty years old and a dog, gassing up.

The eastern end of the Ochoco Forest seems quiet enough, a showcase for the public administration of nature, having narrow roads of unblemished blacktop with level campsites scattered sparsely alongside them. The Rainbow Gathering's website has provided a map leading out toward the wilder part of the mountain and down a dirt road toward a cloud of dust where hundreds of pickups and vans and tiny beat-up cars have parked at the direction of a bunch of wild-looking toothless young pirates with a hand-held radio under a plastic awning and a dirty illegible flag. Even down here, where people wait for the shuttle-vans that take them up the mountain to the gathering or where they shoulder their frame backpacks and start up the hill on foot, all dressed up in the ashes of their most beautiful clothes, in their long skirts and tie-dyed T-shirts, just like the hippies of thirty years ago, even down here there's a feeling of anarchy Third World–style, the pole-and-tarp lean-to, the people with shiny eyes, the lying around, the walking around, the sudden flaring madness, only this is celebratory and happy madness rather than angry or violent. The shuttle-van climbs up past further checkpoints where serious authoritative hippies make sure nobody's just driving up out of laziness to park all over the mountain and get in each other's way. Past the first camp—the A-Camp, the only place where alcohol is permitted, although this segregation has been accomplished voluntarily and nobody would think of enforcing it. Past other camps of teepees, dome tents, shacks of twigs and plastic tarp to where the WELCOME HOME sign stands at the head of the footpath. The path heads into the series of clearings and copses where a whole lot of hippies, nobody can accurately count how many, have come to celebrate themselves, mostly, right now, by walking around and around, up and down the trails, past the kitchens set up under homemade awnings and canvas roofs, food centers staffed by those who want to give to those who need to take. Mike O has instructed me to equip myself with a big enamelware cup, a spoon, and a sleeping bag—to come as a taker, and be confident I won't need more. No money changes hands here, at least that's the idea, everything is done by bartering. But I've brought a couple hundred dollars in my pocket because Joey and I might look for mushrooms and seek some sort of spiritual union together through exotic chemicals like in the old days, and I don't care what they say, I've never seen anybody trade dope for anything except sex or cash.

You hear wildly varying figures, eleven different guesses for everything—4,000 feet elevation, 6,700 elevation, 8,000 elevation. Claims of anywhere from 10,000 to 50,000, as far as attendance. But let's say ten thousand or more hippies touring along the paths here in the American wilderness just as we did up and down Telegraph Ave. in Berzerkely almost thirty years ago. Yes! They're still at it!—still moving and searching, still probing along the thoroughfares for quick friends and high times, weather-burned and dusty and gaunt, the older ones now in their fifties and a whole new batch in their teens and twenties, still with their backpacks, bare feet, tangled hair, their sophomoric philosophizing, their glittery eyes, their dogs named Bummer and Bandit and Roach and Kilo and Dark Star. And as they pass each other they say, "*Loving* you!"—*Loving* you! It serves for anything, greeting and parting and passing, like "aloha," and might burst from a person at any time as if driven by a case of Tourette's, apropos of absolutely jack. Everybody keeps saying it.

Scattered over about one square mile of Indian Prairie in the Ochoco National Forest we have the pole-and-awning kitchens and camps of various tribes and families and impromptu more or less hobo clans: Elvis Kitchen, Twelve-step Kitchen, Funky Granola, Avalon, Greenwich Village. The billboard map near the WELCOME entrance lists and vaguely locates the groups who wish to be located and who have notified someone among the oozing anarchic strata from the Elders down to the children as to where they'd be:

Aloha
Bear Fish
Bliss Rehydration Station

Brew Ha-ha
Cannabis confusion cafe
Carnivores cafe
Cybercamp
Faerie Camp
Eternal Book Assembly
Madam Frog's Dinkytown Teahouse
Northwest Tribe
Ohana Tribe
Ohmklahoma
Shama Lama Ding Dong
Rainbow Solar Bubble
Deaf tribe
Jesus Kitchen
Ida No & Eye Don Kare
Free Family
Sacred Head Church
BC Tribe
Twelve Tribes [w/Star of David]
Thank You Camp
Camp Discordia

. . . and the infamous "A-Camp," the only region whose temporary residents have agreed that among them alcohol shall be one of the chemicals
of happiness.

> *Alcohol: Near the parking area there is a place called "A-Camp."*
> *Rainbow says "We love the alcoholic, but not the alcohol." Personalities*
> *change on alcohol (and hard drugs). Sometimes people can't control them-*
> *selves as well. Therefore you are respectfully asked to leave the alcohol in*
> *A-Camp when you hike in to the main gathering space.*

—so says the Unofficial Rainbow Website. The whole region comman-
deered by the Rainbow tribes, as always without benefit of permits from
the U.S. Forest Service, parking and all, covers about four square miles.
The givers, the ones who hand out food and take care of things to the
extent they're taken care of, the putters-up of portable toilets and showers
and medical stations and crude signs like the directory and map or the
small billboard illustrating how germs get from dogshit to flies to

foodstuff and then to human fingers and mouths, along with advisos to interrupt this process by keeping your hands clean, these who make it all possible arrived and started erecting their camps a week or so before the general celebrants showed up, the takers, the bunch of us who just materialize and stash our stuff under a bush and hold out our blue enamelware cups for hot cereal offered every noon by, for instance, the orange-garbed bald-headed Hare Krishnas, who ladle out three to four thousand such lunches every day of the party.

Joey and I have planned to meet up at the camp of the Ohana tribe, a nomad family of twenty or more who caravan around North America living only in government-owned forests like the Ochoco. I don't find Joey right off and have no real explanation for my presence among them, but the young teenagers who seem to make up the most of the Ohana don't care where I put up my tent and don't seem to hold it against me that I look like somebody from a TV news team, olive shorts, khaki shirt, baseball hat, and jogging shoes. Hey. Even socks. On the other hand nobody seems inclined to talk with me, either. At a glance they see there's no sense asking me for reefer. Ohana means something in Hawaiian, they tell me. Peace. Or Love. They're not sure.

I've located Joey. He looks the same, only older, just as sad or perhaps more so, having lived thirty years longer now and found more to be sad about.

Joey and I sit out front of my tent in the dirt while he tunes up. He's played professionally for decades, and he doesn't do it just for fun very often anymore. But just to oblige me . . . We sing a few of the old ones while the teenage Ohanans get a fire going about six feet away and start good-naturedly hassling whoever wanders past for drugs.

It's the second of July and anybody's who's coming is probably here. The woods aren't quiet. You can hear the general murmur of thousands as in a large stadium, just a bit muted by the forest. The sky turns red and the day dies and Joey has to put away his guitar thanks to competition: Drums start up all around, they call from far and near and not quite anywhere in the forest, they give a sense of its deeps and distances and they sound like thoughts it's thinking.

We stumble through the night amongst them: the drums, the drums, the drums. All through the forest, pockets of a hundred, two hundred dancers gather around separate groups of ten or twenty maniac percussionists with congas and bongos and tambourines and every other kind of thing to whang on loudly, and the rhythm rises up from all directions into the darkness of space, until the galactic cluster at the center of Andromeda trembles. The yellow strobing light of bonfires and the shadows of the dancers on the smoke. Naked men with their penises bouncing and top-less women shaking their beautiful breasts. Every so often when the mood gets them a cry goes up and a hundred voices rise in a collective howling that really just completely banishes gravity for a moment and dies away.

We hear it rained quite heavily two nights ago, but this night is all stars and stillness, the smoke of fires going straight up in the orange light, and the ground isn't particularly uncomfortable, but just the same camping out always feels wrong to me—to sleep outdoors feels desperate, broke, and lonely—brings back those nights under a billboard on Wilshire where Joey and Carter and I found a bush to hide us, panhandler punks moving up and down the West Coast drunk on wine and dreaming of somewhere else, brings back those nights in a bag in the hills above Telegraph Avenue when I literally—literally, because I tried—could not get arrested, couldn't land a vagrancy charge and a bed and a roof and three meals of jail food. In my tent on the earth of the Ochoco Forest I don't sleep right. Neither does Joey. By next day noon we're already talking about finding a motel. The morning's too hot and the party's bumping off to a bad start, we keep running into many more people looking for dope than people who look stoned, and the Krishnas run out of gruel twenty minutes after they start serving. Joey and I join what they call the Circle, about a thousand people sitting in a pack on the ground—no standing up, please—getting fed with one ladleful each of spiceless veggie broth, courtesy, we believe, of the Rainbow Elders.

Once upon a time in the cataclysmic future, according to Rainbow lore, which filters down to us from the ancient Hopi and the Navajo through the cloudy intuitions of people who get high a lot, once upon a time in the future "when the earth is ravaged and the animals are dying," says the Unofficial Rainbow Internet Website, claiming to quote an Old Native American Prophecy, "a new tribe of people shall come unto the earth from many colors, classes, creeds, and who by their actions and deeds shall make the earth green again. They will be known as the warriors of the Rainbow." I see hardly any blacks, hardly any Indians from either continent, but it's astonishing to see so many youngsters on the cusp of twenty, as if perhaps some segment of the '60s population stopped growing up.

The Rainbow Family, consisting apparently of anybody who wants to be in it, not only have a myth but also have a creed, expressed succinctly way back when by Ralph Waldo Emerson in his essay "Self-Reliance": *Do*

Your Thing, and with great reluctance they've allowed to evolve out of the cherished disorganization of these gatherings a sort of structure and an optional authority, that is, an unenforced authority, which defaults to the givers, the ones who actually make possible things like this gathering and many other smaller ones around the country every year since the first one in 1972; and the givers defer to the tribal Elders, whoever they are.

An online exchange of letters headed "God can be found in LSD" winds up urging that those participating in these experiments in spontaneous community-building only

- Be self-reliant
- Be respectful
- Keep the Peace
- Clean up after yourself

and that anything else going on is nobody's business unless someone's getting hurt. "In that event, our system of PeaceKeeping (we call it 'Shanti Senta,' not 'Security') kicks in, and the unsafe situation is dealt with." Speaking as a congenital skeptic, I have to admit that no such situation occurs all weekend, as far as I can learn. And nobody can tell me what Shanti Senta means, either.

I go walking in the woods with Mike O, who's spent the last few days under a tiny awning dispensing information about the Course in Miracles, a heretic sort of gnostic brand of Christian thinking that doesn't recognize the existence of evil and whose sacred text is mostly in iambic pentameter. He's a grizzled old guy, wiry and hairy, lives in the Idaho mountains in an underground house he dug out with a shovel, never wears shoes between April and October. He stops a time or two to smoke some grass out of a pipe, a couple of times also to share a toke with passersby, because Mike is a genuinely unselfish and benevolent hippie, and after that he has to stop once in a while and rest his butt on a log, because he's dizzy. We pass a gorgeous woman completely naked but covered with black mud. She's been rolling in a mudhole with her friends. I guess I'm staring because she says, "Like what you see?"

"In a day full of erotic visions, you're the most erotic vision of all," I tell her. To me it's a poem, but she just thinks I'm fucked.

Somehow these flower people sense I'm not quite there. They see me. And I think I see them back: In a four-square-mile swatch of the Ochoco Forest the misadventures of a whole generation continue. Here in this bunch of 10,000 to 50,000 people somehow unable to count themselves I see my generation epitomized: a Peter Pan generation nannied by matronly Wendys like Bill and Hillary Clinton, our politics a confusion of Red and Green beneath the black flag of Anarchy; cross-eyed and well-meaning, self-righteous, self-satisfied; close-minded, hypocritical, intolerant— *Loving* you!—*Sieg Heil!*

Joey and I have discovered that if we identify ourselves as medical people ferrying supplies, the Unofficials at the checkpoints let us pass and we don't have to bother with distant parking and the wait for one of the shuttle brigade of VW vans and such, and in the comfort of an automobile, Joey's pretty good Volvo, we can come and go as we please. Coming back up from a burger run in town, we pick up this guy hitching. He says he's staying in the A-Camp. "I'm not the big juice-head," he says, "but at least those folks understand I like cash American currency for what I'm selling."

"And what's for sale?"

"'shrooms. Twenty-five an eighth."

I don't ask an eighth of what, just—"How much to get the two of us high?"

"Oh, an eighth should do you real nice if you haven't been eating them as a steady thing and like built a tolerance. Twenty-five bucks will send you both around and back, guaranteed."

And this is why certain people shouldn't mess with these substances: "Better give me a hundred bucks' worth," I say.

It makes me sort of depressed to report that as we accomplish the exchange this man actually says, "Far out, dude."

We now possess this Baggie full of gnarled dried vegetation that definitely looks to be some sort of fungus. Back at my tent I dig out my canteen and prepare to split the stuff, whatever it is, with Joey while he finds his own canteen so we can wash it down quick. And here is why I can't permit myself even to try and coexist with these substances: I said I'd split it, but I only gave him about a quarter. Less than a quarter. Yeah. I never quite became a hippie. And I'll never stop being a junkie.

For a half hour or so we sat on the earth between our two tents and watched the folks go by. In a copse of trees just uphill from us the Ohana group had started a drum-circle and were slowly hypnotizing themselves with mad rhythm. Joey revealed he did, in fact, eat these things once in a while and probably had a tolerance. He wasn't sensing much effect.

"Oh," I said.

In a few minutes he said, "Yeah, I'm definitely not getting off."

I could only reply by saying, "Off."

I was sitting on the ground with my back against a tree. My limbs and torso had filled up with a molten psychedelic lead and I couldn't move. Objects became pimpled like cactuses. Ornately and methodically and intricately pimpled. Everything looked crafted, an inarticulate intention worked at every surface.

People walked by along the trail. Each carried a deeply private shameful secret, no, a joke they couldn't tell anyone, yes, their heads raged almost unbearably with consciousness and their souls carried their bodies along.

"Those are some serious drums."

Anything you say sounds like the understatement of the century. But to get hyperbolic at all would be to hint dreadfully at the truth that no hyperbole whatsoever is possible—that is, it's hopelessly impossible to exaggerate the unprecedented impact of those drums. And the sinister, amused, helpless, defeated, worshipful, ecstatic, awed, snide, reeling, happy, criminal, resigned, insinuating tone of the message of those drums. Above all we don't wish to make the grave error of hinting at the truth of those drums and then, perhaps, give way to panic. Panic at the ultimateness—panic at the fact that in those drums, and with those drums, and before those drums, and above all *because* of those drums, the world is ending. *That* one is one we don't want to touch—the apocalypse all around us. These concepts are wound up inside the word "serious" like the rubber bands packed explosively inside a golf ball.

"Yeah, they sure are," Joey says.

Who? What? Oh, my God, he's talking about the drums! Very nearly acknowledging the unspeakable! He's a mischievous bastard and my best friend and the only other person in the universe.

Loving you!

According to the psychiatrists who have embarked together on a molecular exploration of what they like to call "the three-pound universe" —that is, the human brain—what's happening right now is all about serotonin—5-hydroxytryptamine, or 5-HT for short, "the Mr. Big of neurotransmitters," the chemical that regulates the flow of information through the neural system.

I read this article in *Omni* called "The Neuroscience of Transcendence" that explains the whole thing. Having ingested the hallucinogen psilocybin, quite a bit more than my share, I've stimulated the serotonin receptors and disrupted the brain's delicate balancing act in cycling normal input messages from the exterior world—adding special effects.

At the same time, the messages outward to the motor cortex of the brain are disrupted by the same flood of sacred potent molecules, bombarding key serotonin receptors and sending signals *unprovoked by any external stimulus*. What's happening *in here* seems to come from *out there*. The subjective quality underlying all of experience at last reveals that it belongs to everything. The mind inside becomes the mind all around.

Serotonin and the hallucinogens that act as serotonin agonists—like LSD, mescaline, DMT, and psilocybin—also travel to the thalamus, a relay station for all sensory data heading for the cortex. There, conscious rationalizings, philosophizings, and interpretations of imagery occur. The cortex of the brain now attaches meaning to the visions that bubble up from the limbic lobe—of burning bushes or feelings of floating union with nature. The flow of images is scripted and edited into a whole new kind of show.

EXACTLY!

YES! Bugs Bunny with a double-barreled twelve-gauge shoots you in the head with a miracle.

I watched helplessly as two beings encountered each other on the trail. Two figures really hard to credit with actuality. But they weren't hallucinatory, just very formally and exotically got up as if for some sort of ceremony, covered in black designs and ornamental silver. They greeted each other and transacted. It was brief and wordless with many secret gestures, the most sinister transaction I've ever witnessed, the most private, the most deeply none of my business. Initiates of the utterly inscrutable. My eyesight too geometrically patterned to allow them faces. They had myths instead of heads.

That is very definitely *it* for *me*. I crawl into my tent. It's four feet away but somehow a little bit farther off than the end of time. It's dark and closed and I'm safe from what's out there but not from what's in *here*—the impending cataclysm, the imploding immenseness, the jocular enormity.

It's been somewhere between twenty-five minutes and twenty-five thousand years since I ate the mushrooms, and already we have the results of this experiment. The question was, now that a quarter century has passed since my last such chemical experience, now that my soul is awake, and I've grown from a criminal hedonist into a citizen of life with a belief in eternity, will a psychedelic journey help me spiritually? And the answer is yes; I believe such is possible; thanks; now how do you turn this stuff off?

Because what if the world ends, and Jesus comes down in a cloud, and I'm wrapped in a lowgrade fireball all messed up on chemicals? Is the world ending? God looms outside the playroom. The revelation and the end of toys. The horrible possibility that *I might have to deal with something*.

And the drums, the drums, the drums. Fifty thousand journeys to the moon and back in every beat.

Four hours later I succeed in operating the zipper on my sleeping bag: tantamount to conquering Everest. I got in and held on.

Me and this sleeping bag! People we are going places now!

After several hours I crawled out into the universe and took up my rightful position in outer space, lodged against the surface of this planet. It wasn't raining rain, it was only raining starlight.

This musician friend of Joey's from Austin, this guy named Jimmy G, sits down beside me with a magic-mushroom guitar and serenades me with his compositions until almost dawn. He's about fifty maybe, white-haired, very skinny, with a variety of faint colors washing over him ceaselessly. It's incomprehensible to me that a genius of this caliber, whose rhymes say everything there is to say and whose tunes sound sweeter and sadder and wilder and happier and more melodic than any others in history, should just live in Austin like a person, writing his songs. Songs about getting our hearts right, loving each other, getting along in peace, sharing the wealth, caring for our mother planet.

By then, all over the world, the drums have stopped. Teenage Ohanans in the tent across the trail make tea on a campfire without uttering a word amongst them. Nobody talks anywhere in the Ochoco Forest; it's a time of meditation. Today is the Fourth of July, the focal hour of the Rainbow Family's gathering. Despite all the partying, this is *the day of the party*. The idea is to enter a silence at dawn and meditate till noon. Then get real happy.

Joey and I walk around watching folks start the day without talking. The strange silence broken only by two dogs barking and one naked man raving as if drunk, really raving, feinting and charging at people like a bull, stumbling right through the fire-pit down by the Bartering Circle.

Noon sharp, the howling starts. The wild keening of human hippies emulating wolves. Minutes later, the drums. In the big meadow where the Circle gathers for meals everybody lumps up dancing, some naked, some dressed in clothes, others wearing mud. The sun burns on them as the crowd becomes a mob the size of a football field. A guy pours Gatorade from a jug into people's upturned open mouths, another sprinkles the throng with a hose from a backpack full of water, like an exterminator's outfit—he's a sweatbuster. Higher and higher! I crash under a bush.

Just before sunset I wake up and get back among the Circle and encounter a definite palpable downturn in the vibes. There's not enough food and not enough drugs. The party has scattered among the various camps, the drum-circle that must have included a hundred or so wild percussionists mutters back and forth to itself from just a couple places hidden in the woods.

As the sunset reddens the west, black thunderheads form in the south: a lull, a dead spot, a return of the morning's silence as the Rainbow Family watches a squall gathering, bunching itself together in the southern half of an otherwise clear ceiling.

Then a rainbow drops down though the pale sky.

The sight of it, a perfect multicolored quarter-circle, calls up a round of howling from everywhere at once that grows and doesn't stop, and the drumming starts from every direction. Then it's a double rainbow, and then a triple, and the drums and howls can't be compared to anything I've ever heard, it's a Rainbow Sign from Above—*Loving* you!—then a monster light show with the thunderheads gone crimson in the opposing sunset, the three rainbows, and now forked lightning and profound, invincible thunder, every crooked white veiny bolt and giant peal answered by a wild ten-thousand-voiced ululation—a conversation with the Spirit of All at the Divine Fourth of July Show! Far fuckin out! The Great Mother-Father Spirit Goddess Dude is a hippie!

And this is why a certain type mustn't mess with magic potions: I'm thinking, all through this spectacle, that I should have saved a couple buttons for today, I should be *high* to *dig* this. Forgetting how I dug the starlight last night by zooming around somebody's immense black mind in my sleeping bag and almost never witnessing the sky.

But after the rainbows and the storm the night comes down and we get just a little flashback: I close my eyes and remember that first ride on White Owsley's acid, remember surfacing behind a steering wheel behind which I'd apparently been sitting for some hours, trying to figure out what to do with it; and there was Joey, and Carter B and Bobby Z, the four of us coming back to the barest fringes of Earth, a place we'd never afterward be able to take quite so seriously because we'd seen it obliterated, finding each other in this place now—none of us having ever taken acid before or even really talked to anybody about it, four teenage beatnik aspirants returned from an absurd odyssey for which none of us had been the slightest bit prepared and which we felt we'd just barely survived—remember watching Joey and Carter disappear into an apartment building and remember heading with Bobby, somehow *traveling* through streets like rivers behind this *steering wheel*—five hundred mikes of White Owsley's!—remember steering magnificently through Alexandria, Virginia, in a gigantic teacup that once had been a Chevrolet under streetlights with heads like glittering brittle dandelions, remember letting it park itself and remember floating into a building and down the halls of the Fort Ward Towers Apartments, down the complicated curvature of the halls, and finding, at the end of the palatial mazes, finding—Mom! Mom in her robe and slippers! Her curlers from Mars! Mom from another species! Mom who said It's five in the morning! I nearly called the police! WHERE have you BEEN and remember turning to Bobby Z, who's dead of AIDS, at his funeral I threw dirt onto his coffin while his sister, my old highschool sweetheart, keened and screamed, turned to Bobby Z and said, Where have we been?—and the question astonished and baffled and shocked him too, and we both said, Where have we been? WHERE HAVE WE BEEN?

Bobby them drums are riding themselves up to the very limit and right on through like it was nothing. Where where where have we been?

Where did we go?

MANIFESTO: 1925

Surrealist Declaration
of January 27, 1925

Translated by Richard Howard

With regard to a false interpretation of our enterprise, stupidly circulated among the public,

We declare as follows to the entire braying literary, dramatic, philosophical, exegetical, and even theological body of contemporary criticism:

1. We have nothing to do with literature; But we are quite capable, when necessary, of making use of it like anyone else.

2. *Surrealism* is not a new means of expression, or an easier one, nor even a metaphysic of poetry. It is a means of total liberation of the mind *and of all that resembles it.*

3. We are determined to make a Revolution.

4. We have joined the word *surrealism* to the word *revolution* solely to show the disinterested, detached, and even entirely desperate character of this revolution.

5. We make no claim to change the *mores* of mankind, but we intend to show the fragility of thought, and on what shifting foundations, what caverns we have built our trembling houses.

6. We hurl this formal warning to Society: Beware of your deviations and *faux-pas*, we shall not miss a single one.

7. At each turn of its thought, Society will find us waiting.

8. We are specialists in Revolt.
   There is no means of action which we are not capable, when necessary, of employing.

9. We say in particular to the Western World: *surrealism* exists. And what is this new ism that is fastened to us? Surrealism is not a poetic form. It is a cry of the mind turning back on itself, and it is determined to break apart its fetters, even if it must be by material hammers!

—LOUIS ARAGON, ANTONIN ARTAUD, JACQUES BARON,
J.-A. BOIFFARD, JOË BOUSQUET, ANDRÉ BRETON,
JEAN CARRIVE, RENÉ CREVEL, ROBERT DESNOS, PAUL ÉLUARD,
MAX ERNST, T. FRAENKEL, FRANCIS GÉRARD, MICHEL LEIRIS,
GEORGES LIMBOUR, MATHIAS LÜBECK, GEORGES MALKINE,
ANDRÉ MASSON, MAX MORISE, PIERRE NAVILLE,
MARCEL NOLL, BENJAMIN PÉRET, RAYMOND QUENEAU,
PHILIPPE SOUPAULT, DÉDÉ SUNBEAM, ROLAND TUAL

COURTESY OF THE LIBRARY OF CONGRESS

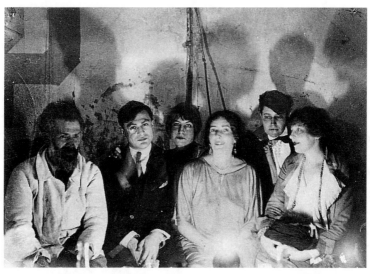

Constantin Brancusi, Tristan Tzara, Mina Loy, and co-conspirators, at Brancusi's studio.

MANIFESTO: 1923

Toward a Constructive Poetry
Theo van Doesburg [I. K. Bonset]
Translated by Claire Nicholas White

Destruction is part of the rebuilding of poetry.
Destruction of syntax is the first necessary preamble to the new poetry.
   Destruction has expressed itself in the following ways:

1. In the use of words (according to their meaning).
2. In atrocity (psychic disturbance).
3. In typography (synoptic poetry).

   In (1) were instrumental: Mallarmé, Rimbaud, Ghil, Gorter, Apollinaire, Birot, Arp, Schwitters, etc. . . .
   In (2) de Sade, Lautréamont, Masoch, Péladan, all religious writings, Schwitters, etc. . . .
   In (3) Apollinaire, Birot, Marinetti, Beauduin, Salvat-Papaseït, Kurt Schwitters, etc.
POETRY IS UNTHINKABLE WITHOUT AN AESTHETIC FOUNDATION
   To take the purely utilitarian as the only general basis of a new artistic expression = nonsense.

$$\left.\begin{array}{l}\text{Utilitarian poetry}\\\text{Utilitarian music}\\\text{Utilitarian painting}\\\text{Utilitarian sculpture}\end{array}\right\} = \text{nonsense}$$

nonsense—nonsense—nonsense etc.

   We are living in a provisional period. We suppose: that there is no difference between the soul and the spinal marrow, between coitus and art.
   But when we make art we use no soap (perhaps the painters do if they have inclinations to cleanliness) and one cannot rise up to heaven on a tomato.
   One cannot brush one's teeth with art. . . .

THE BLOOMSBURY GROUP
LIVE AT THE APOLLO
(*LINER NOTES FROM*
THE NEW BEST-SELLING ALBUM)

Ian Frazier

L ive albums aren't supposed to be as exciting, as *immediate* as the actual stage performances they record, but (saints be praised!) the Bloomsbury Group's newest, *Live at the Apollo*, is a shouting, foot-stomping, rafter-shaking exception to this rule. Anyone who has not seen John Maynard Keynes doing his famous strut, or Duncan Grant playing his bass while flat on his back, can now get an idea of what he's been missing! The Bloomsbury Group has always stood for seriousness about art and skepticism about the affectations of the self-important, and it has been opposed to the avowed philistinism of the English upper classes. *Live at the Apollo* is so brilliantly engineered that this daring Neo-Platonism comes through as unmistakably as the super-bad Bloomsbury beat. A few critics have complained that the Bloomsbury Group relies too heavily on studio effects; this album will instantly put such objections to rest. The lead vocals (some by "Mister White Satin" Lytton Strachey, the others by Clive Bell) are solid and pure, even over the enthusiastic shouts of the notoriously tough-to-please Apollo crowd, and the Stephen Sisters' chorus is reminiscent of the Three Brontës at their best. There is very little "dead air" on this album, even between cuts. On Band 3 on the flip side, there is a pause while the sidemen are setting up, and if you listen carefully you can hear Leonard Woolf and Virginia Stephen coining withering epigrams and exchanging banter with the audience about Macaulay's essay on Warren Hastings. Very mellow, very close textual criticism.

Lytton Strachey, who has been more or less out of the funk-literary picture since his girlfriend threw boiling grits on him in his Memphis hotel room in March of 1924, proves here that his voice is still as sugar-cured as ever. In his long solo number, "Why I Sing the Blues," he really soars through some heartfelt lyrics about his "frail and sickly childhood" and "those painfully introverted public-school years." The song is a triumph of melody and phrasing, and it provides some fascinating insights into the personality of this complex vocalist and biographer.

Much of the credit for the album's brilliance must go to G. E. Moore, who wrote "Principia Ethica," the group's biggest hit, as well as to Lady Ottoline Morrell, their sound technician and roadie. The efforts of professionals like these, combined with Bloomsbury's natural dynamism, have produced that rarest of rarities—a live album that is every bit as good as being there.

II

SAILCAT TURNER REMINISCES ABOUT
THE FOUNDING OF THE BLOOMSBURY GROUP

People will tell you nowadays, "Well, the Bloomsbury Group this or the Bloomsbury Group that," or "Bertrand Russell and Sir Kenneth Clark were members of the original Bloomsbury Group," or some such jive misinformation. I don't pay 'em no mind. Because, dig, I knew the Bloomsbury Group before there ever *was* a Bloomsbury Group, before anybody knew there was going to *be* any Bloomsbury Group, and I was in on the very beginning.

One night in '39, I was playing alto with McShann's band uptown at the old Savoy Ballroom—mostly blues, 'cause we had one of the better blues shouters of the day, Walter Brown—and Dizzy Gillespie was sittin' out front. So after the set Diz comes up to me and he says, "Sailcat, I got this chick that you just *got* to hear. Man, this chick can *whale*." So he takes me over to Dan Wall's Chili Joint on Seventh Avenue, and in the back there they got a small combo—two horns, some skins, and a buddy of mine named Biddy Fleet on guitar. They're just runnin' some new chords when from this table near the stage this chick steps up. She's got what you might call a distracted air. She looks around the room nervous-like, and then she throws back her head and sound comes out like no sound I ever heard before. Man, I sat there till eight o'clock in the morning, listening to her. I asked Diz who this chick was, and he says, "Don't you know? That's little Ginny Stephen." Now, of course, everybody talks about Virginia Woolf, author of *To the Lighthouse*, and so on. When I first knew her, she was just little Ginny Stephen. But man, that chick could *whale*.

I liked her music so much that me and Diz and Billie Holiday and Ginny and Ginny's sister Vanessa started hanging out together. So one day Ginny says to me, "Sailcat, I got this economist friend of mine, he's really outta sight. Would you like to meet him?" So I said sure, and she took me downtown to the Village Vanguard, and that was the first time I ever heard John Maynard Keynes. Of course, his playing wasn't much back then. Truth is, he shouldn't have been on the stage at all. Back then he was doin' "What Becomes of the Broken Hearted," but it sure didn't sound like the hit he later made it into. Back then he was still doin' "What Becomes of the Broken Hearted" as a *demonstration*, with charts and bar graphs. Later, of course, he really started cookin' and smokin'. That cat took classical economic theory and bent it in directions nobody ever thought it could go.

Now, Ginny and John, they were pretty tight, and they had this other friend they used to run with. This was a dude named Lytton Strachey, that later became their lead singer. He also won a wide reputation as an author and a critic. After hours, they used to sit around and jam and trade aphorisms. Me and Cootie Williams and Duncan Grant and Billie Holiday and Leonard Woolf, who later married Ginny, and Ella Fitzgerald, who had just taken over Chick Webb's band, and James (Lytton's brother) and Dizzy and the Duke and Maynard Keynes and Satchmo and Charles Mingus and Theodore Llewelyn Davies and Thelonious Monk and Charles Tennyson and Miles Davis and Ray Charles and Hilton Young (later Lord Kennet) all used to sit in sometimes too. We smoked some reefer. Man, we used to *cook*.

Well, that was the beginning. Later, a lot of people dropped out, and Lytton and Ginny and Vanessa and Maynard and Leonard and Duncan and some of the others started to call themselves the Bloomsbury Group, after their old high school over in England. They asked me and Diz to join, but Diz was supposed to go on tour with Billy Eckstine's band, and as for me, well, I wasn't too crazy about the group's strong Hellenic leanings. Now, of course, I wish I'd said yes.

III

VIRGINIA WOOLF TALKS FRANKLY ABOUT THE BLOOMSBURY GROUP

Being a member of the Bloomsbury Group has brought me out of myself and taught me how to open up to other people. At the beginning, all of us—Leonard, Clive, Vanessa, Lytton, Duncan, Maynard, and me—we were like different states of mind in one consciousness. It was like we each had one tarot card but it didn't make sense until we put all the cards together, and then when we did—it was beautiful. Like in *2001*, when that monkey figures out how to use that bone. Everything was merged.

Of course, we still have our problems. The interpersonal vibes can get pretty intense when we're touring, going from one Quality Court to another and then to another and then another. Sometimes I wonder if I have room to grow as an artist. But usually it works out O.K. Like the time I told Lytton that our new reggae number "Mrs. Dalloway" might work better as a short story or even a novel. We talked it out, and Lytton told me I was thinking too linear. Later, I had to admit he was right.

The hardest thing about being a member of the Bloomsbury Group is learning how to be a person at the same time you're being a star. You've got to rise above your myth. We've reached the point where we're completely supportive of each other, and that's good. But at the same time we all have our own separate lives. I've been getting into video, Maynard recorded that album with Barry White, Duncan's been doing some painting—we have to work hard to keep in touch with each other and ourselves, but it's worth it. The way I figure it, there's really nothing else I'd rather do.

MANIFESTO: 1918

Dada Manifesto
Tristan Tzara
Translated by Mary Ann Caws

*The magic of a word—*DADA*—which has set the journalists at the door of an unexpected world, has not the slightest importance for us. . . .*

There is a literature which doesn't reach voracious masses. A work of creators, the result of a real need of the author, and done for himself. Knowledge of a supreme egoism, where laws fade away. Each page ought to explode, either from deep and weighty seriousness, a whirlwind, dizziness, the new, or the eternal, from its crushing humor, the enthusiasm of principles, or its typographical appearance. Here is a tottering world fleeing, future spouse of the bells of the infernal scale, and here on the other side: new men. Harsh leaping, riders of hiccups. Here are a mutilated world and the literary medicine men with passion for improvement.

I say: there is no beginning and we are not trembling, we are not sentimental. We shred the linen of clouds and prayers like a furious wind, preparing the great spectacle of disaster, fire, decomposition. Let's get ready to cast off mourning and to replace tears with mermaids stretched out from one continent to the next. Pavilions of intense joy, empty of the sadness of poison. ∴ DADA is the signboard of abstraction; advertising and business are also poetic elements. . . .

DADAIST SPONTANAIETY
I call Idon'tgivadamnism the state of a life where each person keeps his own conditions, although knowing how to respect other individuals, if not defending himself, the two-step becoming a national hymn, a whatnot store, a radio playing Bach fugues, neon lights and signs for brothels, the organ diffusing carnations for God, all that together and actually replacing photography and unilateral catechism. . . .

I am writing a manifesto and I don't want anything; I say, however, certain things and I am on principle against manifestos, as I am also against principles (half-pints for judging the moral value of each sentence—too easy;

approximation was invented by the impressionists). I am writing this manifesto to show that you can do contrary actions together, in one single fresh breath; I am against action; for continual contradiction, for affirmation also, I am neither for nor against and I don't explain because I hate common sense.

DADA—now there's a word that sets off ideas; each bourgeois is a little playwright, inventing different dialogues, instead of setting characters suitable to the level of his intelligence, like pupae on chairs, seeking causes or purposes (according to the pyschoanalytic method he practices) to cement his plot, a story which defines itself in talking. Each spectator is a plotter, if he tries to explain a word (knowledge!). From the cotton-padded refuge of serpentine complications, he has his instincts manipulated. Thence the misfortunes of conjugal life.

Explaining: Amusement of redbellies on the mills of empty skulls.

DADA MEANS NOTHING

... DADA was born of a desire for independence, of a distrust of the community. Those who belong to us keep their freedom. We don't recognize any theory. We have had enough of cubist and futurist academies: laboratories of formal ideas. Do you practice art to earn money and fondle the middle class? Rhymes ring the assonance of coins and inflection slides along the line of the tummy in profile. All the groupings of artists have ended at this bank even while they rode high along on diverse comets. A door open to the possibilities of luxuriating in cushions and food.

Here we cast anchor in rich earth. . . .

DADAIST DISGUST

Every product of disgust capable of becoming a negation of the family is *dada*; the whole being protesting in its destructive force with clenched fists: DADA; knowledge of all the means rejected up to this point by the timid sex of easy compromise and sociability: DADA; abolition of logic, dance of all those impotent to create: DADA; of all hierarchy and social equation installed for the preservation of values by our valets: DADA; . . . every object, feelings and obscurities, apparitions and the precise shock of parallel lines, can be means for the combat: DADA; abolition of memory: DADA; abolition of archaeology: DADA; abolition of the prophets: DADA; abolition of the future: DADA; an absolute indisputable belief in each god immediate product of spontaneity:

DADA; elegant and unprejudicial leap from one harmony to the other sphere; trajectory of a word tossed like a sonorous cry of a phonograph record; respecting all individualities in their momentary madness: serious, fearful, timid, ardent, vigorous, determined, enthusiastic; stripping its chapel of every useless awkward accessory; spitting out like a luminous waterfall any unpleasant or amorous thought, or coddling it—with the lively satisfaction of knowing that it doesn't matter—with the same intensity in the bush of his soul, free of insects for the aristocrats, and gilded with archangels' bodies. Freedom: *DADA DADA DADA*, shrieking of contracted colors, intertwining of contraries and of all contradictions, grotesqueries, nonsequiturs: LIFE.

MANIFESTO: 1914–19

Aphorisms on Futurism
Mina Loy

DIE in the Past
LIVE in the Future.

THE velocity of velocities arrives in starting.

IN pressing the material to derive its essence, matter becomes deformed.

AND form hurtling against itself is thrown beyond the synopsis of vision.

THE straight line and the circle are the parents of design, form the basis of art; there is no limit to their coherent variability.

LOVE the hideous in order to find the sublime core of it.

OPEN your arms to the dilapidated; rehabilitate them.

YOU prefer to observe the past on which your eyes are already opened.

BUT the Future is only dark from outside.

Leap into it—and it EXPLODES with *Light*. . . .

NO

Dorothy Gallagher

"**W**hy do you always say no, darling?" my mother used to say. "Someday you'll thank me: Practice the piano . . . don't leave anything on your plate . . . work for half an hour on your handwriting . . . you need a tutor for math . . . make the revolution . . ."

Here we are, Mama and I, on the lawn outside our bungalow at the end of a hot, still afternoon in the second summer of war, face-to-face on the green double glider. (I buried her ashes just about where the glider stood.) Mama is sitting, and I am standing between her knees. Over her shoulder, through the mesh of the screen door into the kitchen, I see my plump aunt Frieda standing at the stove. (In her middle age she will be killed by a runaway car.) To my left, on the porch, my bossy aunt Lily, always a bit sickly, is napping on the swing. (She will live to her dotage and beyond.)

At this moment Mama and I, so often at odds, are in thrilling mutuality. She is painting my face. With her lipstick (Tangee Flame), she makes my mouth feel as heavy as honey. She makes red circles on my cheeks, dusts my nose with powder, ties a flower-printed kerchief over my braids, and holds up the mirror. *Behold!* From memory, she has drawn a Russian peasant maiden. In an hour or two my mother and aunts will watch proudly from the audience, and I, on the stage of the day camp, will

---

Dorothy Gallagher's *How I Came into My Inheritance* was nominated for the 2002 PEN/ Martha Albrand Award for the Art of the Memoir.

swing a wooden scythe and sing "Meadowlands" to celebrate the glory of the Soviet people as they turn the Fascist tide.

And here we all are again, a couple of years later, August, the last summer of war. I am in the bathroom, thrilled at the sight of my first menstrual blood; only ten years old, but I know what's happening. I run to the kitchen to tell Mama. She claps her hands. *Mazel tov!* she cries, and turns to tell my aunts, and my uncles too. Everyone congratulates me. Soon a neighbor comes to our door. *Mazel tov!* he calls. *How does he know?* But his congratulations are for the day's headlines: Russia has entered the war against Japan. History, on two fronts!

When I ask my mother a question about Russia, she says quite severely: "So why do you call it Russia, darling? It's the Soviet Union." Yes, yes I knew that, but I get confused. If I asked, "Where were you born, Mama?" she'd say, "You know where I was born, darling. In Russia." Russian was the language in which she and her sisters told their secrets; Russia—or at least a shtetl in Ukraine—was my heritage. The difference seems to be that while the Russia of my mother's youth was hell on earth, the Soviet Union is the hope of the world.

The ramifications of this Russian/Soviet business radiated through my life. My very name, the "D" of it, honored Georgi Dimitrov, Bulgarian Communist, Comintern leader, hero of the Reichstag trial, the man who brought us the news of the Popular Front. My heart soared to the Red Army Chorus, I knew all the words to "Ballad for Americans," "Meadowlands," "The Banks Are Made of Marble," "The Four Insurgent Generals" before I knew my ABCs. I was in love with Sonny Speisman, who delivered the *Daily Worker* to our house every summer morning; then I was in love with Ernie Lieberman, who played the guitar. Handsome Ernie with the tight brown curls—with his head thrown back, he aimed his sweet tenor at the ceiling: *There once was a Union Maid / Who never was afraid / Of goons and ginks and company finks / And deputy sheriffs who made the raid.* Who was it who said: Beware the movement that makes its own music? Even today the opening notes from any one of those songs will sweep me away. (As for Ernie, decades later I recognize him on the checkout line at Zabar's; to general amusement, I call out, "Ernie! I loved you more than life itself!" He mouths, "Who are *you?*")

Anyway, this is what I take in with my mother's milk, but I am an ignorant, uninstructed child. "Trotskyite" is a well-known curse, but what does it mean? I don't even know that there was such a *person* as Trotsky. It is all as arcane as sex.

Actually, information about sex is easier to come by. From Nina, for example, one of three sisters, who comes running to me and her youngest sister, Irene. "I found prophylactics in the drawer on Daddy's side of the bed."

Irene and I look blank.

"Stupid! The man uses them when they don't want to have a baby." Nina is filled with disgust. "You'd think *three times* would have been *enough* for them!"

Without the picture on the jigsaw-puzzle box, how do you know what the pieces mean? When I think I have an inkling, I test my mother:

"Mama, what's rape?"

"Oh," she says. "It's when a boy kisses a girl and she doesn't want him to."

Is that *all?*

I listen when adults talk. I pick up words and phrases and sentences. I hear "Bolshevik," and "Stalin," and "the Party," and "class struggle," pronounced with reverence. I hear "Trotskyite," and "objectively an agent of Fascism," and "reactionary," and "class enemies" pronounced hatefully. Sometimes people who appeared in earlier conversations as "comrades" become "right-wing deviationists." My mother's cousin Sylvia explains why she will not be going to medical school after all: "They think I can do better work organizing."

Who are *they?*

"What are we, Mama?"

"We're Jewish, darling."

"No, I mean are we Democrats or Republicans?"

"You could say we're progressives."

Is that *it?*

I *love* this place where we spend our summers, and my winter school vacations too. We have an outhouse, no running water, a woodstove. My father, who can do anything, built this house. My real life happens here, sixty miles upstate, at this colony for "Workers and Professionals Only," as it advertises itself, meaning: Nobody is allowed who employs—read "exploits"—labor. (There was a small businessman who misrepresented himself as a worker. He was expelled when it was discovered that he had three employees who were on strike.)

But from September through June, when, during the 1940s, we live at the upper edge of Harlem, my real identity goes into hiding. We still read the *Daily Worker*, but now I have to walk blocks to buy it at a distant newsstand and spend an extra nickel for the *New York Post* to wrap it in for the dangerous walk back home. When Miss Ferguson, my dreadful sixth-grade teacher, tells us to bring in the newspapers our parents read, I hesitate only between the *Post* and *P.M.* and settle on the *Post* as the safer bet.

My classmates are Irish, Italian, Negro: *Americaaaaaan*, as Paul Robeson sang in celebration of premature multiculturalism. On my block—167th Street, between Amsterdam and Edgecombe Avenues—everyone is Italian until suddenly, after a summer away, we return to find that all the Italians have gone and everyone is Negro. At my school—a Gothic fortress on Broadway and 168th Street—almost everyone is some variety of Catholic—or Negro.

Now, I know the story of the Scottsboro Boys. I know that among the oppressed and exploited proletariat (with whom we are as one) the Negro people rank highest and are to be most esteemed. I have heard the talk about Jim Crow and The Negro Question and The Necessity to Root Out White Chauvinism. I have sung the songs of Leadbelly. But here's my problem: Negro children just don't like me. When I was three or four years old and we lived on Stebbins Avenue in the Bronx, my little playmate Shirley announced one day: "My mama says I can't play with you no more because you're white trash."

"Mama, Shirley says I'm white trash."

"That's just an expression, darling."

In fourth grade, May and Edna have the desks on either side of me. On a test day, May goes to the bathroom. An evil breeze blows her test paper to the floor. She comes back, sees her paper, and stares hard at me.

"What?" I whisper.

"You threw my paper on the floor!" she hisses.

"I didn't!"

"You did so. Fuck your mother."

What does this mean? Is it just an expression?

"Same to you," I say.

May and her four friends (her gang; I have no gang) circle me after school.

"She said 'fuck your mother,'" May explains.

I start to run. Edna sticks out her foot. I trip. My hands and knees are scraped raw. Someone shoves me, someone else hits me. I run and run until I run flat into a lady, who puts herself between me and my pursuers and takes me home.

And I tell no one.

"Oh! What *happened* to you?" Mama says.

"I fell, Mama."

"Be more careful, darling."

I just have this feeling that Mama won't take my side, that ideology—though I am years from knowing this word—will interfere with simple justice. I believe that, somehow, Mama will make it my fault. Suppose I had told her the story: the test paper blown to the floor, the words exchanged, etc. I swear she would have said something like: "Darling, you must work to eradicate white chauvinism in yourself; as the vanguard of the working class, we must show the Negro masses how to take their place among the international proletariat."

If you think I'm laying it on too thick, listen to this: I spent my thirteenth and fourteenth summers at Camp Wochica (Workers' Childrens' Camp, in case you thought it was your standard inauthentic Indian name). Our camp song was sung to the tune of "Oh Moscow Mine," and our project was to dig a new cesspool for the camp. (Talk about the theory of surplus value!) I learned to smoke cigarettes during those summers, to wield a shovel, and gratefully, with Karl and Anatole, I learned more about sex. For the same money I had instruction in detecting hidden manifestations of white chauvinism.

Once a week, more often if circumstances demanded, we were subjected to sessions of self-criticism so that we might admit to errors in our behavior and have the opportunity to point out errors in the behavior of our fellow campers. These sessions were led by our counselor, Elsie, in a sort of mini-trial format designed to, as the not-very-catchy slogan went, "root out every manifestation of open or concealed white chauvinism in our ranks."

Elsie to an unwary camper: "Sasha! Did you offer Joan [Negro] a slice of watermelon?"

Sasha: "Well, yes, but we had watermelon for dessert that day . . . "

Elsie: "But Bernie reported that you passed Joan an *extra* slice. Do you admit this?"

Sasha: "She asked me . . . "

Elsie: "So! You blame Joan for her own oppression!"

Poor Joan burst into tears, maybe from embarrassment, or maybe realizing at last the extent of her own oppression. I passed her a tissue.

Elsie: "And you! What right do you have to act as Joan's friend when you have *never* made a special effort to gain her friendship?"

You know what would have happened if I had made such an effort? *A transparent attempt to avoid charges of chauvinism!*

Time passed and I graduated into the Labor Youth League, successor to the Young Communist League. We met in a firetrap tenement on the Lower East Side. At one meeting I got into an argument with our leader, whom we called Rooster (long neck, bobbing Adam's apple). I can't remember what the argument was about: probably something about the wording of one of those jargon-filled leaflets we handed out on street corners to the working class, who (misled by False Consciousness) despised us. I sat in my chair in that cold, badly lit, dirty room, brooding on my grievances. I hated handing out those leaflets to passersby, who at best ignored my out-thrust arm and at worst snarled or even spat at me. I hated being monitored for deviations in thinking and, in turn, being a heresy hunter myself. I was at that moment in a dark, smoky room, and my life was feeling just as airless. I still didn't understand what Trotsky had done that was so horrible, for God's sake! I got up to leave the meeting.

"Sit down!" Rooster called. "A Negro comrade is speaking!"

I was sixteen. It was 1951. The Hollywood writers had been blacklisted; people had informed or refused to inform in front of HUAC; Alger Hiss had been convicted of perjury; the Rosenbergs had been arrested; my English teacher at Seward Park High School had been fired for subversive activities; family friends were being followed by the FBI, whose agents sometimes knocked on our door to try to ask my mother questions. For lack of anyone else to ask, I sometimes asked her questions myself.

"Mama, why did Stalin have Trotsky assassinated?"

"Who says he was assassinated, darling? Some deranged person killed him."

"Mama, why did Stalin sign the pact with Hitler?"

"That was a tactic, darling. To give the Soviet Union more time to prepare for the war."

"Mama, are the Rosenbergs Communists?"

"They're progressives, darling. They're being persecuted because they believe in justice for all people, and because they're Jews."

"Is Alger Hiss a Communist?"

"Of course not. He's a liberal person who's opposed to the warmongers."

"What about Whittaker Chambers? He says *he* was a Communist."

"He's a very sick man."

In this time of trouble, was I a rat leaving a sinking ship? Who was I, if not who I always had been? Who would my friends be? What would we talk about? How would I learn a new vocabulary? And *what* would replace the central mission of my life, to man the barricades when the revolution came?

A few months after my mother died, I dreamed we were together in a foreign country, hurrying along a path toward her childhood home. When we reached the house where she had been born, we found it deserted and derelict: wooden plank walls were splayed apart; the roof gaped; a few half-starved animals wandered around an overgrown yard. In dismay we started back toward the town, hoping to find someone who could tell us what had happened to the inhabitants of the house. The light began to fade. I saw that my mother had crossed the road. She was walking very quickly now, each step leaving me farther behind. I called to her to wait; I was in terror of being left alone in this strange country, where only she knew the language. Then it was pitch-dark. I could not see my mother anymore. I shouted, "Mama! Mama!" but she was gone.

Of course I was dreaming about my mother's death. I was still grief-stricken and bereft. But when the sound of my own voice woke me, I knew in what country she had abandoned me.

And then I remembered that I had first abandoned her.

It was 1948, the year Henry Wallace ran for president. Mama and I were at Madison Square Garden. We were at the very top of the house, looking down on the brightly lit arena. Standing at the center of the stage was Vito Marcantonio, *our* congressman. Oh, he was a *wonderful* speaker, my mother always said, a fiery orator. That man knew how to work a crowd. And as he spoke, his feet stamping, his arms waving, his voice growing louder and more rhythmic as he approached the climax of his speech, the entire audience rose to its feet, chanting with him, roaring approval. And I was on my feet too, transported, at one with the crowd, melted into it, my voice its voice. I was lost.

And suddenly, without willing it, as the crowd still roared, I came to myself. I felt very cold. I looked at Mama, still on her feet, clapping, chanting. *Who was she* now? About Marcantonio, I thought: *He could tell us to do anything now, and we'd do it.* I was out of there. I was history.

No, I said. But not so Mama could hear.

AT THE BALL GAME

William Carlos Williams

The crowd at the ball game
is moved uniformly

by a spirit of uselessness
which delights them—

all the exciting detail
of the chase

and the escape, the error
the flash of genius—

all to no end save beauty
the eternal—

So in detail they, the crowd,
are beautiful

for this
to be warned against

saluted and defied—
It is alive, venomous

it smiles grimly
its words cut—

The flashy female with her
mother, gets it—

The Jew gets it straight—it
is deadly, terrifying—

It is the Inquisition, the
Revolution

It is beauty itself
that lives

day by day in them
idly—

This is
the power of their faces

It is summer, it is the solstice
the crowd is

cheering, the crowd is laughing
in detail

permanently, seriously
without thought

Ultraist Manifesto

Translated by Mary Ann Caws

There are two aesthetics: the passive aesthetic of mirrors and the active aesthetic of prisms. When guided by the first, art transforms itself into an objective copy of its surroundings or of the physical history of the individual. When guided by the second, art frees itself, uses the world as its own instrument, and creates—beyond any spatial and temporal prison—its own personal vision.

This is the aesthetics of Ultra. It wants to create: that is, to impose so far unsuspected ways of seeing on the universe. It demands from each poet a fresh view of things, clear of any ancestral stigmas; a fragrant vision, as if the world were arising like dawn in front of our eyes. And to conquer this vision, it is essential to cast away every aspect of the past. Everything: right-angled classical architecture, romantic exaltation, the microscopic observations of the naturalists, the blue twilights that were the lyrical banners of the nineteenth-century poets. That whole absurd vast cell where the ritualists would imprison the marvelous bird of beauty. . . .

Our audacious and conscious creed is not to have a creed. That is to say, we reject all the recipes and corsets so absurdly proper, leaving them for ordinary minds. Our motto is creation for creation. Ultraist poetry has as much cadence and musicality as any other. It has just as much tenderness. As much visuality and more imagination. What is changed is the structure. Each of its most essential innovations has its root in this: the sensitivity and the feeling will always be the same. We make no claim to modify the soul or nature. What we are renovating is the means of expression.

Our iconoclastic ideology, what sets the philistines against us, is precisely what ennobles us. Every great affirmation takes a negation, as our companion Nietzsche said or forgot to say. . . . Our poems have the freewheeling and decisive structure of telegrams. . . .

—JUAN ALOMAR, FORTUNIO BONANOVA,
JORGE LUIS BORGES, JACOBO SUREDA

YUKIO MISHIMA'S CIVIL WARS

BEAUTY'S KAMIKAZE | JOHN NATHAN

Yukio Mishima's life and death present us with a paradigm of the cultural ambivalence that has beset Japan since the country was opened to the West in the late nineteenth century, after 250 years of isolation. By "cultural ambivalence," I mean the ongoing struggle to find an authentic stance and voice in the modern world by reconciling native values and sensibilities anchored in tradition on the one hand, and Western modes of being in the world on the other. This quest for synthesis of two often irreconcilable cultures has produced a recurrent malaise, akin to a national identity crisis, which continues to shape much of Japanese behavior today. Kenzaburō Ōe, who still hates Mishima implacably, spoke of this dilemma in his 1994 Nobel Laureate address. Ōe said, in English, "My observation is that after 120 years of modernization since the opening of the country, present-day Japan is split between two opposite poles of ambiguity. I too am living as a writer with this polarization imprinted on me, like a deep scar."

Mishima, whose lifestyle was irrepressibly Western, at least on the surface, voiced the same lament in his own way again and again. On November 25, 1970, he delivered cultural ambivalence the final coup de grâce when he committed suicide in the most Japanese way imaginable, by hara-kiri. At 10:50 that morning, he visited the commandant of the Tokyo battalion of a self-defense force, on the pretext of showing him an antique Japanese sword. He was accompanied by four cadets from his private army, the Shield Society, pledged to defend the emperor. At a prearranged signal, the cadets seized and bound the general, and Mishima ordered him to assemble the troops in the courtyard below. Just before noon, he stepped out on the balcony and delivered a short speech, appealing to the soldiers to join him and his men in death as true men and as samurai, in

---

These talks were presented at a PEN Twentieth Century Masters Tribute.

a battle against a postwar democracy that had deprived Japan not only of its army but also of its soul. The soldiers booed and jeered. After seven minutes, Mishima stepped inside again and cut himself open with a sword. At his grunted signal, his second-in-command, who was also his lover, beheaded him and then committed hara-kiri himself.

Mishima's death was problematic, and remains so. In the biography I wrote shortly after he died, I argue that his suicide had been driven by the longing for death that he'd been in touch with, and intermittently terrified by, since his childhood, and that the patriotism he formulated during the last ten years of his life was essentially a sham—a device that enabled him to achieve the warrior's death at the heart of a homoerotic fantasy that he had fully conceived by the time he was twelve. I found evidence to support this view in much of what he wrote, even as a teenager. And I remain persuaded that his final act was, at least in part, private and erotic rather than public and patriotic. That said, having spent time studying Japanese history since I wrote the book, I see now that in my determination to account for the suicide in terms of personal pathology, I failed to see, or to take seriously, its larger social significance.

Mishima's life was flamboyantly Western in style and manners. He dressed in classy Italian suits and smoked Cuban cigars. When he built his house in 1958, he told his architect that he wanted to sit in a Rococo chair in jeans and an aloha shirt. The result was a mélange of Greek statuary and French period furniture that looked like a movie set and disconcerted many Japanese who received invitations to his cocktail parties on Tiffany stationery. One night, soon after we got to know each other, I was sitting in his house late at night and he inquired, somewhat abruptly, if I'd seen Marlon Brando in *The Wild Ones*. When I said yes, he asked me to examine a pair of jeans that he'd been working on with sandpaper and give him a definitive verdict on whether he had achieved the Brando look. He dashed out of his study, leaving me stunned, and returned wearing the jeans; when I told him he was the spittin' image of Marlon, he beamed with a smile of immense pleasure.

Mishima was, in many ways, infatuated with Western styles and modes, and was an avid reader of all kinds of Western writers, including Gide and Cocteau, Novalis, Henry Miller and Fitzgerald, and Truman Capote and Hemingway, both of whom he admired extravagantly, in the kind of paradox for which he was famous. At the same time, he had a prodigious knowledge and understanding of the entire canon of classical Japanese literature, and could write fluently and beautifully in the language of the

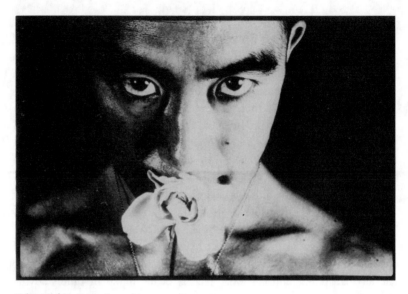

© EIKOH HOSOE

Yukio Mishima, c. 1963.

Heian Court of the medieval period. In fact, by the time he was a teen ager, he had conceived a vision of himself as the final heir to the tradition of classical Japanese beauty. This exalted vision informed a hundred-page story called "A Forest in Full Flower," which he wrote in 1941 at the age of sixteen. It was a dazzling tour de force, written in the elaborate style of *The Tale of Genji*, and it left the adults who were his mentors and champions speechless with admiration. Here is the youthful narrator:

> Now beauty is a gorgeous runaway horse, but there was a time when it was reined in and stood quivering in its tracks, and neighing at the misty morning sky. The horse was clean and pure then, graceful beyond compare. Now severity has let go the reins, and the horse runs headlong, stumbles, its flanks caked with mud. Yet there are times, even now, when a man is endowed with the eyes to see the phantom of an immaculate white horse. It is just such a man that our ancestors are searching for. Gradually, they will come to abide in him.

Mishima was, of course, talking about himself.

The war years, particularly the firebombing of Tokyo in 1944 and 1945, fanned the flames of his fantasy of beauty and death and privileged destiny. As he would later reflect with the wonderful clarity he often had about himself, "The narcissism at the border separating adolescence from adulthood will make use of anything for its own ends. At twenty, I was able to fancy myself as a genius destined for an early death, as a decadent among decadence, even as beauty's kamikaze squad." In 1949, Mishima established himself as a best-selling author with *Confessions of a Mask*, a chronicle of his homosexual awakening, which was in part an attempt to disempower his obsession with erotic death by accounting for it clinically and diagnosing it away. In 1951, he set out on his first trip to the West and embarked on his classical period, a conscious effort, fueled by super-human discipline, to put death behind him once and for all. The first entry in the diary of his journey indicates his determination to become a new man:

Sun, sun, perfect sun, today I did not watch the sunset. Having spent the day gazing lovestruck at the sun, I had no heart to see her in her ancient feeble makeup. In my boyhood, I felt that the sunset was the only justification for the sun's existence. As I bared myself to the sun today, I felt throughout my body the joy of release from the oversensitive stubbornness of my youth.

On his return from this trip, during which he visited New York and Rio (where he misbehaved somewhat) and then finally Greece, Mishima began the regimen of weightlifting that he continued for the rest of his life and that transformed him from a scrawny weakling, whose nickname at school had been Asparagus, into the muscle man that you see in some of Eikoh Hosoe's wonderful photographs.

As evidence of his rehabilitation, Mishima wrote *The Sound of Waves*, his best-selling book ever (from which several films have been made), his only love story that was neither perverted nor sardonic. Ten years later, while I was translating *The Sailor Who Fell from Grace with the Sea* and had the good fortune to spend many evenings at Mishima's home, I began a rhapsody about this book, which I'd just read, running on a bit about the purity and the innocence of the fisher-boy and the diving-girl and so on. I shall never forget how Mishima watched me. When I had finally con-cluded my rhapsody, he said, with a cigarette dangling from his lips, "That was a joke I played on my readers. A lie." And then he closed his eyes and did a sort of gesture as if he were writing the book with his eyes closed. It was a mortifying moment for me. By that time, he was already back in the grip of the death-ridden romanticism he had worked so hard to exorcise, and was moving rapidly in the direction that would end with his suicide. "Today, I no longer believe in that ideal known as classicism," he wrote in his diary in 1963, "and I have already begun to feel that youth, and the flowering of youth, are foolishness. What remains is the concept of death, the only truly enticing, truly vivid, truly erotic concept." For all I know, that twenty-six-year-old, that classicist who felt about himself that he was as close as possible to life, was a dissembler, a fraud.

In July 1968, Mishima published an article entitled "In Defense of Culture," an elaborate disquisition on identity. He argued that the Japanese were Japanese by virtue of Japanese culture, that the emperor was the source of culture, specifically that His Imperial Majesty was the emanating source of *miyabi*, a value in Japanese classical aesthetics that is usually defined as "courtly elegance," as epitomized in *The Tale of Genji*. In Mishima's singular definition, *miyabi* was the essence of court culture and the people's longing for that essence. If the Japanese ever hoped to regain their connection to the aesthetic quality that defined them, he believed they must protect the emperor at any cost. Here, for the final time, Mishima evoked the longing for connection to the cultural past, and specifically to the traditional beauty of the past, which he had first expressed as a young man in "A Forest in Full Flower."

It's important to realize that Mishima was not alone in his sense of discontinuity with a defining past. The terrorism on both the Right and the Left that characterized the 1960s, following the renewal of the U.S.-Japan Mutual Security Treaty, was evidence of a growing national uneasiness in the aftermath of the MacArthur constitution imposed on Japan during the occupation. And if American democracy was proving to be a not entirely satisfactory substitute for wartime values, neither was the frantic pursuit of gross national product that was being promulgated as the new national mission. By the late '60s, Japan's company man, the cog in the wheel of the economic miracle, was tired, hemmed in, too busy to take his annual one-week vacation, and beginning to wonder why life was affording him so little gratification, despite his hard work and new prosperity. Something was missing. The emerging consumer class was finding that the acquisition of wealth and property was not, after all, a goal worth living for. Asked what that goal might be, no one would have answered: "a reconnection with traditional beauty achieved by a warrior's death." Nonetheless, the about his own existence that Mishima increasingly suffered was endemic in Japan. Unquestionably, Mishima's suicide was personal and idiosyncratic, fully comprehensible only in the light of his lifelong erotic fantasies. At the same time, it should be understood as an unbearably lucid and apposite expression of a national affliction: the agony of cultural disinheritance.

One final word about Mishima's place in Japan today. The government and the public were furious and chagrined at the Mishima incident, which came just as Japan was re-emerging on the global scene as a major world economy. By 1980, except by a small number of Mishima worshippers on the far Right, he had been largely forgotten. Recently he has been redis-covered, and there is a full-scale Mishima boom in progress. In November 2000, on the thirtieth anniversary of his suicide, his publisher released the first volume of a new forty-two-volume *Complete Works of Yukio Mishima*. So far, the first fourteen of the major novels have appeared, and each volume has sold between five and six thousand copies at a price of fifty dollars a book. This is an astonishing statistic: book sales in Japan are cur-rently at an all-time postwar low. There's an explanation for this. By 1988, the global economy had created unprecedented affluence in Japan, and the Japanese were disporting themselves like the princes of the known uni-verse. In 1990, the economy took a sharp fall, from which it has yet to recover. By the middle of the decade, familiar troubling questions about identity and the purpose of life were in the air again, and a brash new nationalism was emerging. It seems clear that this environment has Japanese readers to reassess Mishima, and to find meaning for themselves in his work and his final act, evidence that he understood their current plight and might even serve as a beacon to guide them out of confusion and disheartenment toward a rediscovery of self.

THROUGH WESTERN EYES | JAY McINERNEY

Some years ago I interviewed Haruki Murakami, for another PEN event, and inevitably asked him a question about Mishima. His response was a brush-off, as I recall. He said that he wasn't really familiar with Mishima—he'd read him in school, and not at all since. And he made it clear that he didn't really like Mishima. He was annoyed by the question. This is more or less the response that I had been expecting. At least at that time, for many contemporary Japanese, Mishima was an embarrassment. And I suspect he still is. I remember when I first arrived in Japan as a teacher in 1979, partly inspired by my enthusiasm for Mishima, with a copy of *Sun and Steel* in my suitcase, my questions about him were greeted with impa-tience and even irritation by my students. "Why do you *gaijin* always talk about Mishima?" one of them asked me.

Mishima was a very strange Japanese. His ritual suicide, his final call to cast off Western influences and return to traditional Japanese values, including veneration of the emperor, has made him, for a long time, some-thing of a bad joke in his homeland. There is also a touch of parricide in

Murakami's response, which calls to mind the critical dismantling of Hemingway in the '60s and '70s in this country. Mishima was the looming figure in postwar Japanese letters, and nobody likes to be loomed over. Writers such as Murakami and Banana Yoshimoto are from another world, really, a post-Mishima Japan, probably the first generation of Japanese writers since Sōseki Natsume for whom Japan's uniqueness in its relation to the West is not necessarily an explicit theme, is not necessarily *the* theme. Their characters listen to Brahms and the Beatles unselfconsciously, as indeed do most of their contemporaries; they eat miso soup for breakfast and hamburgers for lunch; they wear kimonos to a wedding and Prada to a club. Consciously or not, this newer fiction represents a rejection of Mishima's and Tanizaki's generations.

Mishima, a cosmopolitan figure whose literary influences included Aeschylus and Dostoevsky and de Sade, was one of those rare Japanese of his generation who profoundly understood the West. However, his *seppuku* seems to have made him seem more remote to us, and to the contemporary Japanese, who have turned him into just the kind of oriental hothouse literary exotic that he despised. At the moment, he seems stranded somewhere in the middle of the Pacific. For Americans, he's often a beautiful icon of Japanese exoticism and inscrutability, while for the Japanese, he is sometimes the talented nutcase beloved of the *gaijin*. I remember being indignant when the Kris Kristofferson version of *The Sailor Who Fell from Grace with the Sea* came out, in 1976. You will remember that this is the story of a sailor who gives up the sea in order to marry a widow, and the gang of teenage nihilists who, having admired him as a sailor, decide to murder him once he betrays his lonely destiny and comes ashore. As a fledgling Orientalist back then, I told myself that the story didn't make sense removed from its Japanese context. I haven't seen the movie since it first appeared, but rereading the novel recently, I came to suspect that I was wrong about the cultural specificity of that story. I have to wonder if some young Japanese fan of *Lord of the Flies* would object as strenuously to a Japanese film version of that novel. Which is to say that I think some of Mishima's Western admirers are too content to exoticize him, and to insist upon his citizenship in what he himself contemptuously called the "flower-arranging nation."

No artist embodied the tortured contradictions of postwar Japan as thoroughly as Mishima, the homosexual who worried about Japan's effeminate image, the intellectual who championed the realm of the senses and the physical over the claims of words and ideas, the sickly aesthete who turned himself into a modern-day samurai. At the same time, though, his paradoxes and contradictions—between Apollo and Dionysus, word and world, thought and action—were thoroughly transcended. Or, to put it in the context of the time that I first came under his spell, it was as if he was both William Gass and John Gardner at the same time. For me, in the mid-'70s, he seemed far more vital than any American literary figure.

One of the tasks of reassessing Mishima is to stop seeing him as a representative figure. At the risk of robbing Mishima's life of the perfect shape which he apparently wanted to impose on it, I'm not sure that it would hurt to try to imagine what we would make of his oeuvre if he had, say, died in a car crash, in '68 or '69, or of an aneurysm on his way out the door on that final day in 1970, moments after completing the last installment of The Sea of Fertility. It wouldn't hurt to recall the Mishima that the world knew before he killed himself: an international literary figure, the most successful Japanese literary export of the twentieth century, a writer who has as much in common with Hemingway as he does with Lady Murasaki. We might do well to celebrate Mishima's contradictions rather than seeing them as solved by his death. We need to rescue him from the mists that obscure him; we need to see him in relation to his contemporaries, like his sometimes mentor Yasunari Kawabata, who called Mishima the kind of talent who comes along only once every two or three hundred years. Kawabata was the writer most admired by the *gaijin* in Kyoto in the late '70s—the one who seemed to represent a pure Japanese spirit untainted by Western influence: all those geishas, tea-masters, and Go-masters.

Mishima was a great admirer of Kawabata—although he seems to have written a somewhat unflattering portrait of the master in his novel *Forbidden Colors*—and also saw himself in opposition to Kawabata. Mishima used to rail against the insular aestheticism of much of Japanese literature and culture. Kawabata's aristocratic aesthetes are the epitome of the flower-arranging nation. To Western eyes, some of his books are less novels than series of beautiful tableaux, in the tradition of *The Tale of Genji*. Lady Murasaki's narrative, written some six hundred years before *Don Quixote*, is a weirdly fascinating story of erotic and court intrigue, and represents what Mishima saw as the feminine aesthetic in Japanese literature, the rarefied world of the Heian Court. Mishima eventually seems to have seen himself as resurrecting a more vigorous tradition of martial epic and the samurai ideal, represented by such post-*Genji* works as the *Heike monogatari*, written two hundred years later. But it's important to remember that he also, especially early in his career, acknowledged his debt to Western literary traditions. When asked by an interviewer about the negativity of his protagonists, he put the blame squarely on Western literary models. "We have learned mental disease and shame from the West," he said.

This is a very Japanese statement. His first novel, *Confessions of a Mask*, is a coming-of-age story of a young man discovering his own difference from his peers in the world into which he was born. It fits squarely into the so-called I-novel tradition of Japanese autobiography. But it also records his encounters with Western culture and literature, from the famous picture of Saint Sebastian pierced with arrows, to Greek drama. The epigraph comes from *The Brothers Karamazov*: "Beauty is a terrible and awful thing," it begins, and one wonders what Kawabata would say to that. It continues: "It is terrible because it never has and never can be fathomed, for God sets us nothing but riddles. Within beauty both shores meet and all contradictions exist side by side." This theme reaches its culmination in the great masterpiece of Mishima's middle period, *The Temple of the Golden Pavilion*, in which a young Buddhist priest feels enthralled and enslaved and finally negated by the beauty of the gold-plated temple in Kyoto where he studies and burns it to the ground in order to free himself. Although the story is based on a real incident in Japanese history, it seems to me a direct descendent of Dostoevsky's *Notes from Underground*.

I don't mean to suggest that Mishima is best understood as a Western writer or that we can, or even should, wish away the Japanese context of his work. I'm not sure I want to go back and see the Kristofferson version of *The Sailor Who Fell from Grace with the Sea*; nor do I think we can really pretend that Mishima died in a car wreck. On the other hand, I don't think we should privilege the strange nationalistic rhetoric and political obsessions of his final years, as many have done in order to dismiss him. It's reductive to view Mishima's oeuvre as a suicide note. The novels and stories are stunningly diverse, from the lyrical heterosexual love story of *The Sound of Waves*, through the homoerotic *Confessions of a Mask* and *Forbidden Colors*, to the vast epic of The Sea of Fertility, which I believe to be one of the masterpieces of twentieth-century fiction. The next time I see Haruki Murakami, I'm going to urge him to reread them.

LOST IN TRANSLATION | HORTENSE CALISHER

I was in Japan in 1958, and much later I wrote about it; I'm going to take little passages from that book. In Tokyo, I spent an evening with Yukio

Mishima . . . we got on. The memory must affect what I write here. But that alone does not entitle me to brood on his life and works. His death, however, was a public act, and the work a public offering. The world is invited, commanded, to brood. Place his suicide in a Western context, or in the Japanese one, or in both, where I think it most significantly belongs. Trace his progression toward it. Hear in every book its pure sound. True, only his last act has given us this after-event wisdom. But has he succeeded in that final coincidence of flesh and mind he hoped for?

We had met once before, in New York, at a Gotham Book Mart party for James Baldwin, where Mishima had looked as anyone does under such circumstances: tentative, interestedly afloat on a sea of foreign context. This second time, we did not really talk of literature. He was a handsome man, I thought, with a coherence of face and form. Though I felt very tall in Japan, and he was shorter, he did not appear small. I couldn't tell whether his face seemed as guarded to other Japanese as it seemed to me. Some triangular proportion in it, broad at the brows, made one look at eyes and mouth separately. Hindsight sees how such a face might empathize alternately, as his work did, with the ugly and the beautiful.

We laughed a lot that evening, and most of it was laughter over intramural jokes, not embarrassment or Occidental misinterpretation. Reading the glinting humor of *After the Banquet* five years later, I remember this laughter. When he and his friend kept saying how Oriental I looked, I told them how my daughter's boarding school had surreptitiously asked her if I was Eurasian. We sat, bright-eyed, sympathetically comfortable, and language-hampered. He told me with utter seriousness that he was building a Dutch colonial house. This had its pertinence.

Shortly afterwards, as my journal shows, I was to be sick with what was glibly called "cultural shock." At the time, I knew what it was but hadn't the wit to say. I was smelling the sweat of the dragon-flight, that odor of burnt ideologies, smoked-out shrines, commingled loins, and potsherds, which down the ages must hang invisibly wherever two civilizations are trying to engorge one another. I was seeing how a nation under occupation was dealing with its "conqueror." Mishima, born in 1925, educated at the Peers School, where the Spartan fires of militarism still burned, graduating as its highest honor student, mid-war, spent half his life under the clang of historical glory and all his manhood with the American conqueror standing sentinel at every street corner of Japan's culture.

Grounded deeply in his own literature, Mishima was widely read in Western thought, classical and modern. I told him that in my own country I had never heard a colleague mention the poet Novalis or Amiel, the author of *Journal intime*. But I met their names in his works—particularly, I think, in that strange book called *Sun and Steel*, Mishima's account of a child who refuses to perceive the body and is led into reality through words. In time, words, however useful, become the corrosive evil, and ideas become foreign to that romantic ideality of the body which he craves. In his attempt to straddle and manipulate the two, he becomes the novelist, only increasing further his thirst for reality and the flesh.

In this small book, most certainly a classic of self-revelation, his pursuit of that second language is examined with such dispassion and self-insight that paraphrase would only distort. We are in the range now of a metaphysics where every sentence counts and delivers its poignant message with a shock. "As a personal history, it will, I suspect, be unlike anything seen before," he says, and he is right. In his journey from the black Styx of the inner life to the blue sky of the outer as reflected in ordinary man's eyes, he sees at every point the parable of his own life. He's taking us down that psychic canal in very nearly complete consciousness. In *Sun and Steel*, as in all Mishima's work, one is encountering a mind of the utmost subtlety, broadly educated. The range of that mind may appear terrifying, or cynical, to those who demand of a writer steadily apparent or even monolithically built views. These are there, indeed touchable, at every point in his work; but the variation of surface and seeming reversals of heart, or statement, sometimes obscure this.

Mishima's Western scholarship is touching, all the more so for the possibility that as he rejected words for body, dead literature for live action, or tried to bring the two down to the average coherence, he was also denying the Western impurities that had early ensnared him. For everywhere, his references to our literature, our martyrs, are hallowed, reverent. He takes our classics as seriously as we did once, as a matter of life and death. And death he does illuminate and widen for us, but in a paradox we might well have anticipated, only when he takes his own unique path of learning and experience, not ours. For though he makes analogies with the martyrs of the Christianized West, in the end, the once proud grail of Western existence, addled and dusty as this has come to be, eludes him. What does not occur to him is that the sought death may be as artificial as imagination against the sought life.

Still, he is telling us that death is one of life's satisfactions. We may not be able to believe it, and I wish that death had not so enhanced itself for him. But he tells us how he came to this pass with a sanity that ought to be exquisite enough for our own, and crosses cultures to do it, to tell us how a man bent on *seppuku* might come to it by way of Saint Sebastian. Can Westerners understand such a death, or accept the artist who tosses his life in the balance as easily as they do those who jerk to the very end of the galvanizing money stream, or distill their life knowledge in teaspoonsful for the applause of a coterie?

Mishima is explaining his life and death in admirable style, in words that hold their breath, so that the meaning may breathe, and in a low voice, just short of the humble. Our souls may not be cognate, but he makes us feel again what it is to have one, and understand the persuasion of his. If he had been otherwise in his youth—a porter, a woman, a dancer—the tower of his symbols might have been built another way. But to ask him to break out of the mystic cage of his logic is like asking it of Thomas à Kempis, or Augustine, or to be a Catholic praying for the conversion of the Jews. He is telling us that he is a priori this kind of man, and that insofar as we cannot break out of the cage of our bones, so are we. He is telling us how he was made. To paraphrase him in words not his or with muscles not his is to try to build a China pagoda with a peck of nails. *Sun and Steel*'s power is that it is a book one must experience step by step, led as if by a monk or a great film master, from inner tissue to outer, and back again, along his way. It is not necessary to accept that way, but only the frivolous will not empathize with what is going on here. This is a being for whom life and death too must be exigent, and were.

SUBJECT MATTER | EIKOH HOSOE

I am Eikoh Hosoe, a photographer from Tokyo. It is a great honor for me to speak on this special occasion about my collection of photographs of *Ba-ra-kei*, or *Ordeal by Roses*, and my experience of photographing Yukio Mishima.

Ba-ra-kei began one day in September 1961 as a result of an assignment from the Japanese publisher Kodansha. I was commissioned to photograph Yukio Mishima for the cover of Mishima's book of critical essays, which Kodansha was about to publish.

I knew Mishima by name, but I had never met him. I was curious as to why I had been given such an important assignment and was told by the editor over the phone that I had been chosen at Mishima's special request. I instantly accepted the offer, but the question still remained:

Why had he chosen me?

Soon the editor and I were to meet Mishima, and I hoped to discover the reason for his request and at the same time have an opportunity to photograph him. A taxi was hired to take us to Mishima's house. We drove about thirty minutes from central Tokyo toward Omori Station. The cab suddenly turned in front of a public bathhouse, then followed a narrow path, turned sharply, and brought us in front of Mishima's remarkable house.

Beyond the iron gate, there were a few steps and a straight path about thirty feet long to the front door. To the left was a traditional Japanese house and to the right a flat lawn. In the center of the lawn was a mosaic zodiac made of black and white marble, about five feet in diameter.

On the veranda, Mishima, half-naked and wearing dark glasses, was sunbathing in a white garden chair. On a table, there was a tray with a cup of black tea and a half-finished grapefruit. It appeared that Mishima had just finished breakfast, alone at two o'clock in the afternoon.

After bowing in formal greeting, Mishima began to speak as if he already knew my first question. "I loved your photographs of Tatsumi Hijikata. I want you to photograph me like that, so I asked my editor to call you."

"Mr. Mishima, do you mean I can photograph you in my own way?" I asked.

"Yes, I am your subject matter. Photograph me however you please, Mr. Hosoe," he replied. All my questions and anxiety faded.

Tatsumi Hijikata, one of my great friends, was the originator of Butoh, a form of dance that is now known worldwide. He was devoted to Mishima's writing. In 1959, Hijikata's first major dance performance in Tokyo was based on Mishima's novel *Kinjiki*, or *Forbidden Colors*. Tatsuhiko Shibusawa, a novelist and authority on the Marquis de Sade, was close to both Mishima and Hijikata; he wrote that Hijikata had thrilled Mishima.

The photographs of Hijikata to which Mishima referred were from a thin catalogue for Hijikata's dance performance titled "Eikoh Hosoe's photographic collection dedicated to Tatsumi Hijikata," and it included a number of images of Hijikata selected from the series "Man and Woman" that I photographed between 1959 and 1960.

I soon realized Mishima never wanted a banal portrait of an author. In offering himself as the "subject matter" of my photographs, I thought he might have wanted to become a dancer himself. I was still in my twenties then, so I was naïve. I did not make the distinction between an international literary figure and a dancer.

Mishima's father happened to be watering the garden, so I grabbed his hose, and I wrapped Mishima's entire body in the hose and kept him standing in the center of the zodiac, where he was planning to erect a statue of Apollo.

I asked him to look up and concentrate on my camera, which I was holding from a ladder above. I shouted, "Keep looking at my lens very intensely, Mr. Mishima! Okay, that's great, keep going . . . " He never blinked while I shot two rolls of 35mm film. "I am proud of my ability to keep my eyes open for minutes," said Mishima.

"I have never been photographed like this," he said. "Why did you do it in this way?"

"This is the destruction of a myth," I replied.

"You should wrap the hose around Haruo Satō," he laughed. Haruo Satō was considered a literary giant at that time. But what I really meant was that I wanted to destroy the preconceived ideas about Mishima's image in order to create a *new* Mishima.

After I left, I thought I had gone too far and told Daido Moriyama, who was then my assistant, that I was afraid Mishima would become annoyed with me. I gave the editor ten photographs. Two days later I received a call from the editor saying that Mr. Mishima was very pleased with the photographs and he thanked me very much. Mishima's first book of critical essays was published in November 1961 under the title *The Attack of Beauty*.

The assignment was over, but I continued to be excited. I called Mishima to ask if I could photograph him again. He instantly accepted my offer, asking me, "When is the next session, Mr. Hosoe?"

My shooting sessions continued until the summer of 1962. I had ten sessions in total. In the beginning my ideas were vague, but gradually I came to have a concrete concept that it should be a subjective documentary about Yukio Mishima interpreted dogmatically by Hosoe in devotion to Mishima. How dogmatic? The theme that flows through the entire body of work was ultimately "Life and Death" through Yukio Mishima, borrowing his flesh and using a rose as a visible symbol of beauty and thorns.

Throughout the whole session Mishima was perfect "subject matter," a favorite term of his. He wrote in the preface for my book:

Before Hosoe's camera, I soon realized that my own spirit and the workings of my mind had become totally redundant. It was an exhilarating experience, a state of affairs I had long dreamed of. Hosoe merely explored via the medium of his camera—much as the novelist uses words and the composer sounds—the various combinations in which the objects to be photographed could be placed, and the light and shadow which made these combinations possible. For him, in short, the objects correspond to words and sounds.

One day Mishima showed me many black-and-white photographic prints of Italian Renaissance paintings by artists such as Raphael and Botticelli, and then he showed me several photographs of paintings of Saint Sebastian by Raphael. Mishima said, "How beautiful it is, don't you agree?"

I believe that a person's soul lives in any of his possessions, particularly in art objects, which live together with the artist's soul. Therefore I compounded the Renaissance paintings Mishima most loved into his body. I utilized anything he possessed and anything he had relationships with because *Ba-ra-kei* was meant to be a subjective photographic documentary. Mishima did not have any responsibility at all, except to be the subject.

During the six months I photographed Mishima, he never acted like a literary giant. He always carried a small traveling bag in which he put everything. I never saw him behave arrogantly toward anyone. He was sweet and sincere to those who were serious about things.

I'd like to tell you about an episode I once witnessed. Mishima often held parties at his home for intimate friends, who included writers, editors, and artists. On this occasion I too had been invited. It was the spring of 1965 or 1966. About twenty people were invited, among them a famous leftist writer and a popular novelist whose work Mishima loved. As everyone drank and engaged in lively chatter, the novelist approached Mishima and said loudly, "Teach me how to write a novel, please, Mr. Mishima." Everybody laughed because they thought it was a joke. However, the novelist was serious and Mishima took it seriously, too.

"I had the same experience," said Mishima. "When I was commissioned to write a novel for a newspaper, I asked a veteran novelist to help me. He ignored my request by saying, 'Don't joke.'" Mishima then turned to the popular novelist and said, "Yes, let's talk in the corner." They had a long conversation and I saw the novelist nodding as if he were being given good advice.

Finally, I must mention something about the change of the English title. When the work was initially published in book form in 1963, the title was *Killed by Roses*. Mishima and I chose this title together and the publisher agreed to it. Six years later, at the end of 1969, I suggested to Mishima that we publish a new edition of *Ba-ra-kei*. He agreed and then I proposed that we use the original publisher, who accepted.

All those who were involved in the project—Mishima, Tadanori Yokoo, the designer, the editor, and myself—gathered at Shueisha in the beginning of 1970. The publisher decided to publish an entirely revised bilingual edition in Japanese and English. At the meeting Mishima suggested changing the English title because he said it was not close enough to the Japanese *Ba-ra-kei*, which if translated literally means "punishment of roses."

At first I did not see any reason the original title should be changed just before the bilingual edition was to be published, especially since it was already well known in the world. Mishima was firm, however. He was so particular about his opinion that I finally agreed, and the English title was changed to *Ordeal by Roses*, which I like very much.

On November 25, 1970, Yukio Mishima committed ritual suicide and I understood well why he had been so persistent about changing the English title. *Ba-ra-kei*, or *Ordeal by Roses*, became a requiem to Yukio Mishima, a man of genius and sincerity.

RESTLESS INCARNATION | WILLIAM T. VOLLMANN

Like most novelists, Mishima writes principally about himself. In each volume of his Sea of Fertility tetralogy, which shines ever more obviously as one of the great works of the last century, the protagonist appears to have been reincarnated into a different body. First he is Kiyoaki, a sensitively self-destructive young dreamer who falls in love with the one woman he has been expressly prohibited from loving, and from that love he catches his death at age twenty. Next we see him as a kendo athlete with "a face like new-fallen snow, unaware of what lies ahead," who matures into a right-wing terrorist. In the third novel, he is reborn as a Thai princess who also dies young, of a snakebite; in the last, he's a handsome, cruel young lighthouse keeper. The reincarnated person can always be identified by a certain birthmark, and the identification gets accomplished by the other protagonist, whose name is Shigekuni Honda and who is a judge—perfect profession for a soul whose task it is to decide what might or might not be true and what existence means. In the first novel, he muses about Kiyoaki: "Up until now I thought it best as his friend to pretend not to notice even if he were in his death agonies, out of respect for that elegance of his." In fact, Honda never succeeds in preventing anybody's death agonies. Scrupulous, empathetic, intelligent, aching to understand, and ultimately impotent, Honda might as well be—a novelist. In effect, then, there are two main characters in this long work, the observer and the observed. Is the observed really one soul who comes to life four times, or has Honda deluded himself because he longs for supernatural coherence?

Mishima was both Honda and Kiyoaki, the one and the myriad. As an artist, he could create, but creation can never substitute for action. Action, on the other hand, may be powerful but cannot transcend ephemerality. Action dies, as does Kiyoaki, and as did, ultimately, Mishima himself, whose carefully politicized, aestheticized suicide was not only rabidly observed, but a failure on its own terms; the troops refused to rally to his cause. At least Isao, the kendo athlete of the second book, succeeds in assassinating somebody before he cuts his belly open. Mishima was ultimately more like Honda than like Isao, which is not a terrible thing: while he may be sterile, in the sense that he will not bring about any "great event," his empathy will endure. Honda's seeking, his sincerity, his fidelity to that not necessarily well-founded belief in the reincarnations, these are the strands of perception, conceptualization, and devotion which sustain the patterns of recurrence into something permanent and precious. Without Honda, the young man and the young woman who share nothing but a certain birthmark and a predilection to certain secret self-absorptions would not have added up to any collective thing. Thanks to him, they embody a sacred mystery. That is why Honda can be likened to the immense display case in the Mishima Yukio Literary Museum, where our author's books shine as colorfully frozen as any collection of immaculate butterflies.

So Honda is Mishima, and the butterflies, the various versions of Kiyoaki, are also Mishima, whose strangely plastic features—and this is a quality more often pertaining to women—seem capable of forming themselves into any number of vastly dissimilar faces. Sometimes in the photographs his very head appears elongated, as though he were Cambodian or Vietnamese; at other times it's rounder, like the clay head of some Assyrian idol; that frequently very sensitive and delicate face, that Kiyoaki-face, can on occasion appear bleached and bleak, like an aging prisoner's, or harden into that stereotyped clay vulgarity that I have seen in the attitudes of tattooed Yakuza gangsters who pose for my press camera. (This is, perhaps, an attempt on Mishima's part to embody himself as his Isao, the suicide-terrorist.) We have Mishima the suit-and-tie man, Mishima the flashy dancer caught from above and grainily à la Weegee, Mishima the artful poser in the dark kimono polka-dotted with light. And they are all his expressions of self, his legitimate incarnations. But only the Mishima called Honda sits down to the desk on which the bronze or brass letter opener surmounted with the medallion of a Caucasian's head (a certain Emperor Napoleon, I believe) lies beside a miniature sword; two very Japanese-looking metal fishes and a metal lizard bask eternally by a golden Parker pen. It is Honda who writes in the end of *Runaway Horses*: "The instant that the blade tore open his flesh, the bright disk of the sun soared up and exploded behind his eyelids." This defines Mishima's agony. As he writes in that eerie confession *Sun and Steel*,

> In the average person, I imagine, the body precedes language. In my case, words came first of all; then . . . came the flesh. It was already . . . sadly wasted by words. First comes the pillar of white wood, then the white ants that feed on it. But for me, the white ants were there from the start, and the pillar of plain wood emerged tardily, already half eaten away.

Kiyoaki has the body, of course, and Honda the words. And the words despise themselves, knowing that their own fulfillment necessarily spoils the body with sedentariness. But without the words to define and cohere, the body lapses into its own separate incarnations; and even its most dramatic self-expressions, its mutilations and orgasms, cannot win the *understanding* which words make possible and which will keep the body's consciousness whole. For all his athletic poses toward the end, the mere existence of the Mishima Yukio Literary Museum suffices to prove that the body was not enough for our novelist, that like Kiyoaki he was too restless to stay in one body, that he wanted to be the man of a thousand faces even if the close-cropped hair, the half-smoked cigarette, failed to remove him as much as he thought they did from kinship with a small boy who dresses up as a sailor. Yes, incarnation is restless, and so in some photographs, Mishima, who my own Japanese translator thinks was "definitely gifted, but somehow not really sure how to cope with the 'gift,'" wears a radiant, if at times hysterically radiant, smile, the white teeth tight together; in other images he tries to look stern. In those body-builder portraits, Mishima is rounded and drawn in on himself, transformed into clay, a stolid corporeality that expresses itself more loudly than the inner spirit. But I suspect that the spirit, which accentuated that corporeality because it loathes itself, feels tormented by that loudness and dares not confess it. Could that be one reason that Mishima chose death?

About that death, or at least about its supposed inevitability, a little more should be said. In *Sun and Steel* he bitterly complains about the fact that men cannot objectify themselves, and from the context it's evident that he means *objectify their bodies as women can*. "He can only be objectified through the supreme action—which is, I suppose, the moment of death, the moment when, even without being seen, the fiction of being seen and the beauty of the object are permitted. Of such is the beauty of the suicide squad." Mishima wrote those words in that languorously white house of his, which might be considered a little peculiar for the abode of a Japanese nationalist given its urns, its Greekish statues, and its European horoscope mosaic, that house which serenely bides and forebodes behind its white wall. If anything, it makes me think of the residence of the minister Kuruhara in the second volume of the tetralogy, *Runaway Horses*, whom Isao stabs to death in punishment for the crime of sacrilege. Kuruhara is, among other things, another Honda. The body hates the words (so, at least, the self-hating words say). The body freely, guiltlessly kills and copulates, marches, overthrows, makes history. It can do everything. But what's it made of? The white ants are already eating it. When Mishima, naked but for his loincloth, sits on the tatami mat for yet another photograph (if you knew him only by this image, you wouldn't suspect that he lives amid French engravings of nineteenth-century experimental balloons), when Mishima leans on the staff of his sheathed sword, his face, which to others, including himself, may evince resolution, to me betrays resignation, even vacancy, as if it cannot escape its own clay.

And yet that house with its erotic luxury and its hallmarks of foreign possibilities, that cosmopolitan house which Isao would never live in, that house was a perfect womb for a creative mind. Mishima could have become soft and fat living in that house. In his study stand Japanese brushes in a lacquerware cylinder, an elegantly slender calligraphy box, a block of scarlet ink for what I think is a stamp or seal; with these objects, perhaps, he could have incarnated himself into a living exemplar of the Japanese tradition which he imagined that he had to die for. He could have chosen any number of fates. And it may be significant that the tense, gruesome *Runaway Horses*, whose hero kills himself more or less as Mishima did, is not the final novel of the tetralogy, but the second.

What if Mishima had outlived his own death? Honda is condemned to outlive Isao's *seppuku* for two more volumes, in which nothing nearly as dramatic will occur. In the third novel, *The Temple of Dawn*, Honda witnesses what he thinks is Kiyoaki's reincarnation in the person of that beautiful, mysterious Thai princess. Mishima's mood becomes richly tropical here, and the discourses into Buddhist theology, which irritate some readers, to me evince a last flowering of intellectual excitement on Honda's part as he continues to attempt to find, and Mishima attempts to convey, perhaps to feel, the meaning of existence. But halfway through this novel, the famous aridity has already set in. Lovesickness, ideological rapture, and divine mysteries are done. The final book, *The Decay of the Angel*, exudes a suffocatingly existential quality. It's all about waiting for death—not the joyfully fanatical death of *Runaway Horses*, the death that Mishima tried unjoyfully to die, but the death of the white ants. Reading *The Temple of Dawn* always makes me feel that the tetralogy's end, and Mishima's corresponding finish, were not preordained. The enigmatic little Thai princess offers the prospect of something different, something not only as erotic as suicide, but perhaps more elusive, something worthwhile enough to warrant not killing oneself while one tries to uncover it. Very possibly, if *The Temple of Dawn* is any indication, this something could have been religion or philosophy. I wonder how feverishly Mishima hunted for it in his wood-clad study with its bookshelved walls. He didn't find it, and that is why every year on November 25, the white-clad Shinto priests lay down prayer streamers on the altar, which resembles a tabletop model of round-towered castles, and the blood-red disc of the Hinomaru flag hangs above them in the darkness beside Mishima's portrait.

THE WEIGHT OF WORDS | JOHN NATHAN

Having spent a lot of my time translating Mishima and Kenzaburō Ōe, two diametrically opposed writers, I can contrast them for you in terms of the immense challenge that they present to the translator. Ōe considers himself a liminal writer, working on the periphery of Japan. He's an outsider looking in, and his language accordingly constitutes an assault on everything the Japanese language has inherently and naturally inside itself, as a means of expression. Junichiro Tanizaki, *the* Japanese novelist at one time, reading Ōe, said, "If this is Japanese I am going to kill myself," because it was such a strange and a contorted language, which nonetheless, in Ōe's hands, becomes poetic. It's basically impossible to translate. Each sentence is an agony and an ordeal. Mishima, on the other hand, insisted on his place at the very center of the Japanese tradition of words. That longing for beauty and so on that he took inside himself and embodied was his notion of himself as being inside the language. And as a result, he's much easier to translate, because he was a gorgeous word-master, and he weighed out every word very carefully in a mosaic. And if the translator is able to understand him, and spends enough time looking for the proper stones, it is possible to inlay them into the syntax of an English sentence, paragraph, and book, without breaking the back of that sentence, which is what happens with Ōe, and so it is possible to represent Mishima in English that is at least close to the beauty of language that he achieved.

Talking about Mishima the writer is difficult without invoking Mishima the individual and Mishima the suicide. A lot of what's been said tonight—by me principally—is extratextual. The question is: How important is he? Near the end of his life, Mishima said about himself, in the kind of paradox he learned from Oscar Wilde, "I am a realist who attempts to depict with complete reality a romantic psychology which cannot be found in nature." It's dangerous to take a writer at face value when he's saying something like that, but I think Mishima was telling the truth. He was a man not to be found in nature, in the sense that he built himself into the complex creature he became. Individual works of Mishima are often marred by a kind of contrivance; characters can tend to dangle somewhat helplessly from the strings of a master puppeteer, who has them move in dramas and reveal themselves in ways unfamiliar to us because they're not something we have experienced. The result, I think, is that we can be moved by the gorgeousness of the man's work, which is often gorgeous, and by beautiful and unforgettable scenes, but finally, with some exceptions, we find it hard to identify and hard to feel that this man's art has opened a window for us on a world that we know as our own and shown us something about our own lives.

Still, there are writers about whom it can be said perhaps that their entire oeuvres, their complete works, can be seen as monuments to invention, and diligence, and passion, which are possibly greater and more important than any individual work. Balzac may be such a person, Thackeray may be such a person; certainly Mishima, I believe, was such a person. However, it remains a truth that this man's enormous commitment, and his passion, and his focus, and his invention, move us, even if we are put off by artificiality in some of his works. At the end of his life, he wrote, "If I could remember each hour of my life I spent weighing out words like a pharmacist with his scale, I would surely go mad." Before that kind of passion and artistic commitment, we finally must stand in awe.

SACRIFICE

Yukio Mishima

Translated by John Nathan

That morning, the boys had left the city with packed lunches and gone all the way to Yamauchi Pier in Kanagawa. For a while they had roamed around the railroad siding behind the sheds on the wharf, and then held the usual meeting to discuss the uselessness of Mankind, the insignificance of Life. They liked an insecure meeting place where intrusion was always a possibility.

The chief, number one, number two, Noboru (who was number three), number four, and number five were all smallish, delicate boys and excellent students. In fact most of their teachers lavished praise on this outstanding group and even held it up as an encouraging example to poorer students.

Number two had discovered that morning's meeting place and all the others had approved. In back of a large shed marked "City Maintenance A," a rusty railroad siding, apparently in long disuse, crawled through high wild chrysanthemums and old abandoned tires across an unkempt field. Far away in the small garden in front of the warehouse office, canna flowers were blazing in the sun. They were dwindling, end-of-summer flames, but so long as they were visible the boys didn't feel free of the watchman's eye, so they turned away and followed the siding back from the shed. The track stopped in front of a black heavily bolted warehouse door. They discovered to one side of the warehouse a patch of grass hidden by a high wall of red and yellow and deep-brown drums, and sat down. The garish sun was edging toward the summit of the roof but the little lawn was still in shade.

"That sailor is terrific! He's like a fantastic beast that's just come out of the sea all dripping wet. Last night I watched him go to bed with my mother."

Noboru began an excited account of what he had witnessed the night before. The boys kept their faces blank, but he could feel every eye on him and the straining to catch every word, and he was satisfied.

"And that's your hero?" the chief said when he had finished. His thin red upper lip had a tendency to curl when he spoke. "Don't you realize there is no such thing as a hero in this world?"

"But he's different. He's really going to do something."

"Oh? Like what, for instance?"

"I can't say exactly, but it'll be something . . . terrific."

"Are you kidding? A guy like that never does anything. He's probably after your old lady's money; that'll be the punch line. First he'll suck her out of everything she's got and then, bang, bam, see you around, ma'am—that'll be the punch line."

"Well, even that's something, isn't it? Something we couldn't do?"

"Your ideas about people are still pretty naïve," the thirteen-year-old chief said coldly. "No adult is going to be able to do something we couldn't do. There's a huge seal called 'impossibility' pasted all over this world. And don't ever forget that we're the only ones who can tear it off once and for all." Awe-stricken, the others fell silent.

"How about your folks?" the chief asked, turning to number two. "I suppose they still won't buy you an air rifle?"

"Naw—I guess it's hopeless," the boy crooned to himself, arms hugging his knees.

"They probably say it would be dangerous, don't they?"

"Yes. . . ."

"That's crap!" Dimples dented the chief's cheeks, white even in summer. "They don't even know the definition of danger. They think danger means something physical, getting scratched and a little blood running and the newspapers making a big fuss. Well, that hasn't got anything to do with it. Real danger is nothing more than just living. Of course, living is merely the chaos of existence, but more than that it's a crazy mixed-up business of dismantling existence instant by instant to the point where the original chaos is restored, and taking strength from the uncertainty and the fear that chaos brings to re-create existence instant by instant. You won't find another job as dangerous as that. There isn't any fear in existence itself, or any uncertainty, but living creates it. And society is basically meaningless, a Roman mixed bath. And school, school is just society in miniature: that's why we're always being ordered around. A bunch of blind men tell us what to do, tear our unlimited ability to shreds."

"But how about the sea?" Noboru persisted. "How about a ship? Last night I'm sure I caught the meaning of the internal order of life you talked about."

"I suppose the sea is permissible to a certain extent." The chief took a deep breath of the salt breeze blowing in between the sheds. "As a matter of fact, it's probably more permissible than any of the few other permissible things. I don't know about a ship, though. I don't see why a ship is any different from a car."

"Because you don't understand."

"Is that right? . . ." An expression of chagrin at this blow to his pride appeared between the chief's thin, crescent-shaped eyebrows. Their artificial look, as though they were painted on, was the barber's fault: he insisted, despite the chief's protestations, on shaving his brow and above his eyelids. "Is that right? Since when is it your place to tell me what I understand and what I don't?"

"C'mon, let's eat." Number five was a quiet, gentle boy.

They had just unwrapped their lunches on their laps when Noboru noticed a shadow fall across the lawn and looked up in surprise. The old watchman from the warehouse, his elbows propped on a drum, was peering in at them.

"You boys sure picked a messy place for a picnic." With admirable poise, the chief beamed a scrubbed, schoolboy smile at the old man and said: "Would it be better for us to go somewhere else? We came down to watch the ships, and then we were looking for a shady place to have lunch . . ."

"Go right ahead; you're not doing any harm. Just be sure not to leave any litter around."

"Yes, sir." The smiles were boyish, innocent. "You don't have to worry about that—we're hungry enough to eat the wrappings and everything, right, you guys?"

They watched the hunchback shuffle down the path, treading the border between sunlight and shadow. Number four was the first to speak: "There are plenty of that type around—about as common as you can get, and he just loves 'the youngsters.' I'll bet he felt so generous just now."

The boys shared the sandwiches and raw vegetables and little cakes in their lunches and drank iced tea from small thermos bottles. A few sparrows flew in over the siding and alighted just outside their circle, but no one shared even a crumb with the birds. Matchless inhumanity was a point of pride with every one of them.

These were children from "good homes," and their mothers had packed them rich and varied lunches: Noboru was a little ashamed of the plain-ish sandwiches he had brought. They sat cross-legged on the ground, some in shorts, some in dungarees. The chief's throat labored painfully as he wolfed his food.

It was very hot. Now the sun was flaming directly above the warehouse roof, the shallow eaves barely protecting them.

Noboru munched his food in nervous haste, a habit his mother often scolded him for, squinting upward into the glare as he ate as if to catch the sun in his open mouth. He was recalling the design of the perfect painting he had seen the night before. It had been almost a manifestation of the absolutely blue sky of night. The chief maintained that there was nothing new to be found anywhere in the world, but Noboru still believed in the adventure lurking in some tropical backland. And he believed in the many-colored market at the hub of clamor and confusion in some distant seaport, in the bananas and parrots sold from the glistening arms of black natives.

"You're daydreaming while you eat, aren't you? That's a child's habit." Noboru didn't answer; he wasn't equal to the scorn in the chief's voice. Besides, he reasoned, getting mad would only look silly because they were practicing "absolute dispassion."

Noboru had been trained in such a way that practically nothing sexu-al, not even that scene the night before, could surprise him. The chief had taken great pains to insure that none of the gang would be abashed by such a sight. Somehow he had managed to obtain photographs picturing intercourse in every conceivable position and a remarkable selection of precoital techniques, and explained them all in detail, warmly instructing the boys about the insignificance, the unworthiness of such activity.

Ordinarily a boy with merely a physical edge on his classmates presides at lessons such as these, but the chief's case was altogether different: he appealed directly to the intellect. To begin with, he maintained that their genitals were for copulating with stars in the Milky Way. Their pubic hair, indigo roots buried deep beneath white skin and a few strands already strong and thickening, would grow out in order to tickle coy stardust when the rape occurred . . . This kind of hallowed raving enchanted them and they disdained their classmates, foolish, dirty, pitiful boys brimming with curiosity about sex.

"When we finish eating we'll go over to my place," the chief said.

"Everything's all ready for you know what."

"Got a cat?"

"Not yet, but it won't take long to find one. Nothing will take long."

Since the chief's house was near Noboru's, they had to take a train again to get there: the boys liked this sort of unnecessary, troublesome excursion.

The chief's parents were never home; his house was always hushed. A solitary boy, he had read at thirteen every book in the house and was always bored. He claimed he could tell what any book was about just by looking at the cover.

There were indications that this hollow house had nourished the chief's ideas about the overwhelming emptiness of the world. Noboru had never seen so many entrances and exits, so many prim chilly rooms. The house even made him afraid to go to the bathroom alone: foghorns in the harbor echoed emptily from room to empty room.

Sometimes, ushering the boys into his father's study and sitting down in front of a handsome morocco-leather desk set, the chief would write out topics for discussion, moving his pen importantly between inkwell and copper-engraved stationery. Whenever he made a mistake, he would crumple the thick imported paper and toss it carelessly away. Once Noboru had asked: "Won't your old man get mad if you do that?" The chief had rewarded him with silence and a derisive smile.

But they all loved a large shed in the garden in back where they could go without passing under the butler's eye. Except for a few logs and some shelves full of tools and empty wine bottles and back issues of foreign magazines, the floor of the shed was bare, and when they sat down on the damp dark earth its coolness passed directly to their buttocks.

After hunting for an hour, they found a stray cat small enough to ride in the palm of Noboru's hand, a mottled, mewing kitten with lackluster eyes.

By then they were sweating heavily, so they undressed and took turns splashing in a sink in one corner of the shed. While they bathed, the kitten was passed around. Noboru felt the kitten's hot heart pumping against his wet naked chest. It was like having stolen into the shed with some of the dark, joy-flushed essence of bright summer sunlight.

"How are we going to do it?"

"There's a log over there. We can smack it against that—it'll be easy. Go ahead, number three."

At last the test of Noboru's hard, cold heart! Just a minute before, he had taken a cold bath, but he was sweating heavily again. He felt it blow up through his breast like the morning sea breeze: intent to kill. His chest felt like a clothes rack made of hollow metal poles and hung with white shirts drying in the sun. Soon the shirts would be flapping in the wind and then he would be killing, breaking the endless chain of society's loathsome taboos.

Noboru seized the kitten by the neck and stood up. It dangled dumbly from his fingers. He checked himself for pity; like a lighted window seen from an express train, it flickered for an instant in the distance and disappeared. He was relieved.

The chief always insisted it would take acts such as this to fill the world's great hollows. Though nothing else could do it, he said, murder would fill those gaping caves in much the same way that a crack along its face will fill a mirror. Then they would achieve real power over existence.

Resolved, Noboru swung the kitten high above his head and slammed it at the log. The warm soft thing hurtled through the air in marvelous flight. But the sensation of down between his fingers lingered.

"It's not dead yet. Do it again," the chief ordered.

Scattered through the gloom in the shed, the five naked boys stood rooted, their eyes glittering.

What Noboru lifted between two fingers now was no longer a kitten. A resplendent power was surging through him to the tips of his fingers and he had only to lift the dazzling arc seared into the air by this power and hurl it again and again at the log. He felt like a giant of a man. Just once, at the second impact, the kitten raised a short, gurgling cry . . .

The kitten had bounced off the log for the final time. Its hind legs twitched, traced large lax circles in the dirt floor, and then subsided. The boys were overjoyed at the spattered blood on the log.

As if staring into a deep well, Noboru peered after the kitten as it plummeted down the small hole of death. He sensed in the way he lowered his face to the corpse his own gallant tenderness, tenderness so clinical it was almost kind. Dull red blood oozed from the kitten's nose and mouth, the twisted tongue was clamped against the palate.

"C'mon up close where you can see. I'll take it from here." Unnoticed, the chief had put on a pair of rubber gloves that reached up to his elbows; now he bent over the corpse with a pair of gleaming scissors. Shining coolly through the gloom of the shed, the scissors were magnificent in their cold, intellectual dignity: Noboru couldn't imagine a more appropriate weapon for the chief.

Seizing the kitten by the neck, the chief pierced the skin at the chest with the point of the blade and scissored a long smooth cut to the throat. Then he pushed the skin to the sides with both hands: the glossy layer of fat beneath was like a peeled spring onion. The skinned neck, draped gracefully on the floor, seemed to be wearing a cat mask. The cat was only an exterior, life had posed as a cat.

But beneath the surface was a smooth expressionless interior, a placid, glossy-white inner life in perfect consonance with Noboru and the others; and they could feel their own intricate, soot-black insides bearing down upon and shadowing it like ships moving upon the water. Now, at last, the boys and the cat, or, more accurately, what had been a cat, became perfectly at one.

Gradually the endoderm was bared; its transparent mother-of-pearl loveliness was not at all repellent. They could see through to the ribs now, and watch, beneath the great omentum, the warm, homey pulsing of the colon.

"What do you think? Doesn't it look too naked? I'm not sure that's such a good thing: like it was bad manners or something." The chief peeled aside the skin on the trunk with his gloved hands.

"It sure is naked," said number two.

Noboru tried comparing the corpse confronting the world so nakedly with the unsurpassably naked figures of his mother and the sailor. But compared to this, they weren't naked enough. They were still swaddled in skin. Even that marvelous horn and the great wide world whose expanse it had limned couldn't possibly have penetrated so deeply as this . . . the pumping of the bared heart placed the peeled kitten in direct and tingling contact with the kernel of the world.

Noboru wondered, pressing a crumpled handkerchief to his nose against the mounting stench and breathing hotly through his mouth: "What is beginning here now?"

The kitten bled very little. The chief tore through the surrounding membrane and exposed the large, red-black liver. Then he unwound the immaculate bowels and reeled them onto the floor. Steam rose and nestled against the rubber gloves. He cut the colon into slices and squeezed out for all the boys to see a broth the color of lemons. "This stuff cuts just like flannel."

Noboru managed, while following his own dreamy thoughts, to pay scrupulous attention to the details. The kitten's dead pupils were purple flecked with white; the gaping mouth was stuffed with congealed blood, the twisted tongue visible between the fangs. As the fat-yellowed scissors cut them, he heard the ribs creak. And he watched intently while the chief groped in the abdominal cavity, withdrew the small pericardium, and plucked from it the tiny oval heart. When he squeezed the heart between two fingers, the remaining blood gushed onto his rubber gloves, reddening them to the tips of the fingers.

What is really happening here?

Noboru had withstood the ordeal from beginning to end. Now his half-dazed brain envisioned the warmth of the scattered viscera and the pools of blood in the gutted belly finding wholeness and perfection in the rapture of the dead kitten's large languid soul. The liver, limp beside the corpse, became a soft peninsula, the squashed heart a little sun, the reeled-out bowels a white atoll, and the blood in the belly the tepid waters of a tropical sea. Death had transfigured the kitten into a perfect, autonomous world.

I killed it all by myself—a distant hand reached into Noboru's dream and awarded him a snow-white certificate of merit—*I can do anything, no matter how awful.*

The chief peeled off the squeaky rubber gloves and laid one beautiful white hand on Noboru's shoulder. "You did a good job. I think we can say this has finally made a real man of you—and isn't all this blood a sight for sore eyes!"

From *The Sailor Who Fell from Grace with the Sea*

MANIFESTO: 1914

Our Vortex

I.

. . . The new vortex plunges to the heart of the Present.

The chemistry of the Present is different from that of the Past. With this different chemistry we produce a New Living Abstraction.

The Rembrandt Vortex swamped the Netherlands with a flood of dreaming.

The Turner Vortex rushed at Europe with a wave of light.

We wish the Past and Future with us, the Past to mop up our melancholy, the Future to absorb our troublesome optimism.

With our Vortex the Present is the only active thing.

Life is the Past and the Future.

The Present is Art.

II.

Our Vortex insists on watertight compartments.

There is no Present—there is Past and Future, and there is Art.

"Just life" or soi-disant "Reality" is a fourth quantity, made up of the Past, the Future, and Art.

This impure Present our Vortex despises and ignores.

For our Vortex is uncompromising.

We must have the Past and the Future, Life simple, that is, to discharge ourselves in and keep us pure for non-life, that is Art.

The Past and Future are the prostitutes Nature has provided.

Art is periodic escapes from this Brothel.

Artists put as much vitality and delight into this saintliness, and escape out, as most men do their escapes into similar places from respectable existence.

The Vorticist is at his maximum point of energy when stillest.

The Vorticist is not the Slave of Commotion, but its Master.

The Vorticist does not pander to Life.

He lets Life know its place in a Vorticist Universe!

—R. ALDINGTON, GAUDIER-BRZESKA, E. POUND,
W. ROBERTS, E. WADSWORTH, WYNDHAM LEWIS

ISLANDIA

María Negroni

Translated by Anne Twitty

Sus crónicas contara la alter ego,
su cicatriz que après la lettre no sana,
pero infelice historia que narrara
no aclara razón de sus fatigas
ni afán de citadina lumbre
ni el canvas de su isla donde vive.
A menos que, un snapshot la sorprenda
en gesto de zarpar (rewind: cuestión
dudosa), esperanza no hay.
Tempestad o persecución a posteriori
difícilmente errante iluminarle
puedan su underground. Ella, in rallenti,
se mantiene inmutable: en el punto
cardinal de su aventura, salmodia
—cual si casta fuera o valiente—
¡Santa Escapatoria! (Todo jardín
es tránsito—¡ay!—y ella lo ignora.)

Nadie dijo que la verdadera forma de la isla es el borde. Ni siquiera el perfil
índigo o magenta de los fiordos ni el puerto provisorio ni el viento, soplando
sobre los hombres áridos. Dijo: un cuerpo tibio se parece a la niebla que—como
lo diáfano—desdibuja y configura y es el marco y el objetivo del mar. En un

---

Anne Twitty won the 2002 PEN Award for Poetry in Translation for her rendering of María
Negroni's *Islandia*.

Alter ego would recite her chronicles,
her unhealed scar après la lettre,
but infelice, the tale she'd tell
leaves motive in the dark, obscure
her citified desire, blacked out
the canvas of her island residence.
Unless a snapshot catches her
in act of setting sail (rewind:
remote), there is no hope.
Tardy theatrics, belated inquiry
unlikely to illuminate her tunnel
vagaries. She, in rallenti,
imperturbable, at her adventure's
cardinal point, intones
—as if she valiant were, or chaste—
Holy Moly! (Every garden
transitory—alas!—she doesn't know.)

No one said that the true shape of the island is its edge. Not even the magenta or
indigo outline of fjords nor the provisory port nor the wind, blowing over the
arid men. Said: a warm body resembles fog which—like the diaphanous—blurs
and configures and is the frame and objective of the sea. In a motionless array of

orden inmóvil de barcos perdidos, la felicidad puntiaguda no existe pero simu-
larla es posible. Imantados, como haciendo memoria, los hombres se miraron
entre sí. Condensarse en la frustración (pensaban), hacer un bastión (una intri-
ga larga) de un repertorio de dudas, apostar a un viaje de avatares tortuosos,
atestado de souvenirs y desperdicios. La isla podría ser una forma sutil, feroz, del
sufrimiento . . . como crear . . .

A menos que la percepción los engañe, el miedo a ser engullidos. ¿Son
éstas sus viejas lealtades? ¿Este manojo de sombras representando a sombras que a veces llegan, los visitan? ¿Estas voces que cuesta reconocer?
¿Muecas, manos que se frotan, aluden a una guerra antigua, tejes y mane-
jes, todo el veneno en el cuerpo y debajo nada? A menos que los fantas-
mas sean ellos, ellos ensoberbecidos los que ensanchan la divergencia, los
que habilitan disturbios de la nada. Luna y fogatas encendidas, mientras
piensan. Mientras aducen que otras cosas los urgen, no este rejunte de
corazón y de nervios, esta insolvencia de saber qué sienten. A lo mejor ya
no sufren o es un dolor inútil, ¿a qué conduciría (que no fuera una ligera
cancion, una cínica ligera canción) este cansancio carente de reproches?
¿A qué ventaja, si ni siquiera inflige la autocompasión? ¿A qué licencia, si
no es más que tedio? Pero ¿y si no es así? ¿Si algo se ha despegado? ¿Está
listo para reducirse a un destino? Luna y fogatas encendidas. Temblaban.
Y después no se sabe . . .

La de lilios en la ribera del Hudson,
la homónima niña, incansable huésped,
enlaces entre qué y qué tenderá.
Qué tema intentaría, si la gracia está
en la tonada qué vaina, y no al revés.
Donc, aunque hundiera su embarcación,
la queme en rústico cantar, no importa.
Coplas de su madame, de su dicción
maleva y fuegos de artificio, ha de escribir.
Lástimas no. Que hipotética vida de
santa no contempla su vocación sino
murgas, lentejuelas, el buen arte de velar.
En festival Islandia ha de clavar bandera
y, provisoria, asuntos. En fortaleza
abierta de un plumazo: —¡De aquí,
no me moverán!

lost ships, stabbing joy does not exist but can be feigned. Magnetized, as if trying to remember, the men looked at each other. Cling to frustration (they thought), make a bastion (a lengthy intrigue) out of a repertoire of doubts, wager on a journey of tortuous happenstance, stuffed with souvenirs and flotsam. The island could be a subtle, vicious form of suffering . . . like the act of creation . . .

Unless perception deceives them, the fear of being devoured. Are these their old loyalties? This handful of shadows representing shadows that sometimes arrive, visit them? These almost unrecognizable voices? Grimaces, handrubbing, alluding to an old war, conspiracies, bodies full of venom and nothingness? Unless they are themselves the ghosts, their arrogance widening divergence, they, who conjure riots out of emptiness. Moon and lit fires, while they ponder. While they adduce that other things impel them, not this clutter of heart and nerve, this bankruptcy of consciousness. Possibly they no longer suffer or it is a futile pain, what could this weariness bereft of reproach lead to (besides a light song, a cynical light song)? To what end, if it does not even inflict self-pity? To what license, if it is nothing but boredom? But, what if it is not so? If something has shaken loose? Is ready to be reduced to fate? Moon and lit fires. They trembled. And then who knows . . .

The lily maid on banks of River Hudson,
homonymous, revisitor, now where
to stretch her nets. What theme
try now, and what the hell, since
it's the tone that counts, not vicevers.
Donc, though she sink, or burn
her boats in rustic lay, who cares.
Lady ballads, street argot
and pyrotechnics she'll transcribe.
Not plaints. No hypothesis
of saint, she'll dandle sequins, street
musicians, artful veil. In festival
Islandia her standard plant, also,
for now, her daily grind. In fortress
cloven by a quill: —I
take my stand!

No saber si posponen lo real porque son cómodos e indulgentes o porque les sobra la imaginación, el mero desorden de ideas. Si son juiciosos para llegar más pronto a la lucidez o porque así compensan el asombro que los embargaría o porque no tienen experiencia. Si algo pierden de lo que ven porque lo ven como espectáculo. Si el desprecio que ostentan por lo vulgar es prematuro, usurpa el lugar de algo. Si únicamente la ruindad, a lo sumo una dulzura enconada abre una franja de emoción, sólo entonces el corazón da vuelcos, no se deja confinar, la belleza es asidua, extraviada. No saber si los seres que crean de sí mismos son postizos, apenas una excusa para la conmoción, un hormigueo en frenesí de lenguaje, una enjundia tocada de pasada. Si no atraviesan la obsesión para morirla, y la distancia, las jaulas . . .

Pregones y séquitos y contados
los días de un plazo. La viérades.
Indecisa melisendra, muy más que
prisionera o trunca de su gesta,
begli occhi airada en desenfreno
su entremesil razón de confundida.
Malmaridada, en cancionero sutil
exaspera el recuerdo, lo devora.
¡Qué estelas ha de escribir aún en gráfico
paisaje! ¡Por todo homenaje en su
anonimia, qué pródiga ha de ser!
¡En qué caballerías una sola
página que valga! La viérades:
se mesa los cabellos. Se indaga el
cómo, del cálculo al impulso, volver.

Testamento de escalda: "Sé que no alcanza. Que escribo apenas escrutinios con final, sin arranques, evasiones en círculo a través de la niebla, vestigios de seres humanos, no seres humanos. Que la soledad es aparente. Que no he sabido celebrar. Doy marcha atrás. No quiero la dignidad, ni siquiera una violencia muda que no consigue hacer de mí un nido de repeticiones, una forma vaga como el tiempo. A lo mejor, la malicia no me toque pero la perplejidad sí me tocará (cuando alcance el borde de la ficción). Seré tan intenso que el latido de mi corazón lo inundará todo, entre yo y lo que veo no habrá nada, ninguna multitud, ningún ruido. No sabré seducir pero deslumbraré. (Estaré concentrado en la pena.) Deben esperar. Deben esperar que renuncie a ser tieso, brillante. Que me

Not knowing if they postpone reality because they are idlers and self-indulgent or because they are too full of imagination, the mere disorder of ideas. If they are prudent in order to reach lucidity more quickly or to save themselves from drowning in astonishment or because they lack experience. If some of what they see is lost because they regard it as a spectacle. If their disdain for the vulgar is premature, usurping something else. If only utter wickedness, at most, a rankling sweetness, bares a fringe of emotion, only then the heart somersaults, is uncontainable, beauty is assiduous, astray. Not knowing if those beings they create from themselves are fabrications, no more than a pretext for commotion, an anthill crazed with language, a momentary touch of grandiosity. If they do not travel obsession to put an end to it. It, and the distance, the cages . . .

Street criers, retinue, a few
allotted days. You should see her.
Indecisive Melisande, worse than
prisoner, deprived of geste,
begli occhi furious and wild,
her wits a babbling interlude.
Unhappy ballad wife in subtle song
exacerbates, devours memory.
What wakes will she inscribe on graphic
landscape! Sole homage in obscurity,
how prodigal will be!
Which quests will serve to write
a single worthy page! You should see her
tear her hair. Ask how from rationality
retrace her impulse.

Skald's testament: "I know it is not enough. That I write mere surveys with conclusions, lacking outbursts, circular evasions through the fog, not human beings, only vestiges. That loneliness is illusory. That I have not been able to celebrate. I go backward. I don't want dignity, not even a mute violence that fails to transform me into a nest of repetitions, a form as vague as time. Though malice may not be my portion, perplexity shall be (when I fill fiction to the brim). I shall be so intense that the beating of my heart will flood everything, between me and what I see nothing will remain, no multitude, no sound. I may not know how to seduce but I will dazzle. (Nothing will distract me from pain.) You have to wait. Have to wait for me to renounce (brilliant) rigidity, for me

someta, invisible a mí mismo, a la penumbra del deseo. Con la mitad me bas-
tará. Sólo es perentorio que esperen (. . .)"

Nadie dijo: Habrá para saquear vetas dispersas y un alboroto de escenas
panorámicas como cosecha estruendosa, el futuro llegará a medida que lo
creen, de la mano de un dolor agudo o del silencio o (incluso) de la aver-
sión del amor. No propuso el mundo como peculio de imágenes, ni sugir-
ió que era posible elegir una pena como quien hace ineludible el tiempo,
le cuida los fragmentos, los astilla. Dijo: Hubiera sido mejor ser tardíos. Se
vive siempre lo mismo, momentos perdidos, recaídas. Se gira sobre un
punto muerto, una constante de dolor y de miedo, un boceto que alguna
vez estuvo, un pedacito único, privado. Si se tiene suerte. Después hubo el
silencio, la reacción lenta, los cuerpos deletreando un conflicto, extraña
figura. (Era atroz estar en los comienzos.) Alguien apresuró: La vida es un
trapo entonces donde los hombres estrellan su violencia y tú puedes com-
poner con eso una obra de arte. Era un escalda, inmaduro, que no había
entendido . . .

No volvieron. No volverían nunca. No los vencería la tentación. (No con-
viene mezclar dos lealtades.) Tal vez ya fuera tarde. O se hubieran ido para
despistar. Como si hubieran visto un recuerdo (un destino). Tal vez el viaje
fuera ilícito. Lo afrontaron. Ni más ni menos que otros. Tuvieron lo que
están soñando, todavía, pero sólo a condición de no dejar de imaginarlo, a
condición de coserlo a la desgracia. A lo poco que no quisieron saber.

to submit, hidden from my own eyes, to the shadow of desire. Halfway would be
enough. Your only imperative: to wait (. . .)"

No one said: There will be scattered veins to sack and an uproar of panoramic scenes like thundering harvest, the future will arrive as you create it, hand in hand with a bitter pain and with silence or (even) an aversion to love. No one proposed the world as a peculium of images, nor suggested that it was possible to select a grief like one who makes time inescapable, guards its fragments, splinters them. Said: It would have been better to retard maturity. The same is relived forever, lost moments, relapses. Spinning on a still point, a repetition of pain and fear, a sketch that once existed, a unique, private fragment. With any luck. Afterwards there was silence, sluggish reaction, bodies spelling out conflict, a strange form. (Unbearable, to find they had not moved.) Someone hastily: Life, then, is a cloth where men splatter their violence and from it you can make a work of art. It was a scald, unfledged, who had not understood . . .

They did not go back. Would never go back. They would not succumb to that temptation. (Better not confuse one loyalty with another.) Perhaps it was too late. Or they had gone away to throw others off the scent. As if they had glimpsed a memory (a destiny). Perhaps it was an illicit voyage. They confronted it. No more or less than others. They had whatever they could dream, and live it still, on pain of having to imagine it, fasten it to misfortune. To the little they would not explore.

PISHTACOS

Marie Arana

The corridors of my skull are haunted. I carry the smell of sugar there. The odors of a factory—wet cane, dripping iron, molasses pits—are up behind my forehead, deep inside my throat. I'm reminded of those scents when children offer me candy from a damp palm, when the man I love sighs with wine upon his tongue, when I inhale the heartbreaking sweetness of rotting fruit and human waste that rises from garbage dwellers' camps along the road to Lima.

I am always surprised to learn that people do not live with memories of fragrance as I do. The smell of sugar is so strong in my head. That they could have spent the first years of their lives in places like Pittsburgh or Hong Kong and not gone for the rest of their days with the stench of a steel furnace or the aromas of fungus and salt shrimp tucked into some netherfold of cortex—how is that possible?

I had a friend once, from Bombay, who told how baffling it was to travel this world smelling turmeric, coriander, and cardamom in the most improbable corners of Nantucket or Palo Alto, only to find that they were Loreleis of the olfactory whiffs of his imagination, sirens of his mother's curry wafting in like she-cats, flicking seductive tails.

He chased after those smells, cooking up curries in rented houses in New Jersey, in tidy chalets in Switzerland, in motel rooms along the Shenandoah, mixing pastes from powders out of bottles with Scottish

---

American Chica by Marie Arana was nominated for the 2002 PEN/Martha Albrand Award for the Art of the Memoir.

surnames, searing ghees in Sara Lee aluminum, washing out lunch boxes in Maryland rest stops, trying to bring it back. Bring it back. Up into the sinus, trailing down the throat. He was never quite able to recapture that childhood blend: mashed on stone, dried in a Mahabharatan sun, stuffed into earthenware, sold in an old man's shop, carried home in string-tied packages, measured onto his mother's mortar, locked into the chambers of his heart.

So it has been with me and sugar. I look back and see piles of it, glittering crystals of it—burned, powdered, superfine. I smell sugar everywhere. On whispers, in books, in the loam of a garden. In every cranny of life. And always—always—it is my father's sugar I am longing for: raw, rough, Cartavio brown.

Cartavio was the name of our hacienda: a company town as single of purpose as Akron or Erie or Turin or anyplace where pistons and steel drive residents' lives. It was the mid 1950s, boom days for sugar in Peru, and the American industrial giant W. R. Grace was making the most of it in this remote coastal hamlet, five hundred miles north of Lima. Cartavio was surrounded by fields of sugarcane, fringed by a raging Pacific, and life in it was an eerie mirror of Peru's conquistador past. On one side of the hacienda were the cinnamon-skinned indigenous in a warren of cinder block. On the other, in houses whose size and loveliness depended on the rank of their inhabitants, lived Peruvians of Spanish ancestry, Europeans, North Americans, the elite. There was a church on the square, a mansion for the manager, a Swiss-style guest house, a country club, and a clinic. But in the middle, with smokestacks thrusting so high there could be no doubt as to why the unlikely multitude was there: my father's factories.

Cartavio was nestled in the heart of the nation, just under the left breast of the female torso that Peru's landmass defines. But it was, in many ways, a foreign place, a twentieth-century invention, a colony of the world. Its driving force was industry, and the people who had gathered there were, one way or another, single-minded industrialists. The Americans had come with dollars; the Limeños with political power; the villagers with hands. Although their objectives were shared—a humming production of sugar and paper—Cartavio citizens lived in uncertain harmony. The laborers were willing to surrender themselves to the practicalities of an iron city by day, but under their own roofs by night they returned to ancient superstitions. The Lima engineers were willing to obey the gringo directives, but they suspected they knew a great deal more about those factories than any mahogany-desk boss in New York. The Americans soon learned that if the indigenous believed in ghosts and the *criollo* overlords resented gringo power, then Grace's fortunes turned on such chimeras as phantoms and pride. They understood the social dynamic, used it, and with old-fashioned American pragmatism, made it work for them.

I knew, with a certainty I could feel in my bones, that I was deeply Peruvian. That I was rooted to the Andean dust. That I believed in ghosts. That they lived in the trees, in my hair, under the *aparador*, lurking behind the silver, slipping in and out of the whites of my ancestors' portraits' eyes. I also knew that, for all his nods and smiles at the gringos, my father believed in ghosts, too. How could he not? He faced them every day.

To the hacienda of Cartavio, Papi was *Doctor Ingeniero*, the young Peruvian engineer in charge of the people and the maintenance of this whirring, spewing, United States–owned mill town. He was a sunny man with an open face. Although his hands were small, they were clever. Although he was not tall, his shoulders filled a room. There were photographs my mother would point to when she wanted us to know she thought him handsome, but they were of a man I didn't recognize—gaunt and angular, black wavy hair, eyes as wide as a calf's, mouth in a curl. The Papi I knew was barrel-chested, full-lipped. His hair had receded to a V. His cheeks were cherubic and round. His eyes bulged. In the subequatorial heat, he wore his shirt out, and it flapped in the breeze, revealing skin that was brown, smooth, and hairless. He was not fat but taut as a sausage— *bien papeado*, as Peruvians like to say. Potato-tight. When he laughed, he made no sound. He would lean forward as if something had leapt on his back and held him in an irresistible tickle. His eyes would squint, the tip of his tongue would push out, and his shoulders would bounce vigorously. He'd laugh long and hard like that—silent, save for the hiss that issued from between his teeth—until he was short of breath, red-faced, and weeping. When he wasn't laughing, he was barking orders. When he wasn't doing that, his mouth was ringing a cigarette, sucking hard, his eyelids fluttering in thought.

Papi would not so much walk as strut. Not so much drink as guzzle. Not so much chat with a woman as flirt, wink, and ogle. He was clearly not the slender, soulful man in Mother's photographs. Not anymore. From the moment he registered on my brain, he was straining buttons, *bien papeado*—threatening to burst.

He was a machine virtuoso, improvising ways to go from desert to sugar, from burned plants to Herculean rolls of paper. He could take a field of sugarcane into his steel colossus, shove it through squealing threshers, wet it down with processed seawater, suck it dry of crystals, and feed it onto the rollers to emerge warm and dry from the other end as flying sheets of paper. He could take a faulty German turbine whose only hope for survival was a spare part eight thousand miles away in Stuttgart and, with a knickknack here, a length of wire there, make it hum again. He could pacify the gringos when they came from New York, matching them eye for eye on the intricacies of macromechanics or spherical trigonometry or particle physics. He inspired fervent loyalty from his laborers, striding through his iron city in an impeccably white suit, teaching them the way to an industrial future. The American way.

Every morning he would head for the belching beast long before the whistle sounded. In late afternoons, he returned to survey his pretty wife over lunch and take a brief siesta in his chair. But there seemed to be no end to his work. Even as he walked back through the gate for a late lunch or dinner and the servants fluttered into the kitchen to announce the *señor* was home, he was on call. Ready to pull away.

That he had to work with ghosts was a fact of life and everybody knew it. A worker's hand might be drawn into the iron jaws of the *trapiche* as it gathered cane into its mandibles and pulled the mass into its threshers. A finger, a foot, a dog, a whole man might be lost to that ravenous maw as it creaked and shook and thrashed and sifted everything down to liquid sugar and a fine bagasse.

Los pishtacos, the workers would say to one another whenever such tragedies occurred. *Pishtacos*, their wives and mothers would whisper the next day as they combed the market or polished the silver services on the richly carved *aparadores* of the engineers. Ghosts. Machine ghosts. *Pishtacos norteamericanos*. And as anyone who knew Peruvian *historias* understood: They needed the fat of *indios* to grease their machines.

Our house stood on the corner of prime real estate, behind the offices of head engineers but far enough from the factory to allow us to ignore the less pleasant aspects of a churning industry. Finished in white stucco and shielded by manicured rows of tropical botanica, the house loomed above its compound walls like a castle behind a barricade. Flowers cascaded from its ramparts. In the garden, trees pushed forth pineapples, lucuma, bananas, and mango. An iron gate shut out the world. Behind the gate and the wall and the garden, the house itself was impervious to vendors, to factory workers, to ordinary Peruvians, to the sprawl of humanity that struggled a few hundred feet from its door.

The house was skirted by a capacious veranda. Inside, it was filled with high-ceilinged white rooms, heavy doors, yawning keyholes, arched passageways, Spanish tile. The living room—the *sala*—was dominated by my mother's ornate ebony piano. The master bedroom lay behind it, on the other side of a carved double door, so that when those doors were thrown open, the entire *sala* was surveyable from my parents' bed—a bizarre feature, but houses in outlying haciendas were often capricious and irregular. Through an open arch, you could go from our *sala* to the dining room, which held two massive pieces of furniture—a table and an *aparador*, carved with undulating scallops and garlands. The kitchen was stark, a workroom for servants, stripped down and graceless. A cavernous enamel sink—pocked and yellow—jutted from the wall. There was a simple blue table where we three children and our servants took meals. The kitchen door led to a back atrium garden. On the other side of that, behind a wall, were the servants' quarters, a shabby little building that could sleep six in two spare rooms. There was a stall with a spigot where our *mayordomo* and *amas* could wash, a storage area, and a concrete staircase that led to their rooms. To the left of those stairs, under a shed of bare wood and chicken wire, were the animal cages. At four, I was told very clearly—as my older brother and sister, George and Vicki, had been—that I was not allowed in the servants' quarters. The cages were my demarcation line; they were the point beyond which I could not go.

Our own rooms were upstairs, well away from our parents' bedroom and out of the circuit of revelers when a party was afoot. After dinner, which we regularly took in the kitchen, the *amas* would trot us upstairs and bathe us, struggling with their small arms to balance us in the tubs. We would loll about in our pajamas thereafter. There never seemed any urgency to get us to bed, which was just as well because all three of us were terrified of the dark, afraid to look out the windows at tree branches, so well had our *amas* taught us that *pishtacos* were perched there, slavering and squinting in.

Had we overcome our fears and looked out those windows onto Cartavio's main residential street beyond our own house we would have seen five other houses of the first rank, equally grand, equally walled. Behind them, a row of modest ones for the lesser company families. Our immediate neighbors were the Lattos, freckle-faced Scots whose brogue-filtered Spanish made George and me horselaugh into our hands. Their eight-year-old son, Billy, was the undisputed object of Vicki's affection.

He was a straight, good-looking boy with an easy smile. He would direct his grins freely to Vicki, but George and I—who thought ourselves far more appealing than our prickly sister—had to work hard to draw his charms: We'd stand on our heads, swing from trees, make fools of ourselves if we had to, for the incomparable joy of gazing on his teeth.

As a young child, my days unfolded in the garden. It was, as every garden in that coastal desert is, an artificial paradise: invented, deceptive, precarious. Without human hands to tend it, the lush vegetation would have dried to a husk and sifted down into an arid dune. For years, I did not know how tentative that childhood environment was. Walled in, with green crowding our senses and the deep sweetness of fruit and sugar in the air, I felt a sense of entitlement, as if my world would ever be so richly hung. But it was an illusion, and many had labored to create it: to make us feel as if we were emperors of a verdant oasis on the banks of the Amazon just north of the Andes, where the green was unrestrained.

Fooled, happy, ignorant, George and I would splash in the duck pond our father had built for us. Or we would play with the animals we kept in the cages out back where the servants lived. We'd pet the rabbits, feed them fragrant verbena. We'd put chickens on the backs of goats and shriek with laughter as the bewildered creatures scrambled around in circles, the goats wild-eyed under their unruly riders, the chickens pounding the air.

George was my hero, my general, my god. He was as bright and beautiful as I was fat and slow. He could prance and swagger as well as any cowboy in Mother's storybook litany of Wild West valiants. He would hector; I would follow. He'd do mischief; I'd do cover-up. He'd get caught; I'd confess to everything. He'd be spanked; I'd yank down my pants. He'd yawp; I'd bawl louder. And so we spent our days, crawling under the house, devising schemes to scandalize the *mayordomo*, scare Claudia the cook out of her wits, or pester Vicki, whose prissy ways cried out for redress and revenge. If only to force her to look at us over an eternal rim of books.

After lunch, after my father had come home, gazed at his wife's Hollywood face, dozed off, and gone back to work, Mother came to the kitchen looking for us. First she'd put George in bed for his nap, then she'd lead me to her room for a musical siesta.

My mother did not tell us much about herself beyond the fact that she had been a violinist when she and Papi had met in Boston. She was different, odd, that much I knew: porcelain-fair, near translucent, throwing off a kind of shimmer wherever she went. She spoke a halting Spanish, every bit as strange as that of our Scots neighbors; I recall peering into other people's faces to see if it would make them laugh. Often, it would. But she did not mix much with Peruvians if my father was not about. She was not a social person. She seemed more inclined to spend time with her children than with women her age. Then again, she was so unlike any other woman in Cartavio. What distinguished her most from them was the way she moved, like no Peruvian I'd ever seen—straight ahead, gliding—a motion that led from the rib cage, not the hips. It was the kind of walk that tells you little about a body. Her clothes told less: They were loose and silky, more likely to drape from her shoulders than reveal her essential lineaments. She did not own a tightly belted, bust-hoisting, hip-flaunting dress, like those the Peruvian *señoras* wore.

Very early, somehow—I don't recall exactly why—in the same way that I dared not imagine what was beneath her frocks, I learned not to ask about her life before she married Papi. The sweet mildness of her demeanor, like the silk of her clothes, masked some indeterminate thing beneath. There was a hardness behind her glow. An ice. I felt I could quiz her to my heart's content about music, which came to be the language between us. But beyond that—like the point beyond the animal cages—lay a zone I was not supposed to know.

Her past was the only thing Mother was stingy about. Attentive to her children to the point of obsession, she doted on us, worried about us. Every headache was the start of some dread calenture of the brain. Every bellyache, the possibility that we were teeming with tropical parasites. I could make her ooze with love by telling her that I had eaten a wild strawberry from the roadside: She would be anxious for days that I had contracted some rare, Andean disease, taking my temperature at every opportunity, padding into my bedroom at night to lay a cool hand on my brow. Nowhere was her love more evident, however, than in the way she imparted her music to her children. It was, for her, a constant vocation. Any drama, any spectacle, any mathematical conundrum had a corresponding phrase of music, a melody that might frame it more effectively than words. It was as if she needed to convey the vocabulary and syntax of music to us as urgently as she needed to impart English. She would teach all three of us the language of music to some degree, but with time it became clear that I was the one she had chosen to be the beneficiary of this particular gift, and it was through music that she ultimately spoke to me most directly.

At siesta time, she'd recite long strings of poetry from memory for me. Or she'd try singing me to sleep—hopeless enterprises, since I found her poetry and songs more seductive than any prospect of slumber. Outside her room, I spoke Spanish. But inside, we were range-roving Americans, heirs of the King's English, and Mother unfolded that world in verse: Whitman's *Leaves of Grass*, Coleridge's "Rime of the Ancient Mariner," Gilbert and Sullivan's pirates and maidens, Stephen Foster's dreamers and chariots, Robert Burns's banks and brae, George M. Cohan's flag and salute, Irving Berlin's moon and champagne.

I would lie big-eyed, starstruck, as she spun visions of a faraway country where cowboys reigned, valleys were green, wildflowers sprang from the feet of great oaks, water was sipped—unboiled—from streams, opera houses were lined with red velvet, and sidewalks winked with radiant flecks of mica. "You'll see it all someday, Mareezie," she'd say of her melody-filled *historias*. "You'll see it for yourself."

MANIFESTO: 1913

A Few Don'ts by an Imagiste
Ezra Pound

An "Image" is that which presents an intellectual and emotional complex in an instant of time. I use the term "complex" rather in the technical sense employed by the newer psychologists, such as Hart, though we might not agree absolutely in our application.

It is the presentation of such a "complex" instantaneously which gives that sense of sudden liberation; that sense of freedom from time limits and space limits; that sense of sudden growth, which we experience in the presence of the greatest works of art.

It is better to present one Image in a lifetime than to produce voluminous works. . . .

To begin with, consider the three rules recorded by Mr. Flint, not as dogma—never consider anything as dogma—but as the result of long contemplation, which, even if it is some one else's contemplation, may be worth consideration.

Pay no attention to the criticism of men who have never themselves written a notable work. Consider the discrepancies between the actual writing of the Greek poets and dramatists and the theories of Greco-Roman grammarians concocted to explain their metres.

LANGUAGE

Use no superfluous word, no adjective, which does not reveal something.

Don't use such an expression as "dim lands *of peace*." It dulls the image. It mixes an abstraction with the concrete. It comes from the writer's not realizing that the natural object is always the *adequate* symbol.

Go in fear of abstractions. Don't retell in mediocre verse what has already been done in good prose. Don't think any intelligent person is going to be deceived when you try to shirk all the difficulties of the unspeakably difficult art of good prose by chopping your composition into line lengths.

What the expert is tired of today the public will be tired of tomorrow.

Don't imagine that the art of poetry is any simpler than the art of music, or that you can please the expert before you have spent at least as much effort on the art of verse as the average piano teacher spends on the art of music.

Be influenced by as many great artists as you can, but have the decency either to acknowledge the debt outright, or try to conceal it.

Don't allow "influence" to mean merely that you mop up the particular decorative vocabulary of some one or two poets whom you happen to admire. A Turkish war correspondent was recently caught red-handed babbling in his dispatches of "dove-gray" hills, or else it was "pearl-pale," I cannot remember.

Use either no ornament or good ornament. . . .

COURTESY OF THE LIBRARY OF CONGRESS

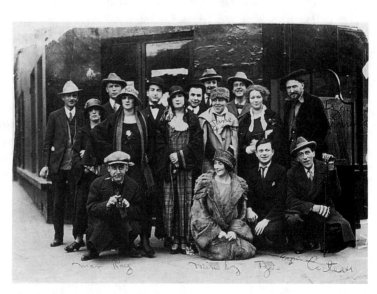

Man Ray, Mina Loy, Tristan Tzara, Jean Cocteau, and Ezra Pound, among others, congregate in Paris.

E-MAIL FORUM

Subject: What's your literary lineage?
From: *PEN America*
To: PEN Members

Seventeenth-century Cavalier poets called themselves the Tribe of Ben, in tribute to the influence of Ben Jonson's work. Some writers continue to define their heritage narrowly (the School of "The Red Wheelbarrow," the Tribe of *The Wretched of the Earth*, the Evil Spawn of *Monty Python*); but modern lists of literary influences tend to be more complex, mixing works and writers that seem to stand for contradictory impulses.

Who and what have helped to make you the writer you are? Are you descended from connoisseurs of silence or of repetition, from realists, surrealists, magic realists, fantasists, ironists, romantics, revolutionaries, clowns? Do you trace your tribal ancestry through Saint Augustine, Lady Murasaki, Rumi, Montaigne, Cervantes, Sterne, Equiano, Austen, Douglass, Woolf, Freud, Kafka, Tagore, Marx (Karl or Groucho), García Márquez? If you claim, say, Joyce or Borges or Rushdie as an ancestor, how do you relate to the multitude of ancestors each of them has already claimed?

The challenge: Can you reduce your lineage to a hyphenated phrase? (An example might be the School of Dickinson-Stevens-Bishop-Ashbery, courtesy of Harold Bloom; perhaps your tribe has a wider cultural and geographical range, perhaps not.) Send us your tribal moniker. We'll run as many as we can fit in the next issue of the journal and post more on PEN's Web site.

—M. Mark

>>>

JOAN SCHENKAR: The Miss Barnes and Mr. Beckett School of (Jacobean-Modernist, Expressionist-Ciceronian, Poststructural Feminist–Alt Rock) Careful Construction and Violent Prose.

STEWART O'NAN: To borrow the format of *The Player*, I'd say my work is more Virginia Woolf meets *Night of the Living Dead*. Or maybe Alice Munro dates the Ramones.

>>>

IRENE TIERSTEN: Pared-down Proust.

>>>

SIMON SCHAMA: Rabelaisiano-Vicovian-Hazlittishy-Carlylian-Dickensiana-Michelettisch-Sveviano-Nabokovian.

>>>

GERALD WEALES: I am by James Whitcomb Riley out of Robert Benchley.

>>>

ROBERT GLUCK: Keats–O'Hara–Proust–Bataille–Language Poetry–Acker–Blanchot.

>>>

ALEKSANDAR HEMON: My father–Flaubert–Joyce–Borges–Schulz–Kiš–Nabokov–Hitchcock–French New Wave–Lennon–McCartney–Bach–Mahler–Sonic Youth–Public Enemy–Sarajevo–Chicago.

>>>

SCOTT SPENCER: My lit lineage gives me the energy to write, supplying not necessarily the how but the why, and it can be short-handed like this: Nabokov-Cain/Chandler/Highsmith-Greene. Considering this little list, I cannot help but wish it were otherwise, but only the very fortunate are immune to the wish to have come from a different family.

>>>

DENISE DUHAMEL: The school is called Dreamers of Jeannie. Our lineage can be traced as Cap'n Crunch–Frank O'Hara–Lawrence Ferlinghetti–SpaghettiOs.

>>>

FENTON JOHNSON: Tribe of Gilgamesh–Homer–Bible (Hebrew and Christian)–Augustine–Jefferson–Lincoln–Faulkner–Welty, with appropriate acknowledgment to the dean of Kentucky writers, Wendell Berry.

>>>

TED SOLOTAROFF: I am descended from the tribe of Yiddish literary journalists. So I have been told and believe, though I don't know Yiddish.

>>>

DEAN KOSTOS: I belong to the unlikely lineage of Hopkins-Breton-Plath-Neruda-Bishop-Oulipo. I love Surrealism and Formalism and find that they overlap in the way constraint triggers the subconscious, hence my interest in Oulipo.

KAREN MALPEDE: *Marjorie Morningstar*, *My Friend Flicka*, Tennessee Williams, Joyce-Bergman-Genet-Faulkner, Aeschylus-Sophocles-Euripides, Woolf–Pat Barker–Sebald.

>>>

DAVID GRIMM: Though descended from the cruel house of Marlowe (by way of the British B-boys—Bond, Brenton, Barker, Barnes), with a streak of the perverse (care of that distant bastard cousin, Orton), it is to that great-grandfather of all dramatists, Bill Shakespeare, that I owe my heart and soul.

>>>

RICK MOODY: School-of-second-wave-experimental-writing-with-predictable-interest-in-Melville-Beckett-Pynchon-Woolf-Gaddis-Nabokov-and-disagreeable-love-of-popular-culture.

>>>

JOHN JAKES: I would say mine is The School of 19th-Century-Triple-Decker-Writers.

>>>

MARY GORDON: On my father's side, it's the line of Ford Madox Ford, passing from him to the women he influenced and often published: Katherine Anne Porter, Jean Stafford, Eudora Welty. On my mother's side, the line of Virginia Woolf, going from her to Katherine Mansfield to Elizabeth Bowen.

>>>

GAIL CALDWELL: Cicero–Song of Solomon–Faulkner–Hank Williams Sr.

>>>

ALFRED CORN: I am a Bible–Homer–Sappho–Dante–Giotto–Shakespeare–Bashō–Vermeer–Bach–Mozart–Wordsworth–Keats–Whitman–Baudelaire–Melville–Dickinson–Tolstoy–Rilke–Matisse–Stevens–Marianne Moore–Joyce–Kafka–Colette–Hart Crane–Langston Hughes–Auden–Borges–Balanchine–Celan–Charlie Parker–Bishop–Miles Davis–Anonymous writer. (Tennyson's Ulysses said, "I am a part of all that I have met," which can mean that a writer learns from every writer she or he has ever read. I have certainly tried to. And I've learned from people I've spoken with who were not artists, represented here in the aggregate term "Anonymous.")

>>>

AMANDA VAILL: I see myself in the tribe of Bloomsbury with a bar-sinister connection to S. J. Perelman. Make of that what you will . . .

>>>

MICHAEL KANDEL: Kafka–Phil Dick Wannabe.

WILLIAM H. GASS: A note in one of Schoenberg's rows
or Arnie's Army

>>>

WILLIAM ALLEN: Homer-Herodotus-Heine-Hölderlin-Hawthorne-Hopkins-Hikmet-Hughes-Hurston-Harjo-Heaney.

>>>

RICHARD KOSTELANETZ: As I work in more arts than writing, J. S. Bach, Charles Ives, John Cage. Otherwise, for essays, George Orwell; for fiction, James Joyce.

>>>

MICHELLE TEA: Charles Bukowski's alcoholica school of hard knocks via Eileen Myles's lesbionic cultural reality check.

>>>

CHRISTOPHER KEANE: The Hemingway–Robbe-Grillet–Salinger school of spunky/spiky realism.

>>>

DELIA SHERMAN: I am of the School of Shakespeare–Morris (William)–Zola–Carter (Angela)–Dunnett.

>>>

ETHAN BUMAS: punk rock cervantes smash the windmill.

>>>

TOM LEWIS: Hammett-MacInnis-Fleming-McDonald-McBain-Higgins.

>>>

CHARLES PATTERSON: School of Amos, Dante, Joyce, and Isaac Bashevis Singer.

>>>

DONALD BRECKENRIDGE: The old school of a winded Emmanuel Bove drinking a six-pack of Rheingold with Alfred Döblin and Claude Simon on Juan Carlos Onetti's stoop while enduring a Brooklyn heat wave.

>>>

HILMA WOLITZER: Before I even learned to read, I belonged to the kitchen table (at and under)–bedroom wall School of Listening and Imagining.

>>>

BEREL LANG: I'm of the Plato-Borgesian tribe.

>>>

BRYCE MILLIGAN: I am a Jack-of-all-Genres-Stateless-Servant-of-the-Muse. JGSSMs are the most common of all the writerly tribes, owing allegiance only to family, food, and creativity.

SAM ABRAMS: School of the Outer Boroughs / Whitman's Brooklyn Section.

>>>

ROBERT KORNFELD (playwright who is a Southerner–New Englander–New Yorker–stranger): As a writer I am a Bardist-Chekhovian-Ibsenesque-Faulknerite.

>>>

KATHARINE WEBER: Maugham-Spark-Hazzard.

>>>

WILLIAM BORDEN: Aristophanes–Cervantes–Rabelais–Fielding–Sterne–Cabell–Donleavy–Henry Miller.

>>>

SANFORD STERNLICHT: A cocktail of G. Manley Hopkins, John Masefield, Padraic Colum, and Henry Roth.

>>>

LISA M. STEINMAN: The School of Stevens-arguing-with-Moore, anticipating Josephine Miles.

>>>

X. J. KENNEDY: a long line of rhymesters and tub-thumpers.

>>>

A. D. WINANS: The school of Blake, William Carlos Williams, Allen Ginsberg, Bob Kaufman, and Charles Bukowski.

>>>

RICHARD J. BRENNER: lyrical-rationalist, rational-lyricist.

>>>

LEONARD S. MARCUS: self-educated (school of Yale).

>>>

HARRIET ZINNES: As a contemporary poet my literary lineage is hardly unusual: School of Dickinson-Pound-Stevens-Bishop-Ashbery-Bernstein.

>>>

MICHAEL LALLY: For prose, Shandy–Joyce–Rilke (that's right, his prose, especially *The Notebooks of Malte Laurids Brigge*)–Rhys–Saroyan (William)–Kerouac! For poetry, Whitman-Williams-Cendrars-Rukeyser-Snyder-O'Hara.

>>>

NILES GOLDSTEIN: The School of Moses–Augustine–Dante–Melville–Hemingway–Faulkner–(Tennessee) Williams–Mishima.

>>>

ARTHUR GREGOR: My lineage is Bach, Stevens, Eliot, Frost, Dickinson, Bishop, and Rilke.

JULES OLDER: I'm a direct descendent of the Joad-Doc-Spenser-Hawk clan.

>>>

HELEN DUBERSTEIN: The tribe of Duras–Joyce–Genet–Woolf–G. Stein.

>>>

EDWARD FOSTER: Emersonian-by-way-of-Spicer-and-Bronk.

>>>

CATHERINE HILLER: Social satirists and sexual explorers: Austin/
Lawrence/McCarthy/Updike—via Erica Jong!

>>>

JOAN CROWELL: Blake, Yeats, Léonie Adams, Szymborska, Billy Collins . . .

>>>

ELINOR LIPMAN: Well . . . modesty aside: The Austen-Algonquin Tribe.

>>>

ELEANOR MUNRO: Waves-out-of-Winesburg: a long Middlemarch-to-
Originals.

>>>

REGINA WEINREICH: Beat generation: Twain-Blake-Dostoevsky-
Burroughs-Ginsberg-Kerouac.

>>>

WIN BLEVINS: I see myself as continuing the work of those twentieth-
century writers who strove best to understand American culture deeply,
Bernard De Voto and Wallace Stegner. If I could find a way to get the spirit
of E. E. Cummings into my prose, I would.

>>>

PATRICIA VOLK: I am a direct literary descendant of Thurber-Melville, who
met cute in Litchfield County. On my father's side, it's Joyce Carey–
Kingsley Amis, despite the fact grandpa hailed from Vilnius.

>>>

LUCY FERRISS: The School of Sappho-Sontag-Simones (Weil and
de Beauvoir, that is)—the literary influences on a woman writer who does
not want to be boxed into the domestic or nonpolitical sphere but seeks
rather a female language of engagement.

>>>

LAURA NEWMAN: Tribe of Global Dreams—Chan-Gordimer-Payer-
Shange-Sebald.

>>>

SAUL BENNETT: As it happens, my second collection was titled *Harpo
Marx at Prayer*, but Groucho has been the driving Marx source for me.
In sum, I'm: The School of Hopkins–Marx (Groucho)–Frank O'Hara.

CATHERINE DALY: anarcho-dada-postmodern-superrealists or perhaps "Third Generation New York School not in New York"-sound poetry.

>>>

DAVID BERGMAN: I consider myself one of the many sons of Howard—Richard Howard, that is, whose generosity, intelligence, and urbanity have inspired several generations. Of course, being a son of Howard means that your genetic material is English, French, and secularly Jewish, as well as deeply American. As his literary child, one finds oneself not "alone with America" but crowded by the world.

>>>

SALLY CHAPPELL: Count me in on the "Midwest Paeans: Cather–Sandburg–Least Heat-Moon tribe." (My latest book is a deep time study—from the Big Bang to the present—of a six-square-mile area in the heart of Illinois. Now a UNESCO World Monument site, this little-known American Indian city was larger than London in 1000 A.D.)

>>>

MARILYN YALOM: feminist scholar.

>>>

TERESE SVOBODA: In fiction: as one of Lish's Ladies, I'm Defoe-Carpentier-Michaux-Spark. In poetry: the conglomerate of Eliot and Walcott (Elicott? or Waliot?) but definitely post-Empire, the tribe of When.

>>>

BETH GUTCHEON: The query, I take it, doesn't allow for wishful thinking—not whom would you like to claim as lineal ancestors, but whose markers are you in fact exhibiting. Unfashionably, I'm afraid, it's Charles Dickens and Scott Fitzgerald, and wouldn't they be surprised to find themselves on a family tree together. (This seems to me to mean accessible social fiction, based on observation, data gathered from both inside and outside the temple but always with the outsider's eye.) As no writer would aspire to the late career of either one, I'm hoping I get to describe my own arc from here on out.

>>>

DENNIS BRIAN BARONE: 1/2/3/ - Charles Brockden Brown - Ralph Waldo Emerson - William Carlos Williams - 1/2/3.

>>>

VINCENT KATZ: I am an Alexandrian-Augustan-Apollinaireian poet.

>>>

WALTER JAMES MILLER: I belong to the One-Man School of Robinson Jeffers/Paul Engle.

LIAM RECTOR: T. S. Eliot's "Four Quartets" meets Byron's "So We'll Go No More a-Roving," with the clean bitterness of Brecht thrown about. The ballad in all its elegiac forms, sung in bed at 3 A.M. on the night before leaving.

>>>

CARMEN BOULLOSA: Pure chance has made me a woman, and my writing isn't marked by it. Still, I am very clear who are my mothers, though my fathers' identities are in doubt: Sor Juana Inés de la Cruz (the father might be Quevedo, or Nezahualcóyotl, or Fray Bernardino de Sahagún, or Góngora), Delmira Agustini (Rubén Darío or Whitman?), Teresa de la Parra (Stendhal or Proust?), Rosa Chacel (Ortega y Gasset or Clarín?), Silvina Ocampo (her close friend Borges, or her husband Bioy Casares?), and Elena Garro (her ex-husband Octavio Paz, or Juan Rulfo?).

I could list more possible fathers. Fate decrees that mothers are clearly visible, and fathers remain blurry.

No tribe. Some brothers (Fabio Morábito, Francisco Hinojosa). No sisters.

>>>

ARNOLD KRAMISH: My grandfather, Abram, was a roofer in Lubartow, then part of czarist Russia. Although illiterate, he was an accomplished fiddler. One day, Cossacks stormed into town, shooting all Jews in sight, including Abram, roofing. Verily, he was the "Fiddler on the Roof"! (The story was family lore long before the musical, and was recently confirmed by Lublin records.) Does this qualify as literary or musical lineage?

To: *PEN America*

Your letter to Chaim Potok arrived at a time shortly before his death. He never saw it. As his wife and amanuensis, I am taking the liberty of responding in his name.

Based on many conversations with, and lectures and articles by, him, I would say that his "hyphenated phrase" would read something like: School of Kafka–Mann–Joyce–Proust–Freud–Maimonides–Ibn Ezra. Though it is now well past your deadline, I am sending this response on to you, in the hope that you might include it.

Sincerely,
Adena Potok

MANIFESTO: 1886

The Symbolist Manifesto
Jean Moréas
Translated by Mary Ann Caws

Like all the arts, literature evolves: in a cycle with its returns strictly determined, complicated by various shifts over time and in the changing climates. It is clear how each new phase in artistic evolution corresponds precisely with the senile decrepitude, the ineluctable end of the school just before it. . . .

So we have been expecting the inevitable manifestation of a new art; it has been hatching for a long time. And all the silly jokes that have so delighted the press, all the concern of the serious critics, all the ill temper of the public surprised in its sheeplike torpor: more and more this all affirms how vital is the present evolution in French writing, so mistakenly called decadence by those in a rush to judge. But notice how decadent literatures are always ambitious and lengthy, timorous and even servile: all Voltaire's tragedies, for instance, are marked with such patches of decadence. And for what could anyone reproach the new school? For its refusal of pompousness; for its strangeness of metaphors, its new vocabulary, where harmonies meld with colors and lines: these are characteristics of every renaissance. . . .

Readers will accuse this aesthetics of obscurity: we aren't surprised. What can you do? Weren't Pindar's *Odes*, Shakespeare's *Hamlet*, Dante's *Vita Nuova*, Goethe's *Faust* Part II, Flaubert's *Temptation of Saint Anthony* said to be ambiguous?

To translate its synthesis exactly, Symbolism needs an archetypal complex style: untainted words, sentences with a central high point alternating with those with highs and lows, meaningful pleonasms, mysterious ellipses, the hanging anacoluthon, and every daring and multiform trope imaginable: the good old language set on a sure footing and modernized—the rich and joyous French language from before writers like Vaugelas and Boileau-Despréaux, the tongue of François Rabelais and Philippe de Commynes, of Villon, of Rutebeuf, and so many other free writers sending out their sharp-tongued darts, as the archers of Thrace sent out their flexible arrows. . . .

CONTRIBUTORS

Pierre Albert-Birot (1876–1967) was a painter, sculptor, and writer. In 1916, he founded the avant-garde review *SIC*. He was the author of the novel *Grabinoulor*.

Meena Alexander was born in India and immigrated to Sudan at age five. At age fifteen, she began publishing poetry in Sudanese newspapers. She has published thirteen books of poetry and prose, as well as a memoir, *Fault Lines*. Her latest novel is *Manhattan Music*, and her most recent volume of poems, *Illiterate Heart*, won the 2002 PEN Open Book Award. She has received a Fulbright Scholar Award and teaches at the Graduate Center of City University of New York.

Sherman Alexie has published fifteen books of prose and poetry. His short-story collection *The Lone Ranger and Tonto Fistfight in Heaven* won the PEN/Hemingway Award for Best First Book of Fiction. His most recent collection of short stories, *The Toughest Indian in the World*, was a PEN Center USA West Fiction Award finalist and the 2001 PEN/Malamud Award winner. Alexie collaborated on the screenplay for the film *Smoke Signals* and held the title of World Heavyweight Poetry Champion from 1998 to 2001.

Marie Arana's memoir, *American Chica*, was a National Book Award finalist. She is the editor of *Washington Post Book World*.

Charles Bernstein has written more than twenty books of poetry, including *Republics of Reality: 1975–1995*, *Dark City*, *Rough Trades*, *The Nude Formalism*, *Stigma*, and *Parsing*. He is also the author of three books of nonfiction: *My Way*, *A Poetics*, and *Content's Dream*. In the 1970s, Bernstein cofounded the journal *L=A=N=G=U=A=G=E*. He has received the Roy Harvey Pearce/Archive for New Poetry Prize and fellowships from the New York Foundation for the Arts, the Guggenheim Foundation, and the National Endowment for the Arts.

Marina Budhos was born in Queens, New York, to an Indo-Guyanese father and a Jewish-American mother. She has published two novels, *The Professor of Light* and *House of Waiting*, and the nonfiction book *Remix: Conversations with Immigrant Teenagers*. She has traveled in India as a Fulbright Scholar and recently received an Exceptional Media Merit Award for her journalistic work on sex tourism in Asia. She lives in New Jersey and teaches at Columbia University.

Hortense Calisher is the author of numerous novels, novellas, and short-story collections. Her *Collected Stories*, the memoir *Herself*, and the novel *False Entry* were all nominated for National Book Awards. She has received a Lifetime Achievement Award from the National Endowment for the Arts and a number of Guggenheim Fellowships. Calisher served as president of PEN American Center from 1986 to 1987 and as president of the American Academy and Institute of Arts and Letters from 1987 to 1990. Her most recent novel is *Sunday Jews*.

Aimé Césaire was born in Martinique and studied at the Sorbonne. He is the author of the nonfiction book *Discourse on Colonialism*, and his books of poetry include *Notebook of a Return to My Native Land* and *Lost Body*. With Léopold Sédar Senghor, he founded the Négritude movement of West Indian and African writers in French.

Sandra Cisneros is the author of the poetry collection *My Wicked, Wicked Ways*, *Woman Hollering Creek and Other Stories*, and the novel *The House on Mango Street*, which won the Before Columbus American Book Award in 1985. She has received a fellowship from the National Endowment for the Arts and has contributed to *The New York Times*, *The Los Angeles Times*, and *The Village Voice*, among other publications.

Sara Crosby grew up in St. Louis, studied at the University of Iowa and the New School, and now lives in New York City.

John D'Agata's *Halls of Fame* is a collection of essays on contemporary American culture. He has an MFA from the Iowa Writers' Workshop and is an associate editor at *The Seneca Review*. D'Agata has received fellowships from MacDowell and Villa Montalvo. He lives in New Hampshire.

Annabel Davis-Goff was born in the south of Ireland. Her novel *The Dower House* was a *New York Times* Notable Book of the Year. Her other books include *This Cold Country* and the memoir *Walled Gardens*. She lives in New York.

Louise Erdrich has published five novels, two collections of poetry, a memoir, and two children's books. Her most recent works include *Master Butchers Singing Club* and the National Book Award Finalist *Last Report on the Miracles at Little No Horse*. Erdrich has received O. Henry Awards and fellowships to the MacDowell and Yaddo colonies. She lives in Minnesota and owns The Birchbark, an independent bookstore.

Ian Frazier's books include *Great Plains, Family, On the Rez, Dating Your Mom*, and *The Fish's Eye: Essays About Angling and the Outdoors*. Frazier is a frequent contributor to *The New Yorker* and *The Atlantic Monthly*. He lives in Montclair, New Jersey.

Lynn Freed was born in South Africa. Her novels include *The Bungalow, The Mirror*, and *House of Women*. Her short fiction and essays have appeared in *The New Yorker, Harper's*, and *The Atlantic Monthly*. She received the inaugural Katherine Anne Porter Award from the American Academy of Arts and Letters and has been awarded numerous grants and fellowships. She teaches at Bennington College and the University of California at Davis.

Samuel G. Freedman's books include *Small Victories: The Real World of a Teacher, Her Students, and Their High School* and *The Inheritance: How Three Families and America Moved from Roosevelt to Reagan and Beyond*, which was a finalist for the Pulitzer Prize. His most recent book, *Jew vs. Jew: The Struggle for the Soul of American Jewry*, won the 2001 National Jewish Book Award. Freedman contributes to *The New York Times, USA Today*, and other publications. He teaches at Columbia University.

Mary Gaitskill has published two collections of short stories, *Bad Behavior* and *Because They Wanted To*, and a novel, *Two Girls, Fat and Thin*. She also writes for a number of magazines and newspapers.

Dorothy Gallagher is the author of *How I Came into My Inheritance, All the Right Enemies: The Life and Murder of Carlo Tresca*, and *Hannah's Daughters: Six Generations of an American Family, 1876–1976*. She lives in New York City.

Amitav Ghosh was born in Calcutta. His books include *The Circle of Reason, Shadow Lines, In an Antique Land*, and *The Glass Palace*, a *New York Times* Notable Book of 2001. *The Circle of Reason* won the Prix Medici Etranger, and *Shadow Lines* won the Sahitya Akademi Award. Ghosh teaches at Queens College in the City University of New York. He lives in Brooklyn.

Wendy Gimbel's first book was *Edith Wharton: Orphancy and Survival*, followed by *Havana Dreams*, which was named a *New York Times* Notable Book of the Year. She has reviewed books and commented on cultural affairs for *The New York Times, The Los Angeles Times, The Nation, Parnassus, Vogue*, and *Mirabella*, among other publications.

Allen Ginsberg (1926–97) was born in Newark, New Jersey. As a student at Columbia University in the 1940s, he began close friendships with William S. Burroughs, Neal Cassady, and Jack Kerouac. His book of poetry *Howl* overcame censorship trials to become one of the most widely read of the century. *Kaddish and Other Poems* was published in 1961. Ginsberg won a National Book Award for *The Fall of America: Poems of These States*.

Francisco Goldman has published two novels, *The Long Night of White Chickens*, which won the Sue Kaufman Prize for First Fiction, and *The Ordinary Seaman*, which was named one of *Hungry Mind Review*'s One Hundred Books of the Century. Both novels were PEN/Faulkner Award finalists. Goldman was raised in Massachusetts and Guatemala City and now divides his time between Mexico City and New York City.

Bessie Head (1937–86) was born in South Africa to a white Scottish mother and a black South African father. She is the author of the novels *When Rain Clouds Gather*, *Maru*, and *A Question of Power*, all of which deal with life in postcolonial Africa. She died in Botswana at the age of forty-nine.

Seamus Heaney was born in Northern Ireland and began to write while a lecturer at St. Joseph's College in Belfast. His collections include *The Spirit Level*, *New Selected Poems 1966–1987*, *Sweeney Astray*, and *Opened Ground*. He has written several volumes of criticism, and his translation of *Beowulf* won the Whitbread Book of the Year Award in 1999. Heaney is a member of the American Academy of Arts and Letters; in 1995 he received the Nobel Prize in Literature. He divides his between Dublin and Massachusetts, where he teaches at Harvard University.

Bob Holman is a poetry activist who has produced the PBS series *The United States of Poetry*. He coedited *Aloud: Voices from the Nuyorican Poets Café*, which won an American Book Award in 1994. His spoken-word CDs include *In with the Out Crowd* and *The Collect Call of the Wild*. Holman has won three Emmys, cofounded a poetry record label, and was the founding editor of the New York *Poetry Calendar*. He is the proprietor of New York City's Bowery Poetry Club.

Eikoh Hosoe was born in Japan. His photography is featured in *Black Sun: The Eyes of Four*, *A Place Called Hiroshima*, and a volume from Aperture's Masters of Photography series. His most recent book, *Ba-ra-kei: Ordeal by Roses*, is a collection of photographs of Japanese author Yukio Mishima.

Langston Hughes (1902–67) was born in Joplin, Missouri, and moved at age thirteen to Lincoln, Illinois, where he began writing poetry. He published his first collection of poetry, *The Weary Blues*, in 1926. His first novel, *Not Without Laughter*, won the Harmon Gold Medal for literature. Hughes produced many children's books, dozens of volumes of poetry and prose, and seven plays. He died in Harlem.

Margo Jefferson is a cultural critic for *The New York Times* and has been a staff reviewer for *Newsweek* and a contributing editor for *Vogue* and *7 Days*. Her reviews and essays have appeared in *Newsweek*, *The Nation*, *Grand Street*, *American Theater*, *The Village Voice*, and *Harper's*. She has received awards from the American Library Association and the Coordinating Council of Literary Magazines. In 1995 she won the Pulitzer Prize for criticism.

Denis Johnson's books include *The Name of the World*, *Already Dead*, and *Jesus' Son*, and his poetry has been collected in *The Throne of the Third Heaven of the Nations Millennium General Assembly*. His most recent work is *Shoppers: Two Plays*. He has received a Lannan Fellowship and a Whiting Writers' Award and was a finalist for the PEN/Faulkner Award. He lives in northern Idaho.

Tony Kushner is the author of *A Bright Room Called Day*, *Angels in America*, *Slavs!*, *Hydriotaphia*, and *Homebody/Kabul*. He has adapted Corneille's *Illusion* and Ansky's *Dybbuk*. Kushner has received the Dramatists Guild Hull-Warriner Award for Best Play, a medal for Cultural Achievement from the National Foundation for Jewish Culture, and the 2002 PEN/Laura Pels Award for Drama. He grew up in Lake Charles, Louisiana, and lives in New York.

Mina Loy (1882–1966) was born in London and lived in Paris, Florence, New York City, and Aspen. Loy has been labeled a Futurist, Dadaist, Surrealist, feminist, conceptualist, Modernist, and Postmodernist. Although her controversial poems were praised by T. S. Eliot, Ezra Pound, and William Carlos Williams, Loy considered herself a visual artist, claiming at the end of her life that she "never was a poet." Her books include *The Autobiography of Mina Loy*, *Insel*, and *The Lost Lunar Baedeker*.

Jay McInerney is the author of several novels, including *Bright Lights, Big City*, *The Story of My Life*, and *Model Behavior*. Selections from his *House & Garden* column, "Uncorked," were recently collected in *Bacchus & Me: Adventures in the Wine Cellar*. He divides his time between New York and Tennessee.

Yukio Mishima (1925–70) was born and lived in Japan. His novels include *The Temple of the Golden Pavilion, The Sailor Who Fell from Grace with the Sea, Thirst for Love, Confessions of a Mask,* and *Forbidden Colors.* He completed the final work of his landmark tetralogy, The Sea of Fertility, in 1970.

Michael Moore is the author of *Stupid White Men . . . and Other Sorry Excuses for the State of the Nation!* and *Downsize This!* and is coauthor of *Adventures in a TV Nation.* Moore is a documentary filmmaker whose company Dog Eat Dog Films has produced fiction and nonfiction films. He established the Center for Alternative Media and served as executive producer and anchor of the award-winning television series *TV Nation.*

Jean Moréas (1856–1910) was the pen name of Yanni Papadiamantopoulos, an Athens-born poet who moved to Paris in 1872. He wrote two volumes of symbolist verse, *Les Syrtes* and *Le Pèlerin passionné.* His later books include *Les Stances.*

John Nathan has translated novels by Kenzaburo Ōe and Yukio Mishima and is the author of *Mishima: A Biography, Sony: The Private Life,* and the forthcoming social chronicle *The Unmaking of Japan.* In 1994, he became the first Takashima Professor of Cultural Studies at the University of California, Santa Barbara.

María Negroni received an Argentine National Book Award for her collection of essays, *Ciudad gótica,* and for her collection of poems, *El viaje de la noche,* published in English as *Night Journey.* She teaches at Sarah Lawrence College.

Frank O'Hara (1926–66) was born in Baltimore, Maryland, and grew up in Massachusetts. His books of poetry include *A City in Winter, Meditations in an Emergency, Second Avenue,* and *Lunch Poems.* In 1973, his *Selected Poems* won a National Book Award. *Standing Still and Walking in New York,* a collection of his essays and notes, was published in 1975.

Willie Perdomo is the author of *Where a Nickel Costs a Dime* and the children's book *Visiting Langston.* His work has been anthologized in *Step into a World: A Global Anthology of the New Black Literature, Listen Up! Spoken Word Poetry, Boricuas: Influential Puerto Rican Writings,* and *Aloud: Voices from the Nuyorican Poets Café.* Perdomo has received a New York Foundation for the Arts Fiction Grant. He lives in New York City.

Ezra Pound (1885–1972) worked to promote the work of James Joyce, Wyndham Lewis, T. S. Eliot, William Carlos Williams, Marianne Moore, H. D., and other Modernists. Among his volumes of poetry are *Canzoni, Lustra, Personae, Ripostes,* and *Hugh Selwyn Mauberley.* His later work, for nearly fifty years, focused on the epic *Cantos.* In 1914 he edited *Des Imagistes: An Anthology.*

Arnold Rampersad is the author of *The Art and Imagination of W. E. B. Du Bois, The Life of Langston Hughes,* and *Jackie Robinson: A Biography,* and is the coeditor of Oxford University's Race and American Culture book series. He has received a MacArthur Foundation fellowship and teaches at Stanford University.

Jacques Roubaud, a writer and mathematician, was born in 1932. His books include *Our Beautiful Heroine, Hortense in Exile, Hortense Is Abducted, Some Thing Black, The Great Fire of London,* and *The Plurality of Worlds of Lewis.*

Edward Said is the author of more than twenty books, including *Orientalism,* which was nominated for a National Book Critics Circle Award; *Culture and Imperialism; Peace and Its Discontents;* and a memoir, *Out of Place.* He teaches at Columbia University.

Lily Saint received her MFA in Poetry from the New School University. She is the editor and publisher of *CROWD,* a journal of literature and art, and her poetry has recently appeared in *swankwriting.com* and *The Monday Poetry Report.*

Sonia Sanchez has written more than a dozen books of poetry, including *Shake Loose My Skin, Like the Singing Coming Off the Drums: Love Poems,* and *Does Your House Have Lions?,* which was nominated for both the NAACP Image and National Book Critics Circle Awards. She has won an American Book Award from the Before Columbus Foundation and a National Endowment for the Arts Award. Sanchez taught at Temple University until 1999. She lives in Philadelphia.

Frederick Seidel is the author of *Final Solutions; These Days; Poems, 1959–1979; My Tokyo; Going Fast; Life on Earth;* and *Sunrise,* which won the Lamont Poetry Selection and the National Book Critics Circle Award in Poetry. His most recent book of poems, *Area Code 212,* completes his trilogy, The Cosmos Poems. He lives in New York City.

Léopold Sédar Senghor (1906–2001) became president of Senegal in 1960, after the country won its independence from France. He wrote several volumes of poetry, including *Songs of the Shadow*, and won the Apollinaire Prize for Poetry in 1974.

Ann Snitow is a professor of literature and gender studies at Eugene Lang College and is a member of the Graduate Faculty of New School University. A literary critic and essayist, Snitow has coedited *Powers of Desire* and, with Rachel Blau Du Plessis, *The Feminist Memoir Project*. She is an activist who has participated in the founding of the Feminist Anti-Censorship Task Force, the action group No More Nice Girls, and the Network of East-West Women (NEWW). Her recent writing and political work concerns women in Eastern Europe.

Tristan Tzara (1896–1963), a Romanian-born French poet and essayist, was the author of *L'Homme approximatif*, *La Premiere Aventure cèleste de Monsieur Antipyrine*, and *Grains et issues*, among many other books. His *Oeuvres complètes* comprise six volumes. Tzara wrote the first Dada texts and the movement's manifestos, *Sept manifestes Dada*.

Theo van Doesburg (1883–1931) was born in Utrecht, the Netherlands. His first exhibition of paintings was held in 1908 in The Hague. In the 1920s he worked with Kurt Schwitters, Jean Arp, Tristan Tzara, and others on the review *Mécano*. He wrote poetry and art criticism and gave lectures on literature in Prague, Vienna, and Hanover.

William T. Vollmann is the author of several volumes of fiction, including *You Bright and Risen Angels*, *Whores for Gloria*, *Butterfly Stories*, *Father and Crows*, and *The Atlas*. His novel *Argall*, about Pocahontas and Captain John Smith, is the third completed volume in his Seven Dreams series, a fictional history of North America.

Anne Waldman has written more than forty books, most recently *Vow to Poetry* and *Marriage: A Sentence*. In the 1960s, she ran the St. Mark's Church Poetry Project in New York's East Village. With Allen Ginsberg, she created the Jack Kerouac School of Disembodied Poetics. She has received the Dylan Thomas Memorial Award, the Poets Foundation Award, the National Literary Anthology Award, and a National Endowment for the Arts grant.

William Carlos Williams (1883–1963) published thirteen volumes of poetry, nine books of prose, and eight collections of letters. His major works include *Kora in Hell*, *Spring and All*, the five-volume epic *Paterson*, and *Pictures from Brueghel and Other Poems*, which won a Pulitzer Prize. In addition to writing, Williams was a physician who practiced medicine in Rutherford, New Jersey, the town where he was born.

C. D. Wright was born in Mountain Home, Arkansas. She has published ten volumes of poetry, including *Steal Away: Selected and New Poems*, *Deepstep Come Shining*, and *String Light*, which won the Poetry Center Book Award. She has won awards from the National Endowment for the Arts, the Guggenheim Foundation, the Bunting Institute, and the Lannan Foundation, as well as the Witter Bynner Prize and the Whiting Writers' Award. In 1994 she was named State Poet of Rhode Island. She teaches at Brown University.

ACKNOWLEDGMENTS

Excerpt from *The Toughest Indian in the World* by Sherman Alexie, copyright © 2000 by Sherman Alexie. Used by permission of Grove Press.

"Ghosts/Pishtacos" from *American Chica* by Marie Arana, copyright © 2001 by Marie Arana. Used by permission of The Dial Press/Dell Publishing, a division of Random House, Inc.

"The Symbolist Manifesto," "Nunism," "Dada Manifesto," "Aphorisms on Futurism," "Our Vortex," "A Few Don'ts by an Imagiste," "Ultraist Manifesto," "Towards a Contructive Poetry," "Declaration of January 27, 1925," "In the Guise of a Literary Manifesto," "Speech and Image," "The Revolution of the Word," "Personism," and "The Conspiracy of 'Us'" from *Manifesto: A Century of Isms*, ed. Mary Ann Caws. Copyright © 2001 by Mary Ann Caws. University of Nebraska Press.

"Those Who Don't" from *The House on Mango Street* by Sandra Cisneros, copyright © 1984 by Sandra Cisneros.

"Living History Hall of Fame, II" and "Museum of American Frontier Culture and Hall of Fame," copyright © 2001 by John D'Agata. Reprinted from *Halls of Fame* with the permission of Graywolf Press, Saint Paul, Minnesota.

Excerpt from "Two Languages in Mind, but Just One in Heart" by Louise Erdrich from *The New York Times*, May 22, 2000. Copyright © 2000 by Louise Erdrich.

"The Bloomsbury Group Live at the Apollo" from *Dating Your Mom* by Ian Frazier. Copyright © 1986 by Ian Frazier. Reprinted by permission of Farrar, Straus and Giroux, LLC.

"No" from *How I Came into My Inheritance* by Dorothy Gallagher, copyright © 2001 by Dorothy Gallagher. Used by permission of Random House, Inc.

"Letter to the Administrators" by Amitav Ghosh, copyright © 2001 by Amitav Ghosh, reprinted from www.amitavghosh.com. Used by permission of the author.

"The Woman from America," copyright © 2002 The Estate of Bessie Head, from *Tales of Tenderness and Power*, Heinemann Educational Publishers, 1989.

Excerpt from "An Open Letter" by Seamus Heaney, copyright © 1983 by Seamus Heaney. Field Day Theatre Company pamphlet 2.

"Final Call," "Juke Box Love Song," "Let America Be America Again," "Letter to the Academy," "My People," "The Negro Speaks of Rivers," "Warning," and "The Weary Blues" from *The Collected Poems of Langston Hughes* by Langston Hughes, copyright © 1994 by The Estate of Langston Hughes. Used by permission of Alfred A. Knopf, a division of Random House, Inc.

"Rock, Church" from *Short Stories* by Langston Hughes. Copyright © 1996 by Ramona Bass and Arnold Rampersad. Reprinted by permission of Hill and Wang, a division of Farrar, Straus and Giroux, LLC.

"To Negro Writers" by Langston Hughes. Copyright © 1935 by The Estate of Langston Hughes. Reprinted by permission of Harold Ober Associates. From *Good Morning, Revolution*, edited by Faith Berry, Carol Publishing Group, 1992.

"Hippies" from *Seek: Reports from the Edges of America and Beyond* by Denis Johnson, copyright © 2001 by Denis Johnson. Used by permission of HarperCollins Publishers.

Act 1, scene 1, and afterword from *Homebody/Kabul* by Tony Kushner, copyright © 2002 by the Author. Published by Theatre Communications Group. Used by permission.

Excerpt from chapter 5 of *The Sailor Who Fell from Grace with the Sea* by Yukio Mishima, translated by John Nathan, copyright © 1965 by Alfred A. Knopf, a division of Random House, Inc. Used by permission of Alfred A. Knopf, a division of Random House, Inc.

Excerpt of "Kill Whitey" from *Stupid White Men . . . And Other Sorry Excuses for the State of the Nation!* by Michael Moore, copyright © 2001 by Michael Moore. Used by permission of HarperCollins Publishers.

Excerpt from *Islandia* by Maria Negroni, translated by Anne Twitty, copyright © 2001 by María Negroni. English translation copyright © 2001 by Anne Twitty. Reprinted by permission of Barrytown/Station Hill Press, Inc.

Excerpt of "On Writing a Memoir" from *The Edward Said Reader* by Edward W. Said and Moustafa Bayoumi, editor, edited by Andrew Rubin, copyright © 2000 by Edward W. Said. Introduction, headnotes, and bibliography copyright © 2000 by Moustafa Bayoumi and Andrew Rubin. Used by permission of Vintage Books, a division of Random House, Inc.

"Bali," "French Polynesia," "The Opposite of a Dark Dungeon," and "Star Bright" from *Life on Earth* by Frederick Seidel. Copyright © 2001 by Frederick Seidel. Reprinted by permission of Farrar, Straus and Giroux, LLC.

"At the Ball Game" by William Carlos Williams, from *Collected Poems: 1909–1939, Volume I,* copyright © 1938 by New Directions Publishing Corp. Reprinted by permission of New Directions Publishing Corp.

WHAT DO THE WINNERS OF

✦ THE 2001 PEN/NORA MAGID AWARD FOR LITERARY EDITING[1]

✦ THE PULITZER PRIZE[2]

✦ THE NATIONAL BOOK AWARD[3]

✦ THE PEN/FAULKNER AWARD[3]

✦ THE PEN/HEMINGWAY AWARD[2]

✦ THE *NEW YORKER* PRIZE FOR BEST DEBUT BOOK[2]

✦ INCLUSION IN *THE BEST AMERICAN SHORT STORIES OF 1999, 2000, AND 2002*[2,4]

✦ INCLUSION IN *THE BEST AMERICAN POETRY OF 2001 AND 2002*[5]

HAVE IN COMMON?

COULD IT BE AGNI?

1. Honoring Founder & Editor Askold Melnyczuk, PEN American Center said *AGNI* "has become a beacon of international literary culture. . . . Around the world, *AGNI* is known for publishing important new writers early in their careers. . . . *AGNI* has become one of America's, and the world's, most significant literary journals." 2. Won by Jhumpa Lahiri for *Interpreter of Maladies* (Houghton-Mifflin, 1999); title story published in *AGNI 47* and in *Best American Short Stories 1999*. 3. Won by Ha Jin for *Waiting* (Random House, 1999), also runner-up for the 2000 Pulitzer Prize. Jin was the Featured Poet in *AGNI 28* in 1989. 4. Won by Carolyn Cooke for "The Sugar-Tit," from *AGNI 53*. 5. Won by Thomas Sayers Ellis *(AGNI 52)*, Linda Gregg *(52)*, John Peck *(51)*, and Ira Sadoff *(53)*.

sample $10 • 1 yr./2 iss. $17, 2 yrs./4 iss. $31 (Canada add $3/yr.; int'l $6)
AGNI • 236 BAY STATE ROAD • BOSTON, MA • 02215
(617) 353-7135 • agni@bu.edu • http://www.bu.edu/AGNI

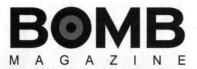

Ortiz-Torres Juan Manuel Echavarria Adelia Prado Mayra Montero Francisco Toledo Juan Formell Susana Baca Guillermo Cabrera Jose Cura Ernesto Neto Claribel Alegria Errol Morris Carlo Ginzburg Raymond Pettibon Judy Pfaff Edward Said Margaret Cezair-Thompson Peggy Shaw Laurie Anderson Chuck D Joseph Chaikin Maryse Conde Robert Altman Ida Applebroog Alvaro Siza Robert Pinsky Peter Campus Alan Warner Scott Spencer Cassandra Wilson Catherine Gund-Saalfield Elevator Repair Service Zoe Wana-maker James Hyde Mary Heilman Simon Winchester Marc Ribot Jenny Diski Janine Antoni Thomas Vinterberg Gary Sinise Simon Ortiz & Petuuche Gilbert Yayoi Kusama Michael Cunningham Ian McKellen Alexander Nehamas Sam Taylor-Wood Mark Richard Geoffrey O'Brien Thomas Nozkowski Yusef Komunyakaa & Paul Muldoon Aharon Appelfeld Stellan Skarsgard Tracy Moffat Jesus Chucho Valdes Richard Powers Maurice Berger & Patricia Williams Eric Kraft Lou Reed Steve Earle Jim Lewis & Dale Peck Gillian Wearing Victor Gar-ber & Alfred Molina Mona Hatoum Martin McDonagh Maureen Howard John Sayles Eliza-beth Murray Olu Dara Phillip Kan Gotanda Anthony Hecht Michael Winterbottom Kerry James Marshall Wong Kar-Wai Martin Sherman Andrew Blanco Rilla Askew Gregory Crewdson Lorna Simpson Rupert Graves Louis Auchincloss Marie Howe Allan Gurganbus Paula Vogel Judy Davis Jane Dickson Peter Greenaway John Lee Anderson David Del Tredici Barry Le Va Roger Guenveur Smith Alfred Uhry David Armstrong Lydia Davis Emmy Lou Harris Wallace Shawn Gilles Peress Tim Roth Christian Wolff George Walker Kendall Thomas Matthew Ritchie Emmet Gowin Donald Atrim Milos Forman Michael Ondaatje Oumou Sangare Ron Rifkin Stuart Hall Marjetica Potc Hilton Als David Robinovich Billy Bob
Michael Winterbottom Kerry James Marshall Wong Kar-Wai Martin Sherman Andrew Blanco Rilla Askew Gregory Crewdson Lorna Simpson Rupert Graves Louis Auchincloss Marie Howe Allan Gurganbus Paula Vogel Judy Davis Jane Dickson Peter Greenaway John Lee A

NEW FROM TCG BOOKS

"Tony Kushner's *Homebody/Kabul* is the most remarkable play in a decade...without a doubt the most important of our time."

John Heilpern, *New York Observer*

Homebody/Kabul
Tony Kushner

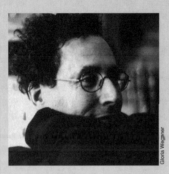

"This compelling evening testifies that Mr. Kushner can still deliver his sterling brand of goods: a fusion of politics, poetry and boundless empathy transformed through language into passionate, juicy theater...a reminder of how essential and heartening Mr. Kushner's voice remains."

Ben Brantley, *New York Times*

"It's impossible not to admire the range, ambition, and rare spirit of generosity that pervades Kushner's work. He makes most other contemporary dramatists look like fussy miniaturists while he sloshes words and ideas around like a theatrical Jackson Pollock. But that analogy won't quite do, because there's nothing abstract about Kushner's writing. He has an old-fashioned relish for a good tale."

Charles Spencer, *The Daily Telegraph*

Also available by Tony Kushner:

Angels in America Part One: Millennium Approaches
Angels in America Part Two: Perestroika
A Bright Room Called Day
Death & Taxes: Hydriotaphia & Other Plays
A Dybbuk (Adaptation)
The Illusion (Adaptation)
Thinking About the Longstanding Problems of Virtue and Happiness

Theater Communications Group

TCG titles are available at fine bookstores or can be ordered directly from TCG's online bookstore at *www.tcg.org* or by calling TCG Customer Service at (212) 697-5230.

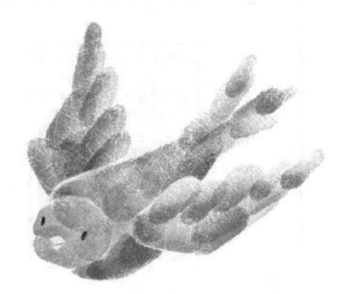

jubilat

poetry

art

interviews

prose

www.jubilat.org

Department of English, Bartlett Hall
University of Massachusetts, Amherst MA 01003

THE KENYON REVIEW

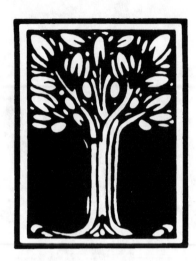

CELEBRATES THE BEST WRITING
FROM AROUND THE WORLD

ESSAYS, FICTION, POETRY, INTERVIEWS,
BOOK REVIEWS, AND MORE

Subscribe for $25,
Two Years $45, Three Years $65

Visit us on the World Wide Web at
kenyonreview.org
E-mail: kenyonreview@kenyon.edu
Telephone: 740-427-5208. Fax: 740-427-5417

The Kenyon Review, 104 College Drive,
Gambier, Ohio 43022-9623

Ploughshares

Stories and poems for literary aficionados

Known for its compelling fiction and poetry, *Ploughshares* is widely regarded as one of America's most influential literary journals. Each issue is guest-edited by a different writer for a fresh, provocative slant—exploring personal visions, aesthetics, and literary circles—and contributors include both well-known and emerging writers. In fact, *Ploughshares* has become a premier proving ground for new talent, showcasing the early works of Sue Miller, Mona Simpson, Robert Pinsky, and countless others. Past guest editors include Richard Ford, Derek Walcott, Tobias Wolff, Carolyn Forché, and Rosellen Brown. This unique editorial format has made *Ploughshares,* in effect, into a dynamic anthology series—one that has established a tradition of quality and prescience. *Ploughshares* is published in quality trade paperback in April, August, and December: usually a fiction issue in the Fall and mixed issues of poetry and fiction in the Spring and Winter. Inside each issue, you'll find not only great new stories and poems, but also a profile on the guest editor, book reviews, and miscellaneous notes about *Ploughshares,* its writers, and the literary world. Subscribe today.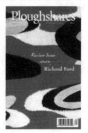

Visit *Ploughshares* online: www.pshares.org

❑ **Send me a one-year subscription for $22.**
I save $7.85 off the cover price (3 issues).

❑ **Send me a two-year subscription for $42.**
I save $17.70 off the cover price (6 issues).

Start with: ❑ Spring ❑ Fall ❑ Winter

Add $12 per year for international ($10 for Canada).

Name_____

Address _____

_____

Mail with check to: Ploughshares · Emerson College
120 Boylston St. · Boston, MA 02116

RATTAPALLAX PRESS

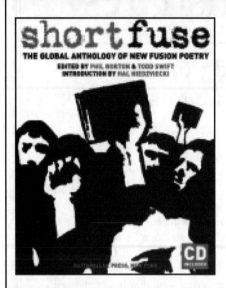

SHORT FUSE
The Global Anthology of New Fusion Poetry

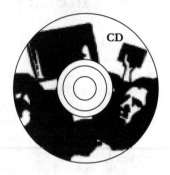

CD

Book with CD & ebook

www.rattapallax.com

Edited by Todd Swift & Philip Norton
Introduction by Hal Niedzviecki
Simon Armitage, Billy Collins, Todd Colby, Patricia
Smith, Bob Holman, Glyn Maxwell, Eileen Tabios,
Robert Priest, Andrea Thompson, Wednesday Kennedy,
Willie Perdomo, Tug Dumbly, Lucy English, Charles
Bernstein, Penn Kemp, Regie Cabico, Edwin Torres,
John Kinsella, Ron Silliman, Peter Finch, Guillermo
Castro, Michael Hulse and many more.

Release Date: Fall 2002

Ram Devineni, Publisher

FENCE 10

Writing by Marjorie Welish, Kenneth Koch, Sam Lipsyte, Norma Cole, Paul Maliszewski, Anne Waldman, David Antin, Andrew Zawacki, Jim Galvin, Tracy Philpot, Joe Wenderoth, Devin Johnston, Peter Gizzi, Leonard Brink, Alice Notley, and a host of others. **Paintings** by Adam Hurwitz.

$14 for one year, $26 for two, or get a special deal: Send in this ad with a check for $10 and we'll subscribe you for one year. Send $20 and we'll subscribe you for two years.

FENCE   14 Fifth Avenue, #1A, New York, NY 10011   **www.fencemag.com**

*FENCE*books **Fall 2002**

Winner of the 2002 Alberta Prize
The Real Moon of Poetry and Other Poems
by Tina Brown Celona

The poet and her poems achieve a plastic, spatial, significant reality on the luxuriously detailed plateau of the natural world: "The cliffs of the/ Seabed the/Poem twisting like a/ Tornado over the/Plains of the interior/Decoration."

ISBN 0-9713189-3-X $12 Paperback
Find it at upne.com or at fencebooks.com

Fence Books Contests

The Alberta Prize November 1-30, 2002

The Fence Modern Poets Series February 1-31, 2003

For required application form and guidelines, visit www.fence-books.com. or send an SASE to: [name of prize]
*FENCE*books
14 Fifth Avenue, #1A, New York, NY 10011

The Academy of American Poets
Poetry Audio Archive

"Hearing these poems from their authors' tongues rather than encountering them on the page, is a revelation."
—The Washington Post

Here is a selection from our growing poetry audio archive, featuring recordings of readings by America's great poets. Tapes cost $10.00 each.

☐ John Ashbery (1994)
☐ Margaret Atwood (1978)
☐ W. H. Auden (1964)
☐ John Berryman &
   Robert Lowell (1963)
☐ Frank Bidart &
   C. K. Williams (1992)
☐ Louise Bogan (1968)
☐ Kamau Brathwaite &
   Allen Ginsberg (1994)
☐ Joseph Brodsky (1980)
☐ Amy Clampitt (1987)
☐ Lucille Clifton &
   Gwendolyn Brooks (1983)
☐ Rita Dove &
   Rosanna Warren (1988)
☐ Alan Dugan (1974)
☐ Robert Duncan (1969)
☐ Carolyn Forché (1975)
☐ Louise Glück (1981/1992)
☐ Robert Graves (1966)
☐ Linda Gregg (1981/1991)
☐ Marilyn Hacker &
   June Jordan (1992)
☐ Donald Hall (1970)
☐ Robert Hass &
   Thom Gunn (1988)
☐ Robert Hayden (1976)
☐ Richard Howard (1994)
☐ Randall Jarrell (1964)

☐ Donald Justice (1982)
☐ Galway Kinnell (1980)
☐ Kenneth Koch (1969/1994)
☐ Yusef Komunyakaa &
   Sharon Olds (1993)
☐ Stanley Kunitz (1991)
☐ Philip Levine (1978/1991)
☐ Audre Lorde (1977)
☐ William Matthews (1988/1992)
☐ Heather McHugh &
   Gerald Stern (1992)
☐ William Meredith (1975)
☐ James Merrill (1992)
☐ W. S. Merwin (1966)
☐ Czeslaw Milosz (1974)
☐ Paul Muldoon &
   Les Murray (1996)
☐ Robert Pinsky (1992/1988)
☐ Charles Simic (1974/1977)
☐ William Stafford (1970)
☐ Mark Strand (1978)
☐ May Swenson (1985)
☐ James Tate (1996)
☐ Quincy Troupe (1990)
☐ Derek Walcott (1964)
☐ Robert Penn Warren (1977)
☐ Richard Wilbur (1989)
☐ Charles Wright &
   Adrienne Rich (1997)
☐ James Wright (1964/1978)

To request a catalog, order by phone with a Visa or MasterCard, or pay by check, please contact the Academy at:

THE ACADEMY OF AMERICAN POETS

POETRY AUDIO ARCHIVE

588 BROADWAY, SUITE 1203

NEW YORK, NY 10012

PHONE: (212) 274-0343 | FAX: (212) 274-9427

www.poets.org

Available now:

CONJUNCTIONS:38
REJOICING REVOICING

*Featuring a special portfolio celebrating
the art of translation*

*Edited by Peter Constantine, Bradford Morrow,
and William Weaver*

Includes new translations of Vladimir Nabokov, Charles
Baudelaire, Miguel de Cervantes, Fyodor Dostoevsky,
Giacomo Leopardi, Maurice Maeterlinck, José Martí, Robert
Musil, Octavio Paz, Marcel Proust, Leo Tolstoy, and others.
Also features new work by Julia Alvarez, Peter Gizzi, Tan Lin,
Rick Moody, James Tate, T. M. McNally, Rikki Ducornet,
Donald Revell, Paul West, and others. 384 pages, $15.

Available in November:

CONJUNCTIONS:39
THE NEW WAVE FABULISTS

*A landmark anthology devoted to
science fiction, horror, and fantasy*

Guest–edited by Peter Straub

New work by John Crowley, Jonathan Carroll, Karen Joy
Fowler, Joe Haldeman, Neil Gaiman, Elizabeth Hand,
Jonathan Lethem, Andrew Duncan, John Clute, Nalo
Hopkinson, M. John Harrison, Kelly Link, John Kessel, China
Miéville, James Morrow, Patrick O'Leary, Geoff Ryman, Gary
K. Wolfe, Peter Straub, and others. 360 pages, $15.

CONJUNCTIONS
Edited by Bradford Morrow
Published by Bard College
Annandale-on-Hudson, NY 12504
(845) 758-1539

Visit www.conjunctions.com

CROWD

Billy Collins
John Gossage
Lyn Hejinian
Barbara Kruger
Joyelle McSweeney
Enrique Vila-Matas
Matthew Zapruder
and more...

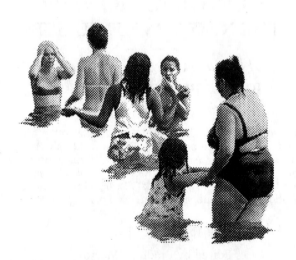

w w w . c r o w d m a g a z i n e . c o m
487   Union   Street,   #3,   Brooklyn,   NY 11231